T5-AFR-184

DISCARD
APR 15 2011
UT Southwestern Library

Shoulder Injuries *in the* Athlete

Surgical Repair and Rehabilitation

Edited by

RICHARD J. HAWKINS, M.D., F.R.C.S.(C)
Clinical Professor
Department of Orthopaedics
University of Colorado School of Medicine
Denver, Colorado
Orthopaedic Consultant
Steadman Hawkins Clinic
Vail, Colorado
Team Physician
Denver Broncos Football Team
Denver, Colorado

GARY W. MISAMORE, M.D.
Clinical Associate Professor
Department of Orthopaedic Surgery
Indiana University School of Medicine
Orthopaedic Surgeon
Methodist Sports Medicine Center
Indianapolis, Indiana

With illustrations by Theodore G. Huff, B.A., M.F.A.

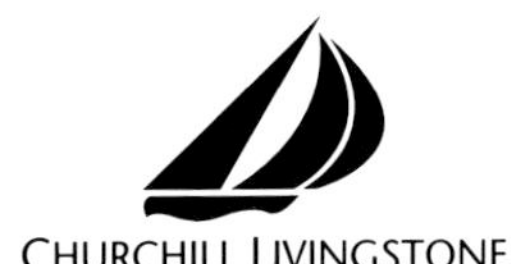

CHURCHILL LIVINGSTONE

New York, Edinburgh, London, Madrid, Melbourne, San Francisco, Tokyo

Library of Congress Cataloging-in-Publication Data

Shoulder injuries in the athlete : surgical repair and rehabilitation / edited by Richard J. Hawkins, Gary W. Misamore ; with illustrations by Theodore G. Huff.
p. cm.
Includes bibliographical references and index.
ISBN 0-443-08947-7
1. Shoulder—Wounds and injuries. 2. Sports injuries.
I. Hawkins, Richard J. II. Misamore, Gary W.
[DNLM: 1. Shoulder—injuries. 2. Athletic Injuries—therapy. WE 810 S55862 1996]
RD557.5.S544 1996
617.5′72044′088796—dc20
DNLM/DLC
for Library of Congress 95-36792
CIP

Distributed in the United Kingdom by Churchill Livingstone, Robert Stevenson House, 1–3 Baxter's Place, Leith Walk, Edinburgh EH1 3AF, and by associated companies, branches, and representatives throughout the world.

Accurate indications, adverse reactions, and dosage schedules for drugs are provided in this book, but it is possible that they may change. The reader is urged to review the package information data of the manufacturers of the medications mentioned.

The Publishers have made every effort to trace the copyright holders for borrowed material. If they have inadvertently overlooked any, they will be pleased to make the necessary arrangements at the first opportunity.

Acquisitions Editor: *Jennifer Mitchell*
Assistant Editor: *Jennifer Hardy*
Production Editor: *David Terry*
Production Supervisor: *Sharon Tuder*
Cover Design: *Jeannette Jacobs*

Printed in the United States of America

First published in 1996 7 6 5 4 3 2 1

Contributors

Jeffrey S. Abrams, M.D.

Attending Orthopaedic Surgeon, Department of Surgery, Princeton Medical Center; Associate Medical Director, Princeton Orthopaedic and Rehabilitation Associates, Princeton, New Jersey

David W. Altchek, M.D.

Assistant Professor, Department of Orthopaedic Surgery, Cornell University Medical College; Assistant Attending Orthopaedic Surgeon, The Hospital for Special Surgery; Medical Director and Team Physician, New York Mets Baseball Team, New York, New York; North American Medical Director, Association of Tennis Professionals, Ponte Verde, Florida

James R. Andrews, M.D.

Clinical Professor, Departments of Orthopaedics and Sports Medicine, University of Virginia School of Medicine, Charlottesville, Virginia; Medical Director, American Sports Medicine Institute; Orthopaedic Surgeon, Alabama Sports Medicine and Orthopaedic Center, Birmingham, Alabama

John Atkins, M.S., A.T.C.

Center Manager, Caremark Sports Center, Steadman Hawkins Clinic, Vail, Colorado

Robert H. Bell, M.D.

Assistant Professor, Department of Orthopaedic Surgery, Northeastern Ohio Universities College of Medicine, Rootstown, Ohio; Orthopaedic Surgeon, CRYSTALClinic, Akron, Ohio

Louis U. Bigliani, M.D.

Associate Professor, Department of Clinical Orthopedic Surgery, Columbia University College of Physicians and Surgeons; Chief, Shoulder Service, New York Orthopedic Hospital, Columbia-Presbyterian Medical Center, New York, New York

N. Douglas Boardman III, M.D.

Resident, Department of Orthopaedic Surgery, University of Pittsburgh School of Medicine, Pittsburgh, Pennsylvania

Martin Boublik, M.D.

Orthopaedic Surgeon, Steadman Hawkins Clinic; Associate Team Physician, Denver Broncos Football Team, Denver, Colorado

James P. Bradley, M.D.

Clinical Assistant Professor, Department of Orthopaedic Surgery, University of Pittsburgh School of Medicine; Director, Sports Medicine Center, St. Margaret Memorial Hospital; Team Physician, Pittsburgh Steelers Football Team, Pittsburgh, Pennsylvania

James D. Cash, M.D.

Orthopaedic Surgeon, Central States Orthopedic Specialists, Inc., Tulsa, Oklahoma

Richard E. Debski, B.S.

Graduate Research Engineer, Musculoskeletal Research Center, Department of Orthopaedic Surgery, University of Pittsburgh School of Medicine, Pittsburgh, Pennsylvania

Mark DeCarlo, M.H.A., P.T., S.C.S., A.T.(C)

Director, Department of Physical Therapy, Methodist Sports Medicine Center, Indianapolis, Indiana

Charles J. Dillman, Ph.D.

Clinical Associate Professor, Department of Orthopaedics and Rehabilitation, University of Virginia School of Medicine, Charlottesville, Virginia; Executive Director, Steadman Sports Medicine Foundation, Vail, Colorado; Consultant, American Sports Medicine Institute, Birmingham, Alabama

Paul A. Dowdy, M.D.
Resident, Department of Orthopaedic Surgery, University of Western Ontario Faculty of Medicine, London, Ontario, Canada

Xavier A. Duralde, M.D.
Orthopaedic Surgeon, Peachtree Orthopaedic Clinic, P.A., Piedmont Hospital, Atlanta, Georgia

Larry D. Field, M.D.
Co-Director, Upper Extremity Service, Mississippi Sports Medicine and Orthopaedic Service, Jackson, Mississippi

Robert E. FitzGibbons, M.D.
Orthopedic Surgeon, Longmont Orthopedic and Sports Medicine Clinic, Longmont, Colorado

Glenn S. Fleisig, M.S.
Director of Research, American Sports Medicine Institute, Birmingham, Alabama

Douglas A. Foulk, M.D.
Orthopaedic Surgeon, Orthopaedic and Sports Medicine Center, Manhattan, Kansas

Peter J. Fowler, M.D.
Professor, Department of Orthopaedic Surgery, and Head, Section of Sport Medicine, University of Western Ontario Faculty of Medicine, London, Ontario, Canada

Hollis M. Fritts, Jr., M.D.
Director of Musculoskeletal Imaging, Center for Diagnostic Imaging, Minneapolis, Minnesota

Freddie H. Fu, M.D.
Blue Cross of Western Pennsylvania Professor of Orthopaedic Surgery, Vice Chairman, Clinical Department of Orthopaedic Surgery, and Chief, Division of Sports Medicine, University of Pittsburgh School of Medicine, Pittsburgh, Pennsylvania

Cooper R. Gundry, M.D.
Director of Osteoradiology, Center for Diagnostic Imaging, Minneapolis, Minnesota

Gene Hagerman, M.D.
Sports Medicine Consultant, Caremark Sports Center, Steadman Hawkins Clinic, Vail, Colorado

Richard J. Hawkins, M.D., F.R.C.S.(C)
Clinical Professor, Department of Orthopaedics, University of Colorado School of Medicine, Denver, Colorado; Orthopaedic Consultant, Steadman Hawkins Clinic, Vail, Colorado; Team Physician, Denver Broncos Football Team, Denver, Colorado

David H. Janda, M.D.
Director, Institute for Preventative Sports Medicine; Associate, Orthopedic Surgery Associates, Ann Arbor, Michigan

Frank W. Jobe, M.D.
Clinical Professor, Department of Orthopaedics, University of Southern California School of Medicine, Los Angeles, California; President and Associate, Kerlan-Jobe Orthopaedic Clinic, Inglewood, California; Orthopaedic Consultant, Los Angeles Dodgers Baseball Team, Professional Golf Association Tour, and Senior Professional Golf Association Tour, Los Angeles, California

John T. Kao, M.D.
Clinical Instructor, Department of Functional Restoration, Stanford University School of Medicine, Stanford, California; Staff Physician, Department of Orthopedics, Kaiser-Permanente Medical Center, San Francisco, California; Consultant, Department of Orthopaedic Surgery, Palo Alto Veterans Affairs Medical Center, Palo Alto, California

Ronald P. Karzel, M.D.
Orthopedic Surgeon, Southern California Orthopedic Institute, Van Nuys, California

Sanford Kunkel, M.D.
Clinical Assistant Professor, Department of Orthopaedics, Indiana University School of Medicine, Indianapolis, Indiana

Robert Litchfield, M.D., F.R.C.S.(C)
Assistant Professor, Department of Orthopaedic Surgery, University of Western Ontario Faculty of Medicine, London, Ontario, Canada

Peter MacDonald, M.D., F.R.C.S.(C)
Assistant Professor, Department of Orthopaedics, University of Manitoba Faculty of Medicine; Head, Section of Orthopaedics, St. Boniface Hospital; Consultant, Pan American Sports Medicine and Surgical Center; Orthopaedic Surgeon, Winnipeg Jets Hockey Club, Winnipeg, Manitoba,Canada

William J. Mallon, M.D.

Assistant Consulting Professor, Division of Orthopaedic Surgery, Department of Surgery, Duke University School of Medicine; Private Practice, Triangle Orthopedic Associates, P.A., Durham, North Carolina

Kathy Malone, M.A., A.T.C.

Research Assistant, Methodist Sports Medicine Center, Indianapolis, Indiana

Anthony Miniaci, M.D.

Associate Professor, Division of Orthopaedic Surgery, Department of Surgery, University of Western Ontario Faculty of Medicine, London, Ontario, Canada

Gary W. Misamore, M.D.

Clinical Associate Professor, Department of Orthopaedic Surgery, Indiana University School of Medicine; Orthopaedic Surgeon, Methodist Sports Medicine Center, Indianapolis, Indiana

Nick Mohtadi, M.D., M.Sc., F.R.C.S.(C)

Clinical Associate Professor, Department of Surgery, University of Calgary Faculty of Medicine; Clinical Associate Professor, Department of Sport Medicine, University of Calgary Faculty of Kinesiology, Calgary, Alberta, Canada

William Morin, M.D.

Clinical Instructor, Department of Orthopaedic Surgery, Uniformed Services of the Health Sciences F. Edward Hébert School of Medicine, Bethesda, Maryland; Director, Sports Medicine Service, Department of Orthopaedic Surgery, Luther-Midelfort Clinic, Eau Claire, Wisconsin; Physician, United States Ski Team

David S. Morrison, M.D.

Director, Shoulder Clinic, Southern California Center for Sports Medicine, Long Beach, California

Jeffrey S. Noble, M.D.

Instructor, Department of Orthopaedic Surgery, Northeastern Ohio Universities College of Medicine, Rootstown, Ohio; Orthopaedic Surgeon, CRYSTAL-Clinic, Akron, Ohio

Steven A. Petersen, M.D.

Orthopaedic Surgeon, Great Lakes Orthopaedics, P.A., Riverside, Illinois

Joshua Port, M.D.

Orthopaedic Surgeon, Blair Orthopedic Associates, Inc., Altoona, Pennsylvania

Mark S. Schickendantz, M.D.

Instructor, Department of Orthopedics, Fairview and Lutheran Hospital; Orthopaedic Consultant, Cleveland Indians Baseball Team, Cleveland, Ohio

Theodore F. Schlegel, M.D.

Orthopaedic Surgeon, Steadman Hawkins Clinic, Denver, Colorado

James F. Silliman, M.D.

Assistant Professor, Department of Orthopaedics, University of Texas Southwestern Medical School, Dallas, Texas

Stephen J. Snyder, M.D.

Orthopedic Surgeon, Southern California Orthopedic Institute, Van Nuys, California

Timothy B. Sutherland, M.D.

Orthopaedic Surgeon, Desert Orthopaedic Center, Las Vegas, Nevada

James E. Tibone, M.D.

Clinical Associate Professor, Department of Orthopaedic Surgery, University of Southern California School of Medicine; Director, Sports Medicine Fellowship, Kerlan-Jobe Orthopaedic Clinic, Inglewood, California

Russell F. Warren, M.D.

Professor, Division of Orthopaedic Surgery, Department of Surgery, Cornell University Medical College; Surgeon in Chief, Department of Orthopedics, The Hospital for Special Surgery, New York, New York

Kevin E. Wilk, M.D.

National Director, Research and Clinical Education, Clinical Director, HealthSouth Sports Medicine and Rehabilitation Center; Director, Rehabilitative Research, Alabama

Mark M. Williams, M.D.

Orthopaedic Surgeon, Florida Sports Medicine and Orthopaedic Center, Panama City, Florida

Savio L.-Y. Woo, Ph.D.

Albert Ferguson, Jr., Professor and Vice Chairman for Research, Musculoskeletal Research Center, Department of Orthopaedic Surgery, University of Pittsburgh School of Medicine, Pittsburgh, Pennsylvania

To our wives, Marla and Susan, and our children, whom we thank for the joy they bring to our lives. Also, to our colleagues and fellow students of the shoulder, with whom we share the pleasure and challenge of exploring the mysteries of the shoulder joint.

Preface

Why create a text on shoulder injuries in athletes? Are athletes different from other patients and do they suffer from different shoulder problems? Should athletes' injuries be treated differently from other patients' and are results of their treatment different? Are there varying standards for measuring success? We have brought together the chapters of this book because the answer to all these questions is *Yes* (or at least a qualified *Yes*).

The pathologic conditions that afflict the shoulders of athletes are not inherently different from the maladies that can afflict all people. However, the way in which these conditions affect athletes is often different. In the athlete, the form of treatment and the outcome may vary from the general population, owing to the demands placed on the shoulder in certain sports, the frequency of certain pathologic conditions in athletes, and the symptoms and disability caused by those conditions.

In some circumstances, certain shoulder problems are seen in athletes more often than in the general population. One example of this is subtle anterior instability secondary to repetitive microtrauma, as seen in baseball pitchers. Another example is suprascapular neuropathy, which affects volleyball players. Both of these conditions are uncommon in nonathletes of similar ages.

In treating athletes, the physician must consider the demands placed on the shoulder as well as the expectations of the athlete. These factors influence the etiology of the injury, the magnitude of disability suffered by the athlete, and the response to treatment. Minor injuries have the potential to cause major disability in athletes, while similar injuries may cause little or no trouble for nonathletes. Accordingly, a nonathlete with a shoulder problem may have a normal vocational and recreational life-style, whereas an athlete's life may be severely affected by the same disorder. Moreover, in athletes, the expectations for recovery time may be much higher. This may be due solely to the personal desires of the athlete, but can also be affected by demands of coaches and teams. For some athletes, there are considerable financial implications associated with injury. For a high school athlete, absence from competition may affect the ability to secure a college scholarship. For collegiate athletes, prospects for professional competition may be an issue. In professional sports, the financial implications are obvious. In many sports, the window of opportunity for competition may be very small. If the athlete misses that opportunity because of an injury, there may be no second chance. Not only must the physician deal with the expectations of the athlete, but in many circumstances our work with these athletes may be viewed and critiqued by many others. Coaches, trainers, fans, and the sports media may all be watching closely.

In this book, we have tried to present an organized approach to the disorders of the shoulder encountered in athletes. Part I provides background information about mechanics and physiology, along with a general overview of the history and physical examination. Part II is an overview of imaging techniques useful in the assessment of athletes with shoulder disorders. Part III covers the basics of shoulder arthroscopy. In Part IV, the specific shoulder disorders commonly encountered in athletes are discussed. Pertinent features of symptoms and examination are reviewed and considerations for treatment decisions discussed. Part IV also focuses on the treatment of these disorders. Special emphasis is directed to surgical intervention, including options and techniques. In many cases, the authors are able to share the details of their preferred technique of surgery. Part V discusses the conditioning and rehabilitation of the shoulder, including both preventive approaches and treatment regimens for presurgical and postoperative rehabilitation. Also, devices useful in preventing and treating shoulder problems are discussed. The chapters in Part VI address specific sports and the injuries that typically occur.

We have called upon many physicians with wide-ranging fields of experience and expertise in an effort to produce a book based on current and established *state of the art* approaches to the shoulder. It is important to recognize that our understanding of the shoulder is changing rapidly and that it is difficult to keep pace with these changes. Students of the shoulder, as we all are, can use this text as a foundation for examining the complex challenges of the treatment of athletes with shoulder problems. We should recognize, however, that this book is simply a foundation upon which to build as our knowledge and understanding grow.

Richard J. Hawkins, M.D.
Gary W. Misamore, M.D.

Contents

CHAPTER ONE

Consideration of the Athlete's Shoulder: How It Differs

Richard J. Hawkins

In a textbook on the challenge of the athlete's shoulder from a surgical and rehabilitative perspective, there are several considerations as to how the athlete's shoulder may differ. One of the concerns relates to the definition of an athlete. Obviously, Orel Herscheiser, pitching for the Los Angeles Dodgers, qualifies, but what about the rest of us? Many of us like to consider ourselves athletes and perhaps we are such, functioning at very different levels and within a varied group of endeavors. Regardless of our definition of an athlete, when we consider the athlete's shoulder and how it differs, we need to analyze it from different viewpoints.

These different viewpoints relate to the level of participation, the sport and position played, the intensity of involvement, motivation, and the age of the athlete. As athletes, we need to consider whether we are recreational, amateurs, or professionals. Also, there are always the financial implications at the professional level. Do athletes have different diagnoses and different pathologies and might therefore have variations in treatment from the normal population? Probably so. When we analyze the outcomes of our treatment for an athlete, should our measurements be different?

If we consider the level of participation, we progress through competition as a youth, recreational, high school, college, and professional athlete and even international in scope. All sports could be considered and related to the athlete's shoulder, but usually the sports that cause shoulder problems particularly relate to an overhead nature such as baseball, tennis, swimming, volleyball, or javelin throwing, among others. Other sports such as football, soccer, and basketball may also result in trauma to the shoulder, resulting in a problem. In the first group of patients, it is an overuse-related situation. The second group of sports represents a traumatic injury. The position played within the framework of a sport may result in different problems within the shoulder. This might be relevant to a baseball pitcher who throws many pitches in a game versus an outfielder who falls on the outstretched arm, injuring the shoulder. Obviously, the intensity of participation and the aggressiveness with which an athlete pursues, particularly the overhead endeavor, may relate to the cause of a painful shoulder.

Athletes have a strong desire to participate. The higher the level at which an athlete participates, frequently the higher the motivation and the greater the desire for normalcy. This all has an effect on the need for early and appropriate diagnosis and aggressive treatment programs. Athletes often may be disabled by problems that may not affect the average sedentary individual. Frequently, the higher the demand in these athletes, the greater the potential for injury.

It is unusual to see problems in very young children who participate in athletic endeavors, even those who play baseball. Progressing through the years, one gets into problems with overuse and tendinosis and may end up as a masters athlete in the older age group with a complete-thickness rotator cuff tear, unheard of in youth.

NAME: ______________________________

DATE: __ __ / __ __ / __ __ Age: __ __ ○ Male ○ Female OCCUPATION ____________

SHOULDER: ○ Right ○ Left HAND DOMINANCE ○ Right ○ Left ○ Ambidextrous

SPORTS PARTICIPATION INFORMATION

Primary Sport ____________ CODE __ __ Years Played __ __ Position Played ____________

What level of intensity is your sport? ○ Recreational Part-time ○ Recreational Full-time ○ High School ○ College ○ Pro-Minors ○ Pro-Majors

At what regional level do you compete? ○ Local ○ Regional ○ National ○ International

INJURY AND TREATMENT HISTORY

What is the primary reason for seeking medical attention?
○ Pain ○ Shoulder coming out ○ Loss of Shoulder function ○ Weakness ○ Stiffness ○ Other ____________

Date of onset of symptoms: __ __ / __ __ / __ __ Did you have an injury? ○ YES ○ NO Sports Related? ○ YES ○ NO

Describe how injury occurred: ______________________________

Is there a worker's compensation claim involved with your injury? ○ YES ○ NO

Have you had supervised physical therapy? ○ YES ○ NO

Did you try other modalities such as: ○ Ultrasound ○ TENS ○ Electical Stumulation ○ Other

Has your shoulder been injected? ○ NO ○ YES **If Yes, how many times?** __ __ __

Thirty minutes after the injection, how much improvement did you have? ○ Worse ○ 0-25% ○ 26-50% ○ 51-75% ○ 76-100%

What was the long-term effect of the injection? ○ Worse ○ 0-25% ○ 26-50% ○ 51-75% ○ 76-100%

Have you had previous shoulder surgery? ○ YES ○ NO If yes, please complete the following list:

Operation	Date	Amount of Maximum Improvement (check one)
____________	__ __ / __ __ / __ __	○ Worse ○ 0-25% ○ 26-50% ○ 51-75% ○ 76-100%
____________	__ __ / __ __ / __ __	○ Worse ○ 0-25% ○ 26-50% ○ 51-75% ○ 76-100%
____________	__ __ / __ __ / __ __	○ Worse ○ 0-25% ○ 26-50% ○ 51-75% ○ 76-100%

PAIN EVALUATION

How bad is your pain at the following times on a scale of 0 to 10 (10 being as bad as it can be)

Today:	○ 0	○ 1	○ 2	○ 3	○ 4	○ 5	○ 6	○ 7	○ 8	○ 9	○ 10
At its	○ 0	○ 1	○ 2	○ 3	○ 4	○ 5	○ 6	○ 7	○ 8	○ 9	○ 10

Is your Pain ○ No Pain ○ Getting Better ○ Staying the Same ○ Getting worse

Do you take narcotic pain medications? ○ YES ○ NO How many pills/day? __ __ Do you take anti-inflammatories? ○ YES ○ NO

Are they benificial? ○ YES ○ NO Are they beneficial? ○ YES ○ NO

How does your pain affect:

your activities of daily living?	○ None	○ Mild	○ Moderate	○ Severe
your function at work?	○ None	○ Mild	○ Moderate	○ Severe
your recreational sporting activities?	○ None	○ Mild	○ Moderate	○ Severe
your sleep?	○ None	○ Mild	○ Moderate	○ Severe

How much pain do you have with your arm at rest by your side? ○ None ○ Mild ○ Moderate ○ Severe

With regard to your sport, how does pain affect:

your endurance	○ None	○ Mild	○ Moderate	○ Severe
your speed	○ None	○ Mild	○ Moderate	○ Severe
your accuracy or agility	○ None	○ Mild	○ Moderate	○ Severe

How does your pain affect your ability to compete?

○ 1 No Pain w/ Competition ○ 3 Mild Pain w/ competition ○ 5 Severe Pain w/ Competition

○ 2 Pain only after Competition ○ 4 Moderate Pain w/ Competition ○ 6 Pain prevents Competition

A

Figure 1-1. **(A & B)** Athlete's shoulder evaluation form. (*Figure continues.*)

SHOULDER INSTABILITY

Have you ever had a shoulder dislocation that someone else had to put back in? ○ Yes ○ No How many? [ ][ ]

How often does your shoulder feel like it will go out? ○ Never ○ Rarely ○ Occaisonally ○ Frequently

Answer the following only if you have this sensation:

Does this instability occur with: ○ Sports ○ Activities of Daily Living ○ Sleep

Which direction does it go out: ○ Front ○ Back ○ Bottom ○ All ○ Unknown

How does your shoulder go back in? ○ By Itself ○ I pull on my arm ○ Someone else assists

How many time does this occur each month? ○ 0-2 ○ 2-5 ○ 5-10 ○ 10-15 ○ more than 15

How is your shoulder instability changing with time: ○ Improving ○ Unchanged ○ Getting Worse

How does your shoulder instability affect your ability to compete in sports?

○ **1** No problems during competition
○ **2** I have instability, but can continue to compete
○ **3** I rarely have to stop competing
○ **4** I occasionally have to stop competing
○ **5** I frequently have instability and have to stop competing
○ **6** I cannot compete due to instability

Does a certain position of your arm interfere with you performance?

○ No ○ Yes, with my arm above my head ○ Yes, with my arm in front of my body

FUNCTIONAL EVALUATION

With regards to your shoulder, at what level can you now participate in Sports?

○ **1** Equal to or above my pre-injury level
○ **2** Slightly below my pre-injury level
○ **3** Moderately below my pre-injury level
○ **4** Significantly below my pre-injury level
○ **5** I cannot compete in my usual sport
○ **6** I cannot compete in any Sports

Describe your current strength or endurance of your shoulder when competing in you usual sport:

○ **1** I have no weakness or fatigue
○ **2** I have mild weakness or fatigue
○ **3** I have moderate weakness or fatigue
○ **4** I have severe weakness or fatigue
○ **5** Weakness or fatigue prevents competition in my usual sport
○ **6** Weakness or fatigue prevents competition in all sports

With regards to your shoulder,at what intensity level do you how compete in your usual sport compared to your pre-injury level?

○ **1** Same or better than my pre-injury intensity
○ **2** 75-100% of my pre-injury intensity
○ **3** 50-75% of my pre-injury intensity
○ **4** 25-50% of my pre-injury intensity
○ **5** <25% of my intensity
○ **6** I can no longer compete at any intensity

B

Figure 1-1. *(Continued).*

DIAGNOSTIC IMPLICATIONS

Problems and diagnoses in the athlete's shoulder may differ from the general population. However, athletes may have exactly the same problem as occurs in the general population, particularly when trauma is involved. If a patient, whether an athlete or not, is involved in a motor vehicle accident, he or she may sustain an acute dislocation of the shoulder. This obviously also occurs in the football lineman who tackles someone. It is important, particularly in the overuse situation, to keep in mind that athletes do have different problems and different diagnoses. For example, the professional baseball pitcher who presents with shoulder pain very often has subtle anterior subluxation and secondary impingement. This might be compared with the 45-year-old nonathlete workman who presents with shoulder pain, who almost never has a diagnosis of anterior subluxation but much more commonly has a diagnosis of impingement degenerative cuff disease. Volleyball players are frequently subject to suprascapular nerve problems. Hockey players very commonly get their shoulders jammed into the boards, resulting in acromioclavicular dislocations. All this suggests that diagnoses may vary, depending on the sport and other features of involvement. In such athletes, it is important to keep in mind an acute injury versus a chronic overuse situation.

CLINICAL EXAMINATION

In the acute injury, the clinical examination after a fracture or an acromioclavicular dislocation or an acute dislocation of the glenohumeral joint is fairly straightforward. These patients present with a painful shoulder with limited range of motion. In many overhead athletes who present with shoulder pain due to overuse, the physical findings vary but frequently consist of limitation of internal rotation and crossed-arm adduction, scapular dysfunction, weakness in certain ranges such as external rotation, instability findings such as excess translation, positive relocation testing, and often impingement signs. Many overhead athletes such as throwers have excess external rotation. This constellation of physical examination signs is frequently found in the high-profile overhead athlete, such as a professional baseball pitcher, but is very rarely found in the general population.

PATHOLOGY

The pathologic findings in the overhead athlete obviously relate to the diagnosis. These athletes can have the same pathology as the general population, such as occurs in an acute anterior dislocation of the shoulder with a Bankart lesion or in a rotator cuff tear of a degenerative nature such as seen in the older individual. In the overuse situation, there is often the aspect of eccentric overload, undersurface rotator cuff irritation, subtle anterior instability, and biomechanical scapular dysfunction. These may eventually lead to a complete rotator cuff tear.

TREATMENT ASPECTS

Rehabilitation and Prevention

Because of their desire, many high-performance athletes gear their rehabilitation program toward performance enhancement. As it relates to this, there is an interest in injury prevention. To achieve these goals, the focus is on eccentric control of the glenohumeral muscles, a stable and efficient scapular platform, elimination of tight posterior capsular structures, and appropriate muscle balance. Velocity and power in performance of an overhead activity come through the kinetic chain from the ground up. The shoulder itself provides only a nominal amount of power for velocity for overhead activities. Nevertheless, the fine-tuning and eccentric control necessary in the glenohumeral joints is important to overhead performance and injury prevention.

Frequently, the athlete who is injured desires an aggressive rehabilitation program to return him or her back to normal, which must address all the biomechanical abnormalities. If the athlete has pain from overuse, then the principles applied in the prevention and performance enhancement arena can be applied in treating the injury.

As one attempts to control the glenohumeral and scapulothoracic articulation, it is important to remember that strength and coordination of the lower extremities and torso are critical.

Implications

Treatment of an athlete's shoulder should differ little from treatment of the normal patient population; however, there are ramifications that may vary. Age alone is an important consideration. For example, a Little League pitcher versus a professional baseball pitcher not only would have a different diagnosis but obviously different treatment programs.

Within the athletic arena, there is a push for aggressive treatment to allow a rapid return to activity. This is the desire of most athletes. There are aspects that have an effect on the treatment programs (e.g., whether an athlete is a professional or an amateur, young versus old, and his or her role within the team make-up). There are financial considerations, particularly at the professional level. The athlete's desire, particularly at a higher level, sometimes is not paralleled in the average individual. Finally, there are parental, coaching, and administrative pressures that occur.

SURGICAL ASPECTS

The surgical goals in the athlete's shoulder are not only to return the athlete to good function but, even greater, to allow performance at the expected and desired level. Frequently, the outcomes after major reconstructions of the shoulder are guarded, particularly in the athlete's functional outcome. Thus, there is perhaps the old adage of the less surgery performed in the athlete's shoulder, the better. The expectation of these athletes for performance constantly challenges us to design the appropriate surgical procedures to address their situation.

If we consider shoulder instability, for example, operations such as the Putti-Platt, Bristow, and Magnuson-Stack have not stood the test of time for high performance in the overhead athlete. The principles now are geared toward lesser surgery and less violation of tissue planes. An example is the recently introduced capsulolabral reconstruction through a subscapular split.

Rehabilitation after surgery in athletes is as aggressive as Mother Nature and the surgery will allow.

EVALUATION AND OUTCOME ANALYSIS

Should we evaluate the athlete's shoulder the same as we do shoulders of nonathletic individuals? It is probable that we need to have a more comprehensive evaluation, looking sometimes at similar but occasionally different parameters. For example, endurance performance in an athlete is critical to the return to desired function. Forms such as the subjective/objective surgical data forms used at the Steadman Hawkins Clinic in Vail, Colorado, are helpful in evaluating the athlete's shoulder (see Figs. 1-1 to 1-4). We have been working with the American Shoulder and Elbow Surgeons and the American Orthopaedic Society for Sports Medicine to develop an athlete's evaluation form.

NAME: DATE: IVY#

INJURED SHOULDER ○ RIGHT ○ LEFT ○ BILATERAL

RANGE OF MOTION	RIGHT		LEFT	
	ACTIVE	PASSIVE	ACTIVE	PASSIVE
FORWARD ELEVATION				
EXTERNAL ROTATION (ARM AT SIDE)				
EXTERNAL ROTATION (ARM 90 ABDUCTED)				
INTERNAL ROTATION (HIGHEST POINT REACHED W/ THUMB) SM=SACRUM LT=LAT. THIGH SI=SI JOINT BU=BUTTOCK, L5-T12				
INTERNAL ROTATION AT 90 DEGREES ABD				

STRENGTH (USE MRC GRADE): 0=NO CONTRACTION 1=FLICKER 2=MOVEMENT W/O GRAVITY 3=MOVEMENT AGAINST GRAVITY 4=MOVEMENT AGAINST SOME RESISTANCE 5=NORMAL

	RIGHT	LEFT
PAIN W/ STRENGTH TESTING	○ NO ○ YES	○ NO ○ YES
FORWARD ELEVATION	○ 0 ○ 1 ○ 2 ○ 3 ○ 4 ○ 5	○ 0 ○ 1 ○ 2 ○ 3 ○ 4 ○ 5
ABDUCTION	○ 0 ○ 1 ○ 2 ○ 3 ○ 4 ○ 5	○ 0 ○ 1 ○ 2 ○ 3 ○ 4 ○ 5
EXTERNAL ROTATION (ARM AT SIDE)	○ 0 ○ 1 ○ 2 ○ 3 ○ 4 ○ 5	○ 0 ○ 1 ○ 2 ○ 3 ○ 4 ○ 5
INTERNAL ROTATION (ARM AT SIDE)	○ 0 ○ 1 ○ 2 ○ 3 ○ 4 ○ 5	○ 0 ○ 1 ○ 2 ○ 3 ○ 4 ○ 5

INSTABILITY 0=NONE 1=MILD (0-1 CM TRANSLATION) 2=MODERATE(1-2 CM OR EQUATOR TO GLENOID RIM) 3=SEVERE(>2 CM OR EQUATOR OVER GLENOID RIM)

	RIGHT	REPRODUCE SYMPTOMS	LEFT	REPRODUCE SYMPTOMS
ANTERIOR TRANSLATION	○ 0 ○ 1 ○ 2 ○ 3	○ YES ○ NO	○ 0 ○ 1 ○ 2 ○ 3	○ YES ○ NO
+ GRIND	○ NO ○ YES		○ NO ○ YES	
POSTERIOR TRANSLATION	○ 0 ○ 1 ○ 2 ○ 3	○ YES ○ NO	○ 0 ○ 1 ○ 2 ○ 3	○ YES ○ NO
INFERIOR(SULCUS)	○ 0 ○ 1 ○ 2 ○ 3	○ YES ○ NO	○ 0 ○ 1 ○ 2 ○ 3	○ YES ○ NO
ANTERIOR APPREHENSION	○ 0 ○ 1 ○ 2 ○ 3	○ YES ○ NO	○ 0 ○ 1 ○ 2 ○ 3	○ YES ○ NO
VOLUNTARY INSTABILITY:				
I. MUSCLE CONTRACTION	○ 0 ○ 1 ○ 2 ○ 3	○ YES ○ NO	○ 0 ○ 1 ○ 2 ○ 3	○ YES ○ NO
II. POSITIONAL	○ 0 ○ 1 ○ 2 ○ 3	○ YES ○ NO	○ 0 ○ 1 ○ 2 ○ 3	○ YES ○ NO
DESCRIBE				
RELOCATION TEST				
+ PAIN	○ 10° ○ 20° ○ 30°	○ YES ○ NO	○ 10° ○ 20° ○ 30°	○ YES ○ NO
+ FOR APPREHENSION	○ 10° ○ 20° ○ 30°	○ YES ○ NO	○ 10° ○ 20° ○ 30°	○ YES ○ NO
LABRAL "CLUNK"	○ NO ○ YES		○ NO ○ YES	

SIGN: 0=NONE 1=MILD 2=MODERATE 3=SEVERE	RIGHT	LEFT
IMPINGEMENT: PASSIVE F.E. IN SLIGHT I.R.	○ 0 ○ 1 ○ 2 ○ 3	○ 0 ○ 1 ○ 2 ○ 3
PASSIVE I.R. IN 90 F.E.	○ 0 ○ 1 ○ 2 ○ 3	○ 0 ○ 1 ○ 2 ○ 3
90 ACTIVE ABD-PAINFUL ARC	○ 0 ○ 1 ○ 2 ○ 3	○ 0 ○ 1 ○ 2 ○ 3
TENDERNESS: SUPRASPINATUS/TUBEROSITY	○ 0 ○ 1 ○ 2 ○ 3	○ 0 ○ 1 ○ 2 ○ 3
AC JOINT	○ 0 ○ 1 ○ 2 ○ 3	○ 0 ○ 1 ○ 2 ○ 3
BICEPS TENDON	○ 0 ○ 1 ○ 2 ○ 3	○ 0 ○ 1 ○ 2 ○ 3
OTHER - LIST:	○ 0 ○ 1 ○ 2 ○ 3	○ 0 ○ 1 ○ 2 ○ 3
CROSSED-ARM ADD. - AC PAIN?	○ 0 ○ 1 ○ 2 ○ 3	○ 0 ○ 1 ○ 2 ○ 3
CERVICAL SPINE SPINOUS PROCESS TENDERNESS	○ 0 ○ 1 ○ 2 ○ 3	○ 0 ○ 1 ○ 2 ○ 3
LOSS OF MOTION	○ 0 ○ 1 ○ 2 ○ 3	○ 0 ○ 1 ○ 2 ○ 3
PAIN WITH STRESSED MOTION	○ 0 ○ 1 ○ 2 ○ 3	○ 0 ○ 1 ○ 2 ○ 3
ATROPHY: LOCATION:	○ 0 ○ 1 ○ 2 ○ 3	○ 0 ○ 1 ○ 2 ○ 3
DEFORMITY: DESCRIBE	○ 0 ○ 1 ○ 2 ○ 3	○ 0 ○ 1 ○ 2 ○ 3
SCAPULA WINGING: STATIC (AT REST)	○ 0 ○ 1 ○ 2 ○ 3	○ 0 ○ 1 ○ 2 ○ 3
DYNAMIC (ACTIVE)	○ 0 ○ 1 ○ 2 ○ 3	○ 0 ○ 1 ○ 2 ○ 3
RESISTED (F.E.)	○ 0 ○ 1 ○ 2 ○ 3	○ 0 ○ 1 ○ 2 ○ 3
ABNORMAL SCAPULAR RHYTHM	○ NO ○ YES	○ NO ○ YES

OTHER FINDINGS	RIGHT	LEFT
CREPITUS: SUBACROMIAL	○ Y ○ N	○ Y ○ N
GLENOHUMERAL	○ Y ○ N	○ Y ○ N
SCAPULOTHORACIC	○ Y ○ N	○ Y ○ N
BICEPS STRAIGHT ARM RESISTED	○ Y ○ N	○ Y ○ N
RESISTED SUPINATION	○ Y ○ N	○ Y ○ N
ABNORMAL LIFT OFF TEST	○ Y ○ N	○ Y ○ N
LIGAMENTOUS LAXITY THUMB TO FORMARM	○ <4cm ○ >4cm	○ <4cm ○ >4cm

INJECTION RESPONSE IMPROVEMENT	
SUBACROMIAL	○ 0-25% ○ 25-50% ○ 50-75% ○ 75-100%
AC JOINT	○ 0-25% ○ 25-50% ○ 50-75% ○ 75-100%

X-RAY FINDINGS	
GLENOHUMERAL JOINT SPACE	○ NORMAL ○ DECREASED ○ ABSENT
HEAD CENTERED	○ YES ○ NO
AC JOINT ACROMION MORPHOLOGY	○ I ○ II ○ III
AC SEPARATION	○ YES ○ NO
AC ARTHRITIS	○ YES ○ NO

DIAGNOSIS ICD-9

Draft

Figure 1-2. Objective shoulder evaluation form.

NAME: ____________________

DATE: [|] / [|] / [|] SHOULDER: ○ Right ○ Left

SPORTS PARTICIPATION INFORMATION

Primary Sport ____________ CODE [|]

What level of intensity is your sport? ○ Recreational Part-time ○ Recreational Full-time ○ High School ○ College ○ Pro-Minors ○ Pro-Majors

At what regional level do you compete? ○ Local ○ Regional ○ National ○ International

INJURY AND TREATMENT HISTORY

SINCE YOUR LAST CLINIC VISIT:

Have you had supervised physical therapy? ○ YES ○ NO

Did you try other modalities such as: ○ Ultrasound ○ TENS ○ Electical Stumulation ○ Other

Has your shoulder been injected? ○ NO ○ YES How many times? [| |]

Thirty minutes after the injection, how much improvement did you have? ○ Worse ○ 0-25% ○ 26-50% ○ 51-75% ○ 76-100%

What was the long-term effect of the injection? ○ Worse ○ 0-25% ○ 26-50% ○ 51-75% ○ 76-100%

Have you had surgery elsewhere? ○ YES ○ NO

Operation	Date	Amount of Maximum Improvement (check one)
____________	[|] / [|] / [|]	○ Worse ○ 0-25% ○ 26-50% ○ 51-75% ○ 76-100%
____________	[|] / [|] / [|]	○ Worse ○ 0-25% ○ 26-50% ○ 51-75% ○ 76-100%
____________	[|] / [|] / [|]	○ Worse ○ 0-25% ○ 26-50% ○ 51-75% ○ 76-100%

PAIN EVALUATION

How bad is your pain at the following times on a scale of 0 to 10 (10 being as bad as it can be)

Today:	○ 0	○ 1	○ 2	○ 3	○ 4	○ 5	○ 6	○ 7	○ 8	○ 9	○ 10
At its	○ 0	○ 1	○ 2	○ 3	○ 4	○ 5	○ 6	○ 7	○ 8	○ 9	○ 10

Is your Pain ○ No Pain ○ Getting Better ○ Staying the Same ○ Getting worse

Do you take narcotic pain medications? ○ YES ○ NO How many pills/day? [|]

Are they benificial? ○ YES ○ NO

Do you take anti-inflammatories? ○ YES ○ NO

Are they beneficial? ○ YES ○ NO

How does your pain affect:

your activities of daily living?	○ None	○ Mild	○ Moderate	○ Severe
your function at work?	○ None	○ Mild	○ Moderate	○ Severe
your recreational sporting activities?	○ None	○ Mild	○ Moderate	○ Severe
your sleep?	○ None	○ Mild	○ Moderate	○ Severe

How much pain do you have with your arm at rest by your side? ○ None ○ Mild ○ Moderate ○ Severe

With regard to your sport, how does pain affect:

your endurance	○ None	○ Mild	○ Moderate	○ Severe
your speed	○ None	○ Mild	○ Moderate	○ Severe
your accuracy or agility	○ None	○ Mild	○ Moderate	○ Severe

How does your pain affect your ability to compete?

○ 1 No Pain w/ Competition
○ 2 Pain only after Competition
○ 3 Mild Pain w/ competition
○ 4 Moderate Pain w/ Competition
○ 5 Severe Pain w/ Competition
○ 6 Pain prevents Competition

A

Figure 1-3. **(A & B)** Return visit shoulder evaluation form. (*Figure continues.*)

SHOULDER INSTABILITY

How often does your shoulder feel like it will go out? ○ Never ○ Rarely ○ Occaisonally ○ Frequently

Answer the following only if you have this sensation:

Does this instability occur with: ○ Sports ○ Activities of Daily Living ○ Sleep

Which direction does it go out: ○ Front ○ Back ○ Bottom ○ All ○ Unknown

How does your shoulder go back in? ○ By Itself ○ I pull on my arm ○ Someone else assists

How many time does this occur each month? ○ 0-2 ○ 2-5 ○ 5-10 ○ 10-15 ○ more than 15

How is your shoulder instability changing with time: ○ Improving ○ Unchanged ○ Getting Worse

How does your shoulder instability affect your ability to compete in sports?

○ 1 No problems during competition
○ 2 I have instability, but can continue to compete
○ 3 I rarely have to stop competing
○ 4 I occasionally have to stop competing
○ 5 I frequently have instability and have to stop competing
○ 6 I cannot compete due to instability

Does a certain position of your arm interfere with you performance?

○ No ○ Yes, with my arm above my head ○ Yes, with my arm in front of my body

FUNCTIONAL EVALUATION

With regard to your shoulder,at what level can you now participate in Sports?

○ 1 Equal to or above my pre-injury level
○ 2 Slightly below my pre-injury level
○ 3 Moderately below my pre-injury level
○ 4 Significantly below my pre-injury level
○ 5 I cannot compete in my usual sport
○ 6 I cannot compete in any Sports

Describe your current strength or endurance of your shoulder when competing in you usual sport:

○ 1 I have no weakness or fatigue
○ 2 I have mild weakness or fatigue
○ 3 I have moderate weakness or fatigue
○ 4 I have severe weakness or fatigue
○ 5 Weakness or fatigue prevents competition in my usual sport
○ 6 Weakness or fatigue prevents competition in all sports

With regards to your shoulder, at what intensity level do you how compete in your usual sport compared to your pre-injury level?

○ 1 Same or better than my pre-injury intensity
○ 2 75-100% of my pre-injury intensity
○ 3 50-75% of my pre-injury intensity
○ 4 25-50% of my pre-injury intensity
○ 5 <25% of my intensity
○ 6 I can no longer compete at any intensity

B

Figure 1-3. (*Continued*).

Is it necessary in the athlete to have a separate system to measure outcome of the various treatment programs, be they operative or nonoperative? The primary goal of the athlete is to return to the previous level of participation or to enhance the performance, allowing him or her to achieve the desired level. Endurance is something that is particularly difficult to measure in these athletes and relates to their ability to participate and perform at a high level. If a scoring system were applied, it would heavily weigh performance and return to activity. There are many scoring systems available for shoulder problems such as the UCLA, the HSS, the ASES, Dr. Rowe's and Dr. Neer's modified system, among others. None of these are geared toward the specific needs and goals of the athlete and frequently fall short.

Athlete's Evaluation Form

We have provided by way of example the athlete's shoulder evaluation forms used at the Steadman Hawkins Clinic. These include a new athlete's evaluation form (Fig. 1-1), an objective athlete's shoulder evaluation form (Fig. 1-2), a return visit evaluation form (Fig. 1-3), and an athlete's scoring system (Fig. 1-4). These are all designed to be put into a scanner and immediately inserted into a computer database. They are therefore easily retrievable. These forms were developed in concert with the American Shoulder and Elbow Surgeons and the American Orthopaedic Society for Sports Medicine with Dr. Russ Warren, Dr. James Tibone, Dr. Peter Fowler, Dr. Jed Kuhn, and myself.

NAME: ______________________

DATE: __ __ / __ __ / __ __ SHOULDER: ○ Right ○ Left

PAIN EVALUATION (10 POINTS)

How does your pain affect your ability to compete?

- ○ 1 No Pain w/ Competition
- ○ 2 Pain only after Competition
- ○ 3 Mild Pain w/ competition
- ○ 4 Moderate Pain w/ Competition
- ○ 5 Severe Pain w/ Competition
- ○ 6 Pain prevents Competition

SHOULDER INSTABILITY (10 POINTS)

How does your shoulder instability affect your ability to compete in sports?

- ○ 1 No problems during competition
- ○ 2 I have instability, but can continue to compete
- ○ 3 I rarely have to stop competing
- ○ 4 I occasionally have to stop competing
- ○ 5 I frequently have instability and have to stop competing
- ○ 6 I cannot compete due to instability

FUNCTIONAL EVALUATION (70 POINTS: PERFORMANCE LEVEL=50; STRENGTH/ENDURANCE=10; INTENSITY=10)

At what level can you now participate in Sports?

- ○ 1 Equal to or above my pre-injury level
- ○ 2 Slightly below my pre-injury level
- ○ 3 Moderately below my pre-injury level
- ○ 4 Significantly below my pre-injury level
- ○ 5 I cannot compete in my usual sport
- ○ 6 I cannot compete in any Sports

Describe your current strength or endurance of your shoulder when competing in you usual sport:

- ○ 1 I have no weakness or fatigue
- ○ 2 I have mild weakness or fatigue
- ○ 3 I have moderate weakness or fatigue
- ○ 4 I have severe weakness or fatigue
- ○ 5 Weakness or fatigue prevents competition in my usual sport
- ○ 6 Weakness or fatigue prevents competition in all sports

At what intensity level do you how compete in your usual sport compared to your pre-injury level?

- ○ 1 Same or better than my pre-injury intensity
- ○ 2 75-100% of my pre-injury intensity
- ○ 3 50-75% of my pre-injury intensity
- ○ 4 25-50% of my pre-injury intensity
- ○ 5 <25% of my intensity
- ○ 6 I can no longer compete at any intensity

RANGE OF MOTION EVALUATION (10 POINTS)

- ○ 1 NO LOSS OF EXTERNAL ROTATION AT 90/90 POSITION, NO LOSS OF ELEVATION
- ○ 2 LESS THAN 5 DEGREES LOSS OF EXTERNAL ROTATION, NO LOSS OF ELEVATION
- ○ 3 LESS THAN 10 DEGREES LOSS OF EXTERNAL ROTATION, NO LOSS OF ELEVATION
- ○ 4 LESS THAN 15 DEGREES LOSS OF EXTERNAL ROTATION, NO LOSS OF ELEVATION
- ○ 5 LESS THAN 20 DEGREES LOSS OF EXTERNAL ROTATION, NO LOSS OF ELEVATION
- ○ 6 MORE THAN 20 DEGREES LOSS OF EXTERNAL ROTATION, ANY LOSS OF ELEVATION

SCORE

EXCELLENT	90-100
GOOD	70-89
FAIR	50-69
POOR	<50

Figure 1-4. Athlete's shoulder scoring system.

CHAPTER TWO

History and Physical Examination

Martin Boublik
James F. Silliman

The successful treatment of a dysfunctional shoulder depends on an accurate diagnosis. This diagnosis can usually be established through a careful history and a thorough physical examination, supplemented by appropriate radiographic and laboratory examinations. Overhead athletes who throw, swim, and serve place extreme demands on their shoulders and are subject to both acute and overuse injuries. This chapter is dedicated to the history and physical examination of the athlete's shoulder.

HISTORY

The patient's chief complaint and age often strongly suggest the correct diagnosis. For example, a 21-year-old complaining of his shoulder "coming out" probably has instability. In the athletic population, additional factors that influence diagnosis are sport and position. A 19-year-old college baseball pitcher who presents with shoulder pain may have anterior subluxation and secondary impingement. A 15-year-old female competitive swimmer with shoulder pain may have tendinitis with underlying multidirectional instability. Similarly, a 68-year-old masters tennis player with shoulder weakness probably has a rotator cuff tear.

It is important, however, to avoid focusing too quickly on the shoulder joint, for fear of missing other disease processes that can present as a shoulder complaint. In addition to the chief complaint, age, sex, handedness, occupation, sports activities, and history of trauma should be documented. Past medical and surgical histories, family and social histories, review of systems, and medication use should also be ascertained.

The format of both the history taking and the physical examination should be organized, comprehensive, and reproducible.

The chief complaint should be elicited at the onset of the interview. This may be related to an acute injury or to a chronic problem and is most commonly pain. In an athletic population, instability is the second most common complaint. Complaints such as weakness, stiffness, crepitus, and deformity are less frequently the presenting complaint but are often secondary symptoms.

The onset of the patient's symptoms should be elicited. This may be spontaneous, it may be due to overuse, or it may be due to a specific traumatic event. In spontaneous or overuse injuries, the patient should be asked about any changes in the pattern, duration, or intensity of activities preceding the injury. In traumatic events, the mechanism and circumstances, including the forces acting on and the position of the shoulder at the time of injury, should be noted. Any previous injury or disability should also be documented.

The progression of the patient's symptoms from onset to presentation should be noted, as well as any intervening treatments and their effect. Improvement, deterioration, or stability of the symptoms should be documented, as well as the degree of disability that this presents to the patient.

With pain as the chief complaint, the patient should be asked about the nature, site, frequency, duration, associated symptoms, and alleviating and aggravating factors. Shoulder tendinitis pain is often dull and diffuse, whereas referred cervical pain may be sharp and radiating in a particular dermatomal distribution. To ascertain the degree of disability that the complaint of pain presents, the patient should be asked about night pain, use of analgesic or anti-inflammatory medications and their effect, and interference with activities of daily living, work, recreation, and sport. The patient should grade the intensity of pain on a scale of 1 to 10.

With instability as a chief complaint, it is important to ascertain onset (traumatic, atraumatic, or overuse), direction (anterior, posterior, multidirectional), degree (dislocation, subluxation), frequency, and disability.[2] In the athletic population, the type of instability pattern found is often related to the specific sporting activity. In contact sports such as football, the most common instability pattern is unidirectional traumatic anterior instability. In noncontact sports such as swimming, one often finds posterior or multidirectional instability.

Most traumatic dislocations are anterior, occur in the provocative position of abduction and external rotation, and require manipulation for reduction. With subsequent dislocations, the amount of trauma required for dislocation typically decreases, and relocation often becomes easier. Most anterior instability patients are apprehensive in or avoid the abducted externally rotated position. With or without a history of dislocation, they may also have episodes of subluxation in which the shoulder subluxes partially out of the joint with a feeling of instability or pain and then spontaneously reduces. The ''dead arm syndrome'' of numbness or tingling probably represents anterior subluxation. Without a positive radiograph or a clear need for manipulation for reduction, it is often difficult to distinguish a history of dislocation and subluxation.

Posterior instability may be traumatic with a posteriorly directed force to the forward flexed and internally rotated shoulder but is more commonly atraumatic and often demonstrable by the patient. It is important to distinguish voluntary and involuntary instability, especially in posterior instability patients. Instability precipitated by arm positioning is considered involuntary, whereas that precipitated by muscular contraction is considered voluntary. There is a subset of voluntary dislocators with personality disorders who may frustrate both conservative and operative intervention.

Posterior instability is often associated with inferior (multidirectional) instability, especially in patients with generalized ligamentous laxity. Multidirectional instability patients usually have an atraumatic onset to their symptoms and present with a chief complaint of pain. They usually also appreciate a ''looseness'' of their shoulders and may have reproduction of their symptoms with inferior traction on the shoulder, such as picking up a suitcase. Subtle shoulder instability in any direction may present with a chief complaint of pain without an appreciation of instability by the patient.

Weakness as a chief complaint may be confusing in the presence of pain. True shoulder weakness is most commonly due to rotator cuff deficiency, or to a neurologic problem. Weakness due to a full-thickness rotator cuff tear may be traumatic or may be due to progression of rotator cuff pathology. In the latter case, it is often preceded by night pain or delayed activity-related pain. Adhesive capsulitis, often seen in middle-aged women and particularly problematic in diabetic patients, may present as a chief complaint of weakness or pain. A feeling of catching may be related to labral injury, loose bodies, instability, or rotator cuff tear or impingement. Deformity is an uncommon presenting complaint but may occur in acute or chronic acromioclavicular joint separation or clavicle fractures.

PHYSICAL EXAMINATION

A comprehensive approach to physical examination of the shoulder is described with particular emphasis on findings pertinent to an athletic population. It should be kept in mind throughout the examination that great variability exists from patient to patient in range of motion, joint laxity, and strength. Certain sports require emphasis on different aspects of shoulder function. For example, weight lifters depend on extreme strength, whereas gymnasts need hypermobility of their shoulders in addition to strength. The format of examination consists of initial impression, inspection, palpation, range of motion and strength testing, stability assessment, and special tests. Also, vascular, cervical, neurologic, and general physical examination can be important components of the evaluation of shoulder problems.

Initial Impression

The physical examination of the patient begins when the patient is first seen by the physician. The setting may be the sidelines of a college football game examining a player with an acute dislocation of the shoulder or at the clinic where a young swimmer presents with shoulder pain. The initial impression is divided into static and dynamic factors. The static factors consider physiologic age and appearance, body habitus, generalized diseases such as rheumatoid arthritis, generalized distress, and distress related to the shoulder. The dynamic factors consider generalized distress with movement, shoulder distress with movement, and the performance of simple tasks such as shaking hands or disrobing. The initial impression suggests which parts of the examination should subsequently receive emphasis.

Inspection

Appropriate exposure of both extremities is necessary for an adequate inspection of the shoulder. Male patients should remove all clothing above the waist. To preserve modesty, female patients might be dressed in a gown that extends to just above the breast line. A methodical inspection is performed, dividing the shoulder into anterior, lateral, posterior, and superior aspects and noting attitude, deformities, swelling, discoloration, and muscle characteristics.

The attitude of the shoulder is noted. A painful shoulder is often held higher than the opposite side. If very painful, it may be held in the ''protected position'' across the abdomen, often supported by the opposite upper extremity. Deformities such as scars, bumps, and bony prominences may be very meaningful. Enlargement of the sternoclavicular or acromioclavicular joints should be noted. A high-riding outer clavicle suggests an acromioclavicular joint dislocation. Squaring off of the shoulder with an anterior prominence of the humeral head suggests glenohumeral dislocation.

Swelling is unusual in most athletic shoulder injuries. Discoloration from bruising may be present from a recent fracture, cuff injury, or biceps rupture.

Muscle symmetry and contours are noted. Wasting of the deltoid is best visualized from the front as squaring off of the shoulder. Excessive prominence of the spine of the scapula is an indication of supraspinatus and infraspinatus wasting. Wasting in the infraspinatus fossa below the scapular spine is a hallmark of a rotator cuff tear or suprascapular neuropathy. A ''Popeye'' appearance of the biceps muscle belly with elbow flexion indicates rupture of the long head of the biceps tendon, often associated with rotator cuff pathology.

Several patterns of scapular winging can be noted, with most of these being associated with some type of glenohumeral pathology. Scapular winging can be due to deformities of the thorax such as scoliosis with rib deformities. Most winging, however, is due to weakness of the major scapular stabilizers, namely, serratus anterior, trapezius, and the rhomboids. The winging due to weakness of the muscular stabilizers typically becomes more evident with motion and stress testing. Minor degrees of scapular asymmetry due to winging can be seen in many people unrelated to glenohumeral pathology. However, this often can be a subtle indicator of an intrinsic glenohumeral problem. Moderate degrees of scapular winging can be seen in association with more pronounced glenohumeral problems, such as posterior subluxation. Severe scapular winging is most commonly related to a neurologic injury, namely, dysfunction of the long thoracic nerve with secondary serratus anterior palsy.

Palpation

The shoulder should regionalized so that the anterior, lateral, posterior, and superior aspects can be palpated. Palpation might be divided into superficial and deep, as well as bone and soft tissue. Features to be considered include tenderness, swelling, temperature changes, deformities, muscle characteristics, and relationships of various structures. The most easily identifiable landmarks are bony prominences and associated joints.

Palpation might begin at the sternoclavicular joint and proceed laterally, palpating specific areas of anatomy, considering common pathologies. Palpation of the supraclavicular region could infrequently reveal anomalous nodes. The clavicle might reveal local deformities and tenderness. The acromioclavicular joint is identified at the lateral end of the clavicle on the superior aspect of the shoulder. Acromioclavicular joint arthritis is unusual without joint tenderness.

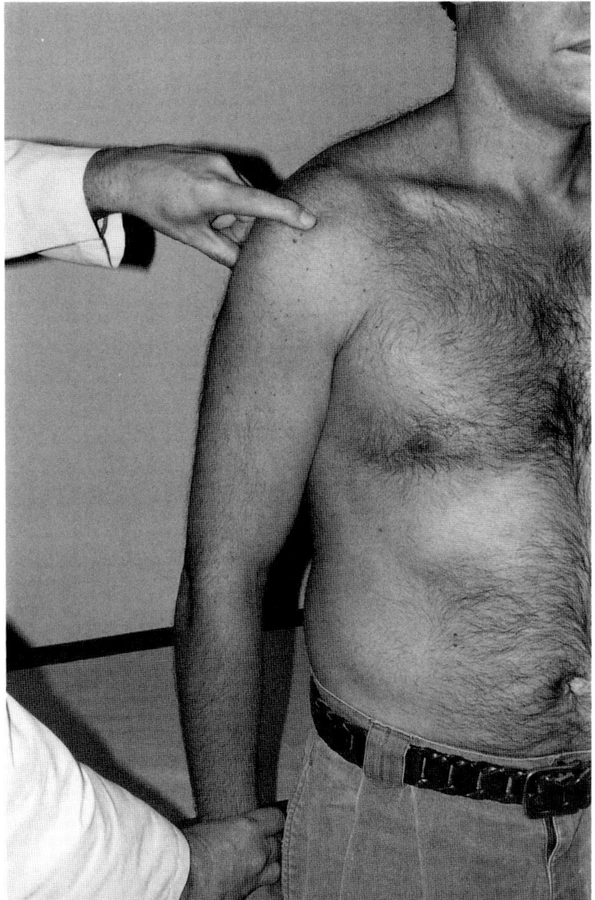

Figure 2-1. Palpation of the supraspinatus portion of the rotator cuff at its insertion into the greater tuberosity.

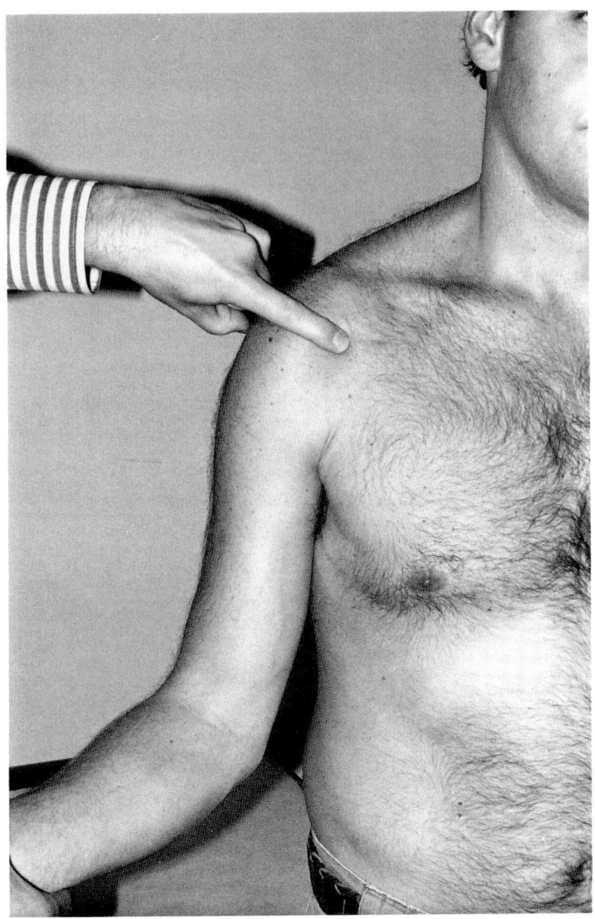

Figure 2-2. Palpation of the subscapularis tendon at its insertion into the lesser tuberosity.

The supraspinatus portion of the rotator cuff at its insertion into the great tuberosity is palpated by extending the arm, bringing the tuberosity from underneath the acromion (Fig. 2-1). The subscapularis tendon insertion into the lesser tuberosity is palpated by positioning the arm in external rotation, bringing the tuberosity lateral to the coracoid (Fig. 2-2). The infraspinatus portion of the rotator cuff is palpated by slightly flexing and internally rotating the arm, bringing the posterior aspect of the greater tuberosity from underneath the acromion (Fig. 2-3). Tuberosity and cuff tenderness may be associated with rotator cuff tendonitis, a rotator cuff tear, or tuberosity fracture.

The biceps tendon is palpated with the arm in the neutral position and is found midway between the apex of the axilla and the lateral border of the deltoid, approximately 1 in. distal to the acromion (Fig. 2-4).

Range of Motion and Strength Testing

The multiplanar range of shoulder motion is primarily from the glenohumeral and scapulothoracic articulations, with additional contributions from the sternoclavicular and acromioclavicular joints. Loss of motion of the shoulder is most commonly due to pain; it is important to determine the degree of pain, as well as the arc of motion in which it occurs. Pain often occurs at the extremes of motion with passive stressing. Disorders of the glenohumeral articulation, such as osteoarthritis or adhesive capsulitis, will increase the relative contribution to motion by the scapulothoracic articulation.

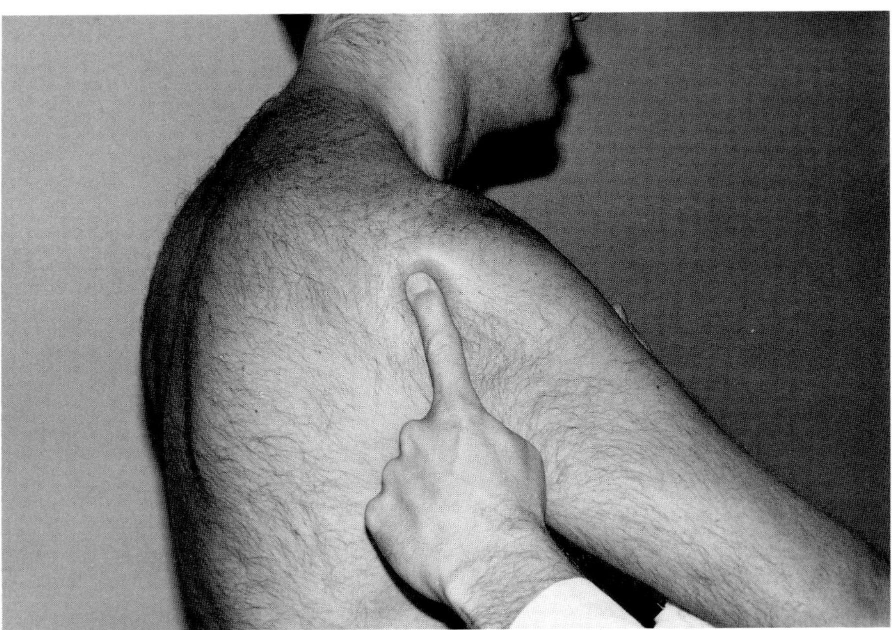

Figure 2-3. Palpation of the infraspinatus portion of the rotator cuff at its insertion into the greater tuberosity.

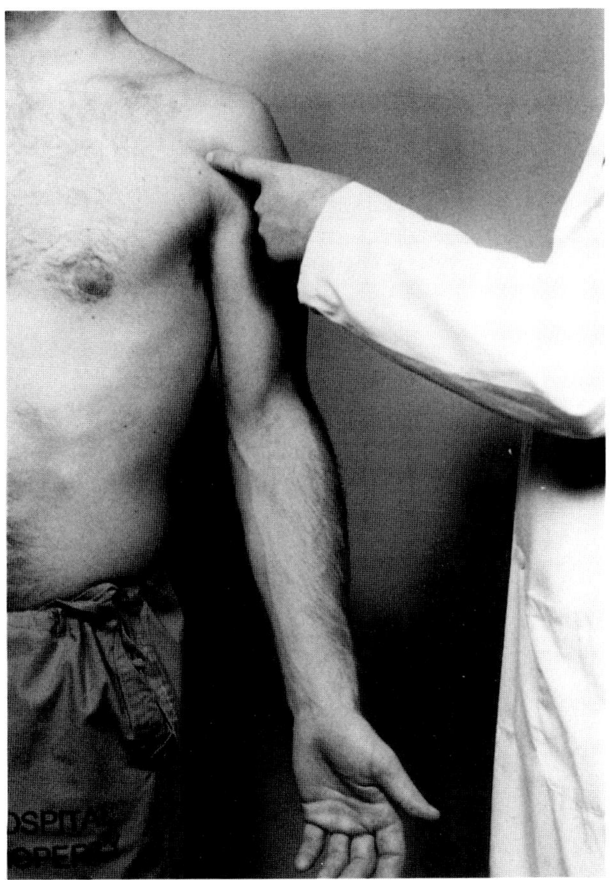

Figure 2-4. Palpation of the bicipital tendon in the intertubercular sulcus.

Rotator cuff tears or labral lesions may cause painful catching and result in hesitant glenohumeral rhythm. Similar types of catching and joint dysrhythmia can be seen with instability as well as with glenohumeral arthritis. Crepitus in the subacromial, glenohumeral, or scapulothoracic region may be palpated during motion. It may be possible to discern the source of crepitus simply by the tactile sensation that it creates. Often, there is a distinct difference between crepitus caused by bone problems such as arthritis, fibrocartilage disorders such as labral tears, and soft tissue disorders such as rotator cuff tears or impingement.

Because of the global nature of shoulder motion, documentation of shoulder movement has often been confusing. The American Shoulder and Elbow Surgeons recommend that four functionally important and reproducible arcs of motion be documented: total elevation (active and passive), external rotation with the arm at the side (active and passive), external rotation in the 90 degree abducted position (passive), and internal rotation (active or passive).

Maximum forward elevation occurs between the coronal and sagittal planes, usually 20 to 30 degrees from the sagittal plane. The angle the arm makes with the thorax should be measured to compensate for body attitude (Fig. 2-5). Total active elevation should be recorded in the upright position, whereas passive elevation can be measured with the patient upright or supine. Typical forward elevation in normal subjects is 150 to 170 degrees.

With forward elevation, the scapulothoracic rhythm should be inspected for winging or dyskinesia, especially with resisted forward elevation. Even in the resting neutral position, with the arms at the side, it is important to examine the scapula for both position and any element of winging that may be present. Winging of the scapula is usually evident at the inferior border but can be along the entire scapula and, rarely, more predominant at the superior border. As the arms are elevated, careful observation should be made in comparing the scapulae throughout the range of motion. Frequently, in instability patients and in overhead athletes, the scapula does not move with its normal rhythm. It may wing very slightly, and it might not move as smoothly on the chest wall. During elevation and, perhaps more importantly, when the arms are brought down from the elevated position, winging becomes obvious. Applying resistance at 60 and 30 degrees of shoulder elevation as the arms are brought down from the elevated position is

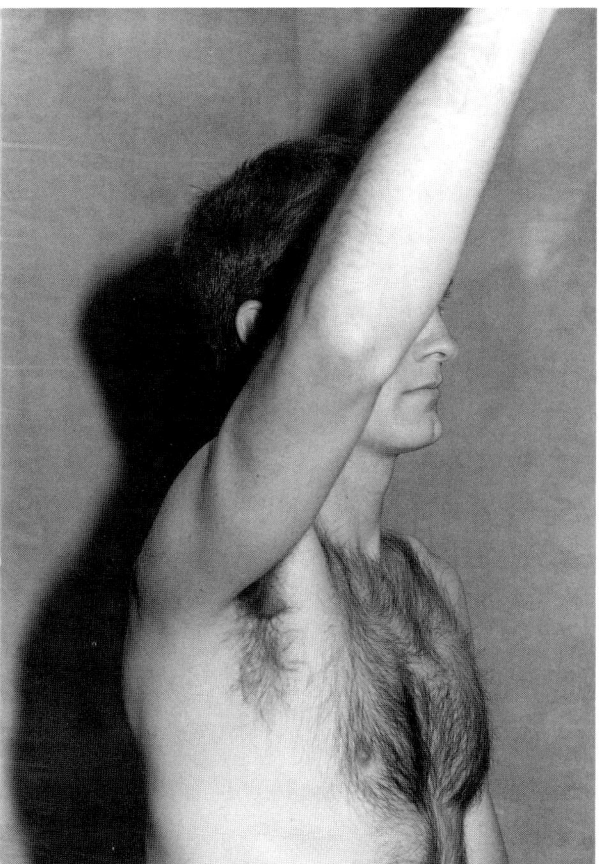

Figure 2-5. Total active elevation of the shoulder.

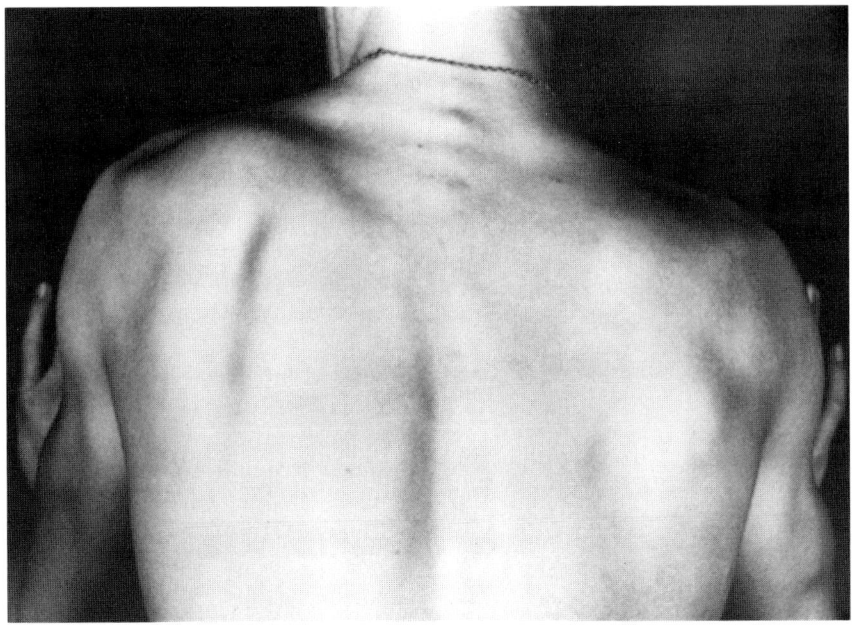

Figure 2-6. Scapular winging demonstrated by a patient pushing against a wall.

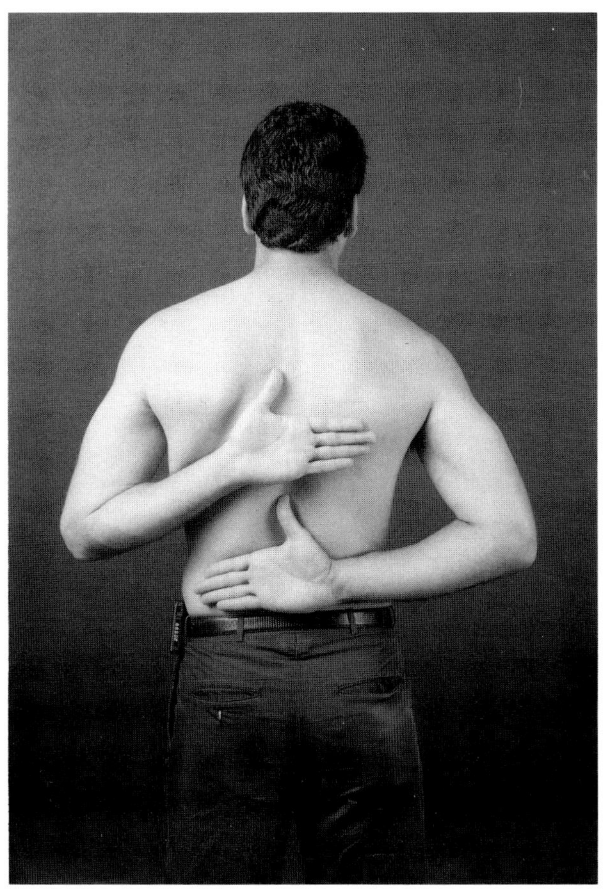

Figure 2-7. Active internal rotation.

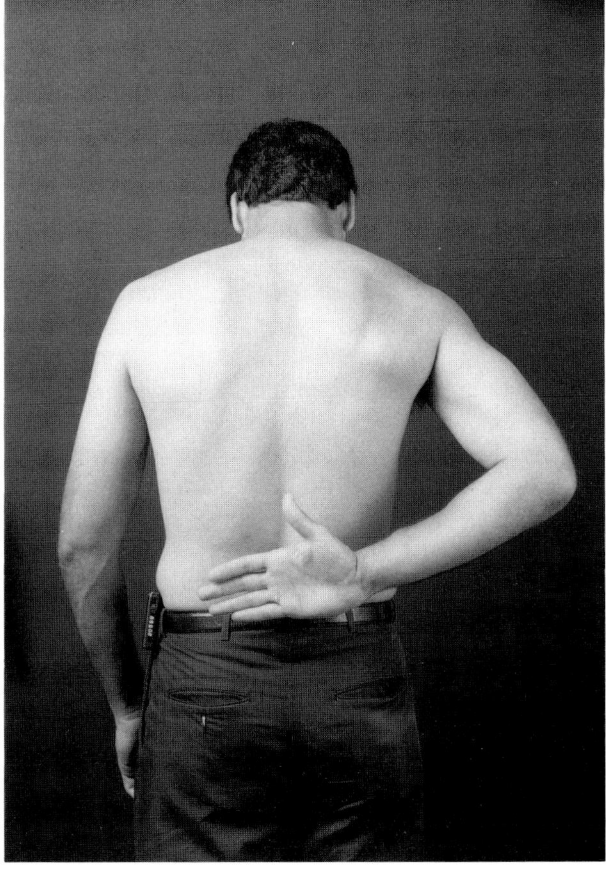

Figure 2-8. Normal lift-off test demonstrating functioning subscapularis muscle.

often the best way to demonstrate scapular winging. Pushing against the wall with outstretched arms or push-ups are standard tests to stress the serratus muscle to demonstrate winging (Fig. 2-6). Visualizing from behind, the distance from the inferior tip of the scapula to the spinous processes on each side can be measured. This should be observed in three positions: (1) with the arms resting at the side, (2) with the hands placed on the hips, and (3) in a 90 degree abducted position. This is an objective measurement of scapular protraction on the chest wall. Winging should be documented relative to the opposite side, and determination should be made of how far away from the chest wall (in centimeters) the scapula moves. Scapular abnormalities are frequently present in athletes, particularly throwing athletes, and may be associated with instability, not only anterior but also multidirectional and posterior. There also may be scapular abnormalities with subacromial impingement and rotator cuff tears.

Measurement of external rotation begins with the arm resting at the side, the elbow flexed 90 degrees, and the forearm in the sagittal plane. To eliminate the effects of gravity, active external rotation should be measured upright, whereas passive motion may be measured upright or supine. There is great variability in total external rotation, and a comparison should always be made with the opposite side. Typical external rotation for normal subjects is 50 to 70 degrees.

If the patient can achieve a 90 degree abducted position, external rotation in this position should be measured. This measurement is meaningful in the presence of previous trauma, such as an old fracture of the greater tuberosity, and is especially important in the overhead athlete. In throwers, excessive external rotation is often present, perhaps at the expense of limited internal rotation, a frequent concomitant finding. Average external rotation in the abducted position for normal subjects is 80 to 100 degrees.

Internal rotation is measured by the position reached by the outstretched hitchhiking thumb up the back in reference to the posterior anatomy (Fig. 2-7). Common reference points include the greater trochanter, buttock, belt line, and the spinous processes of the lumbar and thoracic vertebrae. The lower border of the scapula corresponds to approximately the eighth thoracic vertebra. Limitation of internal rotation is often a manifestation of posterior capsular tightness. An additional technique to assess tightness of the posterior capsule consists of assessing limitation of crossed-arm adduction. Typical internal rotation for normal subjects is T5 to T10. Many subjects will have some asymmetry, with the dominant arm being one to two vertebral levels tighter than the nondominant arm.

A

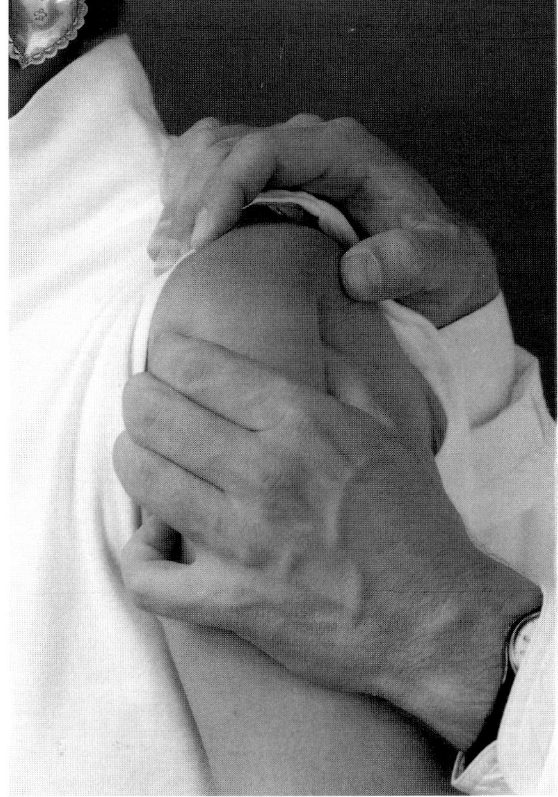

B

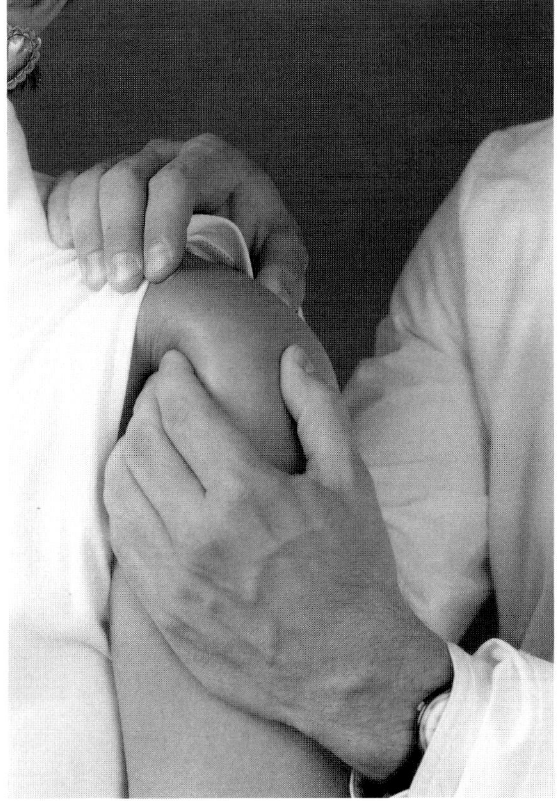

Figure 2-9. "Load-and-shift" test for (**A**) anterior and (**B**) posterior translation determination of the shoulder.

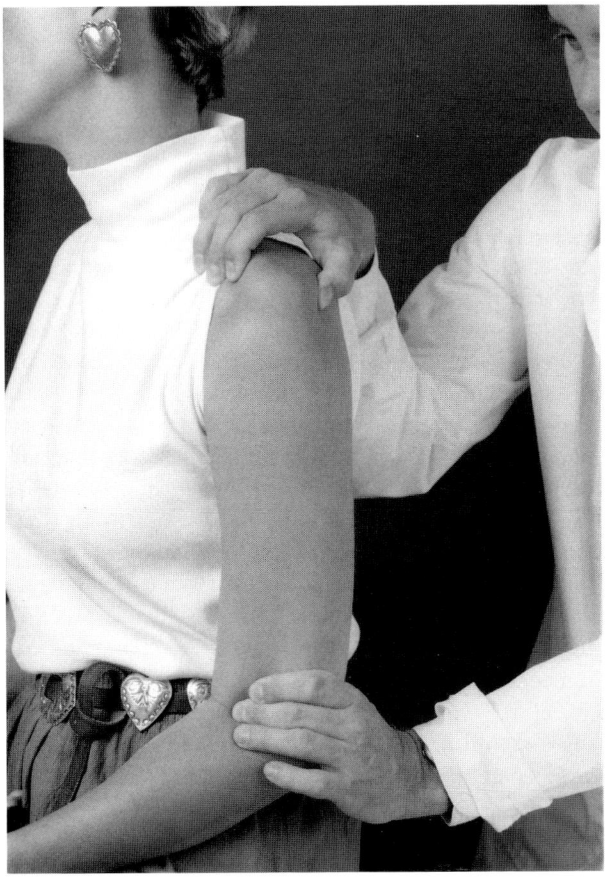

Figure 2-10. "Sulcus sign" with inferior translation of the shoulder.

Muscle strength can be assessed as the shoulder is put through these ranges of motion. The comprehensiveness of strength testing and neurologic evaluation relates to the complaint and general status of the patient. For example, a rheumatoid patient with shoulder pain should have a more extensive examination, including assessment for evidence of long track signs in the lower extremities. A volleyball player with shoulder pain needs careful assessment of the suprascapular nerve, as suprascapular nerve injury is common in these athletes.

Routine strength testing should include the deltoid and the rotator cuff (i.e., forward flexion, abduction, and external rotation). The strength of the anterior deltoid, the chief flexor of the shoulder, is tested by applying a sustained resistance at approximately 90 degrees of active forward elevation. Abduction strength should be tested in the coronal plane to assess the middle deltoid. Hiking of the shoulder with abduction is suggestive of a rotator cuff tear. The infraspinatus and teres minor, the chief external rotators of the shoulder, can be tested by resisted external rotation with the arm adducted and the elbow flexed 90 degrees. Applying resistance to the 90 degrees abducted, 30 degrees forward flexed, and pronated arm tests the strength of the supraspinatus. The ability to actively lift the internally rotated arm off the patient's back is dependent on a functioning subscapularis muscle and is useful in patients suspected of having a massive rotator cuff tear. This is termed the *lift-off test* by Gerber and Krushell[1] (Fig. 2-8).

Muscle strength should be graded 0 to 5 compared with the contralateral side. Unfortunately, manual muscle strength testing is not highly accurate. A great deal of weakness is often necessary before that weakness can be detected by manual testing. More subtle degrees of weakness may need to be objectively measured with isokinetic or isometric strength testing devices.

Instability Testing

Shoulder instability may be anterior, posterior, or inferior (multidirectional), and it may be subtle or obvious. Stability assessment consists of documenting the amount of passive translation between the humeral head and glenoid fossa and attempting reproduction of symptoms of

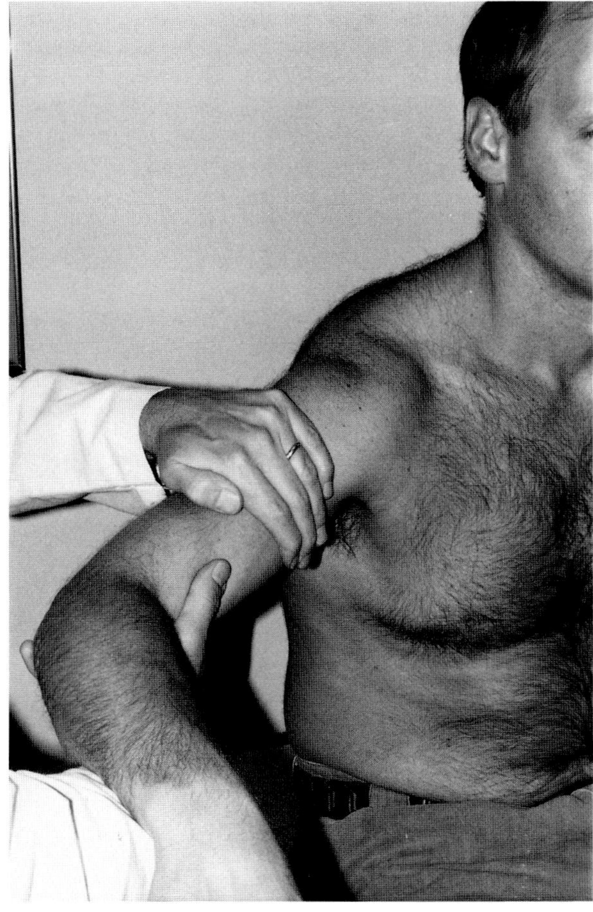

Figure 2-11. Inferior translation with inferior load applied to the abducted proximal humerus.

subluxation, apprehension, or pain by stressing the shoulder.

The stability examination may be performed in the sitting position. The same testing is repeated supine. For anterior and posterior translation measurement, the humeral head is grasped and compressed into the glenoid fossa to ensure its reduction to the neutral starting position. In this "loaded" position, anterior and posterior stresses are applied (Fig. 2-9). This "load-and-shift" test is graded as minimally up the glenoid face, to the glenoid rim (grade I), and over the glenoid run (grade II). Reproduction of the patient's symptoms with anterior, posterior, or inferior translation may confirm the direction of instability.

Inferior translation is measured by grasping the elbow and applying inferior traction to the shoulder. Excessive inferior translation is manifested by a widening of the subacromial space between the acromion and humeral head with dimpling of the overlying skin ("sulcus sign")[4] (Fig. 2-10). Inferior translation is best documented as centimeters of displacement of the humeral head from the acromion (i.e., less than 1 cm, 1 to 2 cm, and greater than 2 cm). Inferior translation should also be measured with the arm

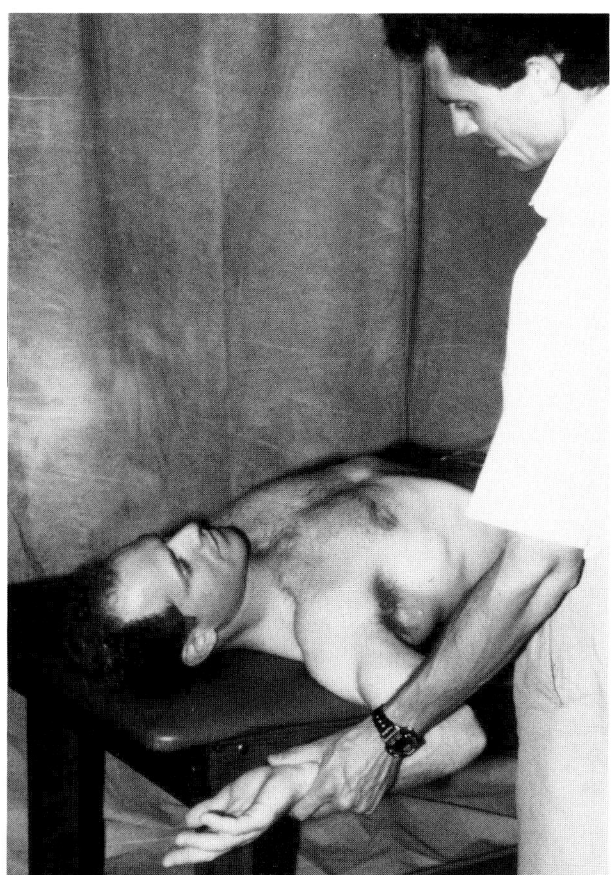

Figure 2-12. "Fulcrum test" for anterior instability in the supine position.

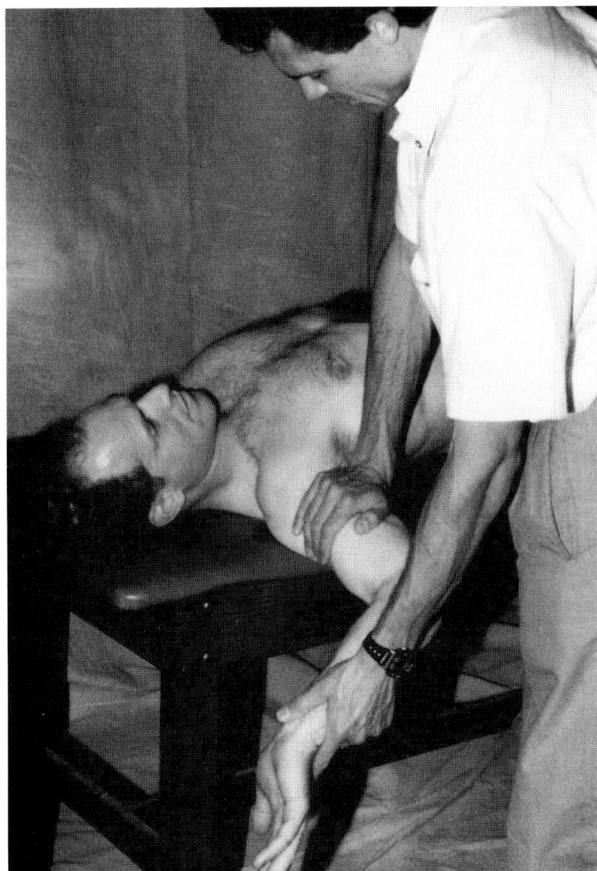

Figure 2-13. "Relocation test." With a posterior stress exerted on the proximal humerus, external rotation is increased.

held in an abducted position by passively abducting the arm and applying an inferior load to the proximal humerus (Fig. 2-11). Reproduction of the patient's symptoms is documented and may be diagnostic of multidirectional instability. A clicking or grinding detected with translation is a nonspecific sign that may suggest labral pathology, such as a Bankart or a SLAP lesion.

The most common direction of instability is anterior, with subluxation or dislocation occurring in the abducted and externally rotated position. To perform the "crank test" for anterior instability, the examiner stands behind the seated patient, raises the arm to 90 degrees of abduction, and externally rotates the shoulder. The examiner's opposite hand is placed with the thumb behind and fingers in front of the humeral head to provide posterior leverage and a restraining force for any sudden instability. An impending feeling of anterior instability is referred to as an "apprehension sign." Pain without apprehension is not a positive apprehension sign, although it is often present and should be recorded.

If apprehension or pain is elicited with the crank test,

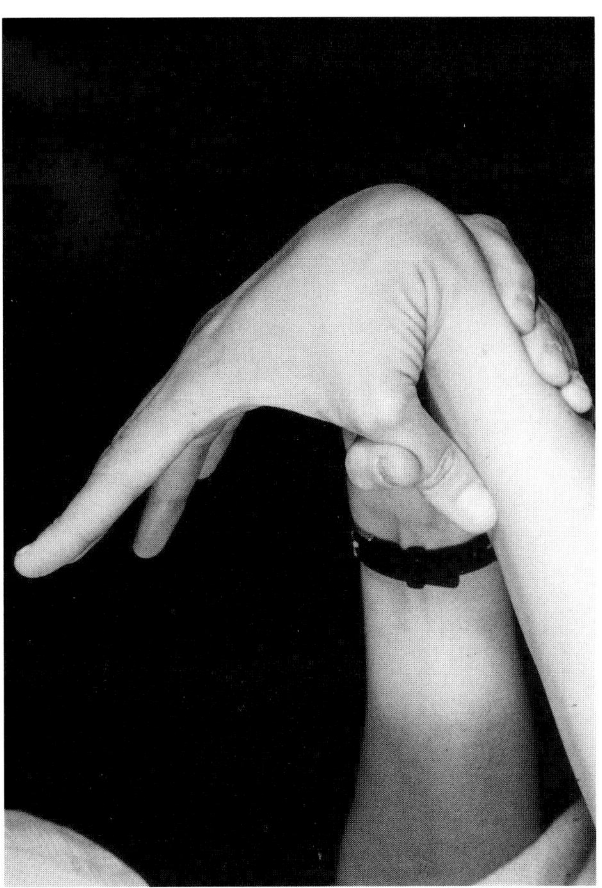

Figure 2-14. Ligamentous laxity in a patient with multidirectional instability of her shoulders.

continued instability testing should be performed in the supine position. In this position, the "fulcrum test" is repeated, using the edge of the examining table as the fulcrum for externally rotating the 90 degree abducted arm (Fig. 2-12). If pain or apprehension is reproduced, a "relocation test" is performed[3] (Fig. 2-13). A posterior stress should be exerted on the proximal humerus. More external humeral rotation being possible before emergence of symptoms constitutes a positive relocation test. Conversely, an "augmentation test" consists of repeating the fulcrum test, with an anterior stress exerted on the proximal humerus. A positive augmentation test allows less external rotation before emergence of symptoms. Both the relocation test and augmentation test can be quantified by the change in external rotation (i.e., increase or decrease of external rotation by 10 degrees, 20 degrees, or 30 degrees). The effect of these two tests on apprehension and pain should be recorded separately.

Historically, the relocation test has been applied in the overhead athlete in whom only pain is produced with external rotation stressing in the abducted position. A diminution of pain with greater external rotation has been termed a positive relocation test, suggestive of anterior subluxation. It is now also applied to "apprehension."

In the supine position, passive anterior, posterior, and inferior translation should be repeated, noting any reproduction of symptoms.

In patients with instability, especially multidirectional instability, generalized ligamentous laxity may be present. The ability to flex the wrist and bring the thumb to the

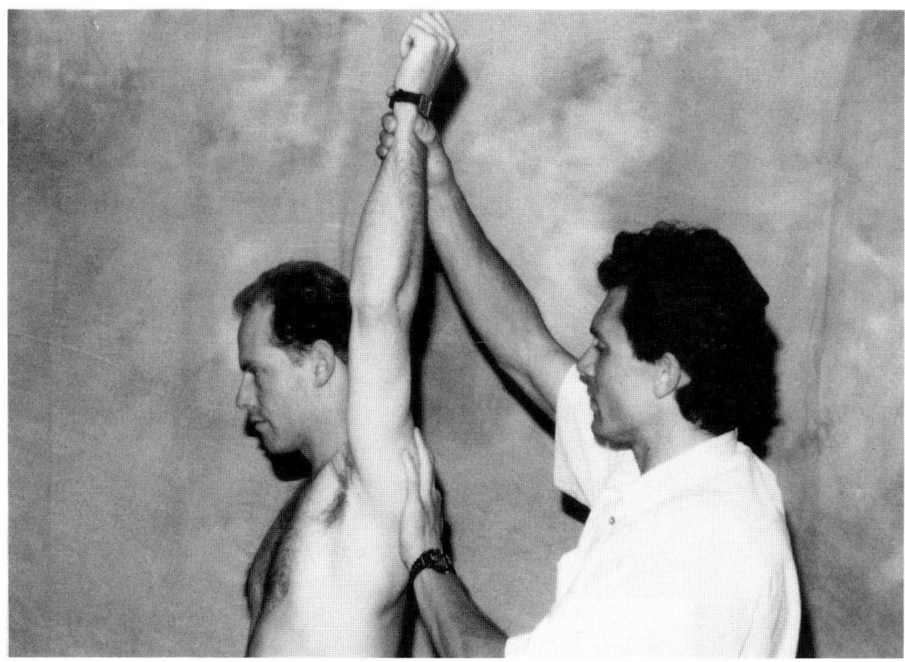

Figure 2-15. "Impingement sign." Pain on forced passive elevation of the shoulder.

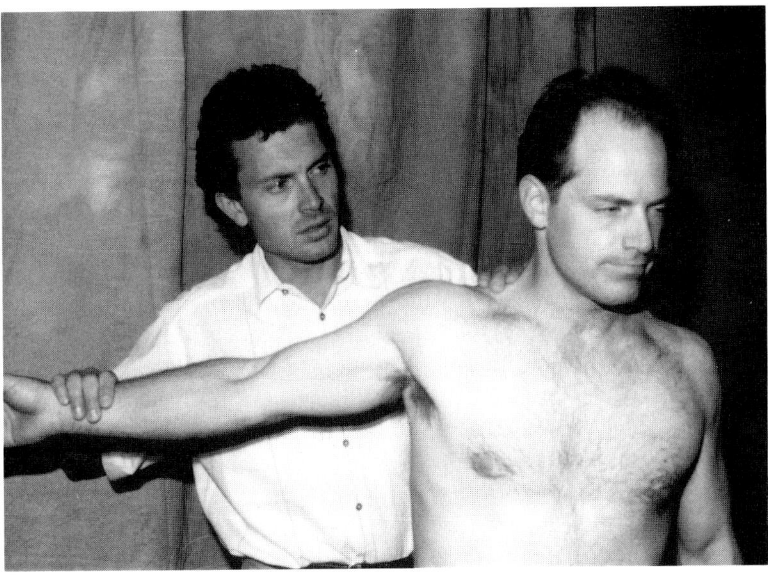

Figure 2-16. "Painful arc." Pain with active resisted abduction just posterior to the coronal plane.

palmar surface of the forearm, metacarpophalangeal hyperextension allowing the fingers to be parallel to the forearm, elbow hyperextension, patellar hypermobility, and the ability to place both hands flat on the floor with the knees straight are all indicative of generalized ligamentous laxity. Perhaps the best indicator of laxity is a thumb-to-forearm distance of less than 4 cm. Many multidirectional instability patients can touch the thumb to the forearm (Fig. 2-14). For all instability testing, it is important that comparison be made with the opposite shoulder.

Special Tests

"Impingement" refers to symptomatic compression of the supraspinatus tendon between the humeral head and the anteroinferior acromion. Forced passive elevation with reproduction of pain constitutes an "impingement sign"[5] (Fig. 2-15). Reproduction of pain with resisted active abduction in or just posterior to the coronal plane constitutes a "painful arc" and is a second test for impingement (Fig. 2-16). Forced internal rotation at 90 degrees of forward elevation in the sagittal plane, driving the greater tuberosity

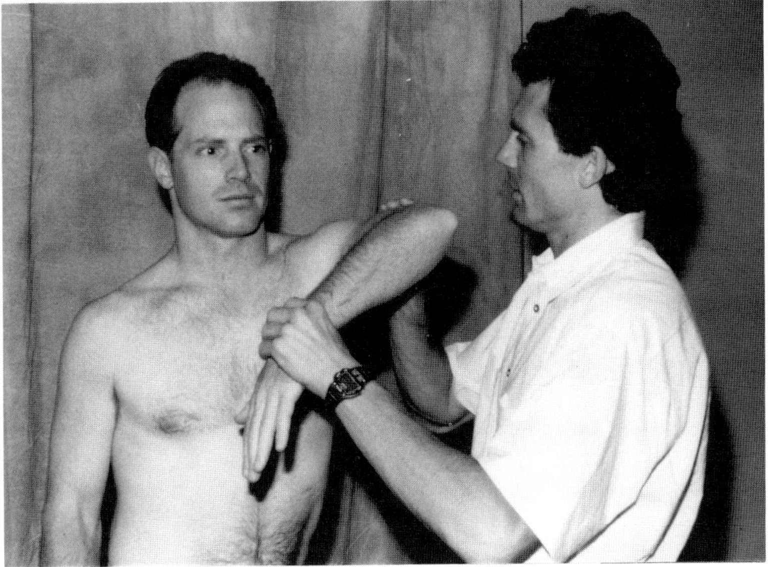

Figure 2-17. Pain with forced internal rotation at 90 degrees of forward elevation, a third sign of impingement.

under the coracoacromial ligament and causing pain, is the third sign of impingement (Fig. 2-17). Stressed crossed-arm adduction at 90 degrees of forward elevation is a test for acromioclavicular joint or sternoclavicular joint pathology (Fig. 2-18). During all impingement and joint stress testing, it is important to ascertain the location of pain reproduced during those maneuvers. Impingement maneuvers are only positive when they recreate pain at the area of impingement, and likewise acromioclavicular and sternoclavicular joint tests are only positive when they recreate symptoms at the affected joint.

As the biceps tendon is usually not palpable, tenderness in the biceps region should be further investigated, using Yergason's and Speed's tests (Fig. 2-19). Yergason's test consists of resisted forearm supination with the elbow flexed to 90 degrees. Speed's test consists of resisted forward elevation of the humerus with the elbow extended and the forearm supinated. Pain with either of these maneuvers is suggestive of biceps tendon irritation. Often biceps pathology is associated with subacromial impingement and disorders of the rotator cuff.

Vascular Examination

A thorough vascular examination is critical in trauma cases and is important in patients complaining of vague achiness, heaviness, or fatigue radiating down the arm. Distal pulses, skin color, temperature, hair growth, and alternation in sensation should routinely be assessed. Provocative tests looking for obliteration of pulses with certain maneuvers and reproduction of symptoms should be performed in all cases of suspected vascular compression about the neck. With Adson's maneuver, the patient is seated, the shoulder extended, the head rotated toward the side being examined, and the pulse taken while the patient holds a deep breath (Fig. 2-20). A modified Adson's maneuver involves rotating the head away from the side being examined. With Wright's maneuver, the arm is abducted and extended and externally rotated[6] (Fig. 2-21). The maneuver can be exaggerated by tilting and rotation of the head and neck to the contralateral side. Any change of radial pulse is recorded during those maneuvers. However, these tests are only considered positive if they reproduce the patient's symptoms of pain or paresthesias.

Inferior traction in patients with vascular compression about the neck may obliterate distal pulses and reproduce symptoms. Overhead exercises with slow repetitive opening and closing of the fingers in the elevated position with reproduction of symptoms is the best provocative test for thoracic outlet syndrome. A bruit under the clavicle may be indicative of vascular compression.

General Physical Examination

A general physical examination is required to complete the overall evaluation of a patient who presents with shoulder complaints. Cervical nerve root compression and many

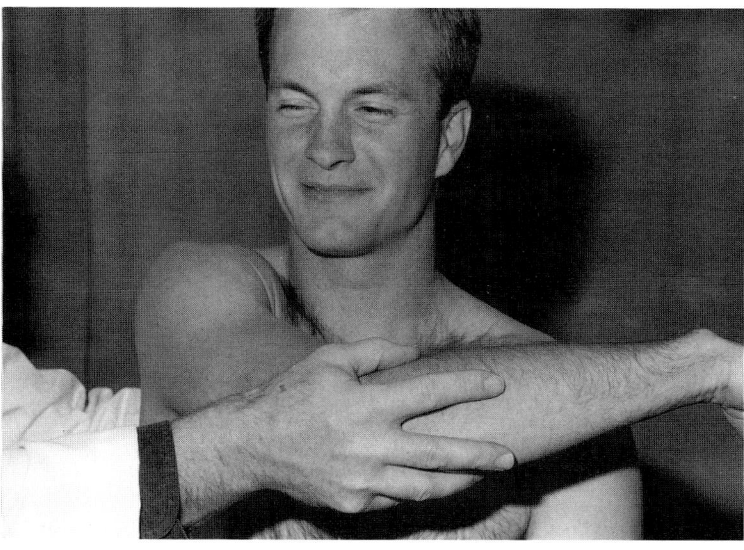

Figure 2-18. Pain with stressed crossed-arm adduction at 90 degrees of forward elevation suggests acromioclavicular joint pathology.

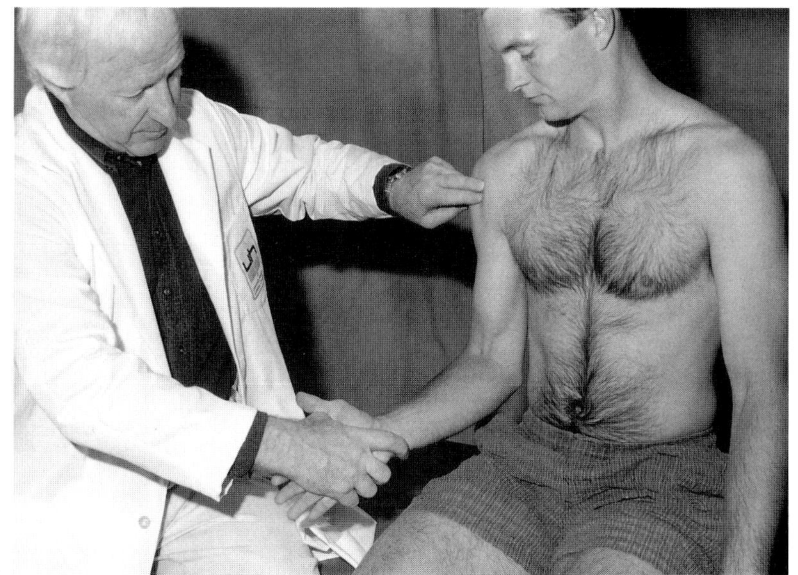

A

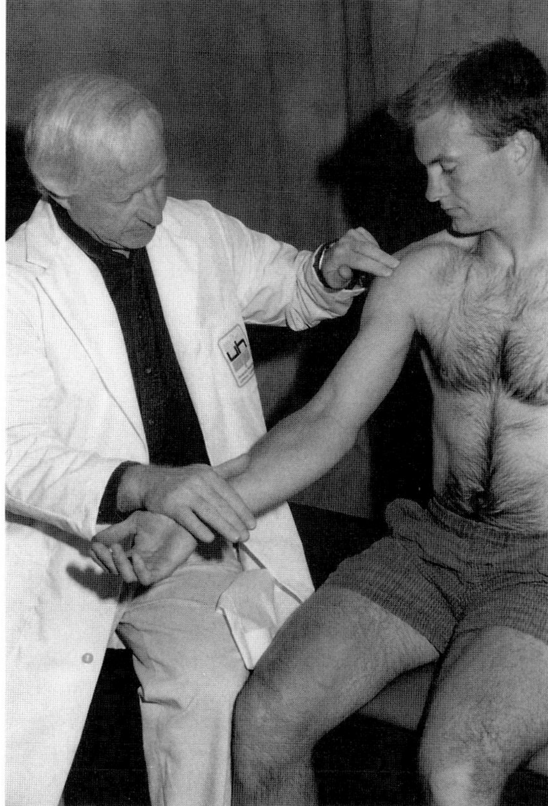

B

Figure 2-19. (**A**) Yergason's and (**B**) Speed's tests for bicipital tendinitis.

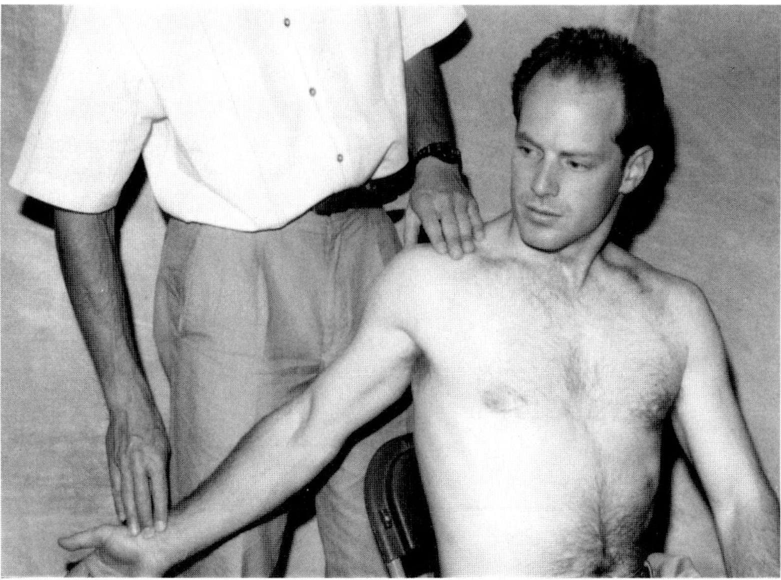

Figure 2-20. Adson's maneuver for vascular compression.

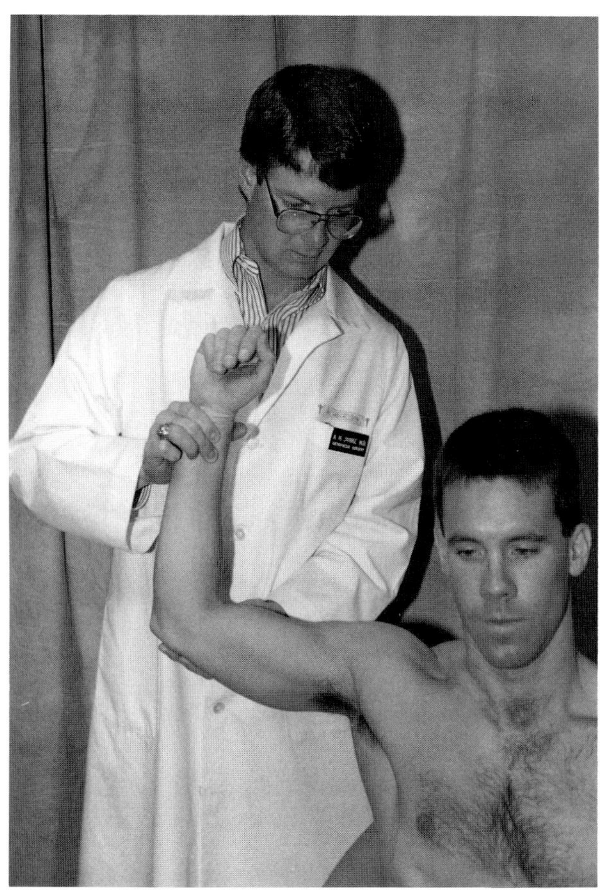

Figure 2-21. Wright's maneuver for vascular compression.

other disease processes, including rheumatoid arthritis, diabetes mellitus, neurofibromatosis, neoplasms, and cardiac disease, can all present with shoulder problems. A general examination is important, and its scope depends on the suspected pathology and clinical presentation.

REFERENCES

1. Gerber C, Krushell RJ: Isolated rupture of the tendon of the subscapularis muscle. J Bone Joint Surg [Br] 73:389, 1991
2. Hawkins RJ, Bokor DJ: Clinical evaluation of the shoulder. pp. 149. In Rockwood CA, Matsen RA (eds): The Shoulder. WB Saunders, Philadelphia, 1990
3. Jobe FW, Bradley JP: The diagnosis and nonoperative treatment of shoulder injuries in athletes. Clin Sports Med 8:419, 1989
4. Neer CS, Foster CR: Inferior capsular shift for involuntary inferior and multidirectional instability of the shoulder. J Bone Joint Surg [Am] 62:897, 1980
5. Neer CS, Welsh RP: The shoulder in sport. Orthop Clin North Am 8:583, 1977
6. Wright IS: The neurovascular syndrome produced by hyperabduction of the arm. Am Heart J 29:1, 1945

CHAPTER THREE

Mechanics of Throwing

Charles J. Dillman
Glenn S. Fleisig
James R. Andrews

Throwing an object illustrates the dynamic capabilities of the shoulder. From an academic point of view, the study of the shoulder in a throwing activity can provide an understanding of the true maximal capabilities of the shoulder complex. This chapter provides a detailed description of the act of throwing that is meaningful for the physician and therapist. The review contains an analysis of movement patterns, muscular involvement, and forces created during the motor act of throwing with emphasis on the shoulder.

PHASES OF THROWING

To understand the mechanics of throwing, it is first necessary to define the movement phases of this skill. These are as follows:

1. Windup—from the initial motion (usually a step backward), through the counter-rotation of the body, to the instant of ball release from the glove (sequences A to D in Fig. 3-1)
2. Stride—from ball release out of the glove until the striding foot has contacted the ground (sequences D, E, and F in Fig. 3-1)
3. Arm cocking—from when the stride foot contacts the ground until the arm reaches maximum external rotation at the shoulder (sequences F, G, and H in Fig. 3-1)
4. Arm acceleration—from maximum external rotation until ball release (sequences H and I in Fig. 3-1)
5. Arm deceleration—from ball release until the arm reaches approximately 0 degrees of internal rotation (sequences I and J in Fig. 3-1)
6. Follow-through—from 0 degrees internal rotation of the arm until the throwing arm crosses over in front of the body (sequences J and K in Fig. 3-1)

It is important to be able to visualize these aspects of the movement pattern because the mechanical factors of the throw are usually described relative to these specific phases.

KINEMATICS OF THE THROWING MOTION

The critical movement features of the throw are the stride toward the plate and the cocking and uncocking of the arm. Figure 3-2 illustrates some of the kinematic descriptions of the stride. A normal stride distance is approximately 87 percent (plus or minus 5 percent) of the body height (front of rubber to middle of foot, length of B in Fig. 3-2). Most highly skilled individuals stride straight toward the target (C in Fig. 3-2), landing the foot in a slightly closed position (Θ in Fig. 3-2). Pitchers who throw at extremely high velocities tend to have a larger stride length (close to 100 percent of body height). However, an extremely open or closed stride for any pitcher would indicate abnormal mechanics relative to our analysis of many highly skilled throwers.

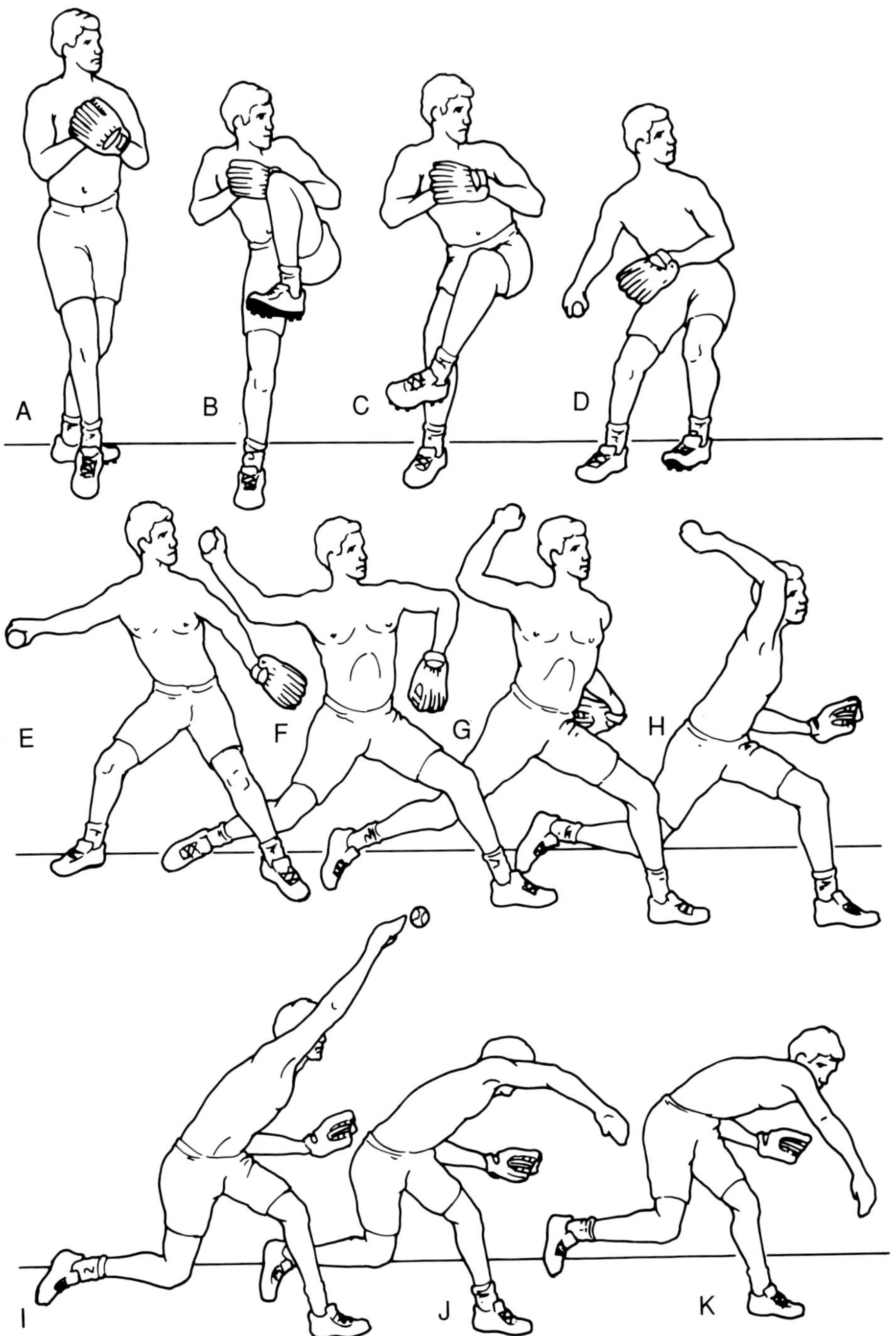

Figure 3-1. **(A–K)** Sequence of critical positions in throwing.

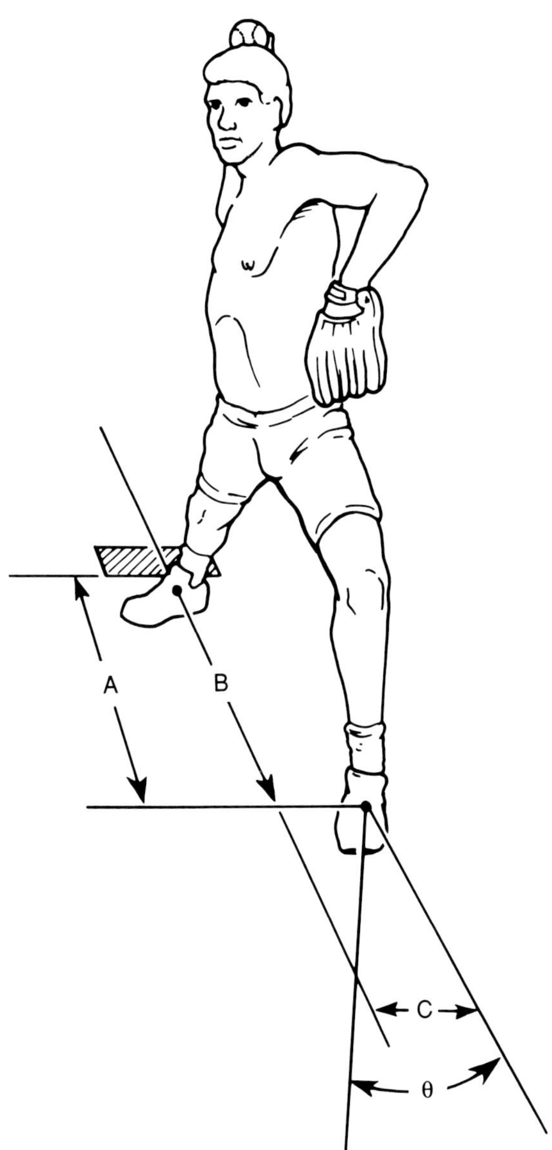

Figure 3-2. Kinematic aspects of the stride in throwing. (For explanation of abbreviations, see text.)

Atwater[1] has illustrated that the arm position relative to the trunk is approximately 90 to 100 degrees of abduction for all throwing and striking activities. Thus, when the arm is elevated up into position before the cocking phase (F in Fig. 3-1), it is generally placed at a 90 degree angle to the trunk and remains in this position during the entire delivery of the throw.

The major kinematic feature of arm cocking and acceleration is the external and internal rotation of the arm about the shoulder. During the cocking phase, from when the striding foot contacts the ground until the arm reaches maximum external rotation (F, G, and H in Fig. 3-1), the arm undergoes a fairly rapid external rotation movement while the hips and trunk are rotating around toward the target. The summation of the glenohumeral, scapulothoracic, and hyperextension of the upper trunk allows the arm to reach a position of 175 degrees of maximal external rotation during this cocking phase (Fig. 3-3).

Generally, maximum external rotation is achieved when the trunk has rotated around and is approximately square to the direction of throwing (H in Fig. 3-1). From the point of maximum external rotation, the elbow begins to extend and the arm undergoes rapid internal rotation, rotating approximately through an angle of 80 degrees in 30 ms (Fig. 3-3, acceleration phase). This is perhaps one of the fastest movements in all of sports. Peak velocities for this motion can reach an astounding value of 7,000 degrees/sec (Fig. 3-4).

Once the ball is released, the arm continues internally rotating, while the shoulder undergoes a rapid abduction (J in Fig. 3-1). This abduction motion is very significant in the throwing act and occurs because the trunk is inclined forward as the ball is released. With a continuing internal rotation, the arm abducts up toward the flexed trunk or in the direction of throwing (Fig. 3-1, I to J). The deceleration of this abduction motion (by the adductors) immediately after release appears to be the main component responsible for the initial deceleration of the arm during this critical period of the throw.

ELECTROMYOGRAPHIC ANALYSIS

Electromyographic evaluation of the muscles involved in a particular activity provides insight into how the muscular system is coordinated to perform a particular motor skill. Fortunately, in the area of throwing, Jobe and colleagues[8-11] have conducted an excellent series of studies that provide detailed insight into which particular muscles are used in the throwing motion.

To provide a reference frame for the measurement of the electrical activity of muscles, a maximum voluntary contraction (MVC) of a specific muscle is evoked before the testing is undertaken. The recording of the MVC is referred to as 100 percent of electrical activity. Thus, the amplitude of a muscular contraction during the performance of a dynamic activity is related to this standard and listed as a percentage of the MVC. This type of analysis provides us with a view of the *relative intensity* of the contractions involved in a skill.

Intervals of MVCs are grouped to provide qualitative descriptors of an electromyographic analysis. For the purposes of our work, we usually describe the ranges of MVCs

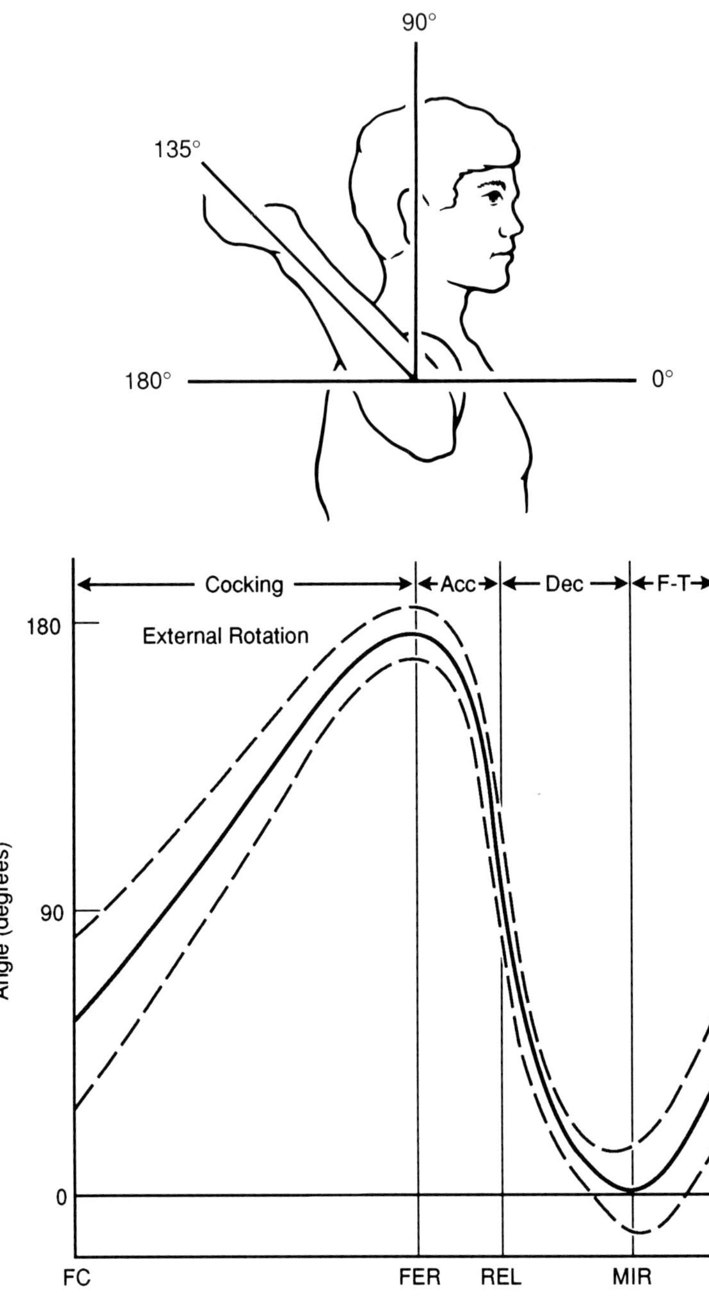

Figure 3-3. External and internal rotation of the arm about the shoulder in throwing. Solid line represents average angular displacement for 29 highly skilled subjects throwing at an average velocity of 85 mph. Dotted line is ±1 SD.

as follows: slight activity (0 to 20 percent MVC); moderate (20 to 50 percent MVC); marked (50 to 100 percent MVC); and greater than 100 percent, a maximal contraction.

If we review the work of Glousman et al[8] for a sample of highly skilled pitchers and rate the muscular activity according to the scheme presented above, the results of the key muscles involved in throwing are tabulated in Table 3-1. The qualitative analysis of the data of Glousman et al[8] in Table 3-1 illustrates that the anterior muscles (subscapularis, latissimus dorsi, and pectoralis major) are highly involved in the throwing act. Conversely, the superior and posterior muscles (supraspinatus, middle deltoid, and infraspinatus) exhibit only slight-to-moderate levels of activity.

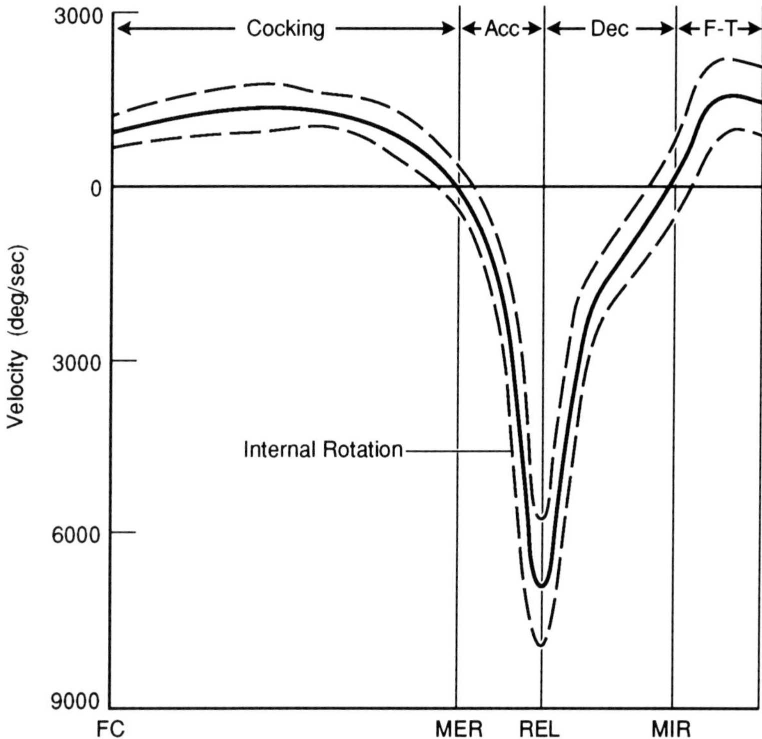

Figure 3-4. Average angular velocity for internal/external rotation of arm about shoulder in throwing. Data are based on 29 highly skilled subjects throwing an average speed of 85 mph. Dotted line is ±1 SD.

The exception to this low level of activity is the infraspinatus firing at a marked amplitude (greater than 50 percent MVC) during the arm cocking phase of throwing.

In addition, Gowan et al[9] has compared the muscular involvement between professional pitchers and amateur throwers. The qualitative levels of muscular involvement are illustrated in Table 3-2 by comparing the professional with the amateur players. The differences in muscular activity between these two groups are highlighted in Table 3-2. The professional throwers seem to have a greater involvement from the subscapularis and latissimus dorsi than the amateurs. However, the amateurs exhibit a greater activity level from the pectoralis major. In terms of the supraspinatus and infraspinatus, the professionals in gen-

Table 3-1. Analysis of Electromyographic Data in Pitching (Normal Subjects)

Muscles	Arm Cocking	Arm Acceleration	Arm Deceleration
Subscapularis	MX	MX	MK
Latissimus dorsi	S	MX	MK
Pectoralis major	MK	MK	MK
Infraspinatus	MK	S	MOD
Supraspinatus	S/MOD	S	MOD
Middle deltoid	S	MOD	MOD

Abbreviations: S, less than 20% maximal voluntary contraction (MVC); MOD, 21 to 50% MVC; MK, 51 to 100% MVC; MX, greater than 100% MVC. (Adapted from Glousman et al,[8] with permission.)

Table 3-2. Analysis of Electromyographic Data in Pitching (Professional versus Amateur) Phases of Throw

Muscles		Arm Cocking	Arm Acceleration	Follow-through
Subscapularis	P	MX	MX	MK
	A	MK	MX	MK
Latissimus dorsi	P	S	MX	MK
	A	S	S	MOD
Pectoralis major	P	MK	MK	MK
	A	MX	MX	MK
Infraspinatus	P	MK	S	MOD
	A	MK	MOD	MOD
Supraspinatus	P	MOD	S	MOD
	A	MK	MOD	MOD
Med. deltoid	P	No comparative data available		
	A			

Abbreviations: P, professional; A, amateur; S, less than 20% maximal voluntary contraction (MVC); MOD, 21 to 50% MVC; MK, 51 to 100% MVC; MX, greater than 100% MVC. (Adapted from Gowan et al,[9] with permission.)

eral have a lower level of activity, particularly during the arm acceleration phase of throwing. The comparative analysis suggests that professionals develop more velocity by using the subscapularis and latissimus dorsi to a greater extent during arm cocking and acceleration and tend to minimize possible antagonistic rotator cuff activity (supraspinatus and infraspinatus) during both of these phases.

FORCES AND TORQUES CREATED DURING THROWING

Recently, in addition to our work, a few other authors have investigated the kinetics of throwing.[2–7] All these studies show remarkable consistency in the findings, given the fact that a kinetic analysis of a human skill provides only estimations of the loads that are created. The basic results of these works illustrate that there are two high loading points during the throwing act. These occur (1) as the arm is approaching maximal external rotation and (2) during the initial period of the arm deceleration after the ball has been released. Figures 3-5 and 3-6 illustrate resultant torques that are created at these two points during the throwing motion.

As the arm approaches maximum external rotation (Fig. 3-5), the internal rotators are being eccentrically stretched, creating a peak muscular torque of 60 Newton-meters (Nm). Also, the horizontal adductors are undergoing eccentric loading equivalent to a torque of 75 Nm. These high eccentric actions are primarily responsible for accelerating the arm rapidly from maximum external rotation to ball release in approximately 0.030 seconds.

Immediately after ball release (Fig. 3-6), two large eccentric actions are once again evoked to decelerate the arm. The first is an eccentric contraction by the shoulder adductors equal to an average torque of 75 Nm to decelerate the rapid shoulder abduction that occurs immediately after the ball is released. The second eccentric torque (average, 80 Nm) is evoked by the horizontal abductors (extension) to control the arm movement across the body during the final stages of arm deceleration. Note that there is a small positive internal rotation torque (10 Nm) in arm deceleration and not a large external rotation torque as

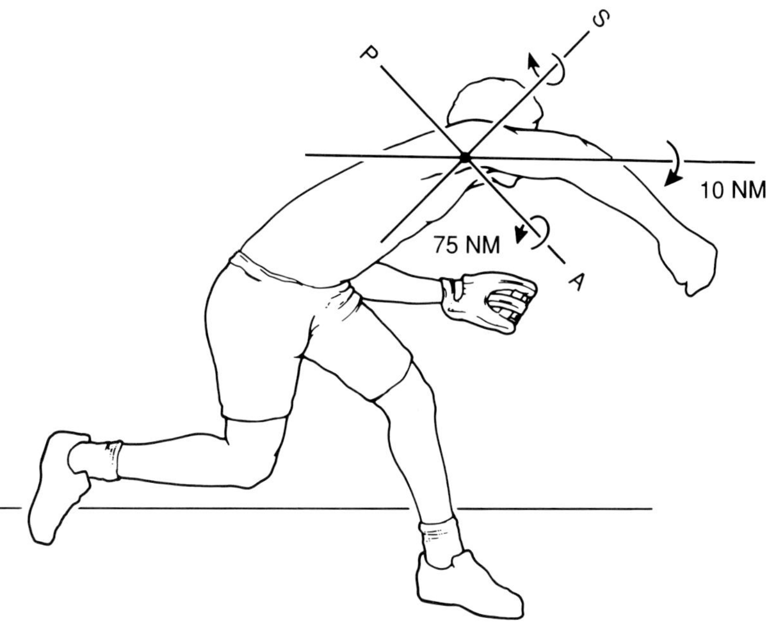

Figure 3-5. Average maximum resultant torques acting about the shoulder as the arm is approaching maximal external rotation. Data are based on 29 highly skilled throwers. 60 Nm, internal rotation torque; 75 Nm, horizontal adduction torque; 35 Nm, shoulder abduction torque.

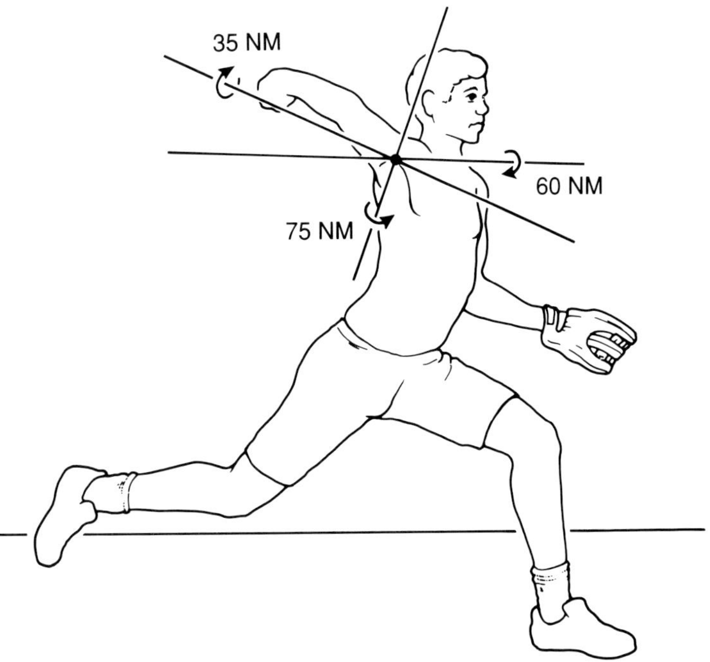

Figure 3-6. Average ($N = 29$) maximum resultant torques occurring during the arm deceleration phase of throwing. 75 Nm, shoulder adduction torque; 80 Nm, horizontal abduction torque; 10 Nm, internal rotation torque.

suggested by many authors. The arm continues to internally rotate after ball release.

The results of this work illustrate that the throwing act is a highly dynamic activity. The forces and torques that are created are relatively large and act over a short period. Thus, in the proper training and rehabilitation of the throwing athlete, the highly rapid dynamic loading of the shoulder complex should be emulated if the proper preparation or rehabilitation is to be achieved with the throwing athlete.

SUMMARY

During the past 5 years, there has been great interest shown by researchers in the three-dimensional analysis of the throwing motion. These relatively new biomechanical investigations have greatly increased our understanding of the movement patterns, muscular involvement, and loads created during throwing. Throwing is one of the most dynamic activities in all of sports. Research results illustrate that the muscles involved have a unique coordination pattern specific to the skill and that there are differences in the muscular pattern between highly and average-skilled throwers. Kinetic analyses of throwing demonstrate that there are very large forces created during this highly dynamic skill but that they are only applied to the body over a short period. The muscular forces that are created seem to be produced primarily in an eccentric manner, both in the acceleration and deceleration phases. These types of high eccentric loading should be simulated both in the preparation and rehabilitation of throwers. This increased understanding of the dynamics of throwing can only lead to improved conservative and surgical treatment for the injured athlete and will certainly aid trainers in the design of better preventative programs for throwers of all ages.

REFERENCES

1. Atwater AE: Biomechanics of overarm throwing movements and of throwing injuries. Exerc Sports Sci Rev 71:43–85, 1980
2. Dillman CJ, Fleisig GS, Andrews JR: Biomechanics of pitching with emphasis upon shoulder kinematics. JOSPT 18:402–8, 1993
3. Dillman CJ, Fleisig GS, Werner SL, Andrews JR: Biomechanics of the shoulder in sports: throwing activities. p. 621–33. In Matsen FA, Fu FH, Hawkins RJ (eds): The Shoulder: A Balance of Mobility and Stability. American Academy of Orthopaedic Surgeons, Rosemont, IL, 1993
4. Feltner ME: Three-dimensional interactions in a two-segment chain. Part II: application to the throwing arm in baseball pitching. Int J Sports Biomechanics 5:420–50, 1989
5. Feltner ME, Dapena J: Dynamics of the shoulder and elbow joints of the throwing arm during the baseball pitch. Int J Sports Biomechanics 2:235–59, 1986
6. Feltner ME, Dapena J: Three-dimensional interactions in a two-segment kinetic chain. Part I: general model. Int J Sports Biomechanics 5:403–19, 1989
7. Fleisig GS, Dillman CJ, Andrews JR: Biomechanics of the shoulder during throwing. p. 335–68. In Wilk KE, Andrews JR (eds): The Athlete's Shoulder. Churchill Livingstone, New York, 1994
8. Glousman RE, Jobe FW, Tibone JE et al: Dynamic electromyographic analysis of the throwing shoulder with glenohumeral instability. J Bone Joint Surg [Am] 70:220, 1988
9. Gowan ID, Jobe FW, Tibone JE et al: A comparative EMG analysis of the shoulder during pitching: professional vs amateur pitchers. Am J Sports Med 15:586–90, 1987
10. Jobe FW, Moynes DR, Tibone JE, Perry J: An EMG analysis of the shoulder in pitching: a second report. Am J Sports Med 12:218–20, 1984
11. Jobe FW, Tibone JE, Perry J, Moynes D: An EMG analysis of the shoulder in throwing and pitching: a preliminary report. Am J Sports Med 11:3–5, 1983

CHAPTER FOUR

Electromyographic Analysis of Shoulder Mechanics

James P. Bradley
James E. Tibone

In 1944, Inman and co-workers[7] presented the first comprehensive biomechanical analysis of the shoulder. A dynamic model of the shoulder was developed using anatomic, roentgenographic, and electromyographic (EMG) analysis systems. Studying muscle activity during motion was a radical new approach in shoulder biomechanics. This new ability to investigate shoulder motion with EMG generated several principles of shoulder biomechanics that are presently accepted. Inman et al[7] described synergistic interaction between different muscle groups, which was termed the *Inman force couple*. Basically, he noted that the supraspinatus muscle acts concomitantly with the deltoid at a single unit throughout abduction and forward flexion during normal arm elevation. Concurrently, the infraspinatus, subscapularis, and teres minor muscles perform as a functional unit depressing and compressing the humeral head during both abduction and forward flexion.

Evaluation of athletic shoulder disorders, however, have clinically demonstrated selective weakness of specific rotator cuff muscles opposed to generalized impairments. These clinical findings were in conflict with Inman's work regarding single-plane motion analysis, prompting investigations into the biomechanics and dynamic EMG analysis of the shoulder during athletic activity. The initial inquiry was whether Inman's conclusions in respect to single-plane motion analysis applied to sport-specific activities. The original findings then spurred investigators to evaluate sport-specific motions on a much broader scale.

Many centers using differing techniques initiated investigations to expand on the role of shoulder biomechanics in sport-specific motions. Much of the EMG nascent work in throwing and related overhead sports was conducted at Centinela Hospital Biomechanics Laboratory. These investigations developed an objective scientific basis for preventive exercises, surgical procedures, and postoperative rehabilitation protocols in overhead athletes.

METHODS

The objective scientific method used was dynamic EMG and high-speed film motion analysis. These were simultaneously applied to identify and isolate the functions of the major muscles controlling the shoulder during normal and sport-specific overhead activities. Subsequently, EMG investigations were expanded to include athletes with specific shoulder injuries and to compare them with normals.

The EMG signal is recorded by using the Basmajian single needle technique in that 50-μm dual-wire electrodes are inserted intramuscularly[1] (Fig. 4-1). Maximal manual muscle testing (MMT) or electrical stimulation is then applied to confirm adequate placement in the selected muscles. The electrodes are connected to a battery-powered transmittal belt pack to obviate restrictions of body movements. EMG signals during the studied activities are telemetered to the computer for conversion to digital signals and quantified by integrating 2,500 samples per second. A peak 1-sec EMG signal during an MMT is selected as

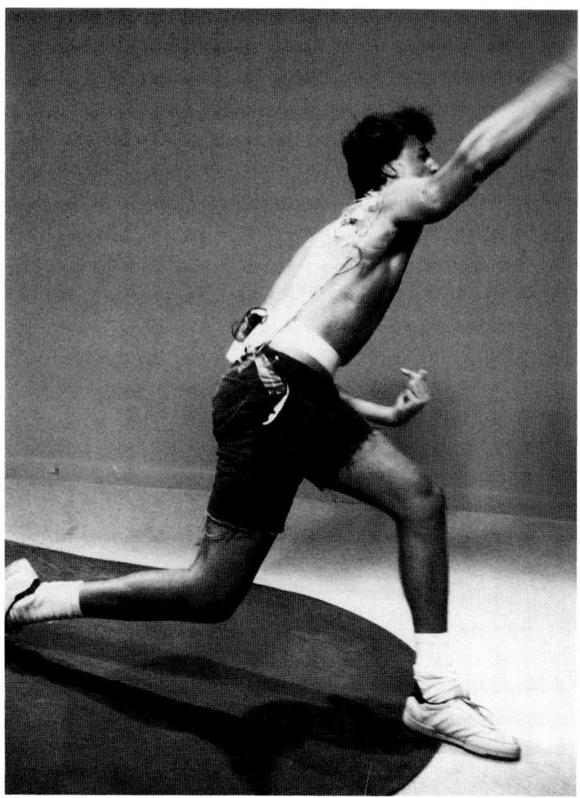

Figure 4-1. Thrower with electrode pack.

a normalizing value (100 percent). Muscular signals are analyzed every 20 ms and recorded as a relative percentage of the MMT. To assist in generalized comparisons, a relative muscle activity scale is used. A range from 0 to 20 percent is considered low activity; 21 to 40 percent, moderate; 41 to 60 percent, high; and greater than 60 percent, very high.[5] A motion analysis system is used to correlate EMG activity with the specific shoulder movements. Multiple 16-mm motion picture cameras are used to film the body movements at a rate of 450 to 1,000 frames per second, depending on the study. Using this system enabled each sport-specific activity to be divided accurately into specific phases. The golf swing, for example, is divided into five separate phases: take-away, forward swing, acceleration, early follow-through, and late follow-through. Synchronization between the phases and the EMG data is accomplished by electronic makers placed on both the motion picture film and the EMG recording. The EMG data is then averaged within each phase of the studied activity for each muscle and each subject. The EMG data collected for each muscle is then averaged among all test subjects and recorded as a mean and a standard deviation.

Assessment of the planar motion in the normal shoulders included elevation of the arm in the coronal, scapular, and sagittal planes with elbow set in 90 degrees of flexion and full extension. EMG and simultaneous motion analysis are used as previously described.

This methodology is the basis of EMG and motion analysis studies of athletic shoulder motion. Information compiled, using this method, has demonstrated that many overhead sports activities (i.e., tennis serve, javelin throw, football pass) are very similar biomechanically to the baseball pitch.[3] Aberrations from the normal EMG activity have lead to suggest problems with specific muscles about the shoulder in certain clinical syndromes. Time-honored shoulder rehabilitation programs have also undergone scrutiny, which has introduced new ideas and concepts concerning proper rehabilitation.

ELECTROMYOGRAPHY OF THE THROWING MOTION

The baseball pitch is the prototype in terms of abundance of EMG biomechanical data and is the benchmark to which studies of other athletic motions are compared. The shoulder musculature supplies two essential functions in pitching biomechanics: activation and stabilization.[14] Activation embodies concentric contraction and energy production, which ultimately results in the ball velocity. Stabilization includes eccentric or isometric contractions and serves to provide dynamic protection to the skeletal linkage system, which bears incredible forces during the transfer of energy.[5] As the transfer of energy emanates from proximal to distal, the body parts energized become smaller. Therefore, the velocity of the body parts must proportionately increase to conserve energy. Accordingly, the timing of the muscular contractions in the upper extremity is just as significant as the absolute force generated. This synchronization of muscular activation is essential to the fluid and safe transfer of energy through the shoulder during the throwing sequence.[5]

The baseball pitch is typically separated into five stages determined by motion analysis and EMGs.[12,14]

Stage I — The wind-up or preparation phase, ending when the ball leaves the glovehand

Stage II — Early cocking, a period of shoulder abduction and external rotation that starts as the ball is released from the nondominant hand and terminates with the contact of the stride foot on the ground

Stage III — Late cocking, the phase that continues until maximum external rotation at the shoulder is evident

Stage IV — Acceleration, a short propulsive phase that starts with internal rotation of the humerus and concludes with ball release

Stage V — Follow-through, the phase that starts with ball release and ends when all motion is complete

Division of the throwing motion into stages permits investigators to compare muscle activity and position of the extremity between normal and injured shoulders in each stage.

Deltoid

The primary motor responsible for arm elevation with active forward flexion and abduction of the humerus is the deltoid.[7,20] The deltoid is divided into anterior, middle, and posterior segments. All three segments of the deltoid attain peak EMG activity in early cocking when the arm is elevated to 90 degrees.[20] This activity decreases during late cocking as the rotator cuff becomes more dominant. This sequential pattern of muscular activity, beginning with the deltoid and concluding with the rotator cuff, contradicts the obligatory "synergy" proposed by Inman et al[7] discussed earlier. The "force couple" mechanism does function in casual elevations of the arc; however, EMG findings have illustrated that the rapid and precise motion patterns that characterize throwing sports demand a more selective muscle action with specific periods of significant intensity.[2]

Biceps Brachii

The biceps activity throwing is relatively low and also predominantly at the elbow during follow-through.[2,6] During late cocking, the biceps reaches its peak EMG activity of only 28 to 36 percent of the MMT. Notably, the biceps and rotator cuff are used during acceleration by amateur pitchers to a much greater extent than by professionals.[19]

Rotator Cuff

The musculature of the rotator cuff exhibits an intricate firing pattern presumably to balance functional mobility while preserving adequate stability (activation and stabilization). The established paradigm is that the supraspinatus muscle helped to initiate humeral abduction.[4,22,26] Interestingly, during pitching, its peak activity was evident in late cocking when the arm is already abducted and exceedingly prone to anterior subluxation.[2] Presumptively, during late cocking, the supraspinatus helped to stabilize by compressing the humeral head toward the glenoid.[22] Supraspinatus muscle activity is significantly greater in amateur pitchers versus professionals, which suggests that at higher levels, rotator cuff function is more selective.[2,19] Because the supraspinatus is used more by amateur pitchers, fatigue causing an overuse syndrome may jeopardize glenohumeral stability. Professional pitchers are much more selective, economical, and proficient in respect to the activity of the supraspinatus and rotator cuff.[19] In normal collegiate and professional pitchers, the type of pitch (i.e., curve-ball, fast-ball, or change-up) does not alter the supraspinatus firing pattern.[17]

External rotation of the humerus is provided by the infraspinatus and teres minor muscles. Apparently, they aid in glenohumeral stability by compressing the humeral head toward the glenoid fossa. Their peak EMG activity is similar and noted in late cocking and follow-through. Both muscles actively lagged behind the supraspinatus temporarily. Different pitches did not affect either muscle's firing pattern.[17]

The subscapularis muscle reaches its peak EMG activity in late cocking when eccentrically contracting. Presumably, it helps to decelerate external rotation of the shoulder and thereby protects the anterior glenohumeral joint, which is under extreme tension.[2,3]

Professional pitchers' use of the rotator cuff differs from amateurs. Electromyographically, they illustrate selective use of individual rotator cuff muscles. Similar patterns of rotator cuff firing are noted during wind-up, cocking, and follow-through stages of both groups. However, the patterns deviate during the acceleration phase as professionals fire the subscapularis selectively over the other cuff muscles.[20] During acceleration, amateurs tended to activate all rotator cuff muscles and the biceps brachii for power.[13] Synchronization of the trunk, shoulder, and elbow obviate the use of the supraspinatus, infraspinatus, teres minor, and biceps muscle for acceleration.[20] Professional pitchers illustrate this principle well. Professional and collegiate pitchers also demonstrate that the type of pitch does not alter the firing amplitude or sequence of the rotator cuff.[17]

Even under ideal conditions, rotator cuff injuries may occur during throwing. The thrower who uses his or her muscles inappropriately or unnecessarily are predisposed to overuse injuries. This principle not only applies to the shoulder but also the trunk and lower extremities.[20,27] Repetitive mechanical training and preventive rehabilitation programs may enhance synchrony of the lower-extremity, trunk, and shoulder precluding injury secondary to overuse.[6,9,10,14]

Pectoralis Major and Latissimus Dorsi

Internal rotation of the humerus is supplied by the pectoralis major and latissimus dorsi. Their activity begins in late cocking when, along with the subscapularis, they eccentrically stabilize the anterior glenohumeral joint.[5,11] As acceleration starts, they are in a prestretched posture, and with concentric contraction, they impel the humerus into rapid internal rotation. The pectoralis and latissimus are the prime muscles responsible for ball velocity. Conversely, the subscapularis acts as a steering muscle to position the humeral head precisely in the glenoid and protect against subluxation of the humeral head.[5,20]

Scapular Rotators

The contribution of the scapular rotators to the throwing motion was initially not appreciated; however, recent work has demonstrated their significance. Scapular motion is controlled by six muscle units: the serratus anterior; upper, middle, and lower trapezius; rhomboids; and levator scapulae. Scapular motion is divided into four basic movements: upward rotation, retraction, protraction, and depression. During the throwing sequence, all four components are apparent.[3]

The main component during throwing is upward rotation in association with arm elevation. The principal upward rotators are the serratus and trapezius. Inman et al[7] reported that only the upper trapezial segment demonstrated consistent activity in both abduction and flexion. This places the major burden of scapular elevation to the serratus anterior; yet, both muscles must be functioning to achieve maximal scapular rotation.[2]

The contributions of the serratus anterior during the throwing motion is confirmed by EMG activity. Normal arm elevation to 90 degrees produces average serratus activity of 41 percent of maximum; continuing to full elevation requires 66 percent of maximum.[20] However, during the throwing motion, a short period exceeding 100 percent of maximum is routinely attained.[20] The EMG activity of the trapezius was consistently lower than the serratus, which only produces 34 to 42 percent of maximum. Anatomically, the two muscles are of equivalent size (12.6 and 12.8 cm^2) and, therefore, should produce similar force potentials.[26,28] Because the serratus anterior withstands greater demand during throwing, selective strengthening is advocated to lessen the threat of overuse injury.[3]

During pitching, it appears that the serratus anterior is the primary muscle controlling the scapula to provide a stable glenoid to serve as a secure platform for the humeral head. This is most obvious during late cocking, when the serratus must produce upward rotation and protraction, therefore allowing the scapula to accompany the humerus, which is horizontally flexing and externally rotating. Conversely, the trapezius demonstrates relatively low activity during both cocking and acceleration. This suggests that the trapezius supplies supplemental scapular stabilization to improve the rotational action of the serratus. The peak activity of the trapezius is recorded during follow-through, where its adduction action helps in deceleration of scapular protraction.[20] Early EMG studies of the throwing motion concentrated on the roles of the deltoid and rotator cuff. Presently, attention has shifted to the function of the scapular rotators in providing a stable platform for the humerus. Jobe and others[3,8,10] have stated that dysfunction of scapular motion exhibited by early serratus fatigue may produce additional stress on the stabilizers of the anterior shoulder and, thus, become a harbinger of injury.

ELECTROMYOGRAPHY OF DIFFERENT PITCHES

Controversy exists concerning the curve-ball's predilection for increasing the risk of injury to the shoulder during pitching. EMG, motion analysis (1,000 frames per second), and radar speed gun analysis of the curve-ball versus the fast-ball, and change-up in professional and collegiate pitches have not demonstrated this problem. Intramuscular EMG analysis of young developing throwers at this time has not been reported.

In high-performance throwers, testing of 29 muscles or muscle bellies of the shoulder girdle and upper extremity illustrates no significant differences in the muscle firing patterns of the three pitches.[17] Three variables were recorded: ball velocity, hand pressure/position, and the timing of radioulnar pronation.

The velocity of the fast-ball was significantly higher (71.4 mph) versus the curve-ball (56.3 mph) or the change-up (56.4 mph). As expected, the acceleration phase of the fast-ball was the shortest (0.05 versus 0.06 second).[17]

Hand position and pressure on the ball varied with each pitch. The fast-ball is gripped across the seams with the index and middle fingers comfortably spread. The curve-ball is gripped with the middle finger extending along the length of the outside seam supported by the index finger, whereas the change-up is gripped deep within the palm with the thumb.

During the fast-ball, the radioulnar pronation of the forearm occurs approximately 10 ms before ball release (causing backspin) compared with the change-up or curve-ball.[17]

In essence, in high-caliber throwers, shoulder muscle firing patterns illustrate no significant differences between pitches; however, young developing pitchers have not been tested using this method.

ELECTROMYOGRAPHY OF BATTING

EMGs of the shoulder during batting shows that the posterior deltoid and biceps are positioners, not power generators, and the supraspinatus and middle serratus did not significantly contribute to the swing.[24] Earlier batting studies used surface electrodes rather than indwelling electrodes, unskilled batters for their subject populations, and a relatively low number of subjects.[15,16] In contrast to the results of earlier studies, the triceps and other muscles of the upper extremity seemed more important in arm positioning rather than power generation. The hamstrings and lower gluteus contributed significantly to a stable base and the power of the thrust from which the torso uncoils during batting. High EMG activity was also noted in the abdominal obliques and erector spinae. It appears that the triceps and other muscles of the upper extremity are more important as positioners, rather than as power generators.

ELECTROMYOGRAPHY OF THROWERS WITH CLINICAL IMPINGEMENT

EMG analysis of throwers with clinical impingement syndrome demonstrated aberrations when compared with normal throwers. Specifically, supraspinatus activity during late cocking is reduced and is associated with a prolongation of deltoid activity during the same phase. Theoretically, impeding the ability of the supraspinatus to aid the deltoid in cocking and affect its ability to compress the humeral head into the glenoid. This reduction in supraspinatus activity is thought to reduce tension on the injured tendon, thereby predisposing the shoulder to a dynamic muscle imbalance during throwing (L. Miller, F. W. Jobe, and D. R. Moynes, unpublished data, 1985).

The most significant variations appeared in the internal rotators, subscapularis, pectoralis major and latissimus dorsi muscles, and serratus anterior. Substantial lower activity in these muscles could allow increased rotation, superior humeral head migration, and impaired scapular rotation, any of which covers, predisposes, or magnifies the impingement process.[20]

This findings may provide evidence that the neuromuscular irregularities recorded may account for the initial and persistent impingement symptoms experienced by throwers.[20]

ELECTROMYOGRAPHY OF THROWERS WITH CLINICAL INSTABILITY

Effective throwing necessitates increased external humeral rotation, force, velocity, and endurance, all of which produce extreme tension on the static anterior stabilizing structures of the glenohumeral joint. Any anomaly in the synchronous firing of the cuff, scapular rotators, or throwing mechanics may jeopardize the anterior stabilizers and lead to the "instability complex."[8,9] The instability complex is a cascade from overuse to instability, subluxation, impingement, and terminally a rotator cuff tear.[8,10]

EMG evaluation of pitchers with isolated anterior instability revealed differences compared with normal pitchers.[6] Supraspinatus activity was elevated during late cocking and acceleration, possibly compensating for lax static restraints. The infraspinatus activity was also elevated during early cocking and acceleration. The elevated activity may draw the humeral head posteriorly, thus resisting anterior humeral translation.[6]

The internal rotators (subscapularis, pectoralis, latissimus) in normal throwers contract eccentrically to dynamically buttress the anterior shoulder. In the subluxators, these muscles illustrate a significant decrease in activity in all stages of throwing. The decreased activity of these muscles may allow accentuated external rotation of the humerus and abrogate their ability to shield the anterior shoulder. These aberrations may be modifiers in perpetuating chronic anterior instability in the throwing athlete.[6,20]

Scapular rotation was also affected in subluxators noted by a significant decrease in serratus anterior activity during late cocking and acceleration. Therefore, scapular rotation and scapular protraction is diminished, thus abating the ability of the scapula to provide a stable platform for the flexing externally rotating humerus. Diminution of scapular rotation and protraction places added stress on the anterior shoulder stabilizer, accentuating the instability.[6]

It is uncertain whether the neuromuscular imbalance in the thrower with instability is a component of the primary pathology or is a secondary phenomenon.

SWIMMING MECHANICS

The shoulder, in swimming, is exposed to significant stress. In particular, the muscular endurance required to swim competitively predisposes the shoulder to high injury rates. Shoulder injuries in competitive swimmers is common and is reported as high as 67 percent.[23]

The swimming shoulder was evaluated using the identical investigative techniques of integrated EMG and motion analysis that were used in the throwing athlete. The major strokes, including freestyle, breaststroke, butterfly, and backstroke, were studied. Both normal and painful shoulders were analyzed. The athletes studied were competitive swimmers including both collegiate and masters level swimmers. The prototype stroke appears to be freestyle.

The freestyle stroke cycle was divided into four specific stages and time intervals using EMG and motion analysis. The four stages and the number of intervals per stage were as follows[21]:

Stage I Early pull-through, which begins with hand entry into the water and ends when the humerus is perpendicular to the axis of the torso (12 intervals)

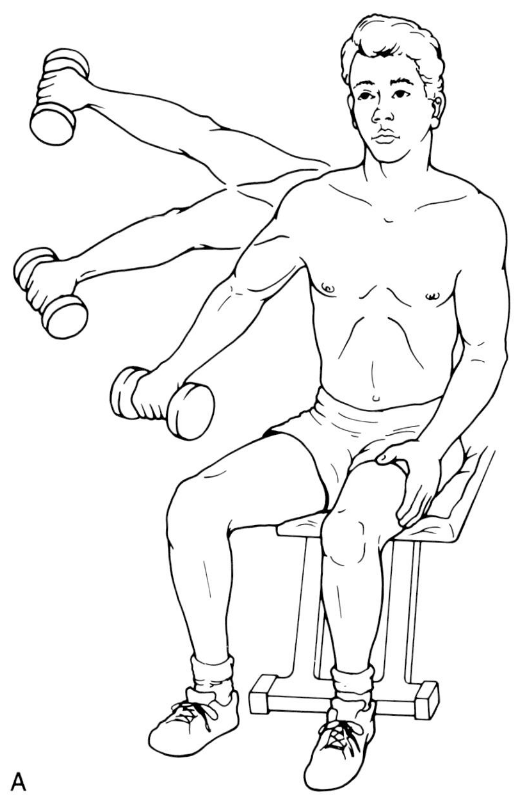

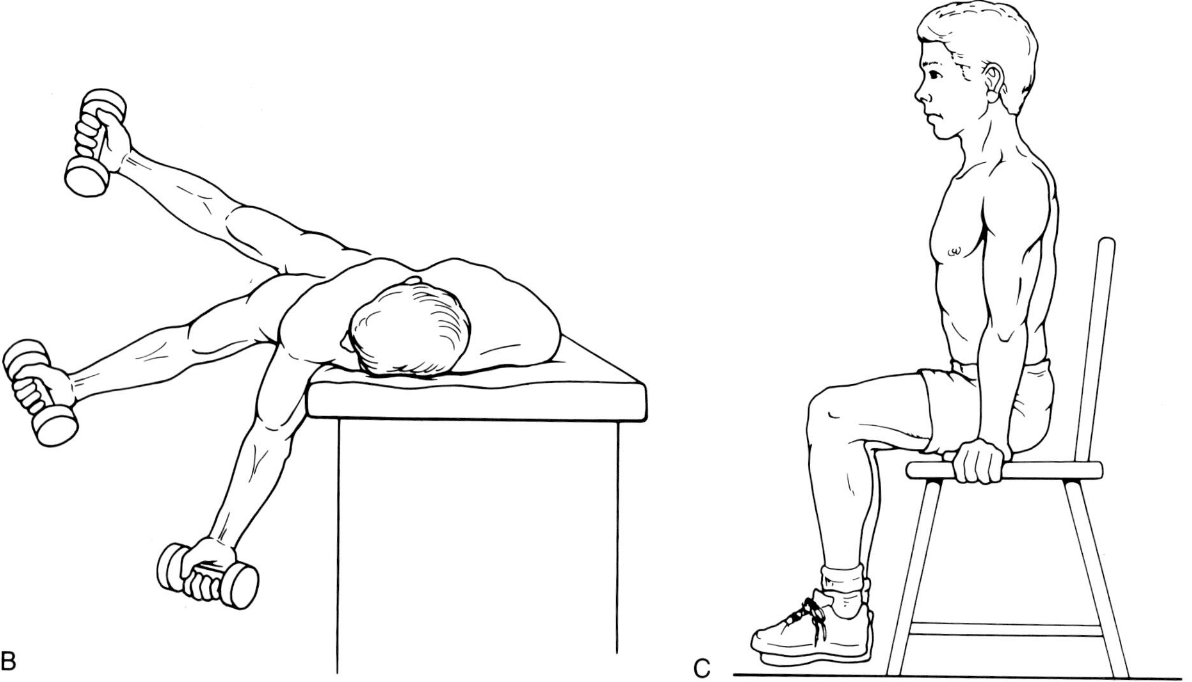

Figure 4-2. (A) Scaption (thumbs down) with internal rotation; **(B)** horizontal abduction in external rotation; **(C)** press-up. (*Figure continues.*)

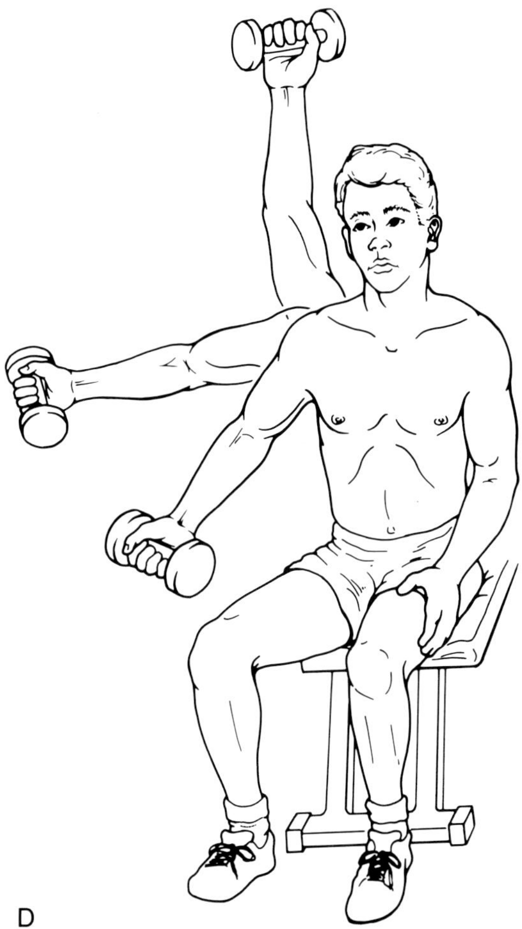

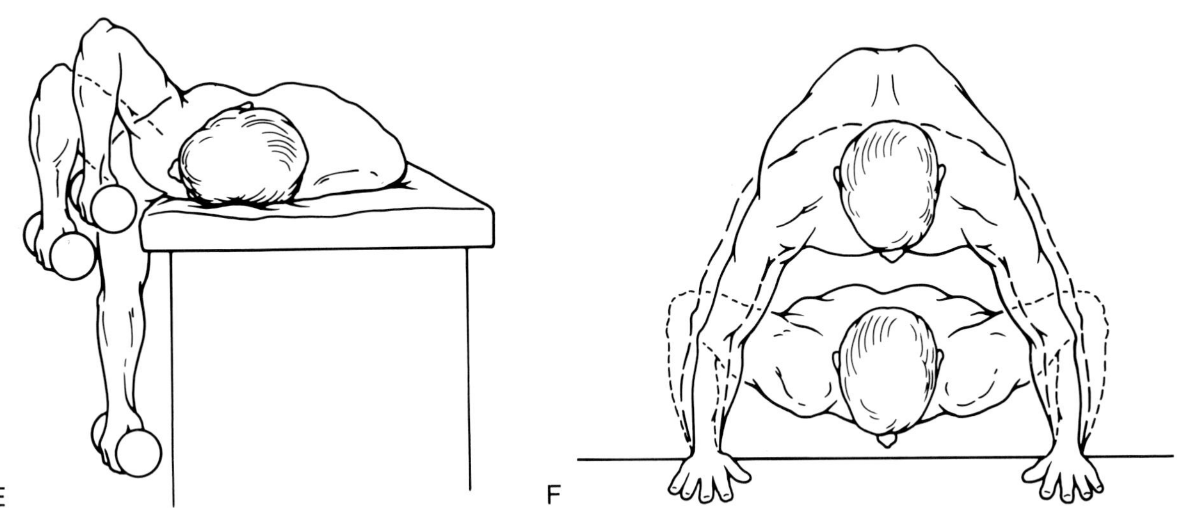

Figure 4-2 (*Continued*). **(D)** Scaption (thumbs up) with external rotation; **(E)** rowing; **(F)** push-ups plus.

Stage II Late pull-through, starting with completion of early pull-through and ending as the hand leaves the water (7 intervals)

Stage III Early recovery, beginning at hand exit and ending when the humerus is perpendicular to the water surface (4 intervals)

Stage IV Late recovery, starting at completion of early recovery and ending at hand entry (2 intervals)

In normal subjects, the findings suggest selective synchrony of the shoulder muscles to allow an effective, efficient stroke. Similar muscle activity patterns were recorded at hand entry and exit. The deltoid (all heads) and the supraspinatus performed in synchrony to position the hand for entry and exit. Simultaneously, the upper trapezius and rhomboids augmented one another in that the upper trapezius upwardly rotated the scapula and the rhomboids retracted the scapula. Each of the four rotator cuff muscles demonstrated a different activity pattern and function throughout the stroke. The supraspinatus achieved peak activity at hand entry (54 percent MMT) and during early recovery (74 percent MMT). The infraspinatus attained peak activity during midrecovery (34 percent MMT). The teres minor illustrated a gradual rise in muscle activity up to mid pull-through (57 percent). The subscapularis was active throughout the cycle, with peaks in late pull-through (64 percent MMT) and early recovery (71 percent MMT). During pull-through (propulsive phase) stage, the pectoralis major (71 percent MMT) and latissimus dorsi (75 percent MMT) exhibited peak activity much like the propulsive phase (acceleration) of the baseball pitch. The serratus anterior muscle demonstrated a constant level of activity throughout the entire stroke cycle, with two peaks recorded at mid pull-through (48 percent MMT) and hand exit (45 percent MMT).[21]

The EMGs invariably documented that the supraspinatus and serratus anterior muscles were constantly operative during the freestyle stroke cycle. These data suggest that both of these muscles may be predisposed to fatigue and therefore susceptible to overuse injury.[21]

Painful Shoulders During Freestyle Swimming

Competitive swimmers with painful shoulders were studied using the same investigative technique. No differences were noted in the muscle firing patterns; however, significant amplitude differences were recorded in 7 of the 12 muscles tested.[25]

Considerably less muscle activity was documented in the rhomboids, upper trapezius, and deltoid at hand entry. During the pulling phase, significantly less activity in the serratus anterior and more activity in the rhomboids were recorded. The subscapularis activity was diminished at midrecovery. No differences were demonstrated in the amplitude of the posterior deltoid, supraspinatus, teres minor, or latissimus dorsi during the stroke cycle.[25]

Basically, the findings show amplitude differences without muscle firing pattern discrepancies between normal and painful swimmers. Future studies will differentiate the specific pathology of the painful swimmers and, it is hoped, uncover the primary muscle aberrations as is demonstrated in throwers.

Painful Shoulders During Breaststroke

Competitive swimmers with painful shoulders were evaluated using the identical technique during breaststroke and compared with normal subjects.[23]

The subscapularis increased its activity and the teres minor decreased its activity during pull-through, resulting in a relative internal rotation of the humerus, which predisposes to impingement in the forward flexed position. During recovery, the middle deltoid, upper trapezius, and supraspinatus considerably decreased their activity. Theoretically, this may disable the deltoid-supraspinatus force-couple during humeral elevation and possibly induce impingement by permitting proximal migration during mid- to late recovery. Once again, the serratus anterior and teres minor were active throughout the breaststroke cycle and possibly predisposed to fatigue.[23]

ELECTROMYOGRAPHY OF THE GOLF SWING

The golf swing was evaluated in 11 professional golfers with normal shoulders. Similar EMG and motion analysis was documented and assimilated as previously described.[13]

EMG and motion analysis allowed division of the swing into five stages similar to throwing and swimming. The five stages included (1) take away, starting at ball address to the end of the backswing; (2) forward swing, from the end of the back swing until the club is horizontal; (3) acceleration, from horizontal club to ball contact; (4) early follow-through, from ball contact to horizontal club; and (5) late follow-through, from horizontal club to the end of motion.[13]

The supraspinatus and infraspinatus muscles work concomitantly at the extremes of shoulder motion as external rotators, abductors, and stabilizers. The subscapularis reaches peak activity during acceleration when the arm is internally rotating. Similar to the baseball pitch and freestyle stroke, the latissimus dorsi and the pectoralis major are the "power drive" muscles during the propulsive stage of the swing. Although the latissimus activates earlier in the cycle, the pectoralis major contributes the most activity of all the muscles studied. Both act to provide rotation and forceful adduction of the arm. The deltoid is comparatively inactive, except for the anterior portion, which elevates and flexes the arm.[13]

The golf swing does not necessitate great shoulder strength or excessive range of motion; however, it does require rapid movement of the shoulder. Nonetheless, the cuff muscles must fire in a concise temporal sequence to permit a coordinated smooth transfer of energy, generating an effective, efficient swing.[13]

ELECTROMYOGRAPHIC ANALYSIS OF REHABILITATION PROGRAMS

Rehabilitation programs to strengthen the muscles about the shoulder typically are based on anatomy, clinical experience, and undocumented EMG data. Although a muscle may anatomically be aligned to perform a specific motion, it may be inactive during execution of that motion.[18] EMGs and motion analysis have helped to isolate muscles that are responsible for humeral head and scapular motion and address how they could be best exercised during a rehabilitation program.

Intramuscular EMGs of 24 normal volunteers performing 17 common shoulder exercises gathered from a shoulder rehabilitation program used by professional baseball teams were evaluated. The EMGs were synchronized with cinematography and averaged over 30 degree arcs of motion. The specific exercise was considered a significant challenge for a muscle if the activation was at least 50 percent of its maximum over three consecutive arcs.

The humeral movers included the three heads of the deltoid, the pectoralis major, the latissimus dorsi, and the rotator cuff muscles. One muscle met the qualifying criteria for 15 of the 17 exercises studied. However, only three of the exercises were consistently graded among the highest two for every muscle tested. Elevation in the scapular plane with interval rotation was the best exercise for the anterior and middle deltoids and subscapularis and the second best for the supraspinatus. Horizontal abduction in external rotation illustrated the highest EMG activity for the infraspinatus and the second best for the teres minor and posterior deltoid. Press-up was the best exercise for both the latissimus dorsi and pectoralis major muscles[26] (Fig. 4-2).

The scapular rotators included the trapezius, the levator scapulae, the rhomboid major, the serratus anterior, and the pectoralis minor. One muscle met the qualifying criteria for 12 of the 16 exercises tested. However, only four exercises were shown to provide substantial activity for the scapular rotators. Scaption (thumbs up), rowing, push-up plus, and press-up all meet the criteria[18] (Fig. 4-2).

Integration of the data from the humeral movers and scapular rotators led to the development of a core shoulder rehabilitation program consisting of the best exercises for each group (Fig. 4-2). Also, an understanding of which exercises should be avoided to protect certain muscles, as well as which exercises should be used to isolate and strengthen individual muscles, was developed. Therefore, exercises can be added or excluded from the core program depending on the diagnosis and the muscles involved.

SUMMARY

Adapting indwelling integrated EMG and motion analysis to study athletic motions has enhanced our understanding of the biomechanics of sports. Generally, three parameters of muscle contractions influence the athlete's ability to maintain efficient, effective shoulder motion: (1) synchrony of firing, (2) strength of contraction, and (3) endurance. Many times, the sequence of events in the shoulder during athletics occurs so rapidly that synchrony of muscular activation is crucial to attain maximal effectiveness while preventing injury.

Muscular synchrony demands a high level of neuromuscular control, which also encompasses the ability to suppress extraneous muscular activity, as well as the ability to recruit salient muscles.[2,5] Performance may also be modified by strength and endurance; deficiencies in either can lead to injury. Therefore, small deficiencies, either skeletal or muscular, can produce a significant and cumulative effect on shoulder function and increase the risk of injury. The information gained from EMG and motion analysis studies has helped in the development of surgical procedures and rehabilitation protocols in the prevention and treatment of shoulder injuries in the athlete.

REFERENCES

1. Basmajian JV, Deluca CJ: Muscles Alive: Their Functions Revealed by Electromyography. Williams & Wilkins, Baltimore, 1985, pp 265–89
2. Bradley JP, Perry J, Jobe FW: The biomechanics of the throwing shoulder. Perspect Orthop 1:49–59, 1990
3. Bradley JP, Tibone JE: Electromyographic analysis of muscle action about the shoulder. Clin Sports Med 10:789–805, 1991
4. Colachis SC, Strohm BR: Effects of suprascapular and axillary nerve blocks in muscle force in the upper extremity. Arch Phys Med Rehabil 52:22–29, 1971
5. DiGiovine NM, Jobe FW, Pink M et al: An electromyographic analysis of the upper extremity in pitching. EMG and motion analysis. J Shoulder Elbow Surg 1:15–25, 1992
6. Glousman R, Jobe FW, Tibone JE et al: Dynamic electromyo-

graphic analysis of the throwing shoulder with glenohumeral instability. J Bone Joint Surg [Am] 70:220–6, 1988
7. Inman VT, Saunders JB, Abbott LC: Observations on the function of the shoulder. J Bone Joint Surg 26:1–30, 1944
8. Jobe FW, Bradley JP: Rotator cuff injuries in baseball: prevention and rehabilitation. Sports Med 6:377–87, 1988
9. Jobe FW, Bradley JP: The diagnosis and nonoperative treatment of shoulder injuries in athletes. Clin Sports Med 8:419–37, 1989
10. Jobe FW, Bradley JP, Pink M: Treatment of impingement syndrome in overhand athletes: a philosophical basis: I. Surg Rounds Orthop 4:19–24, 1990
11. Jobe FW, Bradley JP, Pink M: Treatment of impingement syndrome in overhand athletes: II. Surg Rounds Orthop 4:39–41, 1990
12. Jobe FW, Moynes DR, Tibone JE et al: An EMG analysis of the shoulder in pitching: a second report. Am J Sports Med 12:218–20, 1984
13. Jobe FW, Perry J, Pink M: Electromyographic shoulder activity in men and women professional golfers. Am J Sports Med 17:782–7, 1989
14. Jobe FW, Tibone JE, Moynes DR, et al: An EMG analysis of the shoulder in pitching and throwing: a preliminary report. Am J Sports Med 11:3–5, 1983
15. Kauffman IB, Greenisen MC: An EMG analysis of the validity of warm-up with a weighted bat. In Bleustein JL (ed): Mechanics and Sports. Presented at the Winter Annual Meeting of the American Society of Mechanical Engineers, Detroit, Michigan, Nov. 11–15, 1973, p 247–50.
16. Kitzman EW: Baseball: electromyographic study of batting swing. Res Q 35:166–71, 1964
17. Lowe WR, Jobe FW, Pink M, Perry J: A comparative study of the upper extremity during the fastball, curveball, and change-up baseball pitches. Submitted for publication
18. Moseley JB, Jobe FW, Pink M et al: EMG analysis of the scapular rotator muscles during a shoulder rehabilitation program. Am J Sports Med 20:128–34, 1992
19. Perry J: Anatomy and biomechanics of the shoulder in throwing, swimming, gymnastics and tennis: symposium on injuries to the shoulder in the athlete. Clin Sports Med 2:247, 1983
20. Perry J, Glousman RE: Biomechanics of throwing. p 727–51. In Nicholas JA, Hershman EB (eds): The Upper Extremity in Sports Medicine. CV Mosby, St. Louis, 1990
21. Pink M, Perry J, Jobe FW et al: The normal shoulder during freestyle swimming: an EMG and cinematographic analysis of twelve muscles. Am J Sports Med 19:569–76, 1991
22. Poppen NK, Walker PS: Normal and abnormal motion of the shoulder. J Bone Joint Surg [Am] 58:195–201, 1976
23. Ruwe PA, Pink M, Jobe FW et al: The normal and painful shoulder during breaststroke: an EMG and cinematographic analysis of 12 muscles. Am J Sports Med 22:789–96, 1994
24. Schaffer B, Jobe FW, Pink M, Perry J: Baseball batting an electromyographic study. Clin Orthop 292:285–93, 1993
25. Scovazzo ML, Brown A, Pink M, et al: The painful shoulder during freestyle swimming: an EMG and cinematographic analysis of twelve muscles. Am J Sports Med 19:577–82, 1991
26. Townsend H, Jobe FW, Pink M et al: EMG analysis of the glenohumeral muscles during a baseball rehabilitation program. Am J Sports Med 19:264–71, 1991
27. VanLinge B, Mulder JD: Function of the supraspinatus muscle and its relationship to the supraspinatus syndrome. J Bone Joint Surg [Br] 45:750–9, 1963
28. Watkins RG, Dennis S, Dillin WH et al: Dynamic EMG analysis of torque transfer in professional baseball pitchers. Spine 14:404–8, 1989
29. Weber EF: Uber die Langenverhaltnisse der Fleishfasen der Muskelin and Allegemeninen. Ber Verth K Sach Ges Wissensch, Math-Phys, 1851, p 63

CHAPTER FIVE

Pathophysiology of Injury and Healing

Savio L-Y. Woo
N. Douglas Boardman III
Richard E. Debski
Freddie H. Fu

Injuries about the shoulder girdle represent common occurrences in both the athletic and the lay populations. Indeed, the glenohumeral joint accounts for the greatest percentage of dislocations—and associated soft tissue damage of a tendinous or capsuloligamentous nature—of any major joint in the body.[41] Although a significant subpopulation of those individuals who sustain anatomic damage in either the acute or the chronic setting may remain essentially asymptomatic or functional without therapeutic intervention, many will require operative or rehabilitative measures. Hence, in the aggregate, soft tissue injuries of the shoulder have a significant socioeconomic impact on our society.

The nature of any given injury can obviously vary by the tissue or specific structure involved, the mechanism of injury, and the patient's age and occupation. As the glenohumeral joint lacks inherent bony stability, it therefore relies heavily on the surrounding musculature and capsulogigamentous structures for stabilization[48] (Fig. 5-1). Consequently, the soft tissues are often placed at significant risk for injury. Common lesions of soft tissue around the glenohumeral joint include disruption of the integrity of the rotator cuff, the tendon of the long head of the biceps, the glenoid labrum, and the glenohumeral ligaments. Combined injuries of these structures also occur as it is seen, for example, with bicipital tendinitis or rupture in the context of rotator cuff disease. In this chapter, we first offer a brief synopsis of several types of soft tissue injury to provide some clinical context for a subsequent discussion of the cellular and tissue pathophysiology of soft tissue injury around the glenohumeral joint.

BACKGROUND ON SOFT TISSUE INJURIES

The incidence of rotator cuff tear in the population has been examined in multiple cadaveric models and has been placed at anywhere from 5 percent to greater than 90 percent, depending on the age cohort and the extent of the tendinous insult, whether full or partial thickness.[13,18–20,54,58] Although the prevalence of rotator cuff pathology makes it a significant clinical entity, many patients are asymptomatic—up to 50 percent in some reports—and suffer no pain or functional deficit, even those with relatively large full-thickness tears.[49,58] The incidence of full-thickness tears clearly increases with age and may represent the result of a degenerative aging process, although partial-thickness tears may or may not constitute early forms of the same process producing full-thickness tears.[6,18–20]

Examination of involved tissue reveals that there exists a wide spectrum of pathology exhibited by patients with rotator cuff disease. The exact nature of the tissue involvement may range from tendinous inflammation with little disruption of cuff tissue—calcific tendinitis—to a gross tissue tear involving either a portion or the entire thickness of the cuff tendons.[5,11,57,69] Most commonly, such tears involve the supraspinatus tendon and propagate posteriorly, although a few proceed anteriorly to involve the subscapularis tendon as well. Proposed pathogenetic mechanisms have included such factors as acromial spurring, supraspinatus impingement under the coracoacromial ligament, acromial architecture, and cuff ischemia/hypovascularity in the ''critical zone'' of the supraspinatus tendon near its

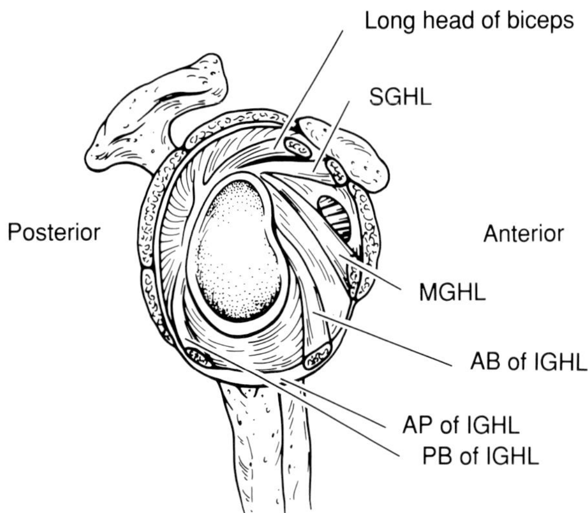

Figure 5-1. Lateral view of the glenoid and capsule with the humeral head removed showing the superior glenohumeral ligament (SGHL), middle glenohumeral ligament (MGHL), and the anterior band (*AB*), axillary pouch (*AP*), and the posterior band (*PB*) of the inferior glenohumeral ligament (IGHL). (Adapted from O'Brien ST et al,[57] with permission.)

humeral insertion.[7,11,44,45,51,53,62] Acute trauma accounts for a few of the injuries seen clinically, although chronic "wear and tear"—so-called repetitive microtrauma—has been implicated as an etiologic factor in the development of rotator cuff disease.[38,39]

On a histologic basis, both full- and partial-thickness rotator cuff tears can exhibit a wide range of associated pathologic findings, with involved tissue seen on microscopic examination to vary in composition from being necrotic and acellular to being neovascularized and hypercellular.[74,75] Calcific tendinitis tends to develop in the relatively hypovascular "critical zone" of the supraspinatus tendon and is characterized by the formation of calcified deposits within the substance of the cuff, which may resorb to varying degrees as a result of the inflammatory and repair response mounted by the body.[70]

Bicipital tendinitis with or without rupture may occur as an isolated finding or in association with other bony or soft tissue pathology at the glenohumeral joint. In particular, biceps tendon pathology tends to be associated with that fraction of rotator cuff tears that extend anteriorly to involve the subscapularis. In such cases, tendon subluxation may occur, with or without some degree of tendon rupture. As with the rotator cuff, the tendon of the long head of the biceps on histologic examination displays varied pathologies from hypercellularity and hypervascularity to frank rupture with fibrous scarring.[5,11,12,18,42,43]

The capsuloligamentous elements of the glenohumeral joint are frequently placed in a position predisposing them to injury, commonly at the extremes of motion such as the combination of extension, abduction, and external rotation, which places the anterior capsule at risk. Such injury may take the form of gross capsulolabral disruption or excessive deformation. The resulting pathology may predispose the patient to recurrent dislocation due to loss of passive restraints to abnormal translation of the humeral head on the glenoid.[52] The glenohumeral capsulolabral complex plays an integral role in enhancing stability, and therefore injury can compromise glenohumeral motion and stability. Indeed, labral tears such as those seen in the classic "Bankart lesion" can result in loss of the multiple-fold increase in glenoid depth provided by the labrum and therefore impair the concavity-compression mechanism. In such cases, the "traumatic, unidirectional, with Bankart lesion, responsive to surgery" (TUBS) instability pattern may present as a direct consequence of an acute soft tissue injury with resultant altered glenohumeral kinematics, which may include recurrent joint dislocation.[47]

In the long term, soft tissue injuries about the glenohumeral joint may, in addition to pain, produce such kinematic alterations that additional degenerative change may arise. Thus, chronic instability with abnormal translation of the humeral head on the glenoid fossa can over time cause the development of such bony changes as osteophyte formation, compromise of articular surfaces of the humerus and glenoid, and eventual bony collapse—the so-called cuff tear arthropathy.[14,32,55] The classic Hill-Sachs lesion may also be seen on the humeral head with recurrent glenohumeral dislocation.[35] In the extreme, severe or repetitive trauma may produce the clinical picture of the "frozen shoulder" due to excessive scarring and soft tissue contracture around the glenohumeral joint capsule. All these clinical entities can severely debilitate a patient and may necessitate surgical intervention.

NORMAL TENDON AND LIGAMENT ARCHITECTURE

To fully appreciate the pathologic and pathophysiologic alterations of soft tissue that occur secondary to injury, we must first review normal tendon and ligament architecture. Normal tendon—connecting muscle to bone—consists of spindle-shaped fibroblasts aligned in parallel within an extracellular proteoglycan matrix in which collagen fibrils are longitudinally arranged. The extracellular matrix comprises the vast majority of the tendon substance, which is relatively hypocellular. Type I collagen constitutes the major component of tendon, with molecules organized into microfibrils, which in turn form subfibrils and fibrils. Fibrils lie embedded within the proteoglycan and glycoprotein extracellular matrix of fascicles. Each fascicle is surrounded by the endotendon, a loose connective tissue envelope. Multiple fascicles are arranged into a tendon,

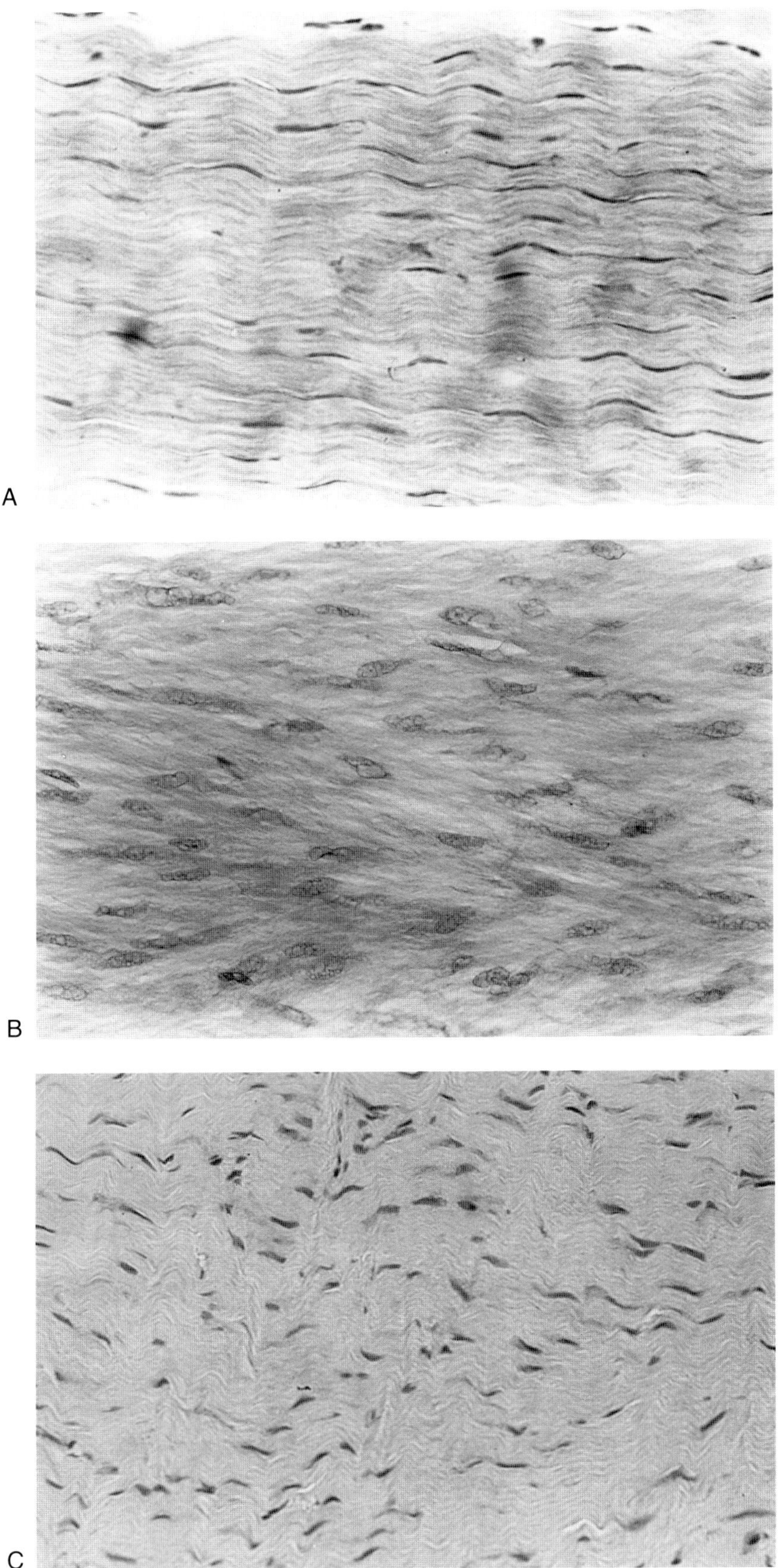

Figure 5-2. Histologic appearance of (**A**) normal ligament; (**B**) ligament at 6 weeks postinjury; (**C**) ligament at 12 weeks postinjury. (H&E, original magnification ×100.)

which is itself bounded by another connective tissue layer, the epitenon (intrasynovial tendons) or paratenon (extrasynovial tendons).

Like tendons, ligaments—typically connecting bone to bone—represent a composite of a fibroblastic cell population lying within an extracellular matrix, and the cells are similarly aligned within that matrix (Fig. 5-2A). Again, type I collagen comprises the bulk of the matrix, with elastin making up a small fraction of the ligament substance. The collagen component is organized into a hierarchical structure comprised of fibrils, fibers, subfascicular units, fasciculi, and the ligament itself. As do extrasynovial tendons, ligaments are surrounded by a loose areolar connective tissue paratenon.

IMPORTANT CONCEPTS OF THE BONE-LIGAMENT-BONE AND MYOTENDINOUS-BONE UNIT

In our consideration of the alterations that occur in soft tissue as a function of an injury, we must examine not only the processes associated with varying degrees of tissue repair but also the implications of those repair processes for the postoperative or postinjury function of the involved tissue. Specifically, with appropriate study designs and tissue preparation, the structural and mechanical properties of both normal and injured tissue may be evaluated in the laboratory with the goal of providing the clinician some insight as to the influences of injury, surgery, and postoperative rehabilitation. Frequently, such testing uses a so-called bone-ligament-bone or myotendinous-bone complex in the assessment of the properties of a given structure—such as the inferior glenohumeral ligament (IGHL) complex—when subjected to a tensile load.[46,79] A brief review of several studies that have assessed normal capsular and ligamentous tissues by this approach should prove beneficial in facilitating our subsequent transition from a histologic and biochemical to a biomechanical examination of the sequelae of soft tissue injury.

The structural properties of a bone-ligament-bone or a myotendinous-bone complex include the response of the constitutive material, geometry, and magnitude and direction of the applied loads and moments. Structural properties reflect the behavior of the complex as a whole, whereas the mechanical properties describe the characteristics of the material itself and depend on its composition, molecular structure, and ultrastructure. The structural properties are represented by linear stiffness, ultimate load, ultimate elongation, and energy absorbed at failure (Fig. 5-3A). Linear stiffness is defined as the slope of the linear portion of the load-elongation curve. Mechanical properties are represented by elastic modulus, ultimate stress, and ultimate

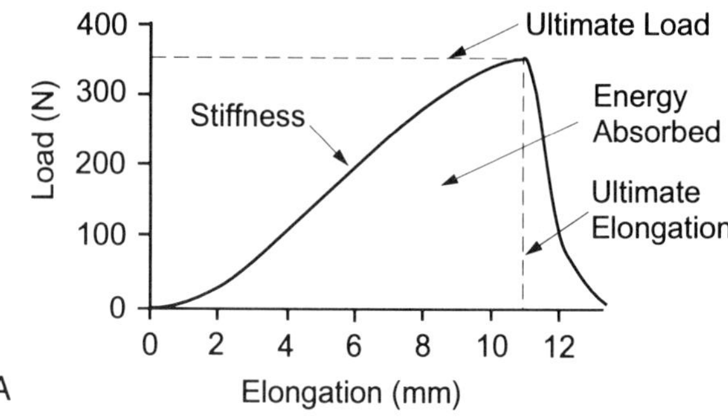

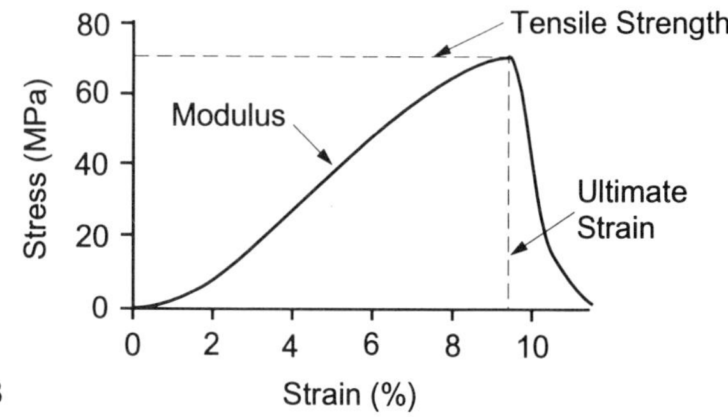

Figure 5-3. (**A**) Typical load-elongation curve for a bone-ligament-bone complex representing its structural properties. (**B**) Typical stress-strain curve for the ligament substance representing its mechanical properties.

strain (Fig. 5-3B). *Stress* is defined as the amount of force acting on a unit area, and *strain* is defined as the local deformation of the material that constitutes a body, quantified as the change in length per original length. Elastic modulus relates the normal stress to the linear strain and is determined from the linear portion of the stress-strain curve. Full understanding of the biomechanical functions of diarthrodial joints requires detailed knowledge of not only the structural properties of the bone-ligament-bone and myotendinous-bone complexes but also the mechanical properties of the tissue substance before and after injury.

Skeletal ligaments and tendons both attach to bone through insertions that allow for the dissipation of forces across the joint and for their distribution over an area of bone. The insertion sites include a gradual transition from ligament/tendon to fibrocartilage to bone. The morphology and properties of the insertion sites and structures as a whole have been shown to be affected by age and levels of stress as well as the mechanism of injury and the healing process.

Reeves[63] determined the tensile strength of the anterior capsular structures through a series of experiments in human cadavers with an age range of 28 weeks to 92 years.[37] Two structures were loaded to failure in a tensiometer at a loading rate of either a "gradually increasing load" or "a sudden load": (1) the subscapularis with humeral insertion and (2) scapula-anteroinferior capsule-humerus complex. Results revealed that 78 percent of the failures occurred at the anteroinferior labral insertion in cadavers between the ages of 10 and 40 years. In cadavers of older subjects, the subscapularis tendon and capsule failed more frequently than the insertion sites.

Kaltsas[40] compared the structural properties of the shoulder and elbow joint capsules as well as their tissue composition and microstructure using electrophoresis and electron microscopy in 24 human cadavers. Each shoulder was dissected down to the joint capsule and mounted in a tensile testing machine with a joint orientation of 90 degrees of abduction. The strength of the joint capsule varied inversely with the age of the cadaver. In all specimens, the anteroinferior capsule ruptured first at an ultimate load of approximately 2,000 N.

Bigliani et al[8] determined the material properties of the IGHL complex during a uniaxial tensile testing procedure. The IGHL complex was divided into three bone-ligament-bone preparations using the regions as outlined by Turkel and co-workers (superior band, anterior axillary pouch, and posterior axillary pouch).[68] Two elongation rates were used: slow (0.4 mm/sec) and fast (4.0 mm/sec). Their results demonstrate that the superior band and anterior axillary pouch have increased strength (62 percent) and higher stiffness (62 percent) at the faster elongation rate. The failure mode of the bone-ligament-bone specimens was also found to differ between the two elongation rates. With the fast rate, 56 percent of the failures occurred in the midsubstance whereas only 35 percent of the specimens tested at the slow rate failed in the ligament substance. The number of humeral insertion site failures also differed between the fast rate (11 percent) and the slow rate (25 percent).

Soslowsky et al[65] compared the geometric and mechanical properties from the coracoacromial ligament in normal shoulders and shoulders with rotator cuff tears. Each ligament was divided into medial and lateral bands, and the cross-sectional area was determined along each ligament's length. The bone-ligament-bone preparations were then tested to failure at a strain rate of 0.001/sec. Differences in ligament width were detected between the medial and lateral bands of the rotator cuff tear specimens only, the lateral band having greater width. No significant differences were found by the tensile testing performed except for modulus, with the modulus of the total specimen in normal shoulders being significantly greater than that of specimens with rotator cuff tears. Their hypothesis that the coracoacromial ligament in rotator cuff tear specimens should be stiffer or stronger was not supported by this study.

The values reported by these studies on the strength and modulus of the glenohumeral joint capsule, glenohumeral ligaments, and coracoacromial ligament are substantially lower than those reported for the ligaments of the knee. For example, the tensile strength of the rabbit medial collateral ligament—up to 80 MPa—is approximately 15 times as great as that reported by Bigliani et al for the IGHL—5.5 MPa.[8,79] Such a relative lack of stiffness and strength in the glenohumeral capsuloligamentous structures underscores the importance of the interaction between the static and dynamic stabilizers of the joint as the passive structures themselves do not possess the structural or mechanical properties to afford sufficient stability through the shoulder's large range of motion.

INJURY AND REPAIR

From both a histologic as well as a biochemical standpoint, the phases of tissue response to injury have been relatively well documented.[76] The recovery of soft tissue from trauma or other insult occurs in a continuum for months after the acute event. Nonetheless, the overall process is described as several overlapping but discrete phases: the acute inflammatory or reactive response phase, the regenerative or repair phase, and the tissue remodeling and maturation phase.[37,64] Although the exact identities and roles of some of the chemical mediators of inflammation remain to be elucidated, many of the individual cellular and molecular interactions responsible for tissue healing are known.

Acute Inflammatory Response

In this phase, the cellular and tissue responses to injury occur within approximately the first 72 hours after a given insult. The classic clinical signs of *rubor* (erythema), *calor* (warmth), *tumor* (hematoma/edema), and *dolor* (pain) represent the results of those humoral and cellular interactions that produce localized reaction to tissue damage and may occur in varying degrees depending on the extent of the injury.

Histologically, with capillary damage and resultant enhanced permeability of involved blood vessels, erythrocytes and inflammatory cells migrate into the tissue defect along with serous exudate that leaks through the injured microvasculature. Neutrophilic and lymphocytic cell populations dominate the white blood cell response during the first few hours, followed by significant populations of monocytes and macrophages that begin active phagocytosis of debris.[22] Concurrently, fibroblastic proliferation occurs, most likely from an undifferentiated mesenchymal precursor population, although the exact precursor cell has not been clearly identified to date.[64] These fibroblasts are responsible for the formation of scar matrix that has been documented via light and electron microscopy to consist of randomly aligned collagen and amorphous ground substance during this early stage of the body's response to injury.

The biochemical alterations and mediators associated with the acute reactive response are both varied and complex. Secondary to direct injury and fibrinic exposure in exudative fluid, localized cellular release of histamine takes place, enhancing capillary permeability and encouraging local vasodilation while stimulating production of additional mediators of inflammation, including serotonin, bradykinins, and prostaglandins.[37] These substances further increase and prolong vasodilation. Bradykinins in particular have been implicated in the enhancement of capillary permeability, contributing to additional exudate and migration of inflammatory cells into the injury site. An additional angiogenesis factor secreted by the macrophagic cell population appears to induce the ingrowth of capillary buds to stimulate early neovascularization.[60]

Clearly and understandably, the biochemical composition of the inflamed tissue differs substantially from the normal during the acute reactive response.[23] The concurrent exudation of serous fluid and early production of extracellular matrix by fibroblasts result in an increased total water content at the injury site as well as an increased total collagen content. However, total collagen concentration is lower than that seen in normal tissue owing to the greater water content in the damaged tissue.[4,17,23] Further, the composition of collagen differs from normal in that the fibroblasts produce predominantly type III collagen in the initial scar matrix formed during the reactive phase.[73] It is this type III collagen that serves as a framework for additional matrix formation that occurs in the reparative and remodeling phases. Also, within the context of the active secretory state of the fibroblastic cell population, increased DNA, fibronectin, and glycosaminoglycan contents are observed relative to normal uninjured tissues.[21,23,37]

Repair and Regeneration Phase

The repair and regeneration phase encompasses those cellular and tissue processes occurring from 48 to 72 hours until roughly 6 weeks postinjury. This time period marks the gradual subsidence of inflammation together with the active commencement of the healing process. Grossly, highly vascular granulation tissue can be seen to form at the site of injury, either filling the tissue defect that had been created or covering the free ends of torn or ruptured tissue.[24]

On histologic examination, cellular and matrix proliferation is observed to take place with the organization of clot that initially formed as a direct result of capillary damage. Fibroblasts become the predominant cell type at the repair site and continue to actively synthesize extracellular matrix. The scar that forms as a result of this fibroblastic activity at this stage is highly cellular, with significant populations of fibroblasts, mast cells, and macrophages found within the matrix (Fig. 5-2B). This matrix becomes progressively more organized with time, although electron microscopy has confirmed that the collagen fibrils laid down by the fibroblasts remain relatively disorganized within an amorphous ground substance. Staining confirms the first appearance of elastin within the scar matrix during this time, whereas the total amount of collagen continues to increase but not to normal concentration levels. Proliferation of capillary buds continues the process of vascular ingrowth in response to the angiogenesis factor secreted by macrophages into the local tissue environment.

From a biochemical perspective, this phase of repair and regeneration marks the peak period of collagen turnover.[4] Although total collagen content within the involved tissue rises, collagen concentration remains relatively low in the face of a persistently elevated water content combined with a concurrently low density of collagen fibrils. Type I collagen now becomes the dominant type found within the evolving scar matrix, as fibroblasts decrease production of type III and switch to preferential production of type I. Levels of DNA and glycosaminoglycans remain elevated due to the persistently high synthetic activity of fibroblasts secreting the scar matrix. These biochemical changes correlate with increasing tensile strength demonstrated by the healing tissue at this point in the reparative process.[23,31,66,67,71,81]

Remodeling and Maturation Phase

Tissue remodeling and scar maturation occur during this phase of recovery, which can last up to 1 year or longer after the time of initial injury. Formation of increasingly organized scar results in continued enhancement of tissue strength. Translucent scar bridging a reparable tissue defect or covering the exposed surfaces of ruptured and separated tissue becomes apparent on gross examination.

Light microscopy reveals decreased cellularity as represented by fewer fibroblasts and macrophages within the scar matrix, along with an overall vascularity of the tissue. The density of the scar increases as the collagen matrix demonstrates enhanced alignment and increased collagen fibril diameter as documented on electron microscopy. Nonetheless, as maturation of the scar progresses, slight disorganization of the tissue does persist relative to normal. Fibroblastic cells become flattened with less rough endoplasmic reticulum and a decreased cytoplasm/nucleus ratio, consistent with their reduced synthetic activity at this stage (Fig. 5-2C).

Biochemical analysis confirms this decreased matrix synthesis and collagen turnover. DNA content reverts back toward normal levels, although a slightly increased proteoglycan content persists. Water content returns to normal levels, and collagen concentration approaches the normal value but remains slightly low. The ratio of type III to type I collagen continues to decline toward normal values as the scar matrix becomes more organized and demonstrates near-normal biochemistry.

Biomechanics of Healing Ligaments

In previous studies examining the healing of the medial collateral ligament (MCL) in rabbit models, the healing tissue was as previously mentioned determined to be clearly abnormal, both biochemically and during mechanical testing.[23,31] The results suggest that the healing tissue may never achieve normal ligament characteristics. On histologic analysis, remodeling was seen to occur in the scar tissue with a decrease in the numbers and size of the fibroblasts. Between 6 and 14 weeks after injury, the cells seemed to align their nuclei longitudinally along the long axis of the ligament. After 14 weeks, few changes were noted.

The geometric, structural, and mechanical properties of the healing ligament were also evaluated. The injury mode selected for this study used a braided steel suture to rupture the ligament. The cross-sectional area of the ligament midsubstance was determined to be significantly increased at all time intervals compared with the normal and sham-operated values. The stiffness, ultimate load, and energy absorbed to failure of the healing bone-ligament-bone complex were all significantly lower compared with normals. The failure modes of these preparations changed over time. Initially, the experimentals failed at the midsubstance, at 6 weeks' failure occurred at the tibial insertion, whereas at periods greater than 14 weeks, midsubstance failure once again occurred. Finally, experimentals demonstrated reduced values for modulus and ultimate stress (40 percent of control). These values reflect the inferior quality of the healed tissue compared with control and correlate well with the previously described biochemical properties of the tissue.

Similar results were obtained in the evaluation of ligament healing in a canine model after sharp transection of the MCL.[78] The influence of mobilization and prolonged immobilization on joint laxity and on ligament structural and mechanical properties was examined. Results reveal that postinjury or postoperative mobilization improved both joint stability and ligament tensile properties, although not to normal levels. For example, linear stiffness in the mobilized groups reached 60 percent of control, whereas ultimate load reached 40 percent of control. The respective values in the group subjected to prolonged immobilization were 36 and 20 percent of control, respectively. These values paralleled the results obtained for joint laxity, whereas the mobilized groups demonstrated only 52 to 61 percent of the laxity of the immobilized group.

More recently, MCL healing was examined using a more physiologic failure mechanism that created a "mop-end" tear of the ligament substance with simultaneous injury to the insertion sites.[72] Two modes of treatment were evaluated using biomechanical and histologic techniques: (1) primary ligament repair and (2) nonoperative treatment. MCL repair did not significantly affect the tensile properties of the femur-MCL-tibia complex (FMTC), although postoperative healing time improved the FMTC properties of both treatment groups. The failure mode of these complexes indicated that the ligament insertion to bone recovered more slowly than the ligament substance after this type of injury.

The healing of soft tissue has been demonstrated to benefit from the application of some degree of stress applied to the healing tissue.[31] Collagen cross-linking in the scar matrix and tensile strength and stiffness of the healing tissue are enhanced by the application of load to the tissue relative to the totally protected/immobilized state. Further, histologic examination confirms the increased formation of adhesions during soft tissue healing in an immobilized joint, predisposing the joint to the development of increased stiffness and decreased function.

Injury and Healing of the Myotendinous Junction

It is important in this context to reiterate that an injury may well not be isolated to one specific tissue or portion of tissue. As documented in the studies cited above, a ligamentous injury may involve the insertion site as well as the midsubstance. Similarly, muscular or tendinous injury may imply some degree of damage to the bony insertion of the tendon or to the myotendinous junction. Since the early work of McMaster, multiple studies using rabbit models have examined the failure modes of myotendinous-bone complexes subjected to tensile loads.[2,3,25,26,50] In virtually all cases, the region of the myotendinous junction represents the weakest link in the system, although McMaster's[50] original report documented failure at the tendinous insertion site and within the muscle substance as well. Interestingly, and in contradistinction to results of bone-ligament-bone testing, the site of failure does not vary with the rate at which the specimens are loaded, as the various investigators have used rates of stretch from 10 to 1,000 mm/min.

Certainly, most myotendinous injuries will not involve

total rupture of the structure. Rather, some degree of incomplete tear—''muscle strain''—will occur. These injuries have also been shown experimentally to disrupt the integrity of the tissue near the myotendinous junction. The work of Nikolaou et al[56] documented reproducible creation of hemorrhage and fiber damage at the myotendinous junction with stretching of rabbit anterior tibial muscles. The inflammatory response resulted in scar formation by the end of the first week postinjury, with gradual return of the muscle's ability to generate normal tension within the same time period. Correlation of computed tomography findings with anatomic dissections has further documented the importance of the myotendinous junction in muscle strain injuries.[27]

CLINICAL IMPLICATIONS FROM BASIC SCIENCE RESEARCH

From a clinical perspective, restoration or maintenance of a patient's functional capabilities necessarily occupies a high priority in the consideration of soft tissue injury and healing. How will limb function be affected? How will the patient compensate for an injury left unrepaired? These issues deserve at least as much attention in clinical practice as do the understanding of the exact mechanisms by which tissue healing occurs. The previously discussed biochemical and biomechanical knowledge generated in the laboratory can provide a scientific basis for a rational approach to soft tissue management in the injured patient.

The benefits of a well-structured rehabilitation program in enhancing the healing process of an injured or postoperative patient are obvious. Basic science data reveal that a combination of controlled mobilization and stress to the healing tissue serves, in essence, a dual function.[31,77,78,80,82] First, as documented in animal models, it enhances the formation of organized scar matrix through improved collagen alignment and cross-linking.[31] The net result of this process will be to improve the strength of the tissue and increase joint stability. This is particularly important in the shoulder, which relies heavily on the soft tissue to maintain stability through a large range of motion. Second, motion/mobilization can reduce the amount of adhesion formation in the surrounding soft tissues and prevent contracture formation. Therefore, joint mobility will benefit, preserving as extensive a range of motion as possible and offering the patient the opportunity to maintain or regain a functional limb.[1,28-30,82] However, more studies are clearly needed to help define and refine programs for postoperative rehabilitation that are solidly founded in basic science.

It should be reiterated that healed tendon or ligament is unlikely to achieve the same quality of tissue (modulus and tensile strength) found in native tissue. In the postoperative or conservatively managed patient, tissue properties will remain relatively low at the injury site for the first several weeks, as the acute inflammatory reaction to injury or surgical repair takes place. As soft tissue repair and remodeling occur over the ensuing weeks, strength improves but never returns to normal. At 1 year, the healing tissue possesses approximately 60 percent of the tensile strength (a mechanical property) of normal tissue. This pattern of recovery should guide postoperative and postinjury rehabilitation programs, such that the remaining strength of the tissue is taken into account in the development of a patient's therapy regimen. Further, in those cases in which surgery is undertaken, the operative approach must also dictate the postoperative plan.

Particularly in the shoulder, the transition from laxity to clinical instability occurs along the spectrum of potential glenohumeral translations. Although diagnosis of glenohumeral instability rests with the clinical presentation, important contributions from basic research have nonetheless taken place in this arena. That there exists a physiologic range of laxity or obligate humeral translation on the glenoid has been clearly documented, establishing a concrete distinction between the basics of glenohumeral and tibiofemoral kinematics.[33,34] In contradistinction to the shoulder, laxity in the knee implies excessive motion. Such a fundamental difference has helped to emphasize that examination of soft tissue restraints at a joint must not focus solely on tissue strength or load-bearing capability. Rather, the nonlinear tensile as well as viscoelastic properties of tendons and ligaments that provide joint stability must remain of paramount concern.

However, even with significant soft tissue damage, joint motion may be preserved due to the patient's ability to compensate for injury. For instance, some patients with even large rotator cuff tears can achieve significant degrees of abduction at the shoulder despite loss of cuff integrity and therefore varying loss of supraspinatus, infraspinatus/teres minor, and subscapularis function. The decrease in relative contribution to motion from the scapulohumeral musculature in these cases can be compensated for by an alteration in the normal relationship between glenohumeral and scapulothoracic motion in producing shoulder abduction. In the normal individual, scapulothoracic motion contributes little to abduction below 30 degrees and then becomes significant up to full abduction, with an overall glenohumeral/scapulothoracic motion ratio of 1.5:1 to 2:1.[61] In the patient with soft tissue injury comprising the glenohumeral contribution, scapulothoracic motion assumes a greater role in both early and total abduction.[36] Thus, patients can achieve good limb function in the face of significant anatomic pathology via this mechanism.

In similar fashion, basic research has enhanced our understanding of the ability of many patients to demonstrate a good clinical outcome after rotator cuff debridement rather than formal repair. For instance, experimental results from our laboratory suggest the importance of maintaining the integrity of the anterior/posterior force couple of the subscapularis/infraspinatus-teres minor to maximize the potential for good range of motion.[16] This correlates well with the clinical conclusions reached by Burkhart.[9,10] Additional kinematic studies in the future are needed to enhance the foundation formed by the biomechanical and biochemical investigations undertaken to date and could offer additional information in aiding the clinicians management of patients after soft tissue injury at the shoulder. Laboratory apparati such as the Pittsburgh Dynamic Shoulder Testing Apparatus[15] can simulate glenohumeral motion using full upper extremities and physiologic muscles forces. Investigations using such equipment can provide relevant information on the effects of various capsuloligamentous and labral injuries at the glenohumeral joint during arm motion as well as the role of the rotator cuff musculature and surrounding muscular envelope in providing joint stability and motion.

REFERENCES

1. Akeson WH, Woo SLY, Amiel D: Rapid recovery from contracture in rabbit hindlimb: a correlative and biochemical study. Clin Orthop 122:359, 1977
2. Almekinders LC, Garrett WEJ, Seaber AV: Histopathology of muscle tears in stretching injuries. Trans Orthop Res Soc 9:306, 1984
3. Almekinders LC, Garrett WEJ, Seaber AV: Pathophysiologic response to muscle tears in stretching injuries. Trans Orthop Res Soc 9:307, 1984
4. Amiel D, Frank C, Harwood FL: Collagen alterations in medial collateral healing in a rabbit model. Connect Tissue Res 16:357, 1987
5. Anderson W, Moor R: Clinico-pathologic study of the shoulder joint, abstracted. Presented at the Second Canadian Conference on Research in Rheumatic Diseases, Toronto, October 28, 1960
6. Bankart ASB: The pathology and treatment of recurrent dislocation of the shoulder joint. Br J Surg 26:23, 1938
7. Bigliani LU, Morrison DS, April EW: The morphology of the acromion and its relationship to rotator cuff tears. Orthop Trans 10:228, 1986
8. Bigliani LU, Pollock RG, Soslowsky LJ, et al: Tensile properties of the inferior glenohumeral ligament. J Orthop Res 10:187, 1992
9. Burkhart SS: Fluoroscopic comparison of kinematic patterns in massive rotator cuff tears. A suspension bridge model. Clin Orthop 284:144, 1992
10. Burkhart SS, Esch JC, Jolson RS: The rotator crescent and rotator cable: an anatomic description of the shoulder's "suspension bridge." Arthroscopy 9:611, 1993
11. Codman EA: The pathology of the subacromial bursa and the supraspinatus tendon. p. 65. In Codman EA (ed): The Shoulder: Rupture of the Supraspinatus Tendon and Other Lesions in or about the Subacromial Bursa. Thomas & Todd, Boston, 1934
12. Codman EA, Akerson IB: The pathology associated with rupture of the supraspinatus tendon. Ann Surg 93:354, 1911
13. Cotton RE, Rideout DF: Tears of the humeral rotator cuff: a radiological and pathological necropsy survey. J Bone Joint Surg [Br] 46:314, 1964
14. Craig EV: The geyser sign and torn rotator cuff: clinical significance and pathomechanics. Clin Orthop 191:213, 1984
15. Debski RE, McMahon PJ, Thompson WO, et al: A new dynamic testing apparatus to study glenohumeral motion. J Biomech, in press
16. Debski RE, Thompson WO, Boardman ND, et al: Rotator cuff function in a variety of deficiency states: a dynamic biomechanical analysis, abstracted. Presented at the American Orthopaedic Society for Sports Medicine Specialty Day Meeting, New Orleans, LA, 1994
17. Delaunay A, Bazin S: Mucopolysaccharides, collagen, and nonfibrillar proteins in inflammation. Int Rev Connect Tissue Res 2:301, 1964
18. DePalma AF: Surgery of the Shoulder. 3rd Ed. JB Lippincott, Philadelphia, 1983
19. DePalma AF, Callery G, Bennett GA: Variational anatomy and degenerative lesions of the shoulder joint. p. 255. In Blount WP (ed): American Academy of Orthopaedic Surgeons Instructional Course Lectures XVI. JW Edwards, Ann Arbor, MI, 1949
20. DePalma AF, White JB, Callery G: Degenerative lesions of the shoulder joint at various age groups which are compatible with good function. p. 168. In Pease CN, Banks SW (eds): American Academy of Orthopaedic Surgeons Instructional Course Lectures XVII. JW Edwards, Ann Arbor, MI, 1950
21. Dunphy JE, Udupa KN: Chemical and histochemical sequences in the normal healing of wounds. N Engl J Med 253:847, 1955
22. Flynn JE, Graham JH: Healing following tendon suture and tendon transplants. Surg Gynecol Obstet 115:467, 1962
23. Frank C, Schachar N, Dittrich D: Natural history of healing of the repaired medial collateral ligament. J Orthop Res 1:179, 1983
24. Frank C, Woo SLY, Amiel D, Akeson W: Medial collateral ligament healing: a multidisciplinary assessment in rabbits. Am J Sports Med 11:379, 1983
25. Garrett WEJ, Almekinders LC, Seaber AV: Biomechanics of muscle tears in stretching injuries. Trans Orthop Res Soc 9:384, 1984
26. Garrett WEJ, Nikolaou PK, Ribbeck BM: The effect of muscle architecture on the failure properties of skeletal muscle under passive tension. Am J Sports Med 16:7, 1988
27. Garrett WEJ, Rich FR, Nikolaou PK: Computed tomography of hamstring muscle strains. Med Sci Sports Exerc 21:506, 1989
28. Gelberman RH, Vandeberg JS, Lundborg GN, Akeson WH: Flexor tendon healing and restoration of the gliding surface: an ultrastructural study in dogs. J Bone Joint Surg [Am] 65:70, 1983
29. Gelberman RH, Woo SLY: The physiological basis for application of controlled stress in the rehabilitation of flexor tendon injuries. J Hand Ther April–June:66, 1989

30. Gelberman RH, Woo SLY, Lothringer K et al: Effects of early intermittent passive mobilization on healing canine flexor tendons. J Hand Surg 7:170, 1982
31. Gomez MA, Woo SLY, Amiel D et al: The effects of increased tension on healing medial collateral ligaments. Am J Sports Med 19:347, 1991
32. Hamada K, Fukuda H, Mikas M, Kobayashi Y: Roentgenographic findings in massive rotator cuff tears: a long term observation. Clin Orthop 254:92, 1990
33. Harryman DT, Sidles JA, Clark JM et al: Translation of the humeral head on the glenoid with passive glenohumeral motion. J Bone Joint Surg [Am] 72:1334, 1990
34. Harryman DT, Sidles JA, Harris SL, Matsen FA: The role of the rotator interval capsule in passive motion and stability of the shoulder. J Bone Joint Surg [Am] 74:53, 1992
35. Hill HA, Sachs MD: The grooved defect of the humeral head: a frequently unrecognized complication of dislocations of the shoulder joint. Radiology 35:690, 1940
36. Inman VT, Saunders JB, Abbott LC: Observations on the functions of the shoulder joint. J Bone Joint Surg 42:1-30, 1944
37. Irvin TT: The healing wound. p. 3. In Bucknall TE, Ellis H (eds): Wound Healing for Surgeons. Bailliere Tindall, London, 1982
38. Jobe FW: Impingement problems in the athlete. p. 205. In Barr JSJ (ed): American Academy of Orthopaedic Surgeons Instructional Course Lectures XXXVIII. American Academy of Orthopaedic Surgeons, Park Ridge, IL, 1989
39. Jobe FW, Kvitne RS: Shoulder pain in the overhead throwing athlete. Orthop Rev 18:963, 1989
40. Kaltsas DS: Comparative study of the properties of the shoulder joint capsule with those of other joint capsules. Clin Orthop 173:20, 1983
41. Kazar B, Relovszky E: Prognosis of primary dislocation of the shoulder. Acta Orthop Scand 40:216, 1969
42. Keyes EL: Observations on rupture of the supraspinatus tendon, based upon a study of 73 cadavers. Ann Surg 97:849, 1933
43. Keyes EL: Anatomical observations on senile changes in the shoulder. J Bone Joint Surg [Am] 17:953, 1935
44. Lindblom K: On pathogenesis of ruptures of the tendon aponeurosis of the shoulder joint. Acta Radiol 20:563, 1939
45. Lohr JF, Uhthoff HK: The microvasculat pattern of the supraspinatus tendon. Clin Orthop 254:35, 1990
46. Lyon RM, Woo SLY, Hollis JM, et al: A new device to measure the structural properties of the femur-anterior cruciate ligament-tibia complex. J Biomech Eng 111:350, 1989
47. Matsen FA, Harryman DT, Sidles JA: Mechanics of glenohumeral instabililty. [Review]. Clin Sports Med 10:783, 1991
48. Matsen FA III, Fu FH, Hawkins RJ (eds): The Shoulder: A Balance of Mobility and Stability. American Academy of Orthopaedic Surgeons, Rosemont, IL, 1993
49. McLaughlin HL: Lesions of the musculotendinous cuff of the shoulder: the exposure and treatment of tears with retraction. J Bone Joint Surg [Am] 26:31, 1944
50. McMaster PE: Clinical and experimental studies on the causes and location of subcutaneous ruptures. J Bone Joint Surg 15:705, 1933
51. Morrison DS, Bigliani LU: The clinical significance of variations in acromial morphology. Orthop Trans 11:234, 1987
52. Moseley HF, Overgaard B: The anterior capsular mechanism in recurrent anterior dislocation of the shoulder: morphological and clinical studies with special reference to the glenoid labrum and the glenohumeral ligaments. J Bone Joint Surg [Br] 44:913, 1962
53. Neer CS: Impingement lesions. Clin Orthop 173:70, 1983
54. Neer CS: Shoulder Reconstruction. WB Saunders, Philadelphia, 1990
55. Neer CS, Craig EV, Fukuda H: Cuff-tear arthropathy. J Bone Joint Surg [Am] 65:1232, 1983
56. Nikolau PK, Macdonald BL, Glisson RR: Biomechanical and histological evaluation of muscle after controlled strain injury. Am J Sports Med 15:9, 1987
57. O'Brien ST et al: Developmental anatomy of the shoulder and anatomy of the glenohumeral joint. p. 1. In Rockwood CA Jr, Matsen FA III (eds): The Shoulder. WB Saunders, Philadelphia, 1990
58. Ozaki J, Fujimoto S, Nakagawa Y: Tears of the rotator cuff of the shoulder associated with pathologic changes in the acromion: a study in cadavera. J Bone Joint Surg [Am] 70:1224–30, 1988
59. Pettersson G: Rupture of the tendon aponeurosis of the shoulder joint in antero-inferior dislocation: a study on the origin and occurrence of the ruptures. Acta Chir Scand Suppl 77:1, 1942
60. Polverini PJ, Cotran RS: Activated macrophages induce vascular proliferation. Nature 269:804, 1977
61. Poppen NK, Walker PS: Normal and abnormal motion of the shoulder. J Bone Joint Surg [Am] 58:195, 1976
62. Rathbun JB, Macnab I: The microvascular pattern of the rotator cuff. J Bone Joint Surg [Br] 52:540, 1970
63. Reeves B: Experiments on the tensile strength of the anterior capsular structures of the shoulder in man. J Bone Joint Surg [Br] 50:858, 1968
64. Ross R: The fibroblast and wound repair. Biol Rev 43:51, 1968
65. Soslowsky LJ, An CH, Johnston SP, Carpenter JE: Geometric and mechanical properties of the coracoacromial ligament and their relationship to rotator cuff disease, abstracted. Trans Orthop Res Soc 18:139, 1993
66. Tipton CM, James SL, Mergner W: Influence of exercise on strength of medial collateral knee ligaments of dogs. Am J Physiol 218:894, 1970
67. Torg JS, Conrad W, Kalen V: Clinical diagnosis of anterior cruciate ligament instability in the athlete. Am J Sports Med 4:84, 1976
68. Turkel SJ, Panio MW, Marshall JL, Girgis FG: Stabilizing mechanisms preventing anterior dislocations of the glenohumeral joint. J Bone Joint Surg [Am] 63:1208, 1981
69. Uhthoff HK, Sarkar K, Matnard JA: Calcifying tendinitis: a new concept of its pathogenesis. Clin Orthop 118:164, 1976
70. Uhthoff HK, Sarkar K, Lohr J: Repair in rotator cuff tendons. p. 216. In Post M, Morrey BF, Hawkins RJ (eds): Surgery of the Shoulder. Mosby-Year Book, St. Louis, 1990
71. Vailas AC, Tipton CM, Matthes RD: Physical activity and its influence on the repair process of medial collateral ligaments. Connect Tissue Res 9:25, 1981
72. Weiss JA, Woo SLY, Ohland KJ et al: Evaluation of a new injury model to study medial collateral ligament healing:

primary repair versus nonoperative treatment. J Orthop Res 9:516, 1991
73. Williams IF, McCullagh KG, Silver IA: The distribution of types I and III collagen and fibronectin in the healing equine tendon. Connect Tissue Res 12:211, 1984
74. Wilson CL: Lesions of the supraspinatus tendon: degeneration, rupture and calcification. Arch Surg 46:307, 1943
75. Wilson CL, Duff GL: Pathologic study of degeneration and rupture of the supraspinatus tendon. Arch Surg 47:121, 1943
76. Woo SLY, Buckwalter JA (eds): Injury and Repair of the Musculoskeletal Soft Tissues. American Academy of Orthopaedic Surgeons, Park Ridge, IL, 1988
77. Woo SLY, Gomez MA, Amiel D: The effects of exercise on the biomechanical and biochemical properties of swine digital flexor tendons. J Biomech Eng 103:51, 1981
78. Woo SLY, Gomez MA, Inoue M, Akeson WH: New experimental procedures to evaluate the biomechanical properties of healing canine medial collateral ligaments. J Orthop Res 5:425, 1987
79. Woo SLY, Gomez MA, Seguchi Y: Measurement of mechanical properties of ligament substance from a bone-ligament-bone preparation. J Orthop Res 1:22, 1983
80. Woo SLY, Gomez MA, Sites TJ: The biomechanical and morphological changes of the MCL following immobilization and remobilization. J Bone Joint Surg [Am] 69:1200, 1987
81. Woo SLY, Inoue M, McGurk-Burleson E: Treatment of the medial collateral ligament injury: II. Structure and function of canine knees in response to differing treatment regimens. Am J Sports Med 15:22, 1987
82. Woo SLY, Matthews JV, Akeson WH: Connective tissue response to immobility: correlative study of biomechanical and biochemical measurements of normal and immobilized rabbit knees. Arthritis Rheum 18:257, 1975
83. Woo SLY, Ritter MA, Amiel D: The biomechanical and biochemical properties of swine tendons: long term effects of exercise on the digital extensors. Connect Tissue Res 7:177, 1980

CHAPTER SIX

Magnetic Resonance and Shoulder Imaging

Hollis M. Fritts, Jr.
Cooper R. Gundry

Despite the availability of many imaging modalities for the evaluation of the shoulder, history and physical examination remain the most important components in the evaluation of shoulder pain and abnormalities. Routine plain films are universally, in conjunction with the clinical examination, providing inexpensive screening for fractures, dislocations, osseous tumors, arthritis, and calcifications. However, plain films are often normal or nondiagnostic in occult osseous or soft tissue injuries. When a thorough clinical examination including radiographs does not provide a specific diagnosis and there is incomplete or no resolution on conservative management, additional imaging may be necessary. In this age of cost-conscious medicine, it becomes even more important to provide an early and definitive diagnosis, thereby allowing a prompt and tailored treatment plan and the most efficient return to sports or the workplace.

SHOULDER IMAGING MODALITIES

Arthrography and Bursography

Until relatively recently, arthrography was the imaging gold standard for evaluation of shoulder pain and impingement syndrome, allowing detection of full-thickness and some deep surface, partial-thickness rotator cuff tears. Reports of the accuracy of arthrography for the detection of full-thickness rotator cuff tears vary from 95 percent to 100 percent.[26,42] However, arthrography is not consistently accurate in estimating the size of full-thickness rotator cuff tears. The accuracy for detection of partial-thickness tears is much less, because only partial-thickness deep surface tears are identified on routine arthrography. Superior surface partial-thickness tears cannot be evaluated by routine arthrography without the addition of bursography.[24,67] These invasive modalities are of limited use in the evaluation of the earlier stages of the clinical impingement syndrome, as neither can detect tendon degeneration or bursitis.

Ultrasound

Sonography has been promoted as a modality to evaluate full-thickness rotator cuff tears and is considered accurate for the diagnosis of full-thickness rotator cuff tears greater than 1 cm in size.[15,20,37,66] Its operator dependency, decreased accuracy for partial-thickness and full-thickness tears less than 1 cm in size, and unreliable depiction of intrasubstance tendon degeneration and bursal changes limit its usefulness in the evaluation of impingement syndrome.[4,71] Ultrasound is unable to evaluate the relationship of the coracoacromial arch to subacromial soft tissues. Also, the proximal aspects of the rotator cuff musculature and the capsulolabral anatomy are not reliably demonstrated.

Computed Tomography and Computed Tomographic Arthrography

Computed tomography (CT) is the modality of choice for depiction of fractures and cortical bone abnormalities. It is also superior in detection of calcification of bony and soft tissue lesions and tumors. CT arthrography does not add significantly to the diagnostic accuracy of arthrography for detection of rotator cuff tears. However, it is excellent for the evaluation of glenoid labrum and capsular abnormalities. In the past, CT arthrography has been the imaging modality of choice for specific evaluation of shoulder instability,[32,57,63,72] although magnetic resonance arthrography is now becoming considered the imaging gold standard in this regard.[11,21]

Magnetic Resonance Imaging

Magnetic resonance imaging (MRI) has become the imaging modality of choice for the evaluation of the painful shoulder beyond initial radiographs in many circumstances. Superior soft tissue contrast and resolution and multiplanar capability allow a global evaluation of all intra-articular and extra-articular soft tissue and osseous structures of the shoulder that is unsurpassed by any other modality. MRI is the only imaging modality that enables detection of the entire pathologic spectrum of the clinical impingement syndrome, from subacromial-subdeltoid bursitis through cuff tendinosis/tendinitis to partial- and full-thickness rotator cuff tears and end-stage rotator cuff arthropathy. It can directly assess the overlying coracoacromial arch morphology, complementing radiographs in the preoperative delineation of its relationship to the underlying subacromial soft tissues. The sensitivity of MRI in the detection of bone marrow and associated pathology allows unparalleled sensitivity and specificity in the visualization of intrinsic bony pathology of the proximal humerus, glenoid, acromion, clavicle, and acromioclavicular joint. MRI noninvasively evaluates the glenoid labrum with accuracy that approaches that of CT arthrography. Surrounding subcutaneous tissues and musculotendinous structures are also visualized, including the biceps tendon and associated abnormalities of degeneration, tear, and displacement. Soft tissue mass lesions including ganglion cysts, which may result in neural impingement, are directly visualized. Other soft tissue injuries deltoid muscle strains and pectoralis major ruptures can also be delineated. Magnetic resonance arthrography, which consists of MRI after intra-articular injection of saline or dilute gadolinium solution, surpasses the CT arthrogram standard for visualization of capsulolabral anatomy and pathology. After dedicated history and physical examination and initial radiographs, MRI is the most global imaging examination of the persistently painful shoulder.

TECHNIQUE

Today's cost-conscious environment requires the maximum amount of information possible in the least amount of time. Two-echo spin-echo imaging with proton density- and T_2-weighted technique in three planes has provided the most diagnostic information per time. After a short axial localizing series using T_1-weighted technique, two-echo spin-echo technique is performed in the oblique coronal, oblique sagittal, and axial planes. Although T_1-weighted images are relatively sensitive for the presence of tendon pathology, they do not provide specificity for differentiation of tendinosis, tendinitis, and tears. T_2-weighted images are critical for this differentiation.[22] T_2-weighted images are also helpful in detection of other soft tissue abnormalities such as bursal hypertrophy or bursal fluid accumulation. Proton density images obtained with two-echo pulse sequences are adequate in providing pseudo-T_1 information for most purposes, including incidental findings of marrow disease. A very short STIR sequence is routinely obtained to screen for subtle marrow edema and pathology.

Typical parameters for shoulder MRI when using a 1.5T scanner are repetition time/echo time of 2,000/20,80 msec, using one-signal excitation with 16-cm field of view. Three millimeter slice thickness with 1-mm gap is used with 192×256 matrix in oblique coronal, oblique sagittal, and axial planes, and the images are filmed with 1.3 to 1.5 magnification. The time of examination from room entry to exit is approximately 35 minutes. Parameters when using a 0.5T scanner are the same except for use of 4-mm slice thickness and a shorter bandwidth. Image presentation on film must provide easy comparison of signal intensity on first and second echo images. We film proton density images on one sheet, with the T_2-weighted images filmed in corresponding order and location on a second sheet.

Magnetic resonance arthrography using a dilute 1 : 250-ml dilution of gadolinium-DTPA is not routinely used for evaluation of the painful shoulder but is becoming established as the imaging modality of choice for the evaluation of capsulolabral anatomy. It is the first choice in evaluation of the painful shoulder of young throwing athletes due to added sensitivity and specificity in the detection of capsulolabral pathology including SLAP lesions, as well as any associated secondary impingement findings. Intravenous gadolinium-DTPA administration is occasionally used when evaluating soft tissue masses.

CLINICAL IMPINGEMENT SYNDROME AND THE CORACOACROMIAL ARCH

Tears of normal rotator cuff tendon tissue are very uncommon.[39] Tears most commonly occur through weakened degenerative tendon tissue, explaining the predominance of rotator cuff tears in older age groups.[12,40] Tears have been thought to be uncommon before the age of 40.[13,48,50] Factors that have been described as contributing to cuff degeneration include normal aging, hypovascularity of the

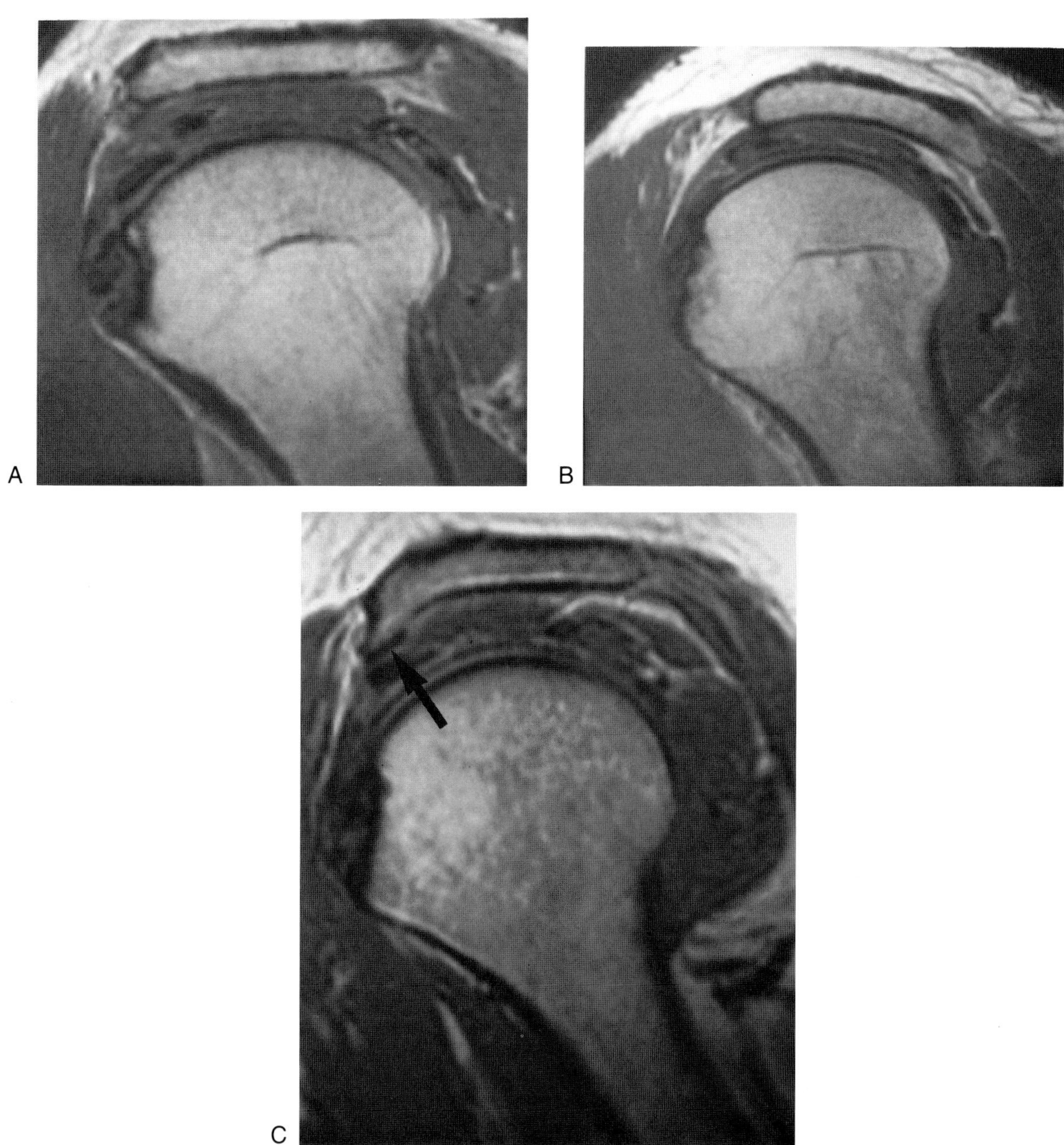

Figure 6-1. Acromion configuration in the oblique sagittal plane. **(A)** Type I acromion has a flat inferior surface. **(B)** Type II acromion has a gentle inferior radius of curvature that approximately parallels the superior surface of the humeral head. **(C)** Type III acromion exhibits a focal decrease in the radius of curvature of the anterior aspect of the acromion (*arrow*), associated with a large subacromial spur underlying the attachment of the coracoacromial ligament.

critical zone, and repeated microtrauma as a result of impingement between the humeral head and the overlying coracoacromial arch. Overuse of the shoulder from athletic or professional activities has also been recognized as promoting rotator cuff injuries. An athletically accelerated aging of the tissue of the rotator cuff has been suggested as a contributory factor in some rotator cuff tears.[16]

Neer[21] popularized the clinical impingement syndrome and proposed a staging classfication based on age, duration of disease process, and response to conservative treatment.

Pathologic changes in stage I impingement, including edema and hemorrhage, evolve into fibrosis and tendon degeneration in stage II and eventually to tear of the tendon in stage III.

Most rotator cuff disorders have been attributed to the clinical impingement syndrome. Impingement syndrome is a clinical diagnosis based on history and physical examination that refers to pain associated with the encroachment of the rotator cuff and associated soft tissues including subacromial-subdeltoid bursa and biceps tendon, between the humeral head below and the overlying coracoacromial arch. The coracoacromial arch consists of the anterior aspect of the acromion, coracoacromial ligament, coracoid process, and the acromioclavicular joint. Impingement by the coracoacromial arch can be secondary to abnormalities involving one or more of these components, resulting in narrowing of the acromiohumeral distance.

Acromion Morphology

Acromial morphology and its relationship to the subacromial space should be noted on every shoulder MRI. Narrowing of acromiohumeral distance can be associated with variations of acromial shape. Bigliani et al[1] described three shapes of the acromion based on lateral outlet plain film analysis. A similar plane of visualization is seen on oblique sagittal MRI, although it must be realized that while radiography represents a summation of the entire morphology on one image. MRI scans are sequential tomographic slices of that anatomy (Fig. 6-1). The type I acromion is relatively flat in its anteroposterior course. The type II acromion curves gently in the anteroposterior dimension, paralleling the superior surface of the humeral head. The type III acromion is associated with a congenital or acquired hook or spur of the distal acromion that focally decreases the radius of curvature of the anterior aspect of the acromion. The latter configuration is specially prone to result in narrowing of the acromiohumeral distance and has been associated with an increased incidence of rotator cuff tears.[44] Epstein and colleagues[18] studied acromial morphology on sagittal oblique MRI of 47 shoulders of a control population, of 30 shoulders of patients with isolated impingement, and of 34 shoulders of patients with full-thickness rotator cuff tears. Patients with rotator cuff tears had a significantly increased prevalence of type 3 acromions compared with control shoulders (62 percent versus 13 percent). Subacromial spur formation may also be seen in the oblique coronal plane (Fig. 6-2).

In the coronal plane, the acromion has a nearly horizontal orientation, similar to that of the distal clavicle (Fig. 6-3). Lateral downsloping of the anterior acromion, which can be seen with or without type 3 acromion shape, is best appreciated on oblique coronal images and can contribute to narrowing of acromiohumeral distance[17,62] (Fig. 6-2).

Os Acromiale

Along with acromial morphology, the presence or absence of an unfused os acromiale should be noted on shoulder MRI. The four types of unfused os acromiale are pre, meso, meta, and basi, from anterior to posterior. The most common is the mesoacromion that comprises approximately 40 percent of all os acromiale. An unfused distal acromial apophysis is commonly mobile and has been associated with an increased incidence of impingement syndrome and rotator cuff tears.[2,45] This may be due to associated inferior bony hypertrophy that narrows the subacromial space. It is also hypothesized that transient inferior displacement of the unstable os acromiale by the attached deltoid muscle with shoulder abduction may lead to a dynamic narrowing of acromiohumeral distance. This variant, which can be seen on axillary plain films, is best detected on axial images (Fig. 6-4). However, its relationship to the subacromial space is best appreciated on coronal and sagittal images in which it can mimic, although be seen separate from, the normal acromioclavicular joint. The presence of fluid-like signal intensity in this defect is suggestive of instability, although absence of this finding does not predict stability at surgery.

Acromioclavicular Joint

Acromioclavicular joint morphology and its relationship to the subacromial space should also be noted. This is best appreciated on oblique coronal and oblique sagittal images in which inferior capsular hypertrophy and osteophyte formation can contribute to narrowing of the subacromial space (Fig. 6-5). Although inferior osteophyte formation may be appreciated on plain films, inferior soft tissue hypertrophy that can only be appreciated on MRI may extend beyond the osteophyte. Symptomatic acromioclavicular joint arthrosis is appreciated not merely by capsular hypertrophy, which is not uncommonly asymptomatic, but also by fluid-like signal in the joint or high signal-intensity marrow edema on T_2-weighted images (Fig. 6-6).

Coracoacromial Ligament

The coracoacromial ligament and its relationship to the subacromial space should be noted. The normal coracoacromial ligament is routinely seen on high-resolution MRI

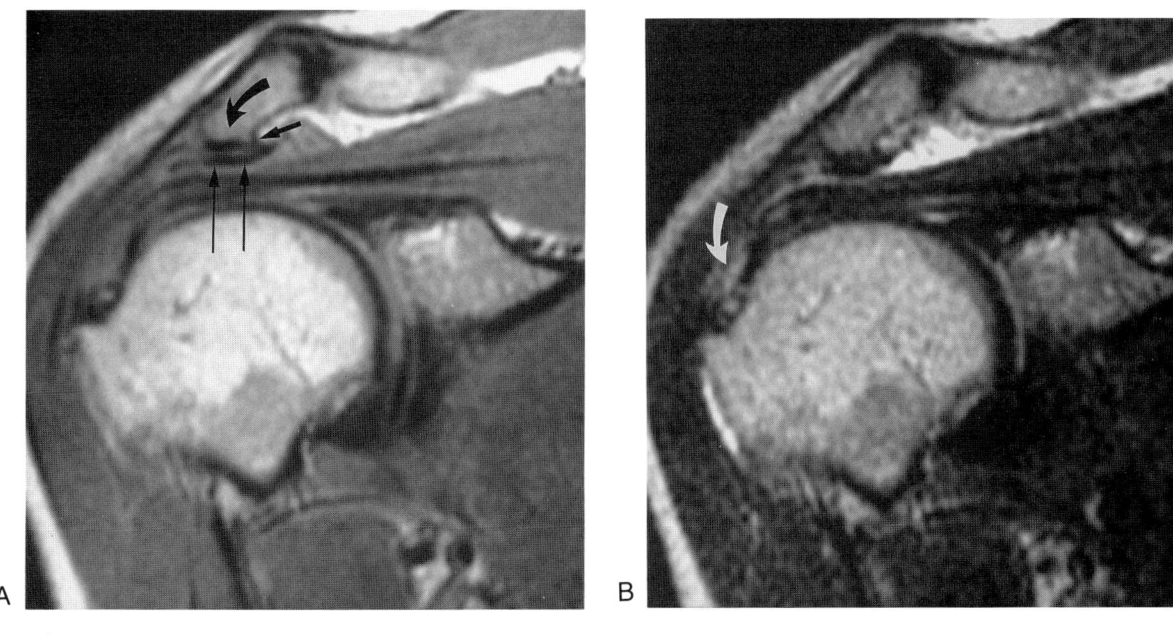

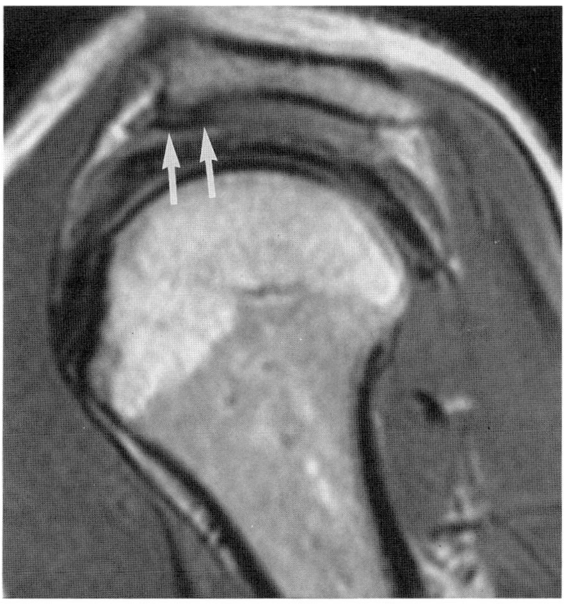

Figure 6-2. Lateral downsloping of the acromion (*curved black arrow*) and thickening of the acromial attachment of the coracoacromial ligament (*long black arrows*) contribute to narrowing of acromiohumeral distance seen on **(A)** proton density- and **(B)** T_2-weighted oblique coronal images. Note the subacromial spur or enthesophyte (*short arrow*) beneath the acromial attachment of the coracoacromial ligament and the superficial partial-thickness tear of the distal supraspinatus tendon (*curved white arrow*). **(C)** Oblique sagittal image also showing prominent coracoacromial ligament (*white arrows*).

as a low signal intensity structure coursing from the coracoid process to a broad-based attachment to the inferior aspect of the acromion on both oblique coronal and oblique sagittal planes (Figs. 6-7 and 6-8). Thickening at its acromial attachment can contribute to narrowing of the subacromial space and associated impingement of underlying soft tissues (Fig. 6-3).

Coracohumeral Impingement

A less common coracohumeral impingement process has been described. This is believed secondary to narrowing of the space between the coracoid process and humeral head, especially prominent in internal rotation position. Bonutti et al[3] have described cine MRI, which consists of

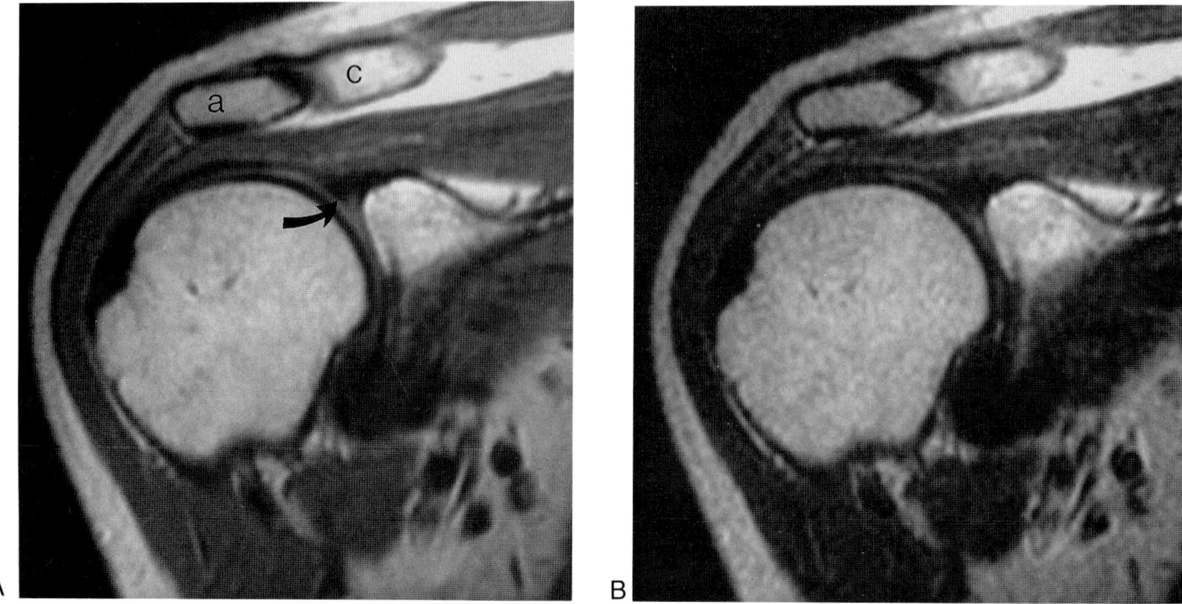

Figure 6-3. Normal shoulder anatomy in the oblique coronal plane on **(A)** proton density- and **(B)** T_2-weighted images. The plane of the acromion (*a*) on coronal images usually closely approximates that of the distal clavicle (*c*). Also note low signal intensity of the normal supraspinatus tendon on proton density- and T_2-weighted images, as well as normal configuration of the superior labrum (*arrow*).

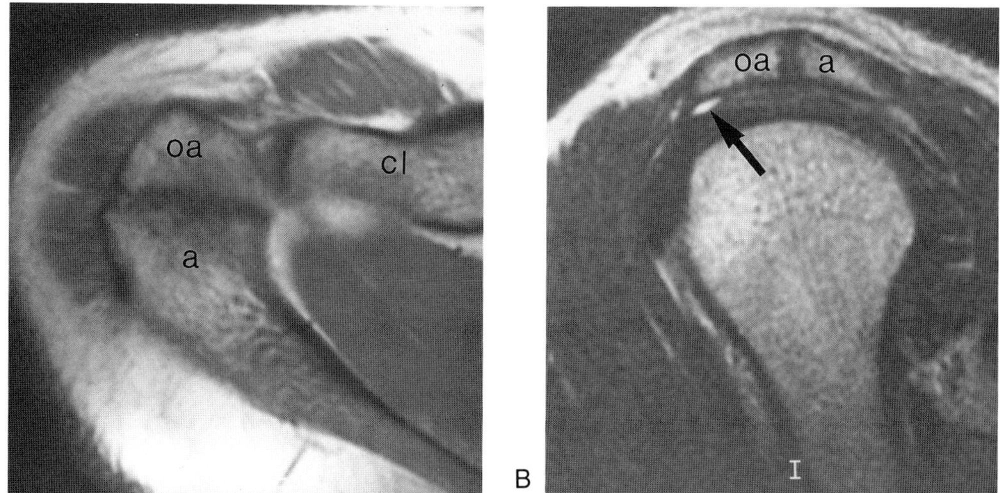

Figure 6-4. MRI of 31-year-old man who presented with 10 months of shoulder pain shows an unfused os acromiale (*oa*) of the mesoacromion type that is best appreciated with respect to the acromion (*a*) and clavicle (*cl*) on the **(A)** proton density axial view. **(B)** Sagittal T_2-weighted image shows small focus of subacromial bursal thickening (*arrow*). Arthroscopic decompression confirmed mobile os acromiale.

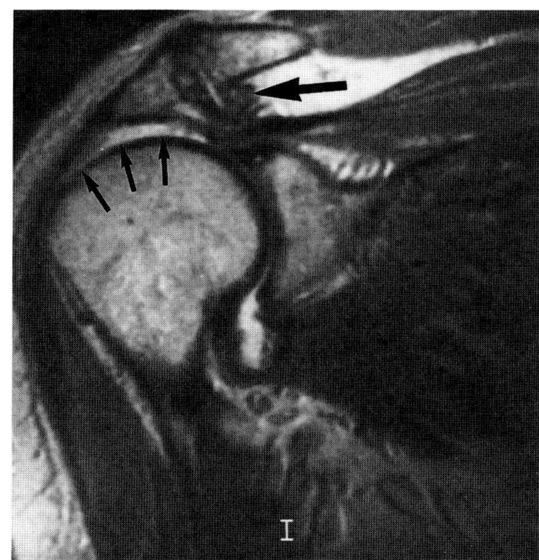

Figure 6-5. Large acromioclavicular osteophyte and large chronic rotator cuff tear. T_2-weighted image reveals large spur (*large arrow*) arising from the acromioclavicular joint that markedly encroaches on subacromial space. High signal intensity subacromial fluid seen replacing large supraspinatus tendon tear (*small arrows*) with marked tendon retraction to the level of the glenohumeral joint.

static imaging of the shoulder joint in the axial plane in incremental degrees of external to internal rotation. The images at a certain level are then played back sequentially in a cine loop, simulating real-time motion. They found that, in the internal rotation position, the normal interval between the lesser tuberosity and coracoid process is greater than 11 mm and that, if this interval is less than 11 mm, coracohumeral impingement is suspected. Occasionally, MRI may detect isolated thickening and signal alteration in the subcoracoid space, which may imply coracohumeral impingement and subcoracoid bursitis (Fig. 6-9).

SOFT TISSUES OF THE SUBACROMIAL SPACE

Soft tissues of the subacromial space include the rotator cuff, biceps tendon, and the subacromial-subdeltoid bursa and surrounding peribursal fat. MRI is the only imaging modality to directly visualize all these soft tissues and their associated pathology.

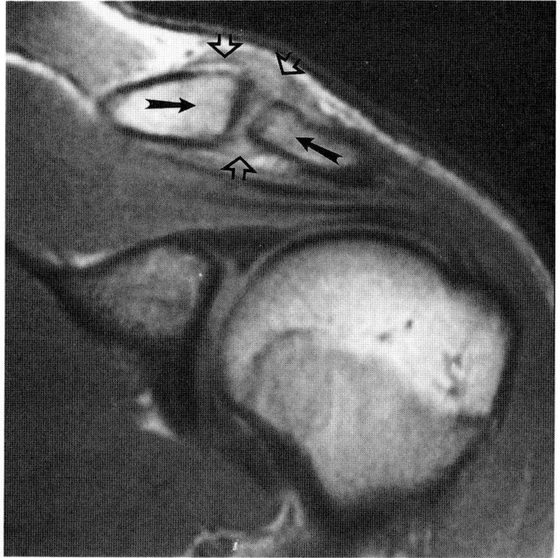

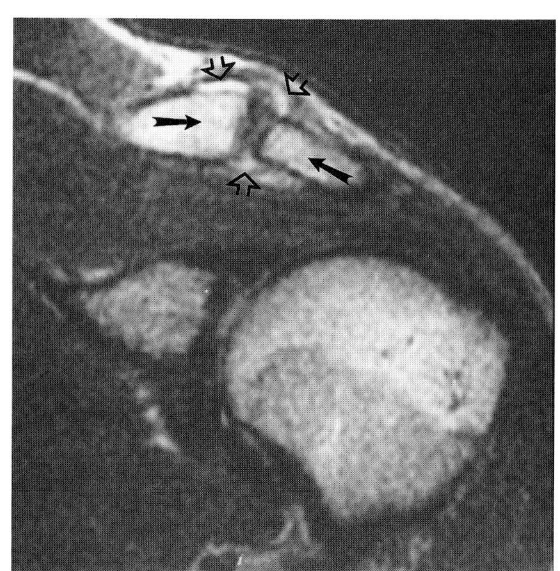

Figure 6-6. Symptomatic acromioclavicular joint arthrosis. This 21-year-old weight-lifting athlete had pain isolated to the acromioclavicular joint. Note capsular hypertrophy (*outline arrows*) as well as decreased marrow signal intensity (*arrows*) on oblique coronal (**A**) proton density-weighted image, both of which increase in signal intensity on corresponding (**B**) T_2-weighted image, reflecting joint fluid and marrow edema. The supraspinatus tendon is normal in signal intensity.

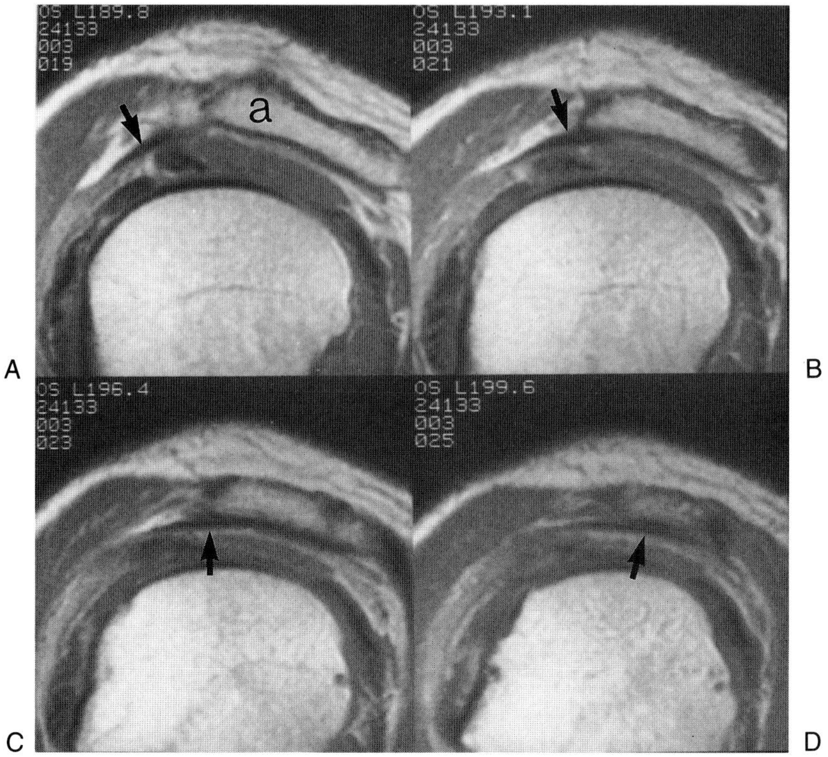

Figure 6-7. **(A–D)** Coracoacromial ligament (*arrows*) seen in the oblique sagittal plane coursing from **(A–D)** the coracoid process to the undersurface of the acromion (*a*).

Subacromial-Subdeltoid Bursa and Peribursal Fat Plane

Codman[12] first described fluid in the subacromial bursa secondary to rupture of the supraspinatus tendon in 1934. With the belief that with the development of a radiographic technique to depict soft tissues, such ruptures would be readily identifiable, he may have anticipated the development of MRI.

The potential space of the subacromial-subdeltoid bursa is seen as a thin line of low signal intensity on proton density- and T_2-weighted images, most commonly normally separated from the overlying deltoid muscle and underlying rotator cuff by the normal subdeltoid peribursal fat plane (Fig. 6-10). In the normal and asymptomatic shoulder, fluid-like signal accumulation in the subacromial-subdeltoid bursa seen on T_2-weighted images is uncommon.[30,43,49] Foci larger than 2×4 mm in thickness may be considered most likely consistent with bursal inflammation or bursal fluid accumulation.

Fluid-like signal seen in the subacromial-subdeltoid bursa has been described as a secondary sign of rotator cuff tears or other cause such as inflammatory arthritis or infection.[75] Others have not relied on this sign as an indication of tear.[5,58] However, pathologic bursal thickening and increased signal intensity can also be seen as the earliest and only sign of an overuse or early impingement process, without underlying tendon pathology (Fig. 6-11), and can be a helpful positive finding for overuse or impingement process in the MRI examination of the painful shoulder.[22]

Bursitis is seen as intermediate-low signal intensity on proton density-weighted images that increases to high signal intensity on associated T_2-weighted images. This high signal intensity on T_2-weighted images may be due to frank bursal fluid accumulation or thickened water-laden bursal tissue. Although bursal thickening may be seen immediately beneath the acromion, the immediate subacromial space is often narrowed due to the associated impingement process, providing little room for bursal tissue accumulation. Bursal hypertrophy therefore tends to accumulate in areas of less confinement anterior and posterior to the acromion, often seen to best advantage on oblique sagittal proton density- and T_2-weighted images. T_1-weighted images alone will not be as sensitive for this finding. Subdeltoid bursal hypertrophy or fluid accumulation may also be seen in the oblique coronal and axial planes next to the lateral aspect of the greater tuberosity (Fig. 6-12). Although bursal thickening and increased signal on T_2-weighted im-

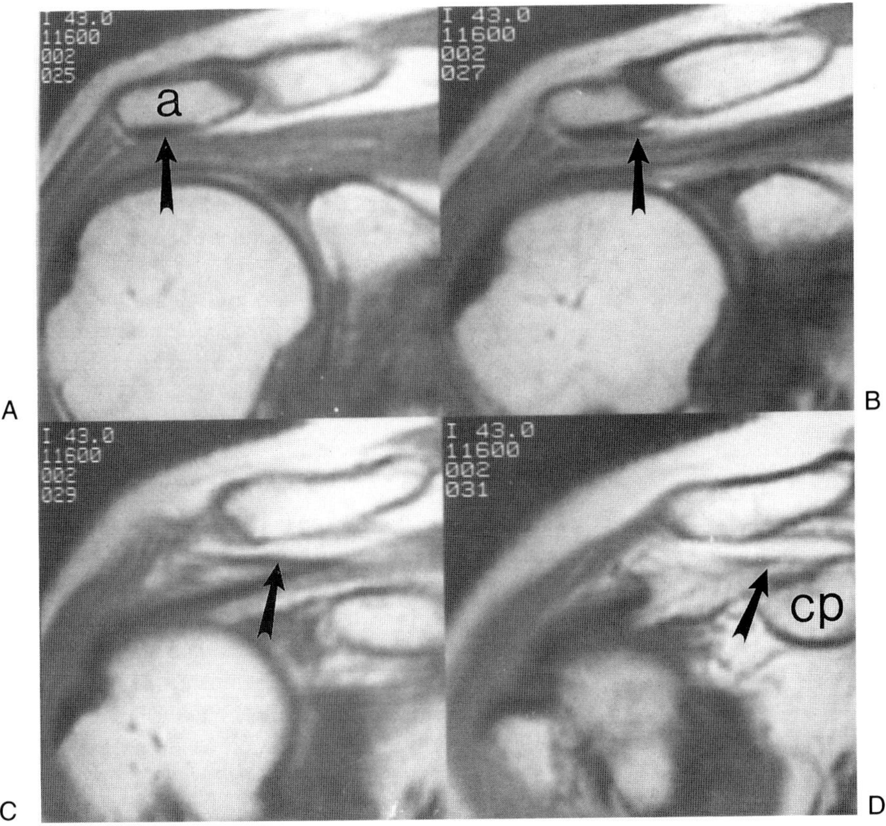

Figure 6-8. Coracoacromial ligament (*arrows*) seen in the oblique coronal plane, coursing from **(A–D)** the acromion (*a*) posteriorly to the coracoid process (*cp*) anteriorly.

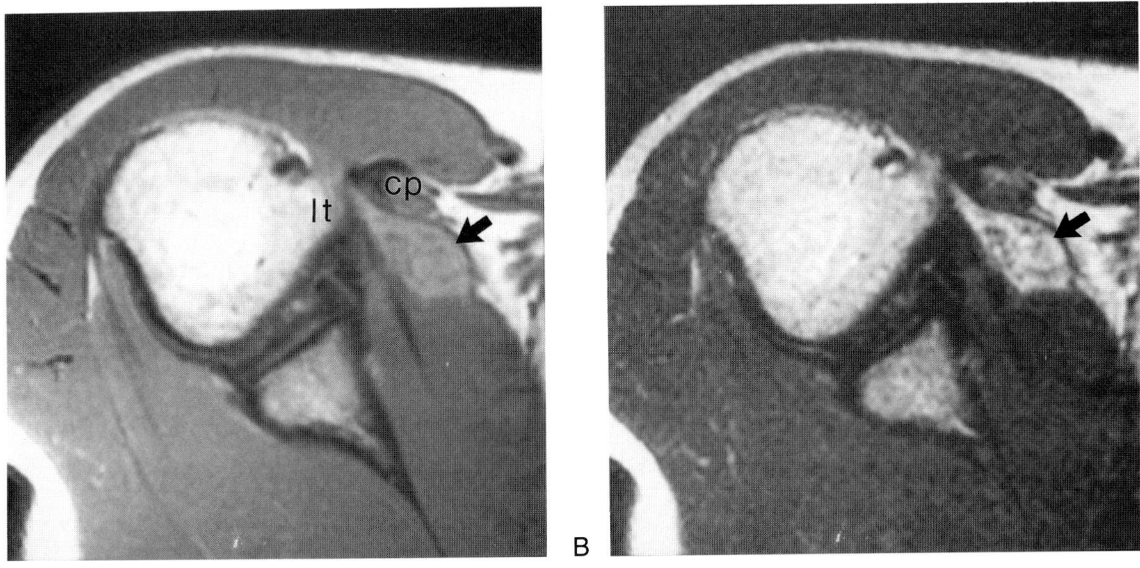

Figure 6-9. Isolated subcoracoid bursitis and suspected coracohumeral impingement. **(A)** Proton density- and **(B)** T_2-weighted axial images show inhomogeneous increased signal intensity confined to the subscapularis recess or subcoracoid bursa (*arrow*), without other joint fluid. Note the narrowed distance between the coracoid process (*cp*) and the lesser tuberosity (*lt*).

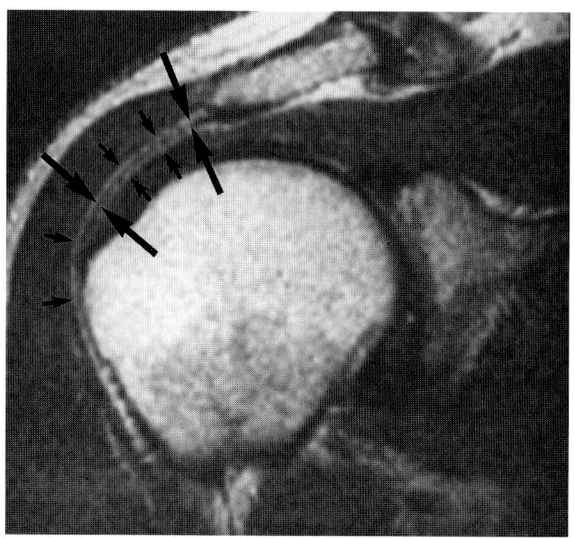

Figure 6-10. The normal subacromial-subdeltoid bursa potential space can be seen on this T_2-weighted oblique coronal image as a line of low signal intensity (*large arrows*) separated from the overlying deltoid muscle and from the underlying rotator cuff by high signal intensity peribursal fat (*small arrows*).

ages is a common finding in individuals with clinical impingement syndrome, the absence of MRI demonstration of pathologic bursal thickening does not exclude clinically significant bursitis and clinical impingement syndrome.

One potential pitfall can be encountered when imaging an individual who recently has had a therapeutic or diagnostic injection, which can mimic bursitis or bursal fluid accumulation. To avert this problem, appropriate history should be obtained at the time of examination, and if injection has been performed recently, a diagnosis of bursitis or bursal fluid must be made with caution. Our institution uses a patient questionnaire that asks if any therapeutic injection has been performed. It has been suggested to delay MRI after diagnostic or therapeutic injection, although for an unspecific time.[61] We recently performed MRI on four asymptomatic volunteers before and after posterior subacromial injections, two with 10 ml of Xylocaine and two with 10 ml of a Xylocaine/cortisone mixture (Wright, Fritts, Buss, and Tierney, submitted for presentation and publication). Imaging was performed within 30 minutes of injection, at 12 hours, and at 24 hours. In all cases, the associated fluid signal intensity was seen primarily posteriorly overlying the distal infraspinatus muscle belly and tendon and was completely gone by 24 hours. Although these results are preliminary, this would suggest that subacromial fluid signal intensity seen on MRI performed more than 1 day after 10 ml of subacromial injection may be considered pathologic rather than iatrogenic.

Normal Rotator Cuff

The normal distal rotator cuff was originally described as uniformly low in signal intensity, perhaps in part due to lower resolution and thicker slice thickness imaging. However, with high-resolution MRI, even the normal distal supraspinatus tendon is not uniformly low on T_1- and proton density-weighted images. Multiple tendinous slips of the distal supraspinatus and a gradual transition of muscle to tendon with muscular fibers routinely extending to within approximately 1 cm of the greater tuberosity contribute to increased signal intensity.[43] A nonfocal configuration and signal intensity identical to that of normal muscle on all pulse sequences, including low signal on T_2-weighted images will suggest that this does not represent tendon pathology (Fig. 6-6).

Uisng both conventional and fat-suppressed two-echo spin-echo technique, Mirowitz[43] described foci of relatively increased signal intensity in the substance of the supraspinatus tendon in all 15 normal subjects. This was described as being present within the substance of the distal supraspinatus tendon, 8 mm proximal to the greater tuberosity. This area of higher intensity was most conspicuous with the fat suppression technique and was visualized less frequently and was less well defined on conventional imaging. This focus was attributed to the critical zone of the rotator cuff, a described site of relative hypovascularity within the supraspinatus tendon that is believed by some to be the initial site of degenerative changes and subsequent tears.[36,59] The possibility of imaging of subclinical degenerative changes in his asymptomatic volunteers with age range of 22 to 54 years and mean of 31.5 years is a real one. This might make an argument against fat suppression imaging, which may be too sensitive and less specific for normal and nonspecific age-related degenerative changes or tendinosis. Conventional spin-echo T_2-weighted images may not be as sensitive for subtle or nonspecific degeneration but may allow any increased signal seen to be more specific for more significant cuff pathology.

Rotator Cuff Degeneration

Tendinitis has been used in the clinical literature as a relatively nonspecific pathologic term including changes associated with tendon degeneration, inflammation, or edema. Because the suffix *-itis* implies an inflammatory response with macrophage infiltration that is not typically seen at histology, the less specific degenerative term *tendinosis* has been proposed as more appropriate.[33] Homogeneous or nonfocal increased signal intensity, especially on T_1- and proton density-weighted images, with otherwise normal tendon morphology may merely reflect nonspecific and asymptomatic tendon degeneration. It is our experience

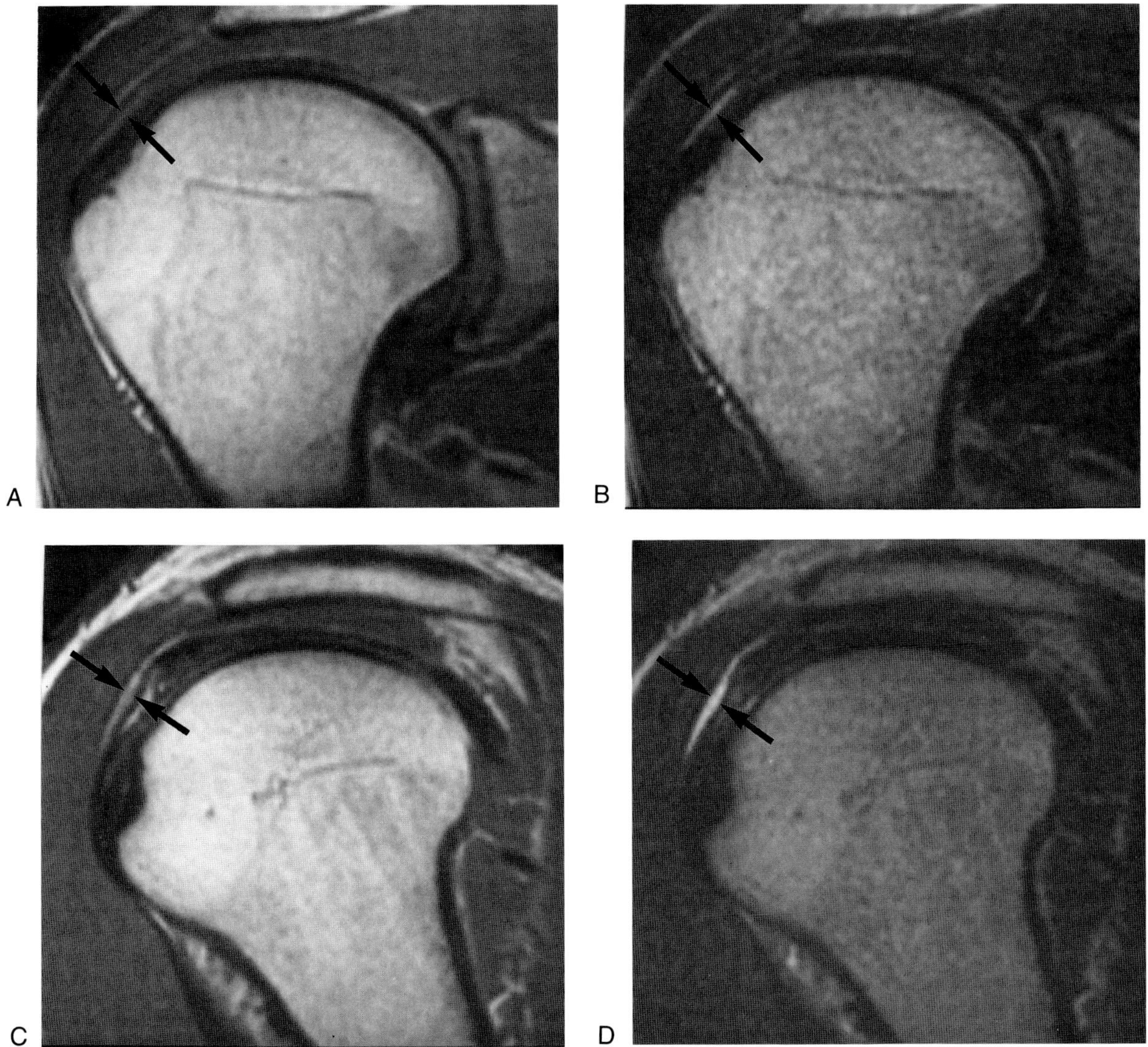

Figure 6-11. Subacromial bursitis without rotator cuff pathology in 24-year-old man with 4 months of persistent shoulder pain. **(A)** Coronal proton density image with a thin layer of intermediate signal intensity that **(B)** increases in signal on corresponding T_2-weighted image (*arrows*). **(C)** Oblique sagittal proton density- and **(D)** T_2-weighted images also show bursal thickening and fluid-like signal intensity (*arrows*) in anterior aspect of the subacromial-subdeltoid bursa overlying the rotator cuff interval.

that with mild nonspecific degeneration this increased signal intensity on proton density-weighted images does not persist on T_2-weighted images. The presence of tendinous enlargement with an inhomogeneous signal intensity including mild-to-moderate increased signal intensity on T_2-weighted images is strongly suggestive of ongoing symptomatic tendinosis/tendinitis (Fig. 6-13). Pathologic thickening and increased signal intensity of the subacromial-subdeltoid bursa would support ongoing and potentially sympatomatic process. Rafii et al[58] noted that some similarity and overlap of signal patterns of partial interstitial tears, tendinitis, and tendon degeneration are observed.

Although predominately a plain film diagnosis, calcium hydroxyapatite crystal deposition (calcific tendinitis) can occasionally be appreciated as a focus of low signal intensity in the rotator cuff tendons on both proton density- and T_2-weighted images (Fig. 6-14). The low signal intensity of small calcific deposits may be difficult to distinguish from the low signal intensity of normal tendon.

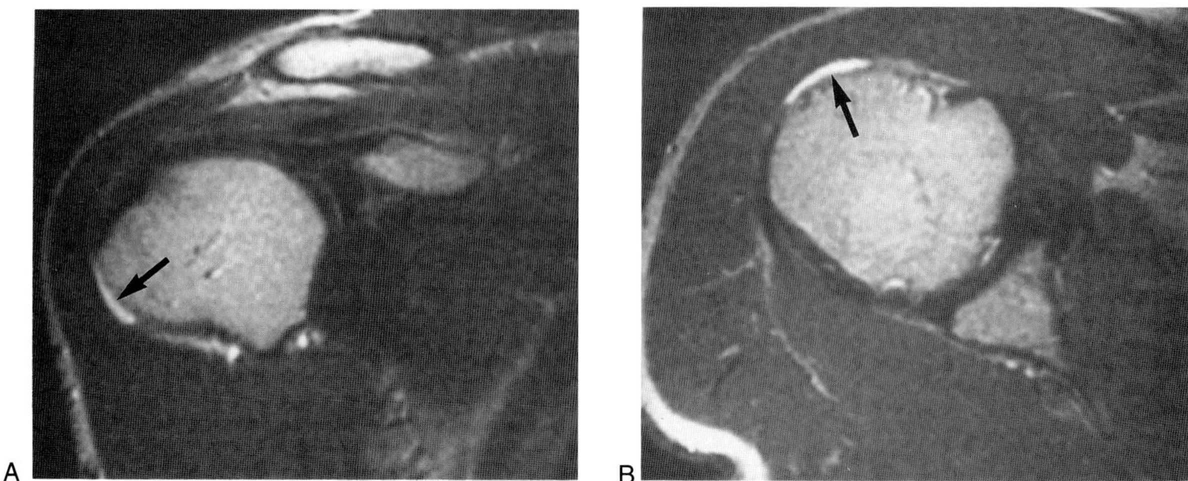

Figure 6-12. Subdeltoid bursitis or bursal fluid accumulation (*arrow*) overlying the lateral aspect of greater tuberosity. High signal intensity similar to fluid is seen in T_2-weighted **(A)** oblique coronal and **(B)** axial images.

Supraspinatus Rotator Cuff Tears

The value of detection and subsequent repair of full-thickness rotator cuff tears has been documented. Some also believe it is useful to distinguish between partial-thickness tears and a degenerative cuff. Partial-thickness cuff tears are commonly found in patients with impingement who fail conservative management. Open surgical techniques have probably missed many undersurface partial-thickness tears in the past, so the clinical significance of such partial tears needs further study. Although yet to be proved, it is widely believed that a partial-thickness tear represents an intermediate stage of an evolving process that, with continued impingement, leads to increased incidence of development of full-thickness tear. It is also believed, although not yet proved, that if intervention occurs early, such as with anterior acromioplasty for subacromial decompression, the progressive degenerative process may be arrested or slowed, leading to an improved outcome. This speculation into the evolution and pathogen-

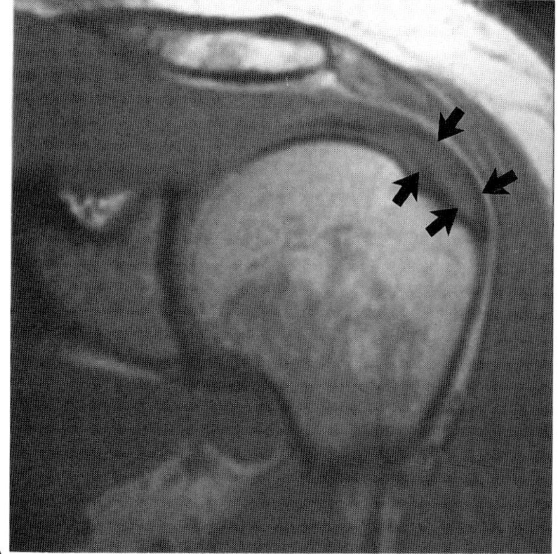

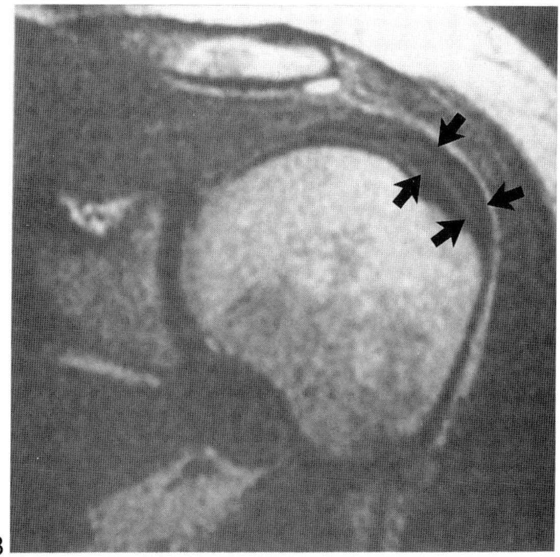

Figure 6-13. Moderate intrasubstance degeneration/tendinosis (''tendinitis'') of the supraspinatus tendon. Moderate fusiform tendon thickening (*arrows*) associated with ill-defined increased signal intensity on **(A)** proton density- and **(B)** T_2-weighted axial images.

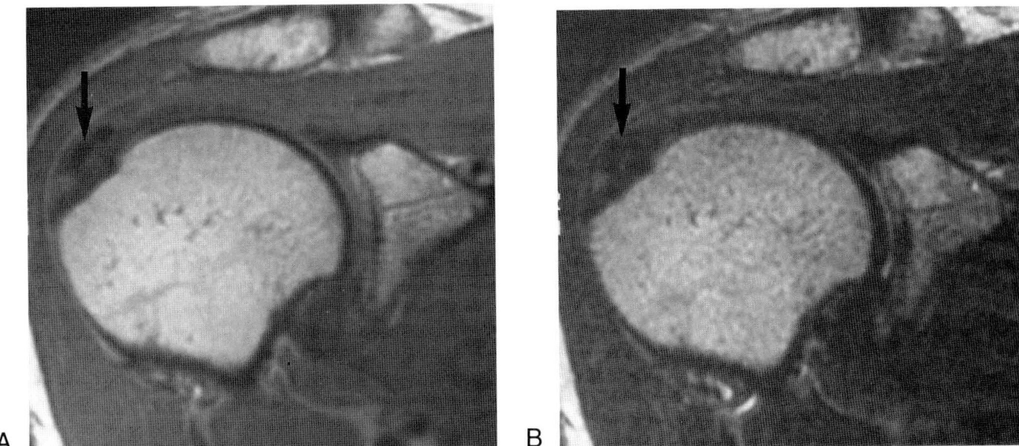

Figure 6-14. Calcific tendinitis of the supraspinatus tendon without tear. **(A)** Proton density- and **(B)** T_2-weighted oblique coronal images show a focal collection of decreased signal intensity within the superficial aspect of the distal right supraspinatus tendon (*arrow*), representing calcium hydroxyapatite crystal deposition.

esis of rotator cuff tears fosters continued attempts of early diagnosis of subacromial space pathology including tendinitis and partial-thickness tears before the development of full-thickness tears.

Rafii and colleagues[58] studied the signal intensity patterns of rotator cuff lesions at MRI in 80 patients who had surgical correlation, as well as in 13 asymptomatic individuals. The accuracy of MRI in detection of 31 full-thickness tears was 95 percent and of 16 partial-thickness tears was 84 percent. The most common and most accurate diagnostic findings of partial- and full-thickness tears were regions of increased signal intensity on T_2-weighted images, indicating fluid or fluid-laden bursal tissue in the cuff defect (Fig. 6-15). This was seen in 22 of the 31 full-thickness tears. High signal intensity on T_2-weighted images was the most accurate, although less common, finding in 7 of 16 partial-thickness tears.

In seven of the full-thickness tears, the diagnosis was

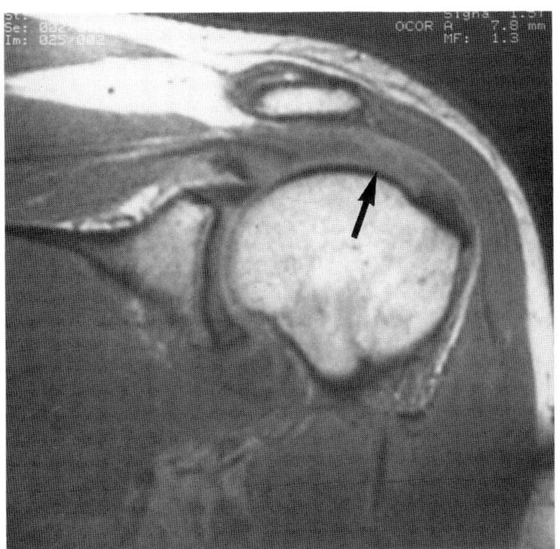

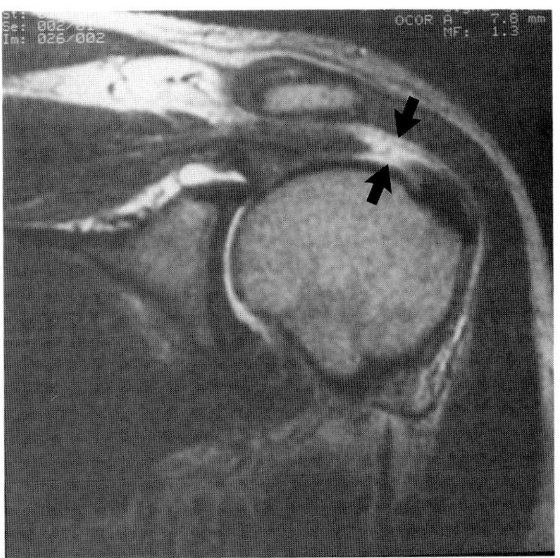

Figure 6-15. Full-thickness supraspinatus tendon tear. **(A)** Proton density coronal images reveals abnormal signal intensity (*arrow*) but poor definition of tear. **(B)** T_2-weighted image shows high signal intensity fluid (*arrows*), which better defines the size of full-thickness rotator cuff tear.

made in absence of high signal on T_2-weighted images. The abnormality was seen as low or moderate signal intensity on proton density and T_2-weighted images. This represented a severely degenerated tendon, a low signal intensity of intact bursal or synovial surface, or perhaps granulation or scar tissue that replaced the region of torn tendinous fibers and, in some, maintained the continuity of the tendinous margins. The diagnosis was made on the basis of alteration of normal morphology and contour as well as secondary signs such as subacromial-subdeltoid bursitis, retraction of the musculotendinous junction, and muscle belly atrophy. Rafii et al[58] suggest that the appearance of tendon tear replaced by connective tissue showing moderate signal intensity may simulate the appearance of tendinitis. They further surmise that, in fact, partial interstitial tears and tendinitis may represent the same pathologic entity.

All errors in the diagnosis of full-thickness tears (one false-negative and two false-positive) were in cases with low signal intensity cuff defects. Two false-positive cases were reported as tears with scar formation. Arthroscopy revealed marked tendon scarring without defect. Part of the difficulty in correlation of MRI findings and surgical findings may be inherent in difficulties at documentation of tendon pathology at arthrography or surgery. The same difficulty encountered in MRI diagnosis of older or chronic partial- and full-thickness tears that are filled or replaced with low signal intensity scar tissue can result in false-negative arthrography and potentially false-negative surgical exploration unless all portions of the cuff are probed and explored. This observation has been described by Skinner[64] as retracted tendons remaining concealed by intact synovial and bursal layers. Obscuration of cuff tear by scar or granulation tissue in a subacute stage has been recognized as a cause of infrequent false-negative arthrography.[56,60]

Traughber and Goodwin[46] reported a comparison of preoperative MRI findings and careful arthroscopic inspection of both sides of the rotator cuff in 28 patients. MRI correctly identified all five of the full-thickness tears for a sensitivity and specificity of 100 percent. However, only five of nine partial-thickness tears were diagnosed on MRI. The combined sensitivity and specificity for diagnosis of both partial- and full-thickness tears were 71 and 93 percent, respectively. It was their impression that STIR sequences improved tear conspicuity.

Histologic differences between the bursal- and joint-side layers of the supraspinatus have been described in a cadaveric study by Nakajima et al.[46] They further noted different biomechanical properties of these two layers and concluded that the joint-side layer is more vulnerable to a tensile load than the bursal-side layer. The bursal-side layer, which was composed primarily of tendon bundles, increased in length to a tensile load but was resistant to rupture. The joint-side layer was a complex of tendon, ligament, and joint capsule that elongated more poorly but tore more easily. This may be hypothesized to contribute to the observation by others that joint-side partial-thickness tears are more common than bursal-side tears. Although not specifically addressed by those authors, one might further speculate that a different degree of tendon lengthening on tensile loading between the superficial and deep layers might contribute to a shearing force between the two layers. This shear force in an already intrinsically weakened tendon may lead to horizontal and lamellar separation between the joint- and bursal-side layers. Horizontal separation of tendon fibers can be seen histologically in intrasubstance partial-thickness tears.[70] Extension through the deep surface of the tendon may further allow joint fluid to extend into this delamination, perhaps contributing to its propagation.

An appreciation of differences between the joint- and bursal-side layers of the rotator cuff can be seen on MRI of the pathologic rotator cuff tendon. First, lamellar orientation of abnormal increased signal intensity between superficial and deep layers of the rotator cuff is not infrequently observed. Most commonly, this delamination between the superficial (bursal-side) and deep (joint-side) layers is seen adjacent to a partial- or full-thickness rotator cuff tear as a variable degree of moderate increased signal intensity on both proton density- and T_2-weighted images. However, differentiation of this surgical alteration from the lower signal intensity of the adjacent layers is most often best seen on T_2-weighted images (Fig. 6-16). This delamination process is documented at surgery as ext nsion into the margins of a partial- or full-thickness rotator cuff tear. Recognition of this anatomy may be helpful in preoperative planning of rotator cuff tear repair.

Superficial (bursal-side) (Fig. 6-2) and deep (joint-side) (Fig. 6-17) partial-thickness tears can be seen as interruption of the normal morphology or signal intensity on proton density- and T_2-weighted images. Perhaps the most difficult superficial tear to visualize is the shallow abrasion or fraying occurring proximally beneath the overlying acromion. Fluid or fluid-laden bursal tissue in the subacromia-subdeltoid bursa can increase the conspicuity of a bursal-side partial-thickness tear. However, without bursal thickening or with the more common situation of chronic bursal adhesions and scarring, which may be intermediate or intermediate-low in signal intensity, these superficial partial tears of abrasions can be obscured or difficult to appreciate.

Subscapularis Tendon Tears

Subscapularis tendon tears are most commonly associated with supraspinatus tendon tears and have been described as occurring only rarely in isolation.[38] However, it

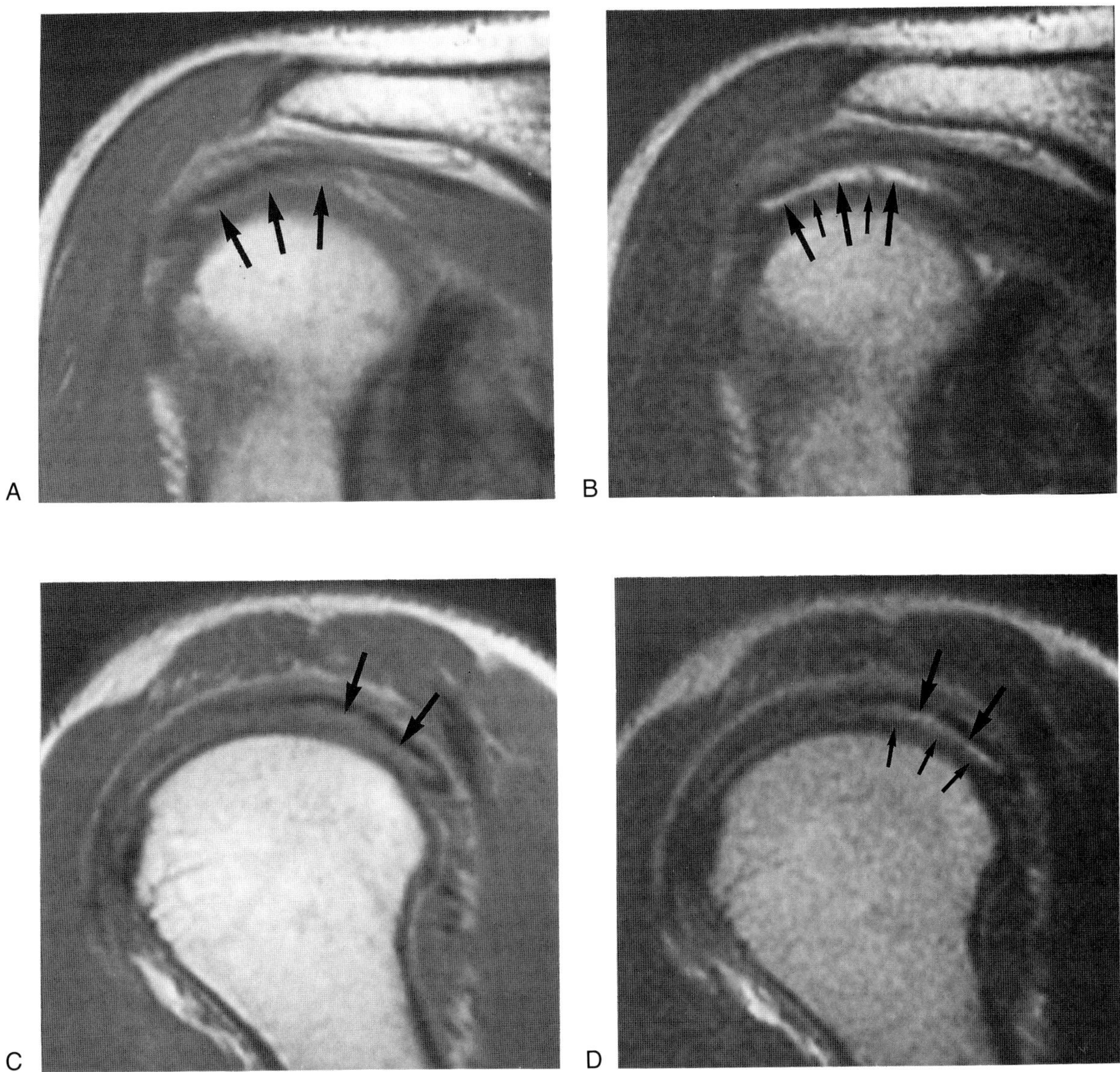

Figure 6-16. Intrasubstance delamination partial-thickness tear between superficial and deep layers of the infraspinatus tendon. Oblique coronal (**A**) proton density- and (**B**) T_2-weighted images, as well as oblique sagittal (**C**) proton density- and (**D**) T_2-weighted images through the infraspinatus tendon, show lamellar increased signal (*large arrows*) between superficial and deep layers (*small arrows*).

is our experience that MRI has increased the detection of subscapularis tendon abnormalities and that isolated subscapularis tendon tears are perhaps not as infrequent as originally thought.

Patten[53] reported MRI findings in nine patients with surgically confirmed rotator cuff tears solely or predominantly involving the subscapularis tendon, representing 6 percent of 149 rotator cuff tears found in 571 patients who had MRI over a 3-year period. The MRI appearance of subscapularis tendon tears is similar to that previously described for

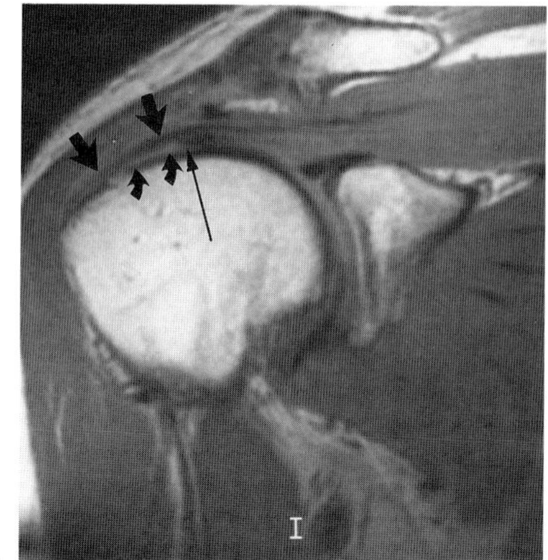

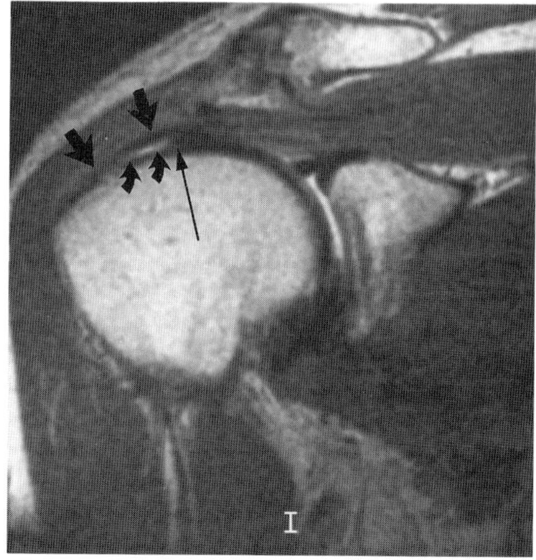

Figure 6-17. Deep surface partial-thickness tear with retraction of torn edge of deep layer on **(A)** proton density- and **(B)** T_2-weighted image. Ridge of low signal intensity at 12:00 position (*long arrow*) represents the torn edge of the deep tendon layer of the supraspinatus. The superficial layer remains intact (*straight arrows*), whereas there is absence of the distal aspect of the deep layer (*curved arrows*) seen as increased signal intensity on T_2-weighted image.

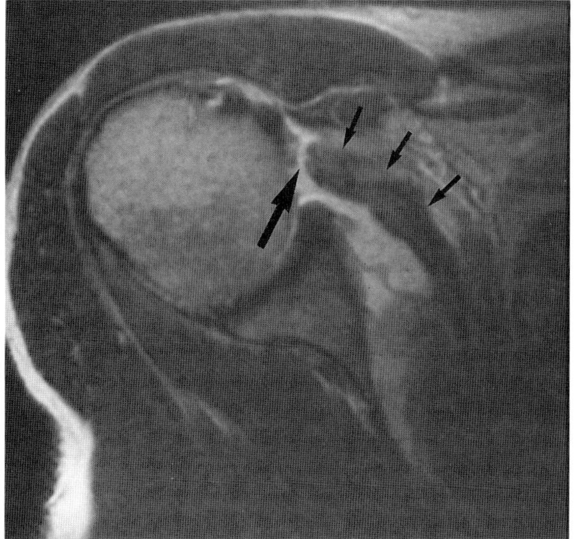

Figure 6-18. Isolated full-thickness tear of the subscapularis tendon. T_2-weighted axial image shows high signal intensity fluid in full-thickness tear (*large arrow*) interrupting the low signal intensity of the distal subscapularis tendon (*small arrows*).

supraspinatus tears, including areas of abnormal and disorganized tendon morphology and abnormal increased signal intensity on all pulse sequences. As in supraspinatus, tears are best appreciated when comparing proton density- and T_2-weighted axial images (Fig. 6-18), which are preferable to T_1-weighted or gradient echo T_2*-weighted images for best tear conspicuity and specificity.

Infraspinatus and Teres Minor Tendon Tears

Infraspinatus tendon tears are most commonly associated with supraspinatus tendon tears. Isolated full-thickness infraspinatus tears are relatively uncommon (Fig. 6-19). Full-thickness tear of the entire teres minor tendon is very uncommon, even with massive full-thickness tears involving the rest of the rotator cuff. We have not noted an isolated teres minor tendon tear, although isolated teres minor muscle belly edema representing strain can occasionally be seen. Isolated teres minor muscle atrophy has been reported to be associated with impingement or denervation of the axillary nerve in the quadrilateral space[35] (Fig. 6-20).

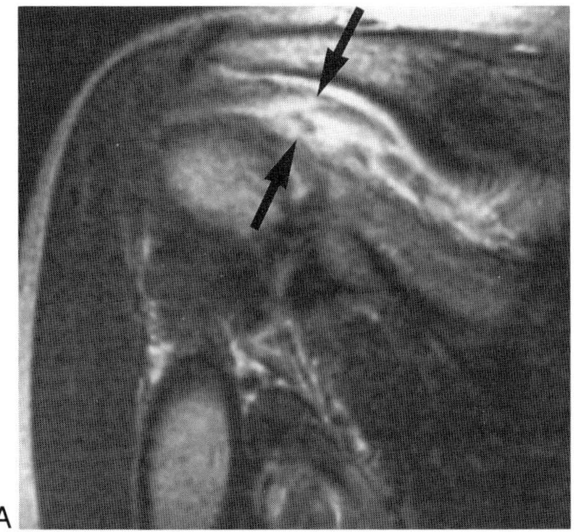

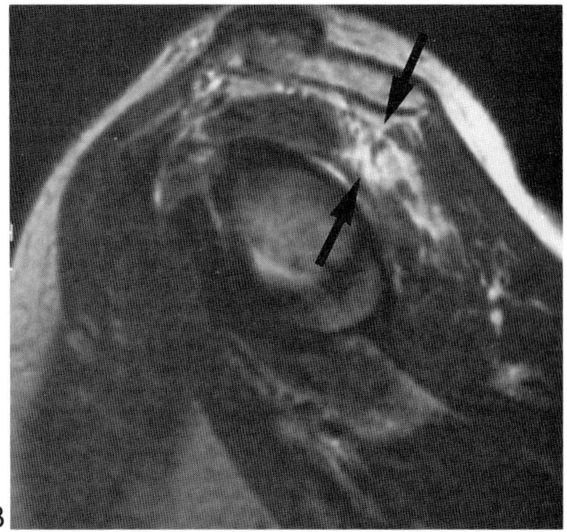

Figure 6-19. Isolated tear of infraspinatus at its musculotendinous junction. **(A)** T_2-weighted oblique coronal and **(B)** oblique sagittal images show high signal intensity representing fluid and hemorrhage at the site of infraspinatus tear (*arrows*).

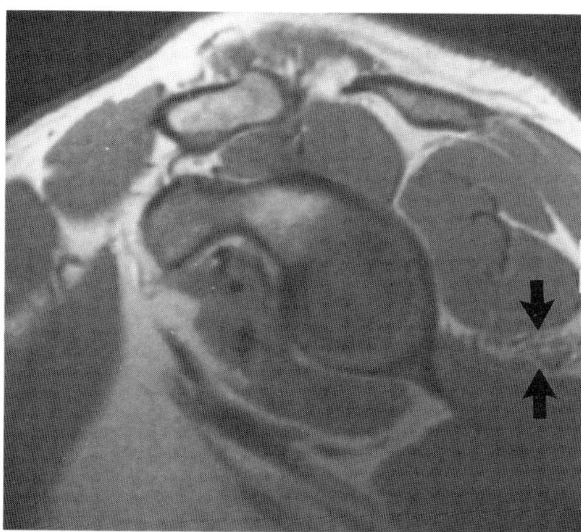

Figure 6-20. Isolated teres minor muscle belly atrophy without tendon tear. Note atrophic teres minor muscle with marked fatty infiltration (*arrows*). Although this has been proposed to represent the result of denervation of the branch of the axillary nerve supplying this muscle, no abnormality was seen involving the quadrilateral space.

MAGNETIC RESONANCE IMAGING OF THE BICEPS TENDON

The entire complex course of the biceps tendon is visualized at MRI. Erickson et al[19] described the normal MRI appearance of the biceps tendon and illustrated associated pathologic conditions. Biceps tendon medial dislocation and subluxation are commonly associated with subscapularis tendon pathology and tears. MRI is not only excellent for noninvasive diagnosis and localization of biceps tendon ruptures (Fig. 6-21) but can be used in preoperative planning in cases in which biceps tendon repair is contemplated. Lesser degrees of biceps tendon pathology can also be appreciated on MRI, including tendinosis/tendinitis, partial-thickness fraying, and longitudinal splitting.

Intrinsic Abnormalities of the Biceps Tendon

Oblique sagittal and axial planes are obligatory for optimal evaluation of the biceps tendon, with oblique coronal images providing an ancillary role. Although axial images are best for visualization of the biceps tendon at the level of the bicipital groove, the proximal biceps tendon and abnormalities associated with the clinical impingement

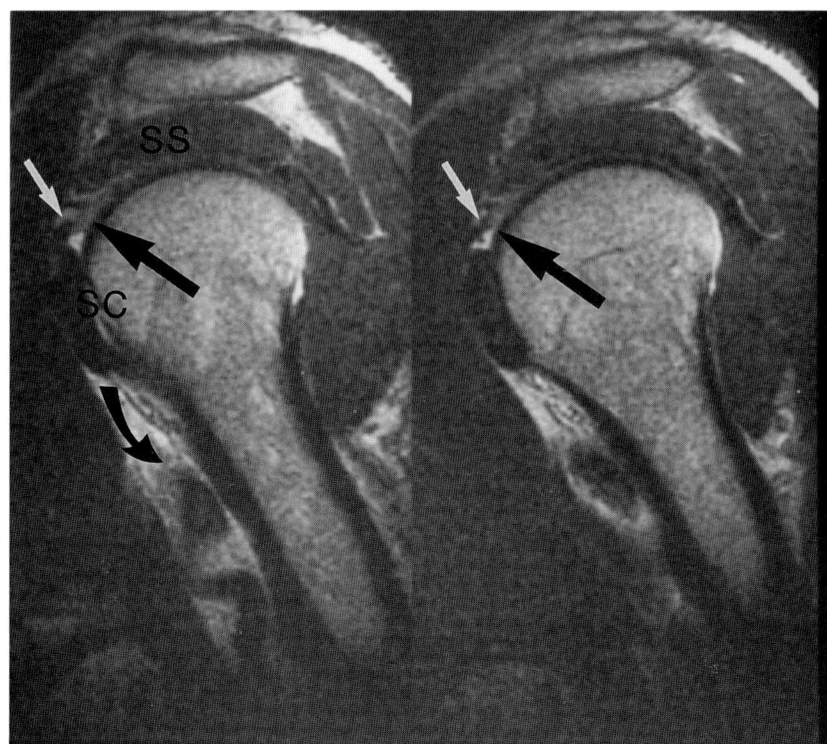

Figure 6-21. Isolated biceps tendon rupture. Two consecutive T_2-weighted oblique sagittal images show the proximally torn biceps tendon as a serpiginous structure retracted distally to a level below the bicipital groove (*curved arrow*). The biceps tendon is not seen in the rotator cuff interval (*large arrow*) between the supraspinatus (*ss*) and subscapularis (*sc*) tendons, although the coracohumeral ligament (*white arrow*) may simulate the biceps tendon in the interval.

syndrome can be best appreciated on oblique sagittal images. Here, the intra-articular portion of the tendon is seen in cross section within the rotator cuff interval, underlying the coracohumeral ligament. In this location, the normal biceps tendon is relatively flat or slightly ovoid in configuration and very low in its signal intensity on proton density- and T_2-weighted images (Fig. 6-22). Biceps tendinosis/tendinitis is seen as abnormal thickening with pronounced ovoid or round cross section and increased signal intensity on proton density-weighted images that may decay or persist in signal on associated T_2-weighted images, depending on the degree of tendon degeneration (Fig. 6-23). Care must be taken when evaluating the biceps tendon at the distal rotator cuff interval as it courses through the cuff. In this location, the course of the tendon will commonly subtend an angle of 55 degrees with respect to the direction of the magnetic field of the magnet, Bo, which has been called the "magic angle."[19] This can lead to artifactually increased signal intensity on T_1- and proton density-weighted images. This artifactual increased signal will decrease in signal on T_2-weighted images. Persistence of increased signal intensity on T_2-weighted images suggests tendon pathology rather than magic angle effect. When thickening or irregularity of the tendon is seen, a diagnosis of biceps tendon pathology can be ensured. Such irregularity, consistent with fraying, as well as longitudinal splitting can occasionally be appreciated (Fig. 6-24). Superior labrum tears or separation can be seen associated with proximal biceps tendon pathology in SLAP lesions.[9,65]

Positional Abnormalities of the Biceps Tendon

A strong association of subscapularis tendon tears with biceps tendon positional abnormalities has been noted.[10,53] Abnormalities range from complete medial dislocation anterior to the glenohumeral joint to incomplete medial subluxation. Five of nine (56 percent) of Patten's series of subscapularis tendon tears were associated with medial dislocation of the biceps; two of nine (22 percent) were associated with partial or complete biceps tendon tears.[53] Cervilla and associates[10] described the MRI appearance of six patients with medial dislocation of the biceps tendon

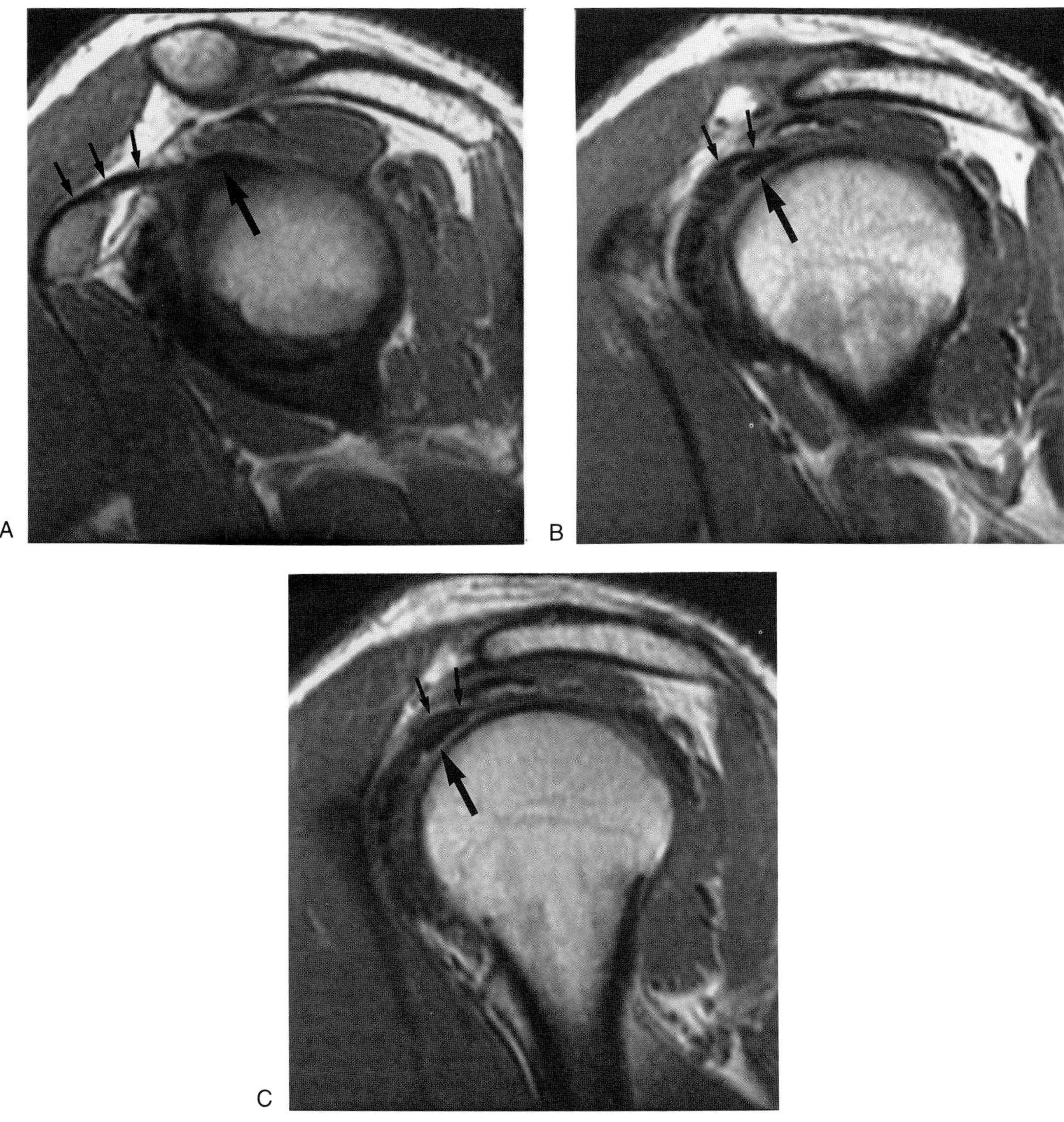

Figure 6-22. Normal biceps tendon at the level of the rotator cuff interval. Oblique sagittal proton density images at the rotator cuff interval progressing from **(A–C)** medial to lateral show the biceps tendon to have a relatively flat cross section and low signal intensity (*large arrow*). Note the smaller low signal intensity coracohumeral ligament (*small arrows*) passsing immediately superior to the biceps tendon as it contributes to the joint capsule.

that were seen to be of two types. Five of the dislocations were markedly dislocated to a position anterior to the glenohumeral joint and associated with full-thickness subscapularis tendon tears. One was only mildly dislocated from the groove into degenerated and partially torn subscapularis tendon fibers.

Although complete medial biceps tendon dislocation is most commonly seen associated with full-thickness subscapularis tendon tears (Fig. 6-25), it is not uncommon to observe a completely medially dislocated biceps tendon with superficial fibers of the subscapularis tendon remaining intact on both MRI and at open surgery (Fig. 6-26).

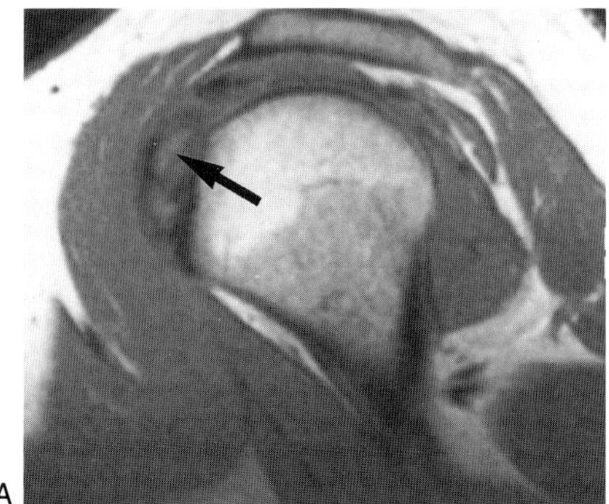

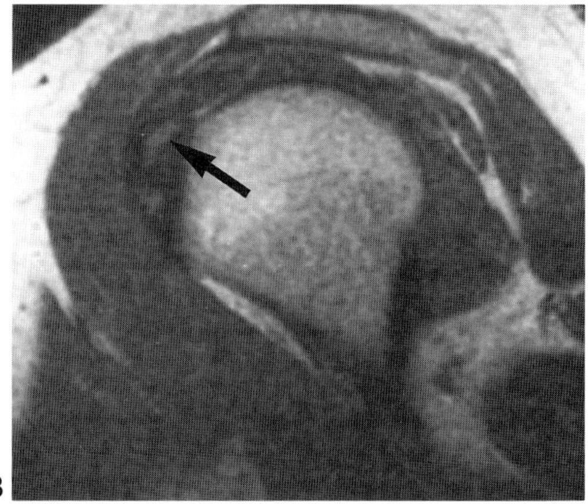

Figure 6-23. Marked biceps tendinitis. Marked thickening and increased signal intensity of the biceps tendon *(arrow)* in the rotator cuff interval on oblique sagittal **(A)** proton density- and **(B)** T_2-weighted images is consistent with severe intrasubstance tendon degeneration, without rupture.

This may at first seem a paradox but can be explained with an understanding of the anatomy and relationship of the subscapularis tendon and the transverse humeral ligament. Superficial fibers of the subscapularis tendon contribute to the transverse humeral ligament, which then attaches to the greater tuberosity at the lateral aspect of the bicipital groove. The medial tendinous wall of the bicipital groove represents intrasubstance and deep surface fibers of the distal subscapularis that acts as the primary restraint preventing medial displacement of the biceps tendon from the bicipital groove. Recognizing this anatomic relationship, one can now appreciate how intrasubstance and deep surface degeneration and tears of the subscapularis tendon can allow the biceps tendon to dislocate medially beneath the intact transverse humeral ligament and superficial subscapularis tendon without full-thickness interruption of this ligament and tendon. In this instance, open surgical inspection of the outer surface of the subscapularis will be normal, and the deep surface partial-thickness subscapularis tendon tear and biceps tendon dislocation may not be recognized. Arthroscopic evaluation may more easily detect this abnormality. In 1986, Petersson[54] described surgically proven cases of biceps tendon medial dislocation with intact external fibers of the subscapularis tendon merging into the superficial fibers of the transverse humeral ligament.

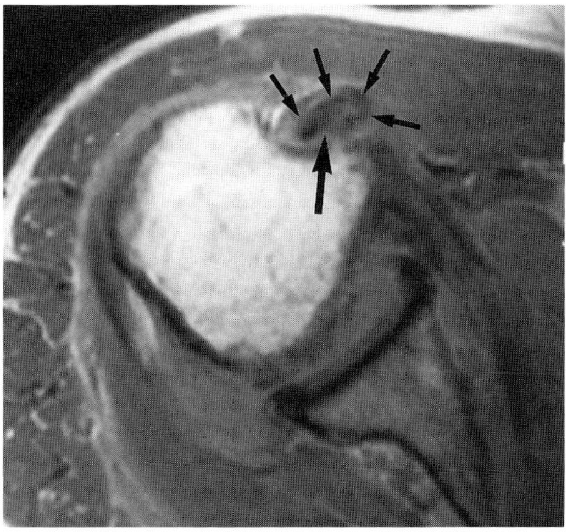

Figure 6-24. Marked degeneration including longitudinal splitting of the biceps tendon, without complete rupture. Proton density axial image just below the level of the rotator cuff interval showing longitudinal linear increased signal intensity *(large arrow)* within the biceps tendon *(small arrows)*.

Medial dislocation of the biceps tendon superficial to an intact subscapularis tendon is less common. Petersson described only one case of medial dislocation superficial to an intact subscapularis tendon. This injury is most likely associated with disruption of the transverse humeral ligament.

Incomplete dislocation or subluxation of the biceps tendon may be appreciated. One of the patients in Cervilla's series had incomplete medial dislocation of the tendon into partially disrupted fibers of the subscapularis tendon.[10] This likely reflects an earlier stage of subscapularis tendon de-

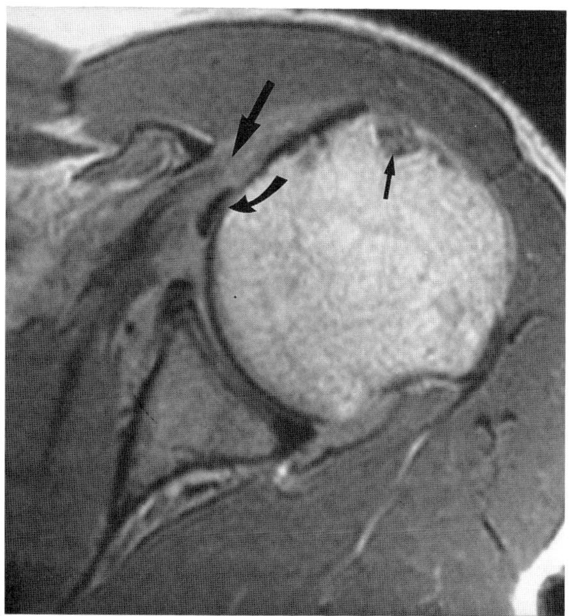

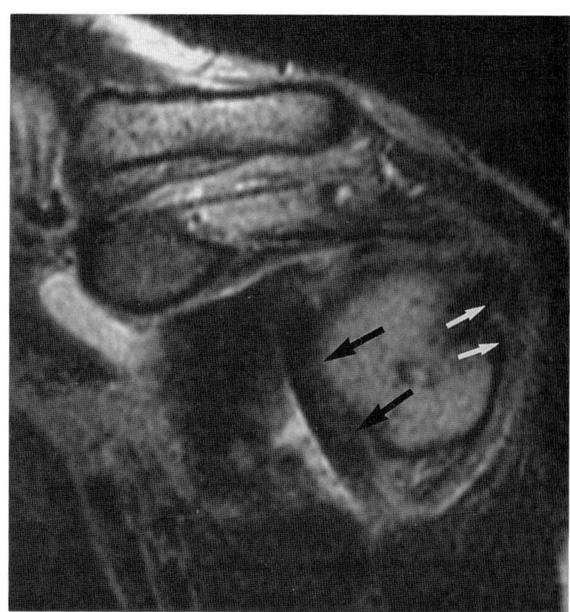

Figure 6-25. Medial dislocation of the biceps tendon from the bicipital groove associated with full-thickness subscapularis tendon tear **(A)** Proton density axial image shows subscapularis tendon tear and retraction (*large arrow*). The bicipital groove is empty (*small arrow*), due to medial displacement of the biceps tendon (*curved arrow*) to a location anterior to the glenohumeral joint. **(B)** T_2-weighted coronal image through the anterior humeral head also visualized the medially dislocated biceps tendon (*black arrows*) and the empty bicipital groove (*white arrows*).

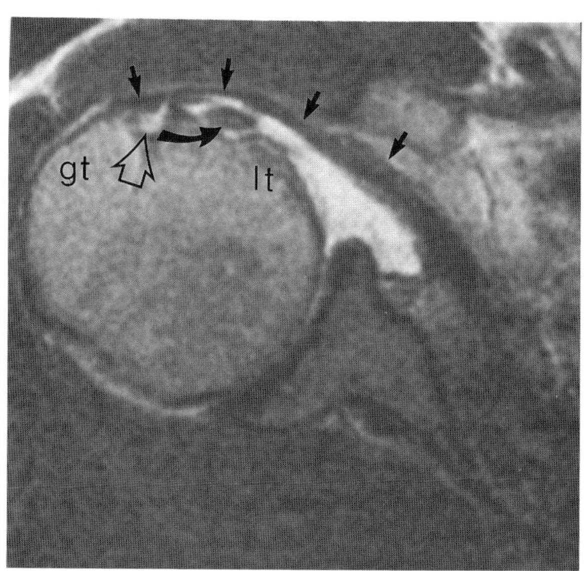

Figure 6-26. Medial dislocation of the biceps tendon (*curved arrow*) beneath intact superficial fibers of the subscapularis tendon. T_2-weighted axial image shows that the deep layer of the subscapularis tendon is torn from the lesser tuberosity (*lt*), whereas the superficial layer and its contribution to the transverse humeral ligament (*small arrows*) remain intact to the greater tuberosity (*gt*) at lateral aspect of the bicipital groove (*open arrow*).

generation involving its intrasubstance fibers and their contribution to the medial tendinous wall of the bicipital groove. The biceps tendon may then sublux or mildly dislocate into an intrasubstance partial-thickness tear. If entirely intrasubstance, this abnormality may not be appreciated at open or arthroscopic surgery.

MAGNETIC RESONANCE IMAGING OF THE POSTOPERATIVE ROTATOR CUFF

Persistent or recurrent shoulder pain and symptoms after shoulder surgery are not uncommon and can be a difficult diagnostic challenge. Differential diagnosis includes recurrent rotator cuff tear, persistent subacromial impingement, deltoid detachment and deficiency, residual or recurrent instability, and nerve injury.[55] Plain radiographs can be of help in the evaluation of residual subacromial bony impingement but are not sensitive for recurrent cuff tears. Arthrography is rendered less useful due to common occurrence of normal leakage of contrast through the repair site into the subacromial space.[8] Interpretation of shoulder ultrasound is also more difficult due to distortion of cuff anatomy and echo patterns.[14] Interpretation of MRI of the shoulder after surgery is also, in general, more difficult than that of the nonoperated shoulder.[27,51] Findings that may be diagnostic of pathology in the unoperated shoulder may be expected after surgery. Knowledge of the type of surgery that has been performed and of what is normally expected as a result of that surgery is essential.

Technical parameters that we use for evaluation of the postoperative shoulder and rotator cuff are the same as our routine shoulder MRI technique: proton density- and T_2-weighted 3-mm oblique coronal, oblique sagittal, and axial images. We routinely use 16 field of view and 192 × 256 matrix with one signal excitation and do not routinely use fat suppression.

Normal Postoperative Shoulder

Ferromagnetic surgical hardware will cause a component of signal-void artifact in the immediate vicinity and, if nearby, can obscure the area of interest. Titanium surgical hardware causes minimal artifact due to its nonferromagnetic nature. Even if no metallic surgical hardware is left behind, it is very common to see punctate foci of micrometallic signal-void artifact in the area of surgery that represent microparticles of metal not visible on plain film radiographs (Fig. 6-27). Because gradient-echo images are more susceptible than spin-echo images to metallic signal-void artifact, an argument can be made to avoid gradient-echo imaging in the postoperative shoulder.

Subacromial Decompression

Neer[47] popularized the concept of the clinical impingement syndrome and advocated anterior acromioplasty for surgical decompression of the narrowed subacromial space, with or without rotator cuff repair. A common procedure performed in combination with both open and arthroscopic acromioplasty for shoulder decompression is resection of the subacromial bursa. Resection of the peribursal fat layer, as well as fibrosis and scarring, commonly result in the postoperative appearance of obscuration of the subdeltoid fat plane, a normal postoperative MRI finding. Either by open or arthroscopic approach, the anteroinferior aspect of the anterior acromion is resected in a wedge-like fashion, with the greatest resection anteriorly and tapering posterolaterally. The aim is to surgically convert a Bigliani type 2 or type 3 acromion to a type 1 configuration. MRI appearance of postsurgical results can be best evaluated on oblique sagittal images (Fig. 6-28). This resection typically includes division or resection of a portion of the acromial

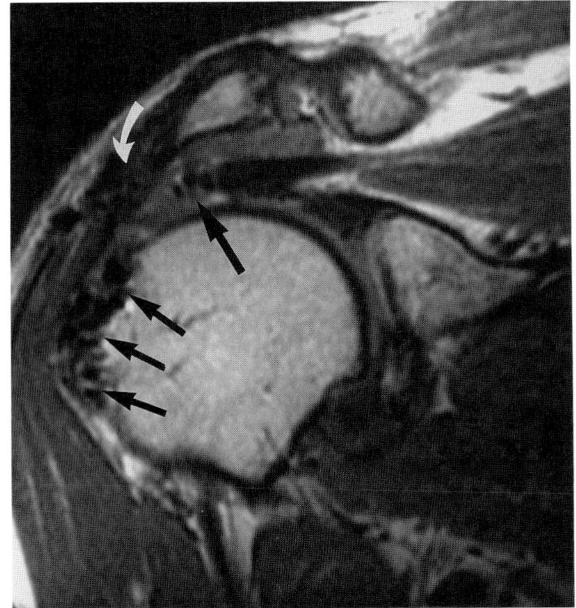

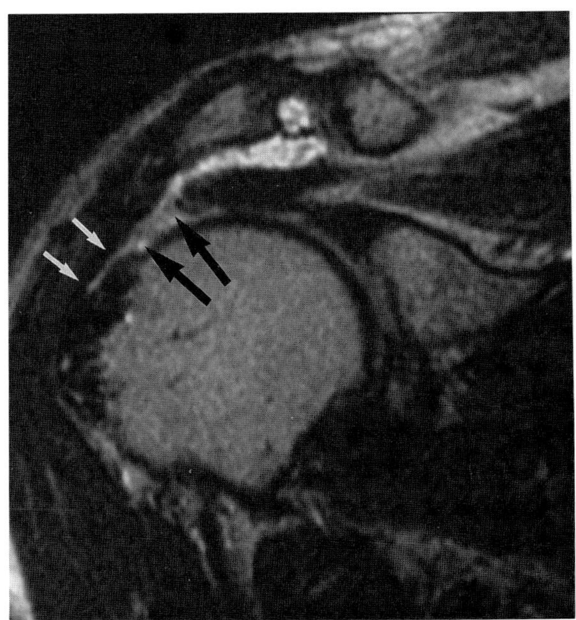

Figure 6-27. Recurrent supraspinatus tendon tear in an individual with history of open subacromial decompression and rotator cuff repair. **(A)** Proton density coronal image shows punctate micrometallic artifact and fibrosis involving the subacromial space from anterior acromioplasty (*curved arrow*). Artifact is also seen at the site of trough creation and suturing of the sulcus (*small arrows*) of the humeral head, as well as involving the proximally retracted supraspinatus tendon (*large arrow*), reflecting retear of the repair site. **(B)** Corresponding T_2-weighted image better shows the high signal intensity fluid (*arrows*) interrupting the supraspinatus tendon and repair. Incidental note is made of a central tendon slip (*small white arrows*) of the overlying deltoid muscle that can falsely mimic an intact superficial layer of the supraspinatus.

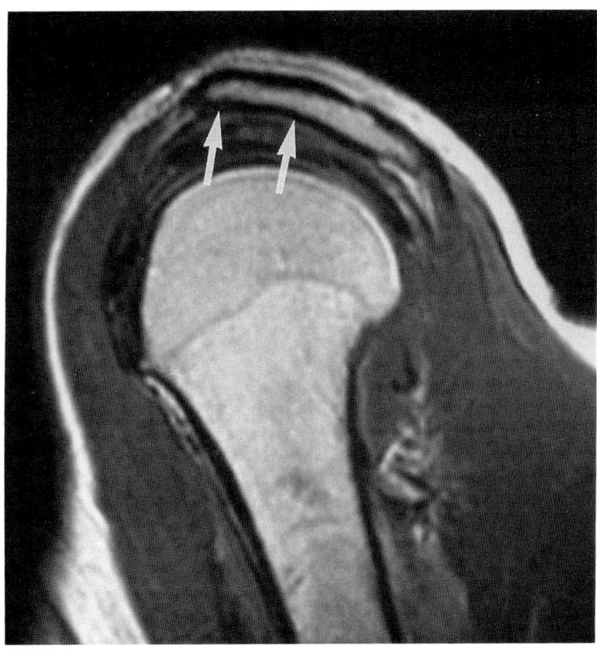

Figure 6-28. Adequate subacromial decompression including anterior acromioplasty. Proton density oblique sagittal image shows residua of anterior acromioplasty with resultant Bigliani type I to II acromion morphology (*arrows*).

attachment of the coracoacromial ligament. If inferiorly hypertrophic, the distal clavicle and acromioclavicular joint may be resected.

Owen et al[56] found postoperative MRI to be 64 percent sensitive and 82 percent specific in predicting residual subacromial impingement. Factors contributing to persistent narrowing and associated persistent impingement include inadequate acromial resection and failure to address inferior hypertrophy of the acromioclavicular joint. Another cause of continued or recurrent pain is development of rotator cuff tear or retear.

Rotator Cuff Repair

Rotator cuff repair is most commonly performed openly, although increasingly more common for small tears is an arthroscopically guided mini-open incision. The margins of the tear are usually debrided to good viable tissue. Small tears may be sutured in a side-to-side fashion, although larger tears generally require creation of a bone trough in the humeral sulcus or more proximal aspect of the head down to bleeding bone followed by suture fixation of the torn tendon edge into the trough.

The normal postoperative MRI appearance after rotator cuff tear repair includes findings seen after anterior acromioplasty, discussed previously. A shallow defect or trough is often seen in the humeral sulcus.

Full-thickness high signal intensity on T_2-weighted images or nonvisualization of a portion of the cuff is diagnostic of full-thickness recurrent tears (Fig. 6-27). Owen[51] reported an overall accuracy of 90 percent in the diagnosis of recurrent full-thickness rotator cuff tears. Recurrent tears can occur not only in the location of the repair but also tear in a different location of the cuff, presumably due to additional stress put on adjacent degenerated tendon tissue.

A potential imaging pitfall can occur when imaging the patient who has had repair of a very large or massive chronic cuff tear, in which attempted mobilization of the cuff may have been inadequate to provide enough length to bring the tendon to the humeral sulcus without undue tension on the repair. In this instance, a trough may be created in a more proximal portion of the humeral head rather than in the humeral sulcus, thereby allowing function but minimizing stress on the repair site. At postoperative MRI, this can result in the absence of visualization of cuff tissue more distally at the greater tuberosity and sulcus, falsely simulating a full-thickness rotator cuff tear.

Fluid-like signal intensity in the subacromial-subdeltoid bursa on T_2-weighted images is even less specific than in the unoperated shoulder. Not only can this be present as bursal inflammation with an intact cuff, but cuff repair may not produce a watertight seal of the cuff.[8] This could result in bursal fluid collection that may be expected to be difficult to differentiate from a pathologic recurrent subacromial-subdeltoid bursitis or hematoma/seroma.

MRI can detect and delineate the extent of deltoid deficiency, a clinical condition consisting of deltoid detachment from the acromion that can occasionally result from a postoperative injury or inadequate reattachment of the deltoid to the acromion after open surgery. Deltoid deficiency is a severe complication that can lead to a flail shoulder and chronic pain that may require glenohumeral arthrodesis.[55]

CAPSULOLABRAL STRUCTURES AND PATHOLOGY

Glenoid Labrum Tears

Several imaging modalities have been used to evaluate the capsulolabral pathology of the shoulder, including arthrography, CT arthrography, MRI and magnetic resonance arthrography. Until recently, CT arthrography has been the imaging modality of choice based on several studies showing high sensitivity and specificity.[7,57,63,72]

MRI has proved to be useful for visualization of the soft tissues of the capsulolabral complex including labral anatomy and labrum tears (Figs. 6-29 and 6-30). The reported sensitivity for detection of labrum tears ranges from 44[25] to 95 percent.[34] However, pitfalls in interpretation of MRI outnumber those of CT arthrography, resulting in greater inter- and intraobserver variability.

Flannigan et al[21] correctly diagnosed nine labral tears in 23 patients, whereas only three of the nine were diagnosed by conventional MRI. Chadnani et al[11] compared conventional MRI, magnetic resonance arthrography, and CT arthrography to surgical findings in 28 patients with a mean age of 27 years. Their findings were that magnetic resonance arthrography is more sensitive than CT arthrography or conventional MRI in detection of abnormalities of the labrum. These patients were selected for diagnostic imaging because of signs and symptoms consistent with shoulder instability or shoulder pain of unexplained origin. Labral tears were found at surgery in 26 of the 28 patients. Conventional MRI, magnetic resonance arthrography, and CT arthrography found 93, 96, and 73 percent of these tears, respectively. A surgically proven detached labral fragment was found in 46, 96, and 52 percent, respectively. Labral degeneration consisting of fraying or attenuation was found in 11, 56, and 24 percent, respectively. Capsular injuries can occasionally be demonstrated, especially in acute injuries (Fig. 6-31).

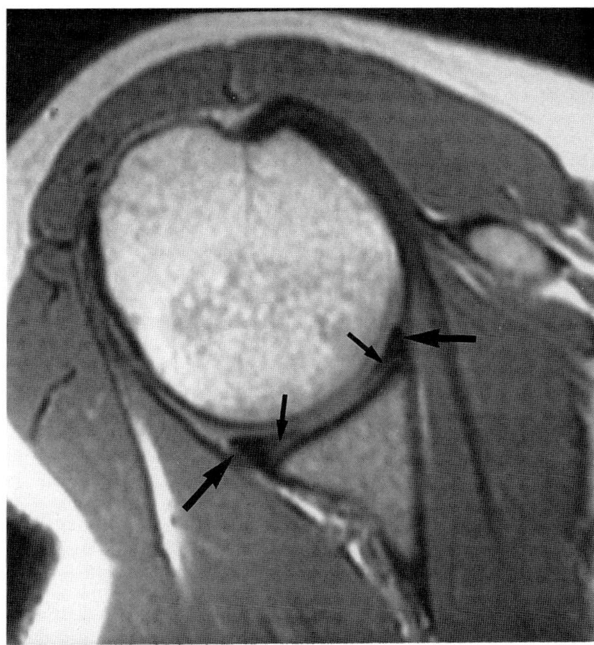

Figure 6-29. Normal glenoid labrum. Proton density axial image shows uniformly low signal intensity of the anterior and posterior glenoid labrum (*large arrows*). Note the linear increased signal intensity on proton density images at the base of the labrum that represents the normal hyaline articular cartilage of the glenoid on which the fibrous labrum attaches (*small arrows*). This is not to be mistaken for a labrum tear.

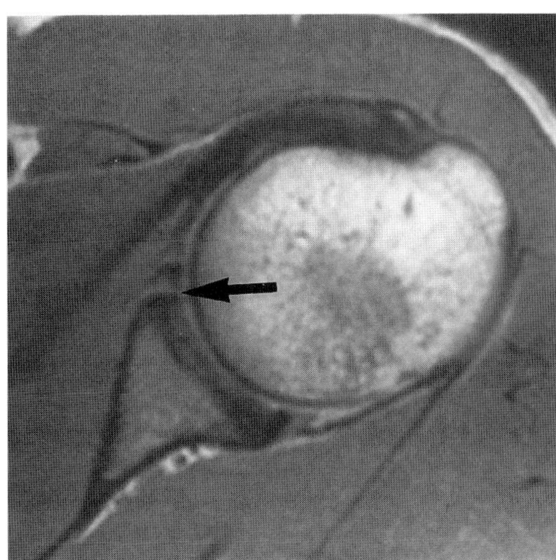

Figure 6-30. Isolated anterior glenoid labrum tear. This 20-year-old water polo player suffered a hyperextension injury when trying to block a shot. Persistent pain prompted MRI, which revealed an anterior glenoid labrum tear (*arrow*) without demonstration of medial capsular stripping or Hill-Sachs deformity.

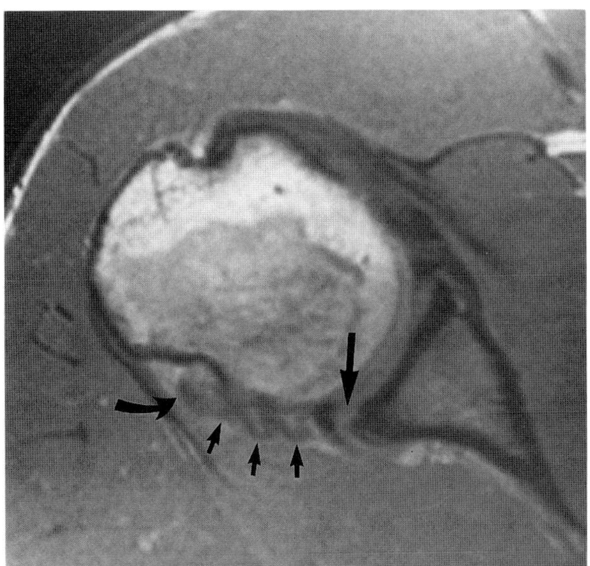

Figure 6-31. Acute posterior labrum tear and avulsion of the posterior capsule off the humerus. This 18-year-old man had a shoulder injury 3 days prior to examination. Proton density axial image shows posterior labrum tear (*large arrow*) as well as posterior capsule detachment from the humerus (*curved arrow*) and abnormal undulation (*small arrows*).

Anterior Instability

Hill-Sachs deformity represents a compression fracture of the posterosuperior aspect of the humeral head caused by impaction of the head into the inferior glenoid at the time of dislocation. It can be detected on plain films including internal rotation anteroposterior, axillary, and Stryker notch views. However, smaller lesions can be detected with greater sensitivity and specificity on axial CT and MRI.[73] Bankart lesions, including anteroinferior labrum tears and associated capsulolabral injuries, can be detected, as can medial capsular stripping after acute or subacute anterior dislocations (Fig. 6-32). Chronic thickening of the medial capsule can be seen as residua of more chronic anterior dislocation injury.

Posterior Instability

Posterior shoulder dislocation injuries are much less common than anterior dislocation injuries. However, posterior subluxation/dislocation episodes are not rare among football players, particularly linemen. MRI can similarly detect posterior labrum tears and reverse Hill-Sachs deformities (Fig. 6-33). Posterior glenoid rim fractures can be differentiated from posterior labrum tears (Fig. 6-34).

Superior Labrum Tears (SLAP Lesions)

There has been increasing interest of arthroscopists and sports medicine clinicians in superior labral injuries. In 1990, Snyder et al[65] described the SLAP lesion, an eponym that stands for superior labrum, anterior to posterior, including the origin of the biceps tendon. This injury may occur after acute trauma sustained during a fall on an outstretched arm, during traction of the biceps tendon by a sudden traumatic pull, or with repetitive stress in throwing athletes. Hurley and Anderson[29] noted an association between superior labral tears and the impingement syndrome in a population of athletes and raised the possibility of secondary impingement caused by instability. This interest has prompted radiologists to pay more attention to diagnostic imaging of the superior labrum.

Although these superior labrum tears can be detected at CT arthrography,[28] the ability of MRI to obtain direct coronal images, which are optimal for evaluation of the superior labrum and biceps tendon anchor, MRI better evaluates these lesions (Fig. 6-35). The addition of intra-articular saline or dilute gadolinium solution adds to the accuracy of MRI by providing an intra-articular contrast material that, like CT arthrography, imbibes into the abnormal labrum and labral tears (Fig. 6-36). Magnetic resonance ar-

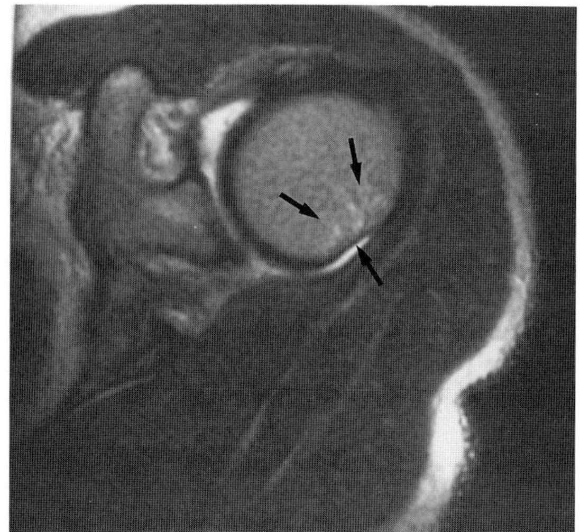

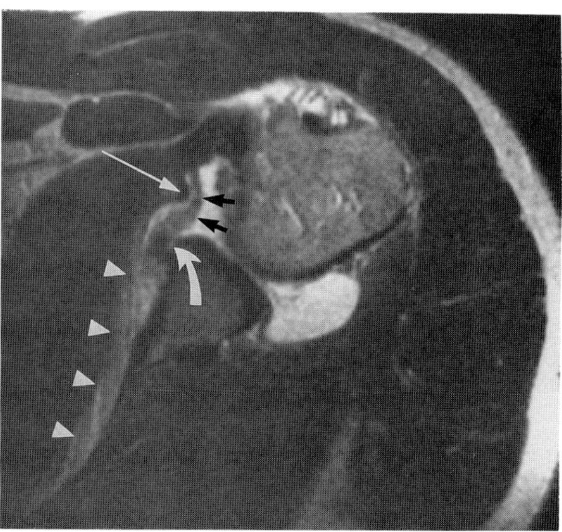

Figure 6-32. A 22-year-old man with recent shoulder injury and MRI findings consistent with residua of anterior shoulder dislocation injury. **(A)** T_2-weighted axial image showing small and shallow Hill-Sachs deformity with underlying marrow edema/hemorrhage (*arrows*). **(B)** T_2-weighted axial image through the level of the inferior glenoid shows Bankart lesion with displaced anterior labrum tear (*curved white arrow*), associated with injury and thickening of the inferior glenohumeral ligament (*small arrows*) and mild medial capsular stripping with dissection of extracapsular fluid between the subscapularis and bony scapula (*arrowheads*). The middle glenohumeral ligament can be seen as a thickening of the anterior capsule (*long white arrow*).

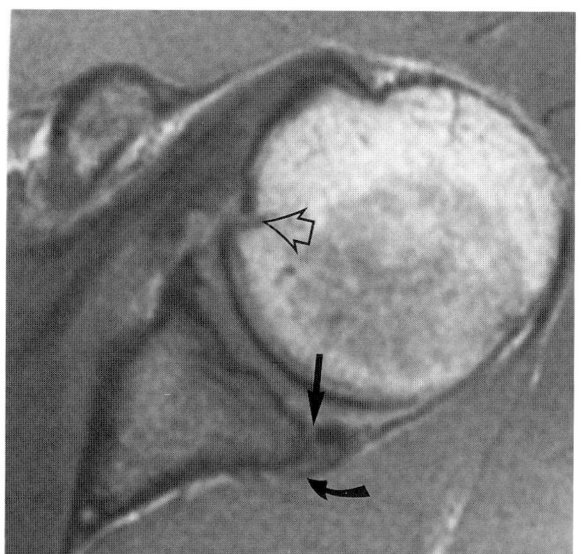

Figure 6-33. Posterior glenoid labrum tear (*arrow*) seen with posterior capsular stripping (*curved arrow*) and small reverse Hill-Sachs deformity of the anteromedial humeral head (*open arrow*) are findings consistent with residua of posterior shoulder dislocation inury.

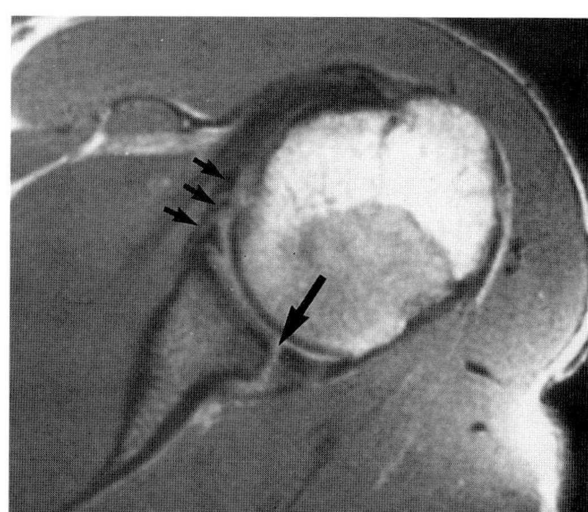

Figure 6-34. A 17-year-old high school football lineman with persistent pain when pushing off. Proton density axial image shows posterior glenoid rim fracture (*arrow*) and posterior labrum otherwise intact to the posterior fragment. Anterior capsule and glenohumeral ligaments (*small arrows*) are intact.

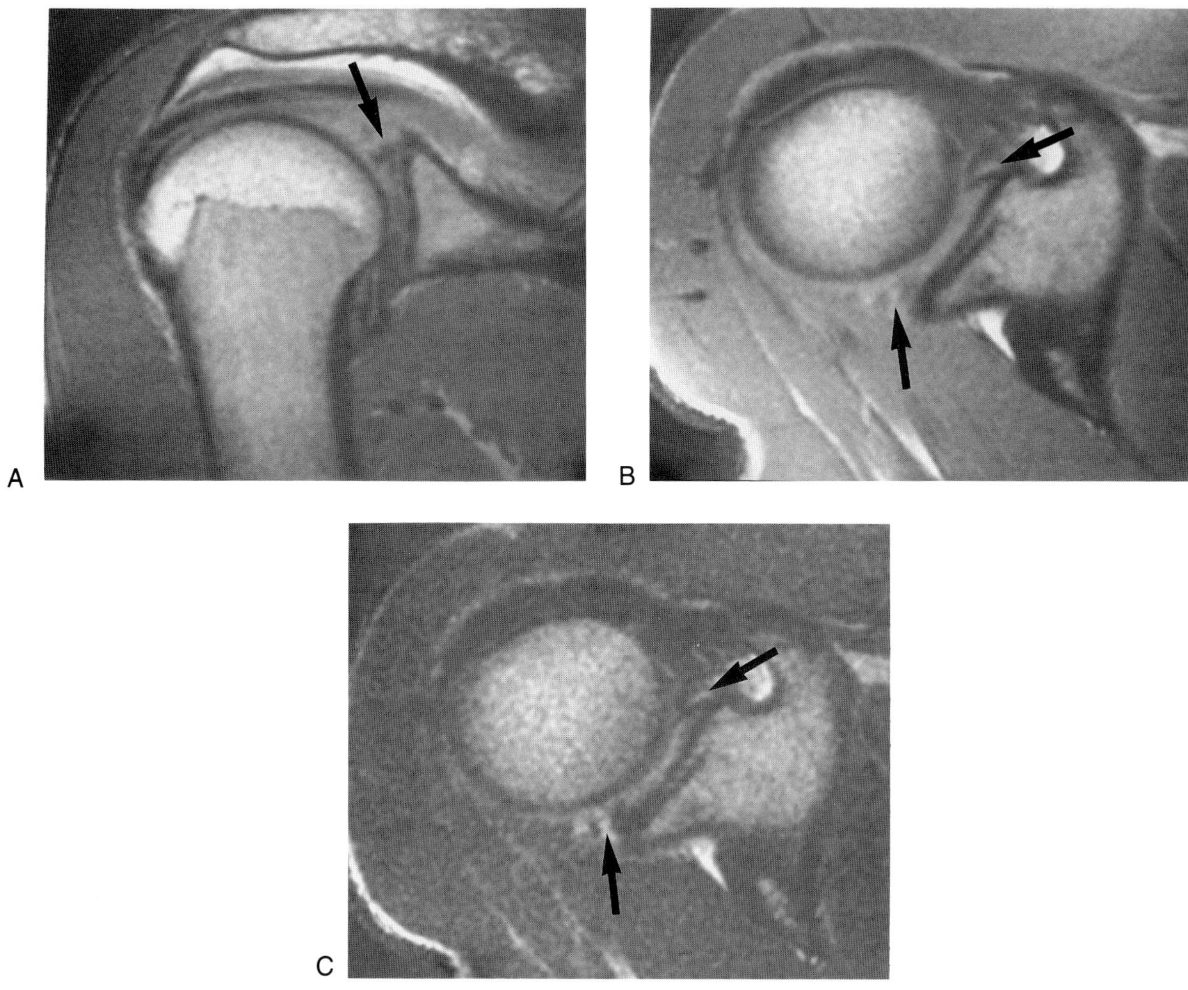

Figure 6-35. A 19-year-old throwing athlete with persistent shoulder pain especially with throwing motion and clinical examination consistent with impingement syndrome. **(A)** Proton density oblique coronal image shows linear increased signal intensity (*arrow*) involving the superior glenoid labrum. Superior labrum tear is seen to better advantage on axial **(B)** proton density- and **(C)** corresponding T_2-weighted images as linear foci of increased signal intensity (*arrows*) through the normally low signal intensity superior labrum. A SLAP lesion was documented at arthroscopic surgery.

thrography has now been established as the imaging modality of choice for detection of these lesions.[11,31,52,68]

OSSEOUS CHANGES

MRI can be used to detect occult osseous injuries of the glenohumeral joint and shoulder including radiographically occult fractures and bone contusions, which represent bone marrow trabecular microfractures with associated marrow edema/hemorrhage with or without cortical infractions. The sensitivity of MRI to marrow edema and pathology combined with its tomographic capability allow sensitivity approaching that of bone scintigraphy while providing greater specificity and better anatomic detail.

Burk and associates,[6] in a study of MRI of 10 symptomatic professional baseball players and 1 asymptomatic player, described cortical irregularity or subchondral cyst formation at the posterior aspect of the greater tuberosity near the insertion of the infraspinatus tendon in five of

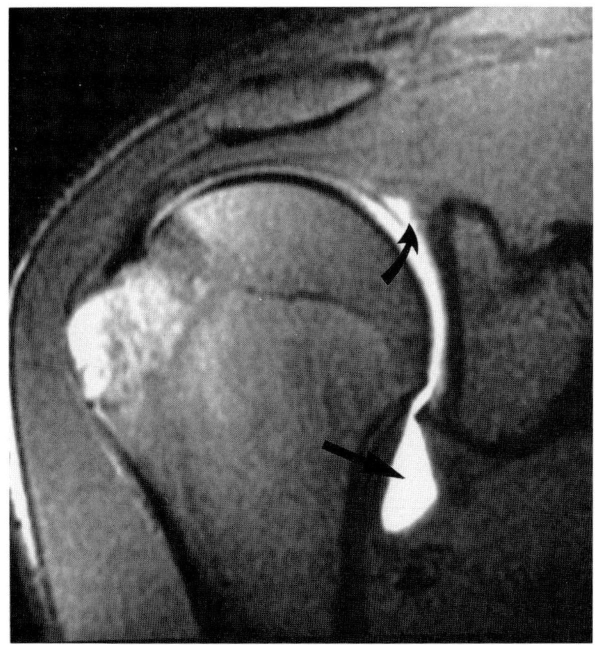

Figure 6-36. Magnetic resonance arthrogram showing SLAP lesion in this 21-year-old pitcher with persistent shoulder pain, especially with throwing motions. High signal intensity contrast extends into the axillary recess (*arrow*) and a superior labrum tear (*curved arrow*) on this T_1-weighted fat saturation coronal image.

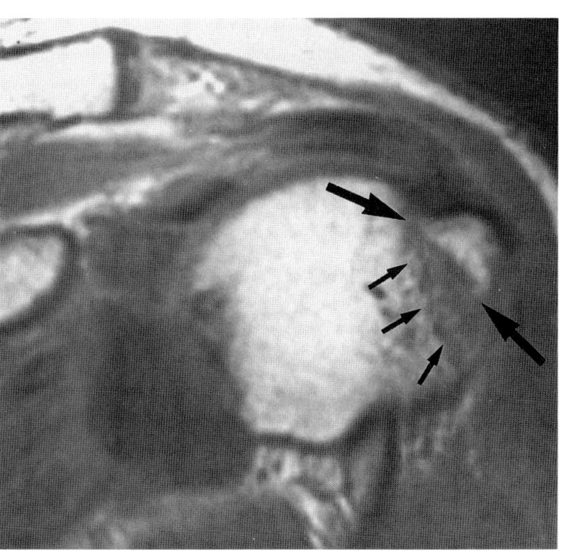

Figure 6-37. Radiographically occult greater tuberosity fracture. This 37-year-old male cross-country skier fell onto an abducted shoulder when descending a hill 3 weeks previously. Initial radiographs were negative. Persistence of pain and weakness prompted MRI examination to rule out rotator cuff tear. Proton density image shows minimally elevated fracture line (*large arrows*) and surrounding intermediate signal intensity marrow edema/hemorrhage (*small arrows*), as well as intact rotator cuff. Pain and weakness gradually resolved over the course of 2 months.

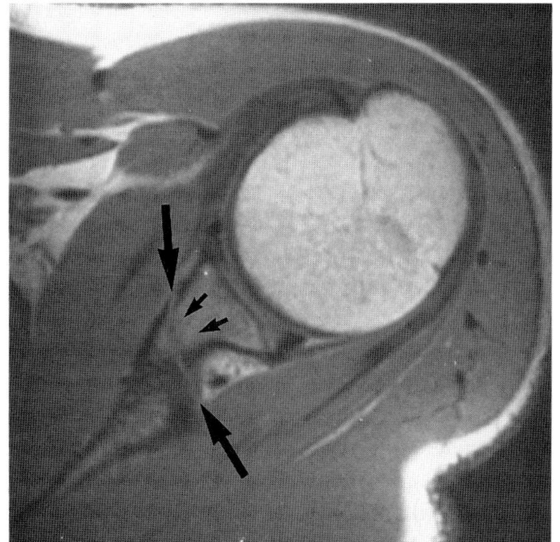

A

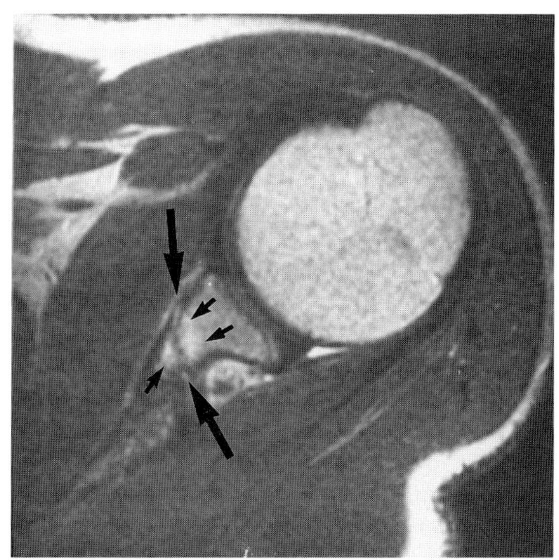

B

Figure 6-38. Nondisplaced scapular fracture. A 21-year-old snowboarder with persistent shoulder pain after fall. **(A)** Proton density- and **(B)** T_2-weighted axial images reveal nondisplaced fracture line (*large arrows*) and surrounding marrow edema/hemorrhage (*small arrows*).

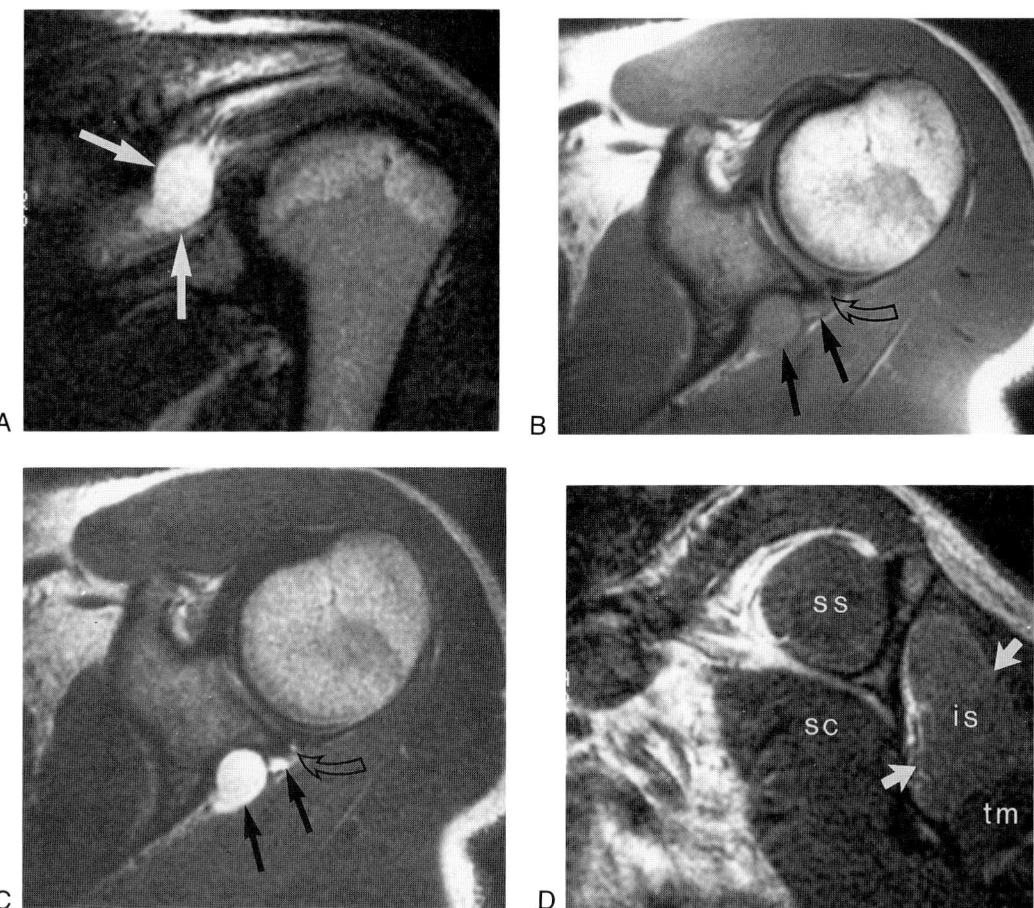

Figure 6-39. Large posterosuperior ganglion cyst with impingement on the infraspinatus branch of the suprascapular nerve in the spinoglenoid notch, associated with denervation signal change in the infraspinatus muscle. **(A)** T_2-weighted coronal image shows ganglion cyst (*arrows*) in the spinoglenoid notch. **(B)** Proton density- and **(C)** T_2-weighted axial images show ganglion cyst and associated slender neck (*arrows*) extending through posterior component of superior labrum tear (*curved open arrow*). **(D)** T_2-weighted sagittal image shows generalized increased signal intensity of the infraspinatus (*is*) muscle belly (*arrows*) relative to the supraspinatus (*ss*), teres minor (*tm*), and subscapularis muscles (*sc*), reflecting denervation signal alteration.

seven players with rotator cuff tears. These findings were thought to represent chronic avulsion changes resulting from the deceleration stresses of the follow-through motion. However, similar findings were noted in the asymptomatic volunteer and one of the three players without cuff tear. Such findings of signal alteration of subcortical marrow at the posterior aspect of the humeral sulcus are common, increasing in frequency with age, although not uncommon in the 20- to 40-year age group. It is not our experience that this finding is necessarily associated with cuff pathology or confined to throwing athletes. This is the location of the anatomic humeral bare area, an intra-articular portion of the humerus that is not covered by articular cartilage. Lack of protective articular cartilage is expected to lead to increased incidence of erosions and subchondral cyst formation in this region. These erosions have been documented at arthroscopy without being seen to be intimately related to the infraspinatus insertion.

Occult osseous injury of the greater tuberosity, including bone contusion and radiographically occult fracture of the greater tuberosity, is a cause of persistent shoulder pain and weakness after trauma to the shoulder (Fig. 6-37). This may occur from a fall directly onto the shoulder or on an outstretched arm. Although most common in the elderly population, we have seen six cases sustained by younger cross-country and downhill skiers during a fall. It is most commonly seen as an incidental finding on MRI examination that was performed to rule out rotator cuff tear. MRI is useful to rule out rotator cuff tear and establish a diagnosis that may be expected to resolve without sequelae with further conservative management.

Overt greater tuberosity fractures can also be evaluated preoperatively for determination of the degree of fracture displacement or elevation, as well as allowing detection of any associated rotator cuff tears. Occasionally, an occult or unsuspected scapula fracture can be identified as a result of shoulder trauma (Fig. 6-38). MRI is not considered ideal for evaluation of fracture healing and CT examination is still considered modality of choice in that regard.

GANGLION CYSTS AND SUPRASCAPULAR NEUROPATHY

MRI is the modality of choice for evaluation of clinical suspicion for suprascapular neuropathy.[23,74] Differential diagnosis includes posterosuperior ganglion cysts that, if large enough, can encroach on branches of the suprascapular nerve. If extending into the supraspinatus foss or suprascapular notch, encroachment on the suprascapular nerve with denervation atrophy of both supraspinatus and infraspinatus can occur. Extension into the spinoglenoid notch can encroach on the suprascapular nerve branch to the infraspinatus muscle, resulting in denervation with isolated infraspinatus atrophy and weakness (Fig. 6-39). In a recent study (Moore, Buss, and Fritts, submitted for publication), 14 patients with MRI findings of posterosuperior ganglion cysts were identified. All except one were found to have a labrum tear, usually a SLAP lesion, at arthroscopy. That one patient had a primary excision of the cyst. Arthroscopy performed 2 years later for recurrent pain and ganglion cyst showed a very small SLAP lesion that, retrospectively, is thought to have been missed at initial arthroscopy. Therefore, all 14 had associated labrum tears. Intramuscular cysts are seen occasionally. They are usually associated with

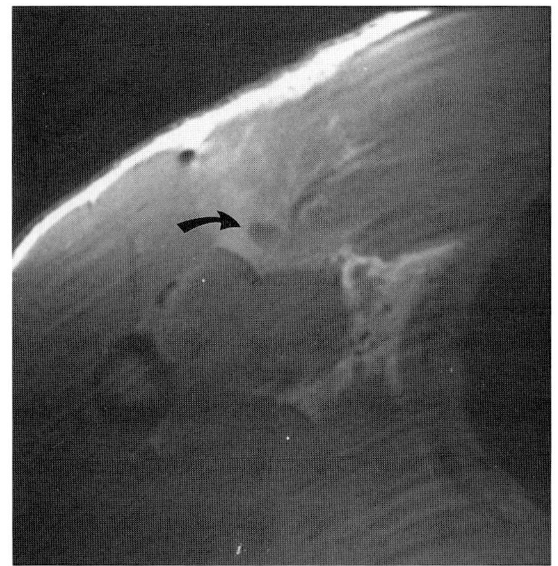

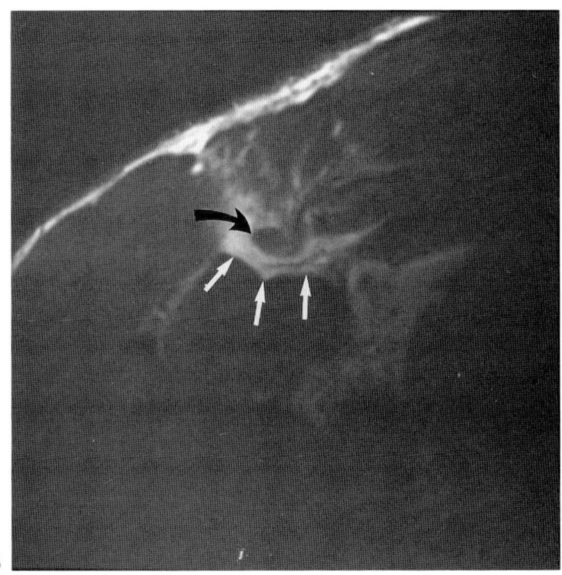

Figure 6-40. Professional football player who sustained a forced external rotation injury of the right upper extremity and shoulder against resistance and full-thickness pectoralis major tendon rupture. **(A)** Proton density- and **(B)** T_2-weighted axial images show rupture and retraction of the pectoralis major tendon (*curved arrow*), surrounded by edema/hemorrhage (*straight arrows*). Tear was surgically documented and repaired.

intrasubstance or deep surface degeneration and partial-thickness tears. Fluid may be forced along the course of tendon fibers into the distal aspect of the muscle belly, where there is less external compressive force by the overlying coracoacromial arch.

OTHER MUSCULOTENDINOUS INJURIES

MRI can also be useful in the evaluation of other musculotendinous injuries about the shoulder. One of the most useful is the detection and evaluation of the extent of pectoralis major injuries. Pectoralis major ruptures typically occur at the distal musculotendinous junction proximal to the tendinous attachment to the medial aspect of the proximal humerus and can be repaired acutely and chronically with high success rate.[41] Pectoralis injuries can be best appreciated on proton density- and T_2-weighted axial images (Fig. 6-40). Because the area of interest is inferior to that generally included for a routine shoulder MRI, any clinical suspicion for pectoralis injury must be relayed to the MRI technologist and radiologist to ensure inclusion of the area of interest. Injuries of the deltoid and coracobrachialis muscles can also be detected.

CONCLUSION

MRI of the shoulder is considered the imaging modality of choice in the evaluation of shoulder pain, injuries, and the clinical impingement syndrome. It directly evaluates all the soft tissue structures of the subacromial space, as well as the relationship of the overlying osseous and soft tissue structures of the coracoacromial arch. Information is also obtained regarding the capsulolabral anatomy and, with the addition of magnetic resonance arthrography, is becoming recognized as the imaging modality of choice for instability workup, especially in the young throwing athlete with the possibility of a SLAP lesion. Detection and evaluation of soft tissue injuries and masses of the shoulder are unsurpassed. MRI evaluation, when combined with the always important clinical history, physical examination, and radiographs, provides the referring clinician and orthopaedic surgeon the most anatomic and pathologic information possible. This, in turn, allows the most informed decision making possible regarding conservative management or surgical treatment presurgical evaluation.

REFERENCES

1. Bigliani LU, Morrison, D, April EW: The morphology of the acromion and its relationship to rotator cuff tears. Orthop Trans 10:228, 1986
2. Bigliani LU, Norris X, Fischer J et al: The relationship between the unfused acromial epiphysis and subacromial impingement lesions. Orthop Trans 7:138, 1983
3. Bonutti PM, Norfray JF, Friedman RJ, Genez BM: Kinematic MRI of the shoulder. J Comput Assist Tomogr 17:666, 1993
4. Brandt TD, Cardone BW, Grant TH et al: Rotator cuff sonography: a reassessment. Radiology 173:323, 1989
5. Burk KL, Karasick D, Kurtz AB et al: Rotator cuff tears: prospective comparison of MR imaging with arthrography, sonography, and surgery. AJR 153:87, 1989
6. Burk, DL, Torres JL, Marone PJ et al: MR imaging of shoulder injuries in professional baseball players. J Magn Reson Imaging 1:385, 1991
7. Callaghan JJ, McNeish LM, Dehaven JP et al: A prospective comparison of double contrast computed tomography (CT) arthrography and arthroscopy of the shoulder. Am J Sports Med 16:13, 1988
8. Calvert PT, Packer NP, Stoker DJ et al: Arthrography of the shoulder after operative repair of the torn rotator cuff. J Bone Joint Surg [Br] 68:117, 1986
9. Cartland JP, Crues JV, Stauffer A: MR imaging in the evaluation of SLAP injuries of the shoulder: findings in 10 patients. AJR 159:787, 1992
10. Cervilla V, Schweitzer ME, Ho C: Medial dislocation of the biceps brachii tendon: appearance at MR imaging. Radiology 180:523, 1991
11. Chandnani VP, Yeager TD, DeBarardino T et al: Glenoid labrum tears: prospective evaluation with MR imaging. AJR 161:1229, 1993
12. Codman EA: The shoulder, Thomas Todd, Boston, 1934
13. Cofield RH: Current concepts review rotator cuff disease of the shoulder. J Bone Joint Surg [Am] 67:974, 1985
14. Crass JR, Craig EV, Feinberg SB: Sonography of the postoperative rotator cuff. AJR 146:561, 1986
15. Crass JR, Craig EV, Feinberg SB: Ultrasonography of rotator cuff tears: a review of 500 diagnostic studies. JCU 16:313, 1988
16. Craven WM: Traumatic avulsion tears of the rotator cuff. p. 129. In Andrews JR, Wilk KE (eds): The Athlete's Shoulder. Churchill Livingstone, New York, 1994
17. Crues JV, Fareed DO: Magnetic resonance imaging of shoulder impingement. Top Magn Reson Imag 3:39, 1991
18. Epstein RE, Schweitzer ME, Frieman BG et al: Hooked acromion: prevalence on MR images of painful shoulders. Radiology 187:479, 1993
19. Erickson SJ, Fitzgerald SW, Quinn SF et al: Long bicipital tendon of the shoulder: normal anatomy and pathologic findings on MR imaging. AJR 158:1091, 1992
20. Farin PU, Jaroma H, Soimakallio S: Shoulder impingement syndrome: sonographic evaluation. Radiology 176:845, 1990
21. Flannigan B, Kursunoglu-Brahme S, Snyder S et al: MR arthrography of the shoulder: comparison with conventional MR imaging. AJR 155:829, 1990
22. Fritts HM, Craig EV: MRI of the shoulder. Semin USG CT MR 15:341, 1994
23. Fritz RC, Helms CA, Steinbach LS et al: Suprascapular nerve entrapment: evaluation with MR imaging. Radiology 182:437, 1992

24. Fukuda H. Mikasa M, Yamanaka K: Incomplete thickness rotator cuff tears diagnosed by subacromial bursography. Clin Orthop 223:51, 1987
25. Garneau RA, Renfrew DL, Moore TE et al: Glenoid labrum: evaluation with MR imaging. Radiology 179:519, 1991
26. Goldman A, Ghelman B: The double-contrast shoulder arthrogram: a review of 158 studies. Radiology 127:655, 1978
27. Haygood, TM, Oxner KG, Kneeland JB et al: Magnetic resonance imaging of the postoperative shoulder. Magn Res Imag Clin North Am 1:143, 1993
28. Hunter JC, Blatz DJ, Escobedo EM: SLAP lesions of the glenoid labrum: CT arthrographic and arthroscopic correlation. Radiology 184:513, 1992
29. Hurley JA, Anderson TE: Shoulder arthroscopy: its role in evaluating shoulder disorders in the athlete. Am J Sports Med 18:480, 1990
30. Kaplan PA, Bryans KC, Davick JP et al: MR imaging of the normal shoulder: variants and pitfalls. Radiology 184:519, 1992
31. Karzel RP, Snyder SJ: Magnetic resonance arthrography of the shoulder: a new technique of shoulder imaging. Clin Sports Med 12:123, 1993
32. Kieft GJ, Bloem JL, Rozing PM, Obermann WR: MR imaging of recurrent anterior dislocation of the shoulder: comparison with CT arthrography. AJR 150:343, 1987
33. Kjellin I, Ho CP, Cervilla V: Alterations in the supraspinatus tendon at MR imaging: correlation with histopathologic findings in cadavers. Radiology 181:837, 1991
34. Legan JM, Burkhard TK, Goff WB et al: Tears of the glenoid labrum: MR imaging of 88 arthroscopically confirmed cases. Radiology 179:241, 1991
35. Linker, CS, Helms CA, Fritz RC: Quadrilateral space syndrome: findings at MR imaging. Radiology 188:675, 1993
36. Lohr JF, Uhthoff HK: The microvascular pattern of the supraspinatus tendon. Clin Orthop 254:29, 1990
37. Mack LA, Gannon MK, Kilcoyne RF, Matsen FA: Sonographic evaluation of the rotator cuff: accuracy in patients without surgery. Clin Orthop 234:21, 1988
38. McAuliffe TB, Dowd GS: Avulsion of the subscapularis tendon: a case report. J Bone Joint Surg [Am] 69:1454, 1987
39. McMasters PE: Tendon and muscle ruptures: clinical and experimental studies on the causes and location of subcutaneous ruptures. J Bone Joint Surg[Am] 15:705, 1933
40. Meyer AW: The minute anatomy of attritional lesions. J Bone Joint Surg[Am] 13:341, 1931
41. Miller MD, Johnson DL, Fu FH et al: Rupture of the pectoralis major muscle in a collegiate football player. Am J Sports Med 21:475, 1993
42. Mink GH, Harris E, Rappaport M: Rotator cuff tears: evaluation using double-contrast shoulder arthrography. Radiology 157:621, 1985
43. Mirowitz SA: Normal rotator cuff: MR imaging with conventional and fat-suppression techniques. Radiology 180:735, 1991
44. Morrison DS, Bigliani LU: The clinical significance of variations in acromial morphology. Paper presented at ASES 3rd Open Meeting, San Francisco, 1987
45. Mudge MK, Wood VE, Frykman GK: Rotator cuff tears associated with os acromiale. J Bone Joint Surg [Am] 66: 427, 1984
46. Nakajima T, Rokuuma N, Hamada K et al: Histologic and biomechanical characteristics of the supraspinatus tendon: reference to rotator cuff tearing. J Shoulder Elbow Soc 3:79, 1994
47. Neer CS II: Anterior acromioplasty for the chronic impingement syndrome in the shoulder: a preliminary report. J Bone Joint Surg [Am] 54:41, 1972
48. Neer CS II: Impingement lesions. Clin Orthop 173:70, 1983
49. Neumann CH, Holt RG, Steinbach LS: MR imaging of the shoulder: appearance of the supraspinatus tendon in asymptomatic volunteers. AJR 158:1281, 1992
50. Nevaiser JS: Ruptures of the rotator cuff. Clin Orthop 3:92, 1954
51. Owen RS, Iannotti JP, Kneeland JB et al: Shoulder after surgery: MR imaging with surgical validation. Radiology 186:443, 1993
52. Palmer WE, Brown JH, Rosenthal DI: Labral-ligamentous complex of the shoulder: evaluation with MR arthrography. Radiology 190:645, 1994
53. Patten RM: Tears of the anterior portion of the rotator cuff (the subscapularis tendon): MR imaging findings. AJR 162:351, 1994
54. Petersson CJ: Spontaneous medial dislocation of the tendon of the long biceps brachii: an anatomic study of prevalence and pathomechanics. Clin Orthop 211:224, 1986
55. Post M: Complications of rotator cuff surgery. Clin Orthop 254:97, 1990
56. Preston BJ, Jackson JP: Investigation of shoulder disability by arthrography. Br J Radiol 28:259, 1977
57. Rafii M, Firooznia H, Golimbu C et al: CT arthrography of capsular structures of the shoulder. AJR 146:361, 1986
58. Rafii M, Firooznia H, Sherman O et al: Rotator cuff lesions: signal patterns at MR imaging. Radiology 177:817, 1990
59. Rathbun JB, Macnab I: The microvascular pattern of the rotator cuff. J Bone Joint Surg[Br] 52:540, 1970
60. Resnick D: Shoulder arthrography. Radiol Clin North Am 19:243, 1981
61. Seeger LL: Magnetic resonance imaging of the shoulder. Clin Orthop 244:48, 1989
62. Seeger LL, Gold RH, Bassett X et al: Magnetic resonance imaging of glenohumeral joint disease. Invest Radiol 23:650, 1988
63. Singson RD, Feldman F, Bigliani L: CT arthrographic patterns in recurrent glenohumeral instability. AJR 149:749, 1987
64. Skinner HA: Anatomical considerations relative to rupture of the supraspinatus tendon. J Bone Joint Surg[Am] 19:137, 1937
65. Snyder SJ, Karzel RP, Del Pizzo X et al: SLAP lesions of the shoulder. Arthroscopy 6:274, 1990
66. Soble MG, Kaye AD, Guay RC: Rotator cuff tear: clinical experience with sonographic detection. Radiology 173:319, 1989
67. Strizak AM, Danzig L, Jackson DW: Subacromial bursogra-

phy: an anatomical and clinical study. J Bone Joint Surg[Am] 64:196, 1982

68. Tirman PF, Applegate GR, Flannigan BD et al: Magnetic resonance arthrography of the shoulder. Magn Res Imag Clin North Am 1:125, 1993
69. Traughber PD, Goodwin TE: Shoulder MRI: arthroscopic correlation with emphasis on partial tears. J Comput Assist Tomogr 16:129, 1992
70. Uthoff HK, Sardar K: Pathology of rotator cuff tendons. p. 259. In Watson MS (ed): Surgical Disorders of the Shoulder. Churchill Livingstone, New York, 1991
71. Vick CW, Bell SA: Rotator cuff tears: diagnosis with sonography. AJR 154:121, 1990
72. Wilson AJ, Totty WG, Murphy WA et al: Shoulder joint: arthrographic CT and long-term follow-up with surgical correlation. Radiology 173:329, 1989
73. Workman TL, Burkhard TK, Resnick D et al: Hill-Sachs lesion: comparison of detection with MR imaging, radiography, and arthroscopy. Radiology 185:847, 1992
74. Zeiss J, Woldenberg LS, Saddemi SR et al: Case report: MRI of suprascapular neuropathy in a weight lifter. J Comput Assist Tomogr 17:303, 1993
75. Zlatkin MB, Ianotti JP, Roberts MC et al: Rotator cuff tears: diagnostic performance of MR imaging. Radiology 172:223, 1989

Color Plates

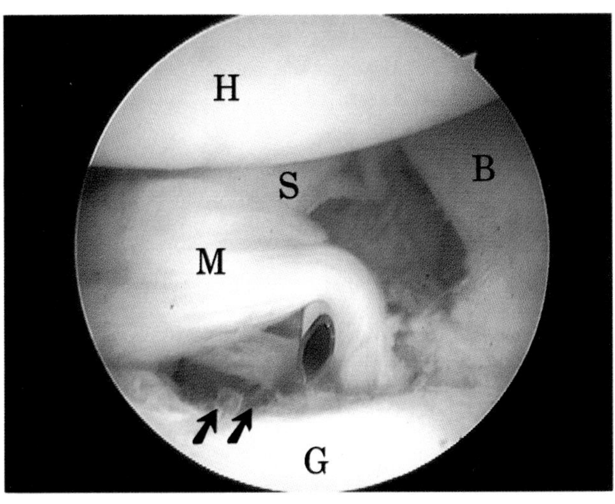

Plate 7-1

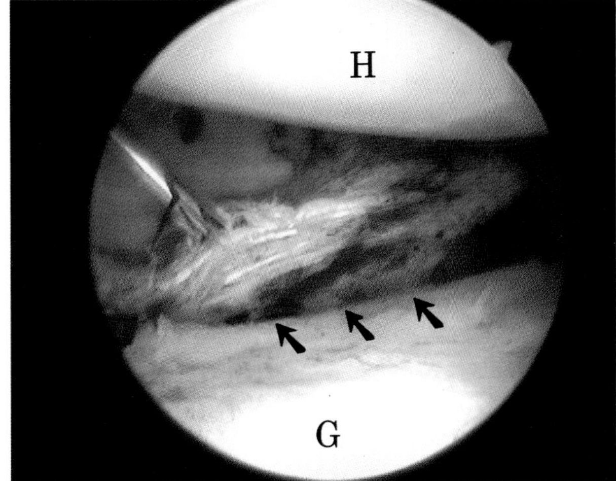

Plate 7-2

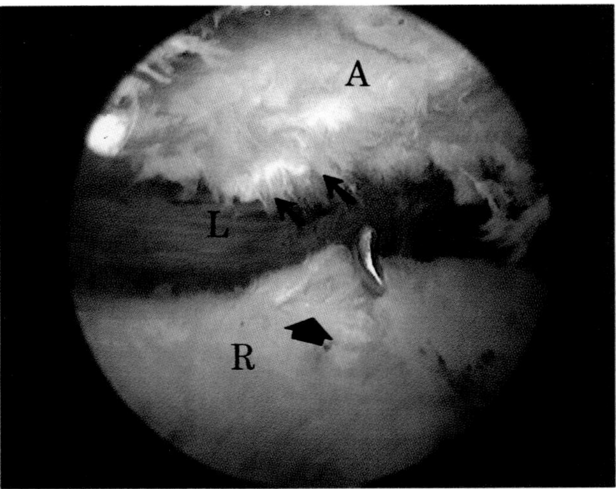

Plate 7-3

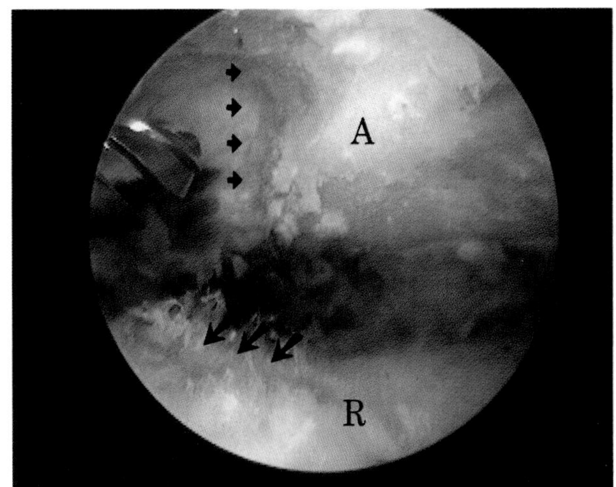

Plate 7-4

Plate 7-1. Normal glenohumeral anatomy. H, humeral head; B, biceps tendon; G, anterior superior glenoid rim; S, subscapularis tendon; M, middle glenohumeral ligament. Arrows indicate a normal sublabral foramen; this is a normal anatomic variant above the equator of the glenoid and it not a Bankart-type lesion.
Plate 7-2. Bankart lesion. H, humeral head; G, anterior inferior rim of the glenoid. Arrows point toward the Bankart lesion with the avulsed inferior glenohumeral ligament; the needle points toward the ligament.
Plate 7-3. Subacromial impingement syndrome. A view of the subacromial space from posterior looking anterior. R, superficial surface of the rotator cuff with a probe sticking through a superficial partial thickness rotator cuff tear (*large arrow*); L, coracoacromial ligament; A, anterior lateral corner of the acromion showing abrasion and wear of the anterior lateral attachment of the coracoacromial ligament (*arrows*).
Plate 7-4. Subacromial decompression. A, anterior acromion (small arrows point to the area that has already been removed by the burr on the left); R, rotator cuff (large arrow indicates superficial partial thickness rotator cuff tear).

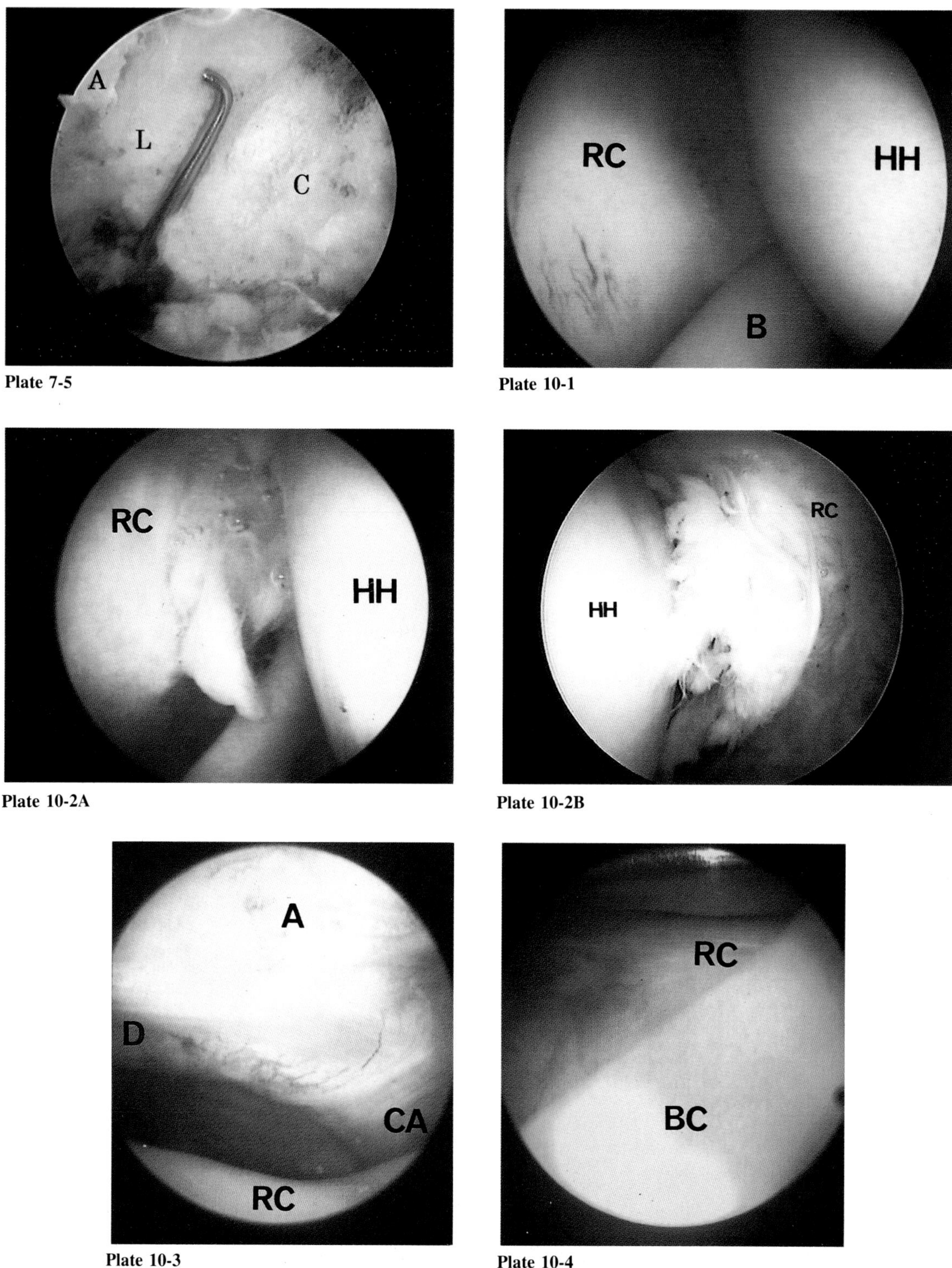

Plate 7-5. Arthroscopic excisional arthroplasty of the acromio-clavicular (AC) joint. C, remaining distal clavicle; A, acromial articulation of the AC joint; L, superior acromioclavicular ligaments being probed by a 4-mm arthroscopy probe. Width of resection is approximately 1 cm.

Plate 10-1. Normal articular surface of supraspinatus tendon (*right*). RC, rotator cuff; HH, humeral head; B, biceps tendon.

Plate 10-2. **(A)** Mild fraying of the articular surface of the supraspinatus tendon (*right*). **(B)** Significant partial thickness tear on the articular surface of the supraspinatus tendon (*left*). RC, rotator cuff; HH, humeral head.

Plate 10-3. Normal subacromial space (*left*). A, acromion; D, deltoid fascia; CA, coracoacromial ligament; RC, rotator cuff.

Plate 10-4. Posterior bursa curtain obscuring the rotator cuff. A trocar is seen anteriorly against the coracoacromial ligament (*right*). BC, bursal curtain; RC, rotator cuff.

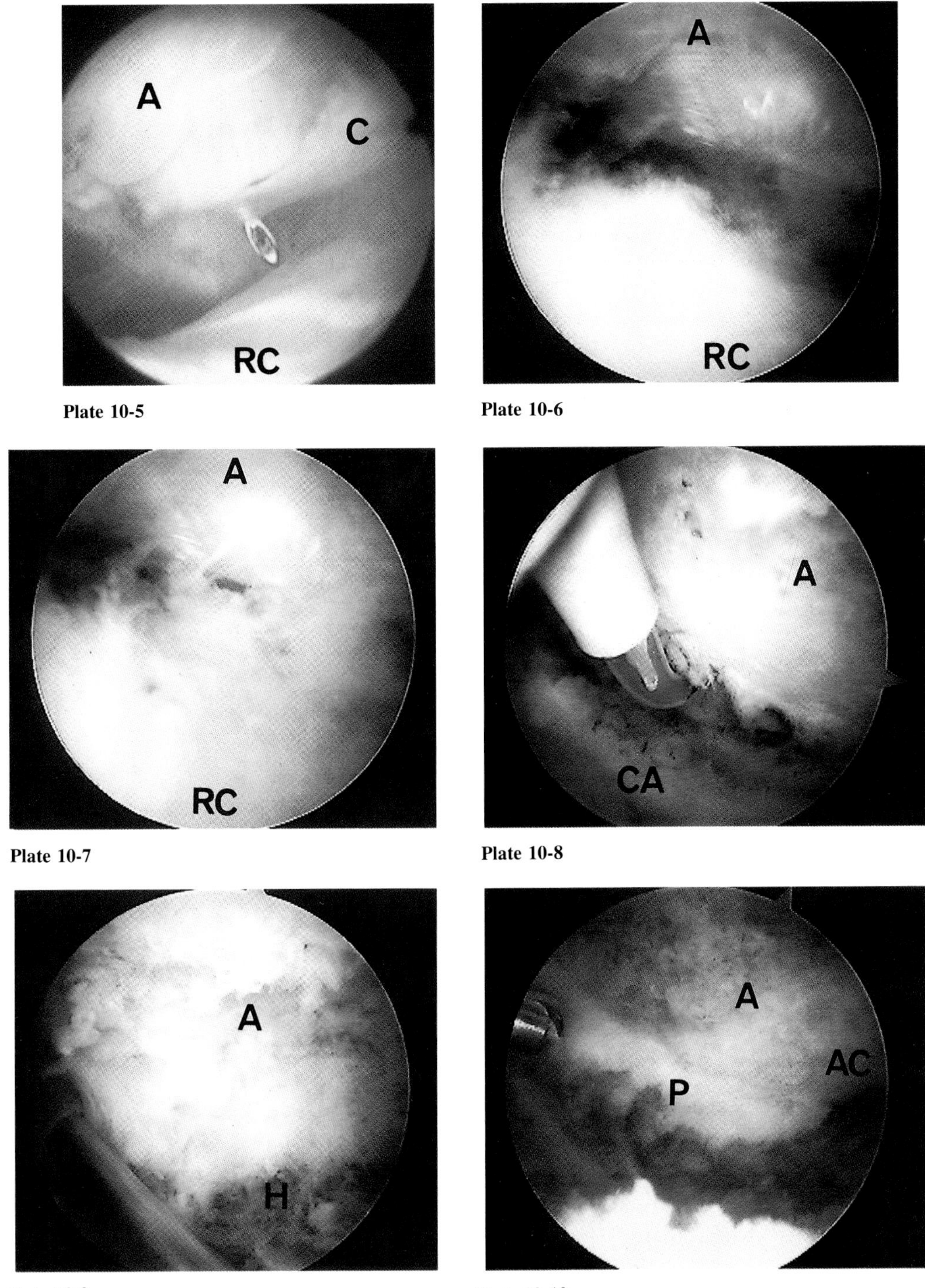

Plate 10-5

Plate 10-6

Plate 10-7

Plate 10-8

Plate 10-9

Plate 10-10

Plate 10-5. Subacromial space with needle inserted through the acromioclavicular joint. Note the overlying fat pad at the joint (*left*). A, acromion; C, clavicle; RC, rotator cuff.

Plate 10-6. Abrasion of undersurface of acromion at the anterolateral corner and fraying of the bursal surface of the supraspinatus tendon (*right*). A, acromion; RC, rotator cuff.

Plate 10-7. Abrasion of bursal surface of the supraspinatus tendon. Prominence of the anterior acromion is due to the presence of an anterior acromial hook (*left*). A, acromion; RC, rotator cuff.

Plate 10-8. Use of the electrocautery on the anterior acromion to release the coracoacromial ligament and for hemostasis (*left*). A, acromion; CA, coracoacromial ligament.

Plate 10-9. Anterior acromial hook debrided of soft tissue (*left*). A, acromion; H, acromial hook.

Plate 10-10. Appearance after acromioplasty. Note anterior periosteal sleeve (*left*). A, acromion; AC, acromioclaviclar joint; P, periosteal sleeve.

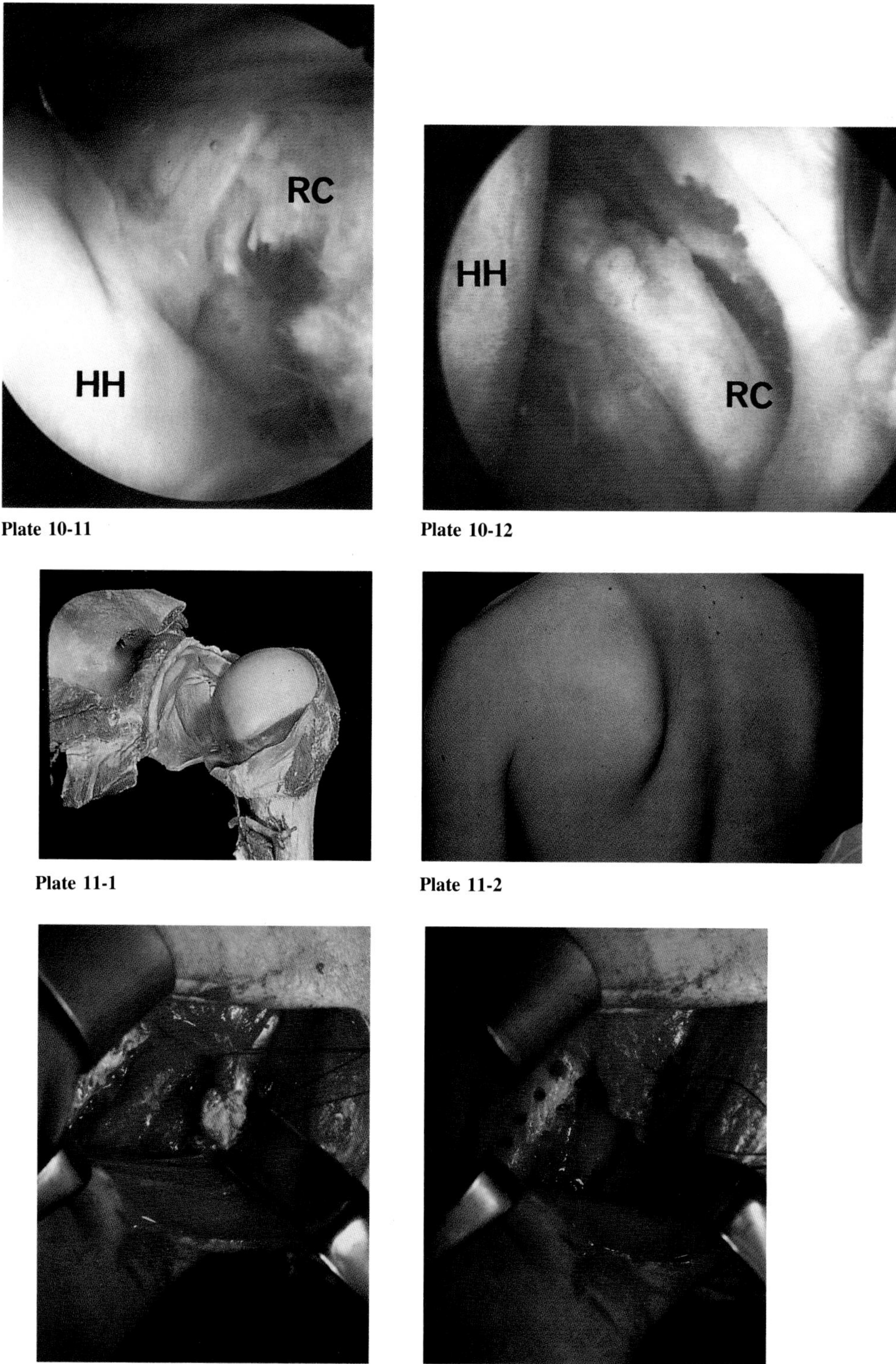

Plate 10-11

Plate 10-12

Plate 11-1

Plate 11-2

Plate 21-1

Plate 21-2

Plate 10-11. Small full-thickness tear of the supraspinatus tendon (*left*). RC, rotator cuff; HH, humeral head.

Plate 10-12. Long-standing massive tear of the rotator cuff (*left*). RC, rotator cuff; HH, humeral head.

Plate 11-1. Ligaments of shoulder viewed from behind showing superior, middle, and inferior glenohumeral ligament and an inferior pouch.

Plate 11-2. Scapular dysfunction, common in the athlete's painful shoulder.

Plate 21-1. Intraoperative photograph demonstrating avulsion of the right pectoralis major tendon from its insertion. Patient was an Olympic gymnast.

Plate 21-2. Intraoperative photograph of the patient seen in Plate 21-1 demonstrating the double row of cortical holes fashioned in the intertubercular groove of the humerus.

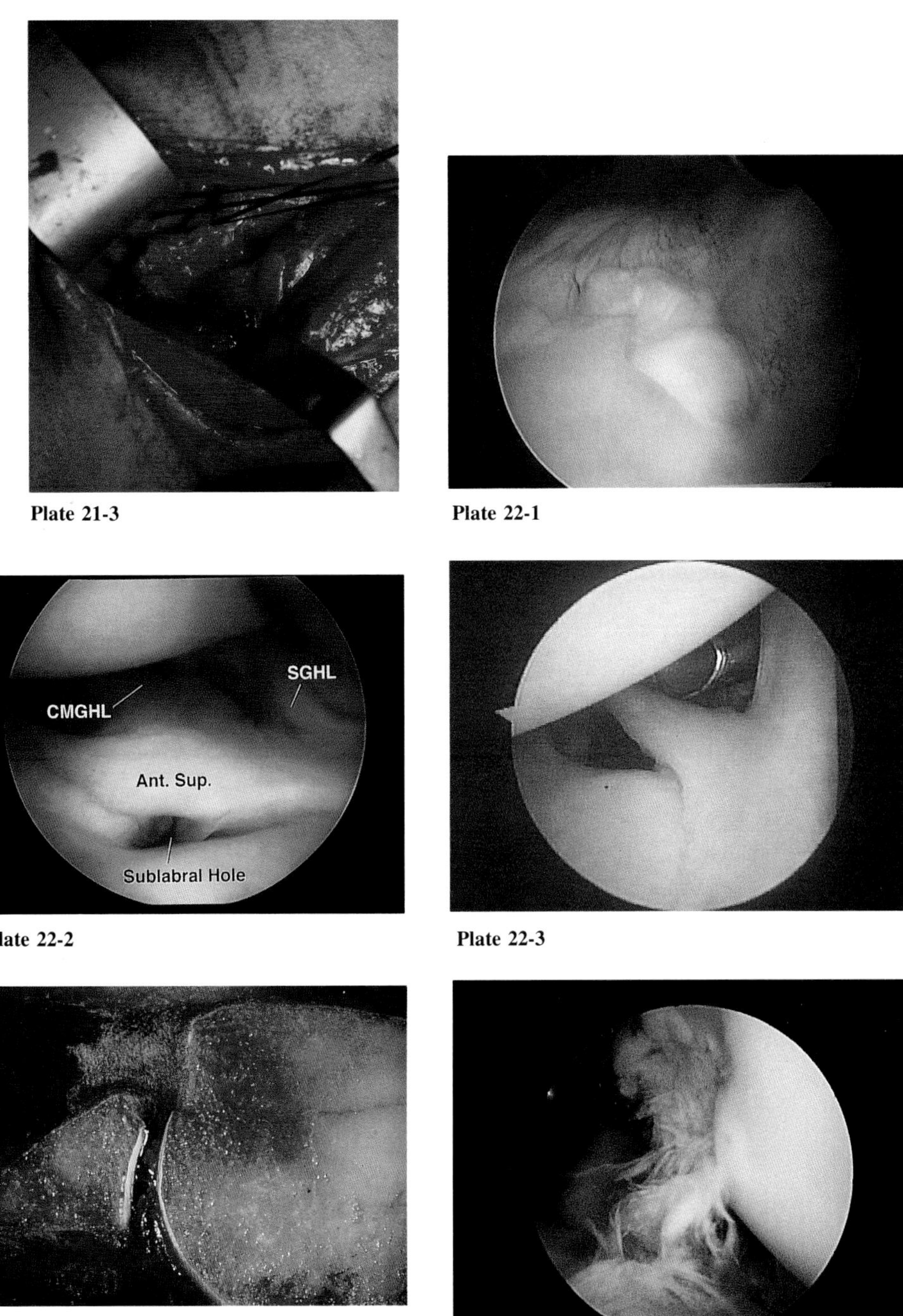

Plate 21-3

Plate 22-1

Plate 22-2

Plate 22-3

Plate 22-4

Plate 22-5

Plate 21-3. Intraoperative photograph of sutured pectoralis major tendon after passage of the sutures.

Plate 22-1. A free central edge of the labrum is a normal variant that appears meniscoid. This superior labrum should not be confused with pathologic detachment.

Plate 22-2. Normal sublabral hole in the left shoulder. In this case, it is associated with a cordlike middle glenohumeral ligament (CMGHL) attaching to the anterosuperior labrum (Ant. Sup.). A normal superior glenohumeral ligament (SGHL) is present.

Plate 22-3. Buford complex. There is a cordlike glenohumeral ligament and absent anterosuperior labral complex.

Plate 22-4. The posterior labrum and cuff may be compressed between the bony glenoid and greater tuberosity when the arm is placed in the throwing position, as seen in this cadaver specimen. (Courtesy of Christopher M. Jobe, M.D.)

Plate 22-5. A humeral head chondromalacic ''kissing lesion.'' Such lesions occur secondarily as a result of labral degeneration.

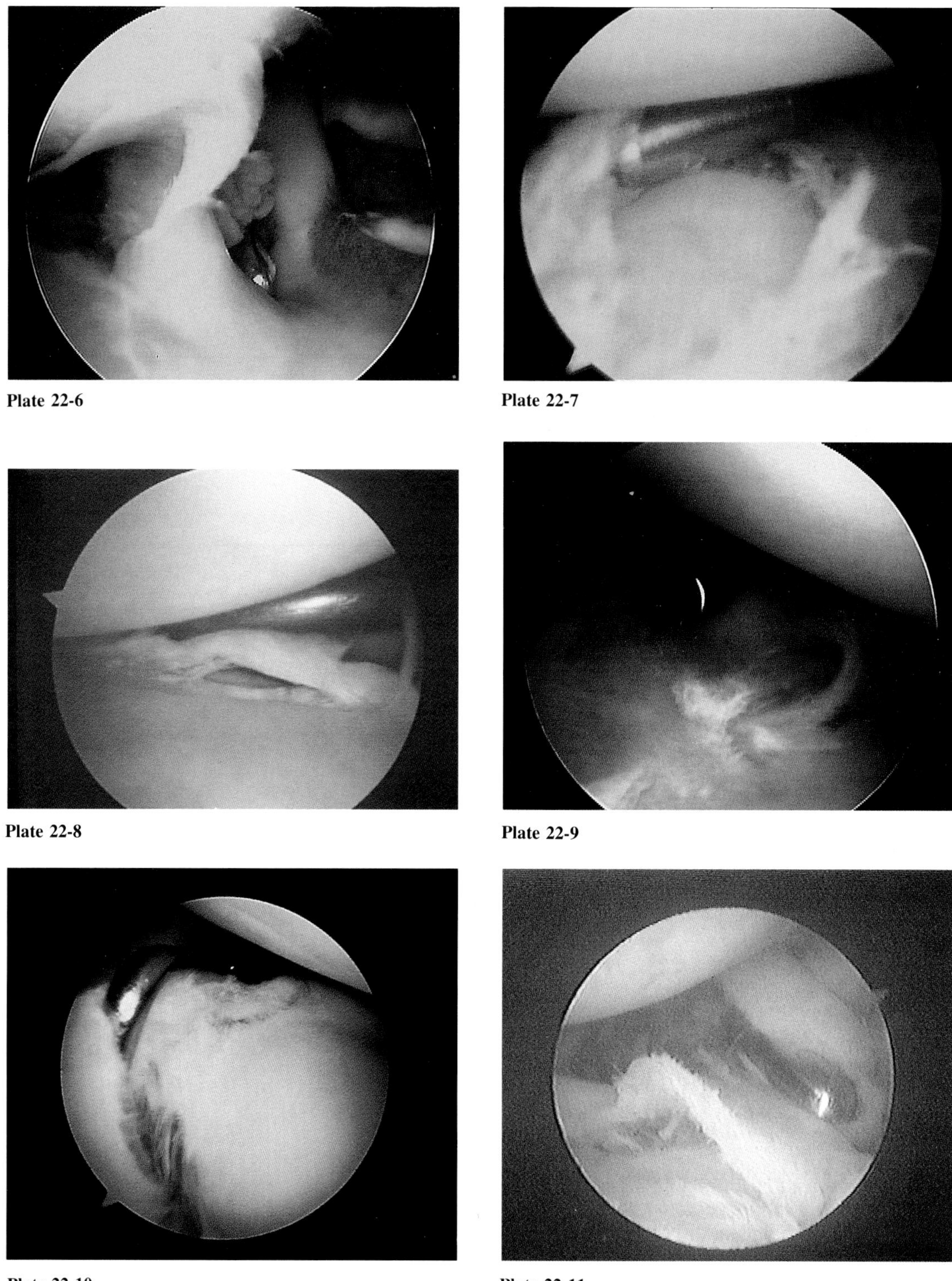

Plate 22-6

Plate 22-7

Plate 22-8

Plate 22-9

Plate 22-10

Plate 22-11

Plate 22-6. Significant anterosuperior labral flap tear. An isolated labral tear may be associated with glenohumeral instability.
Plate 22-7. Anteroinferior glenoid labral tear and articular defect (GLAD lesion).
Plate 22-8. Bucket-handle labral tear. Such tears are rare and may cause considerable mechanical symptoms without true instability.
Plate 22-9. SLAP type I lesion. (See Plate 22-4.)
Plate 22-10. SLAP type II lesion. (See Plate 22-7.)
Plate 22-11. Normal variant of meniscoid superior labrum. Such variants may have the appearance of a type II SLAP lesion.

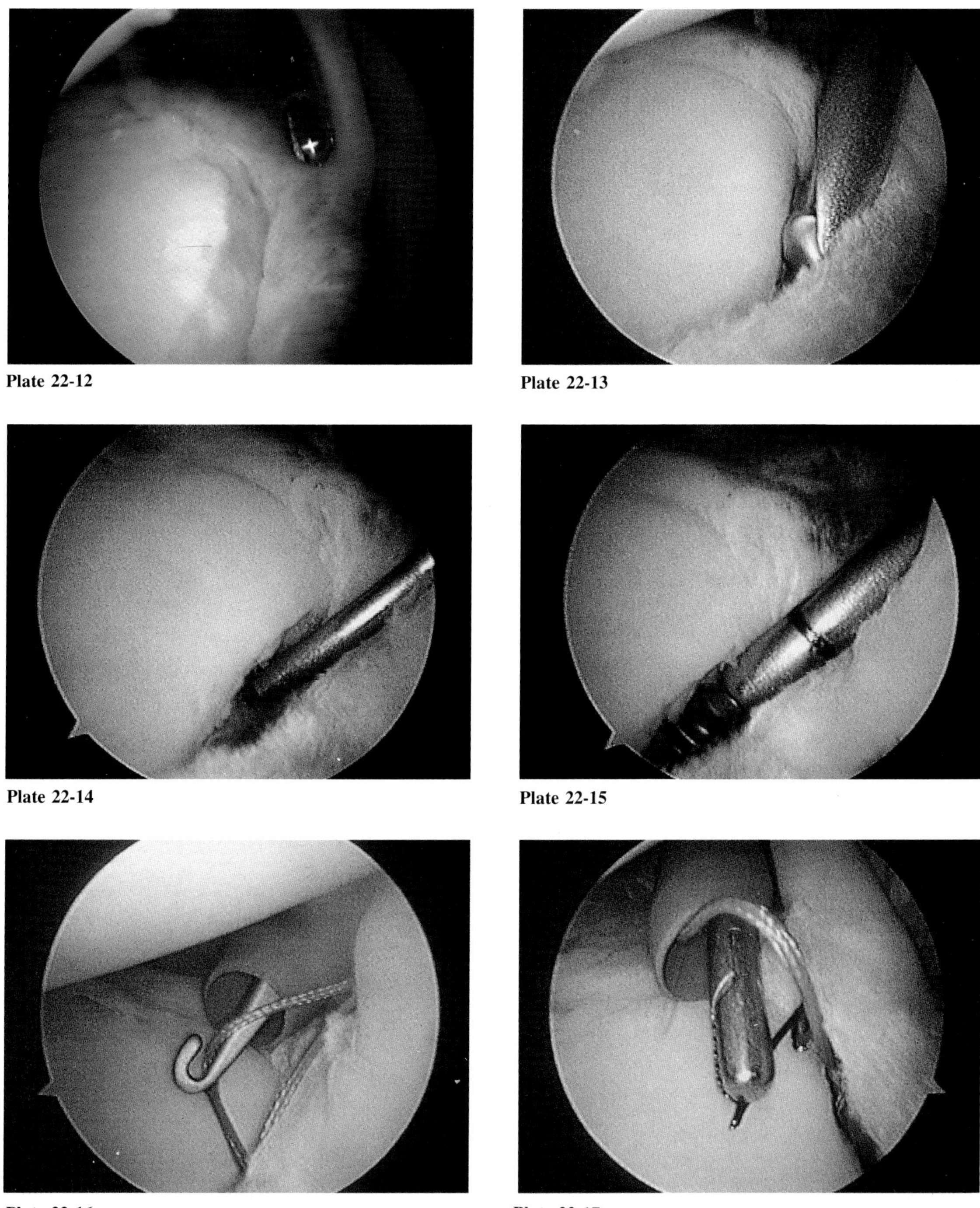

Plate 22-12 Plate 22-13

Plate 22-14 Plate 22-15

Plate 22-16 Plate 22-17

Plate 22-12. A type II SLAP lesion that arches away greater than 3 to 4 mm from the underlying glenoid. This is consistent with pathologic detachment.
Plate 22-13. A 4.0-mm ball-shaped burr is helpful in decorticating the exposed bone beneath the biceps tendon anchor.
Plate 22-14. A drill or a punch is inserted through the anterior superior portal and maintained at a 45-degree angle to the articular surface.
Plate 22-15. A suture anchor device, loaded with a #2 braided permanent suture, is passed through the anterosuperior cannula into the prepared hole below the biceps anchor.
Plate 22-16. One limb of the suture is then retrieved through the anterior midglenoid portal.
Plate 22-17. A 6-inch 17-gauge epidural needle is inserted through the anterosuperior cannula to pierce the labrum and biceps anchor. A suture Shuttle Relay (Linvatec Inc., Largo, FL) is then passed through the tissues and retrieved with a grasper through the anterior midglenoid portal.

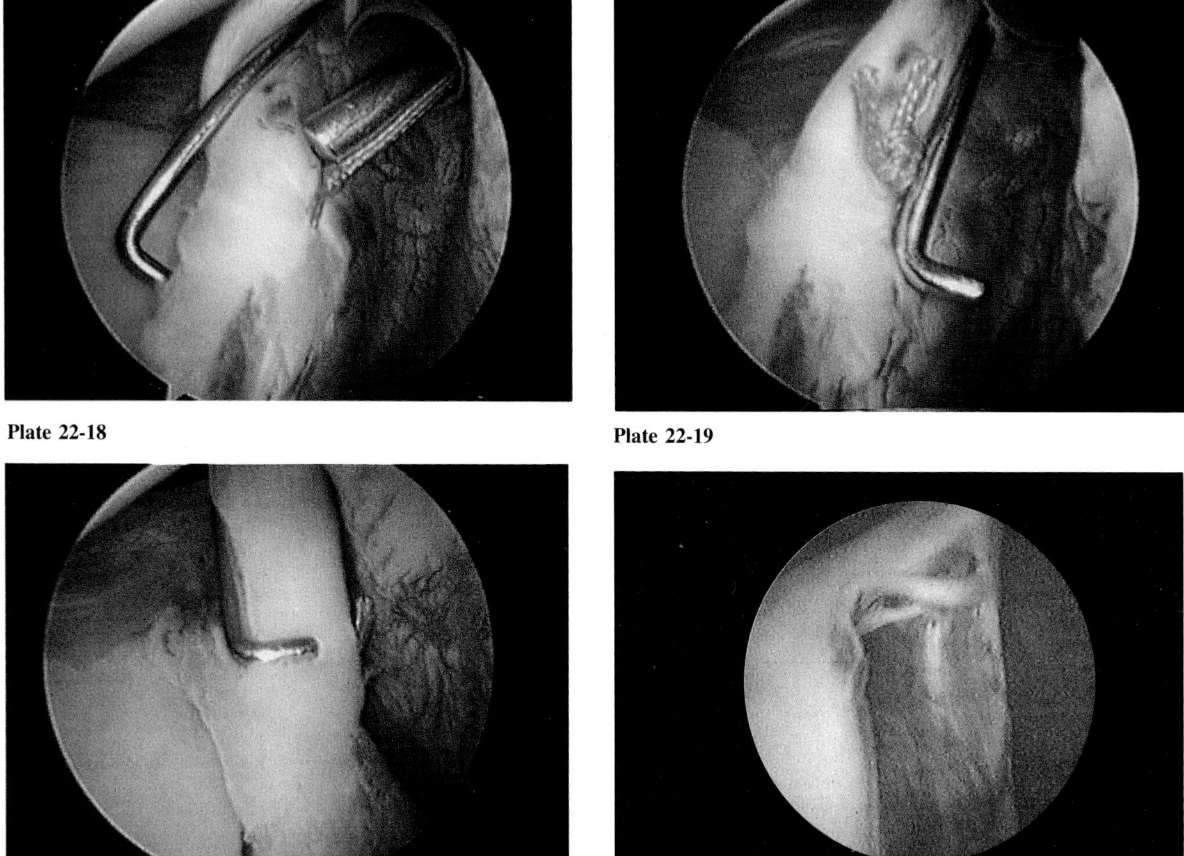

Plate 22-18

Plate 22-19

Plate 22-20

Plate 22-21

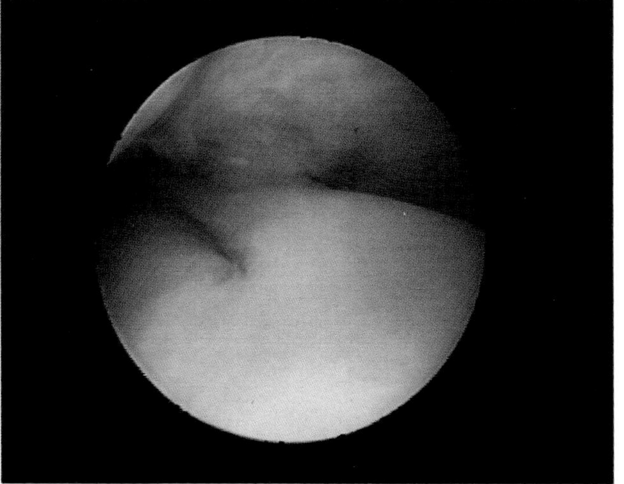

Plate 28-1

Plate 22-18. The two limbs are tied with a knot-pushing device, while a probe is used to hold the labrum and the biceps anchor is reduced.
Plate 22-19. The final appearance of the SLAP lesion repair is shown here after cutting the suture tails.
Plate 22-20. A palpating probe should be used to test the integrity of the repaired SLAP lesion.
Plate 22-21. A type IV SLAP lesion with greater than 30 percent of the biceps tendon involved should be evaluated for repairs or tenodesis.
Plate 28-1. Arthroscopic findings of internal impingement with undersurface partial rotator cuff tear associated with a ''kissing lesion'' on the posterosuperior glenoid labrum.

CHAPTER SEVEN

Basics of Shoulder Arthroscopy

David S. Morrison
Joshua Port

Diagnostic and surgical arthroscopy of the shoulder are well-established but continually evolving procedures. The history of diagnostic arthroscopy dates back to 1931 when Berman viewed cadaveric shoulders.[3] Clinical arthroscopy of the shoulder was first reported in 1965 by Andren and Lundberg.[2] In the past 15 years, the popularity of shoulder arthroscopy has increased, as have the number of operative procedures technically feasible. As with the knee, there is a learning curve in the application of arthroscopic techniques to the shoulder. A thorough knowledge of the anatomy and pathologic processes about the shoulder are necessary to obtain good results. All the approaches to the shoulder require perforating at least one muscle and one tendon or two muscles before the capsule is entered. The arthroscopic instruments, even properly placed, are never more than a few centimeters from the many neurovascular structures that supply the shoulder girdle and upper extremity. Complications associated with arthroscopic surgery about the shoulder are infrequent provided the surgeon knows the anatomic landmarks, positions the patient and extremity appropriately, and adheres to basic surgical principles.

SET-UP

Most arthroscopic shoulder surgeries are performed with the patient in the lateral decubitus position on the operating table. Support in this position can be achieved with a beanbag or kidney rest. A strip of 4-in. adhesive tape running from the side rails of the bed and across the upper chest can be used to further stabilize the thorax. Appropriate padding of the axilla and peroneal nerves as well as a pillow between the legs minimizes pressure injuries to the skin and neurovascular structures. We prefer to use general endotracheal anesthesia. Anesthesiologists who are familiar with the operation assist in managing the head and shoulder position during surgery. Arthroscopy of the shoulder has been performed under local or interscalene block anesthesia; however, the lateral decubitus position is fairly uncomfortable, and should intubation become necessary in the midst of the procedure, it is likely to be difficult and require repreparing and redraping. A large self-adhesive U-drape is applied along the spine, up over the neck, and down the sternum anteriorly. This keeps the patient and anesthesiologist dry and separated from the operative field. We use an inflatable glove that encloses the hand for traction attachment. This device distributes pressure evenly and avoids radial or ulnar nerve injury. The amount of traction varies between 5 to 15 lb depending on body habitus and ligamentous laxity. Caution should be used when greater weights are applied, as transient traction palsies to the brachial plexus and musculocutaneous and radial nerves have been reported. The position is adjusted to place the arm in 20 degrees of abduction and 15 to 20 degrees of forward flexion. This position may be used for diagnostic and operative arthroscopy of the glenohumeral joint as well as the subacromial space (Fig. 7-1). It provides distraction and inferior subluxation of the glenohumeral joint. Fine adjustments during the procedure can be achieved by having an assistant manipulate the arm. Klein et al[6] in a cadaveric model compared visibility versus

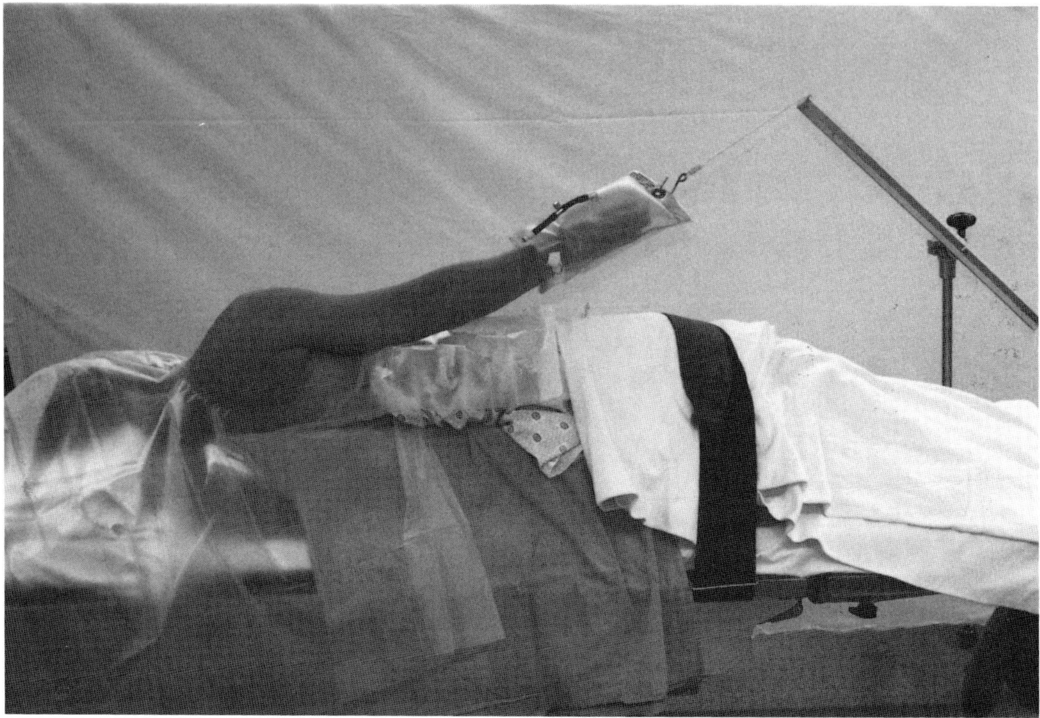

Figure 7-1. The modified lateral decubitus position for shoulder arthroscopy. The patient is supported on a deflatable beanbag. The head, axilla, and trunk are isolated from the operative field by waterproof drapes. Traction is applied via an inflatable glove. Initially, 5 to 10 lb of traction is usually sufficient but may vary due to body habitus.

brachial plexus strain in the lateral position with arm traction. Strain was maximal with 0 degrees of flexion and 10 degrees of abduction. Ninety degrees of flexion and no abduction minimized strain, but the visibility was poor. Our position is a compromise between these two extremes and has resulted in our experience of more than 1,000 consecutive shoulder arthroscopies, with excellent visualization and no neurovascular complications. Traction is applied when the surgeon is ready to make his skin incision. During preparing and draping, we prefer the arm to be held by an assistant. Should joint distraction be necessary during surgery, traction can be applied perpendicular to the midshaft of the humerus. The patient should be positioned on the table such that the glenoid is parallel to the floor, approximately 45 degrees posterior of vertical. This position allows for ease of instrumentation from either the anterior or posterior portal.

Shoulder arthroscopy may also be performed in the "beach chair" position in which the operating table is flexed to 45 degrees and the knees flexed for comfort. A towel or sandbag is placed behind the operative shoulder to bring it forward and clear of the operating table. A Mayfield headrest is used to facilitate access to the posterior aspect of the shoulder. The patient is first placed supine, and interscalene block or general endotracheal anesthesia is administered. The table is then adjusted by flexing at the waist and then at the knees. The head of the table is elevated to at least 60 degrees. This must be done slowly and the patient's blood pressure monitored as orthostatic hypotension, especially in the elderly patient, has been reported. Preoperative loading of the intravascular volume reduces the likelihood of orthostasis. Advantages of the beach chair position are that there is less bleeding and easier access to the rotator cuff should open or limited open operative repair be necessary. Surgery can often be performed without the use of added traction because the weight of the arm alone will open the subacromial space. Also, the capsular anatomy is not placed under nonanatomic stretch. The arm is free to be manipulated to allow a more thorough review of the intra-articular and subacromial anatomy. The beach chair position allows manipulation into internal rotation and easy access to the anterior glenoid for arthroscopic stabilization procedures.[16] The major disadvantages are the increased time to set up and fogging of the arthroscope secondary to irrigation fluid leaking out the posterior portal and onto the instrument due to its dependent position. Also, the beach chair position is somewhat awkward for performing a standard arthroscopic subacromial decompression.

EQUIPMENT

A 4 mm, 30 degree oblique arthroscope is preferred for shoulder arthroscopy. The entire joint can be visualized using this arthroscope and manipulating the arm. The 70 degree arthroscope can be useful in certain instances, especially for visualizing the anterior glenoid and inferior glenohumeral ligament during arthroscopic stabilization procedures. Standard intra-articular arthroscopic instruments used in the knee are appropriate for the shoulder, especially a probe, full-radius resector, arthroscopic burr, pituitary forceps, a tissue grasper, and a wide Shutt resector. To minimize soft tissue trauma due to reinsertions, it is preferable to maintain portals once they have been established. Thus, an interchangeable cannula system is recommended to allow passage of both the arthroscope and the motorized instruments through the same cannula. The cannula is equipped with rubber diaphragms that close while changing instruments and thus help to maintain intra-articular irrigation pressure and joint distention without removal or plugging of the cannulas. The importance of a constant and adequate flow of irrigation fluid during shoulder arthroscopy cannot be overstated. The shoulder region is quite vascular, and because no tourniquet can be used, positive intra-articular pressure aids in visualization. In some cases, it is difficult to control bleeding by increasing the intra-articular fluid pressure, and a good flow of irrigation and directed use of the electrocautery will be beneficial. Extravasation of fluid into soft tissues may be pronounced if care is not taken to establish and maintain portals in a precise position. We use glycine irrigation fluid for shoulder arthroscopy because it allows the use of the electrocautery without changing irrigant. Unlike the urologic literature, no reports of adverse reaction to glycine have been recorded for shoulder arthroscopy. We have used it for several years and hundreds of patients without complications. All shoulder arthroscopy should be performed with controlled blood pressure. True hypotensive anesthesia is not usually necessary, but if the systolic pressure is allowed to rise to more than 120 mmHg, bleeding may be so severe as to require abandonment of the procedure. This is especially critical during subacromial decompression. The topic of hypotensive anesthesia is discussed in more depth in the section discussing arthroscopic acromioplasty.

SURFACE ANATOMY AND PORTALS

Four basic portals are used in shoulder arthroscopy, three for the glenohumeral joint and one additional for the subacromial space. It is helpful to maintain these portals with a cannula or instrument. Because we are passing through as much as 5 to 7 cm of tissue and as many as seven anatomic planes, the chance of re-establishing an identical portal after it has been lost is remote. Establishing a new portal causes unnecessary tissue damage. It is important to palpate the surface anatomy such as the scapular spine, acromion, clavicle, acromioclavicular joint, and the coracoid. Early on, it is sometimes helpful to mark the surface anatomy on the skin. There are four primary arthroscopic portals in the shoulder (Figs. 7-2 and 7-3). Their placement and use are presented in the following sections.

Posterior Portal

The primary portal of entry is posterior and is located 2 cm below and 1 cm medial to the posterolateral corner of the acromion. This portal is the most commonly used one in the shoulder, allowing adequate visualization of most of the joint and facilitating the placement of other portals. Your left hand should be placed on the top of the shoulder with the thumb palpating the "soft spot" and thus the posterior glenohumeral joint line. Then, the index or middle finger is used to palpate the coracoid process. A 5-mm incision is made through skin only, not into the deltoid muscle because this can cause excessive bleeding. A blunt tipped changing rod or trocar is passed through

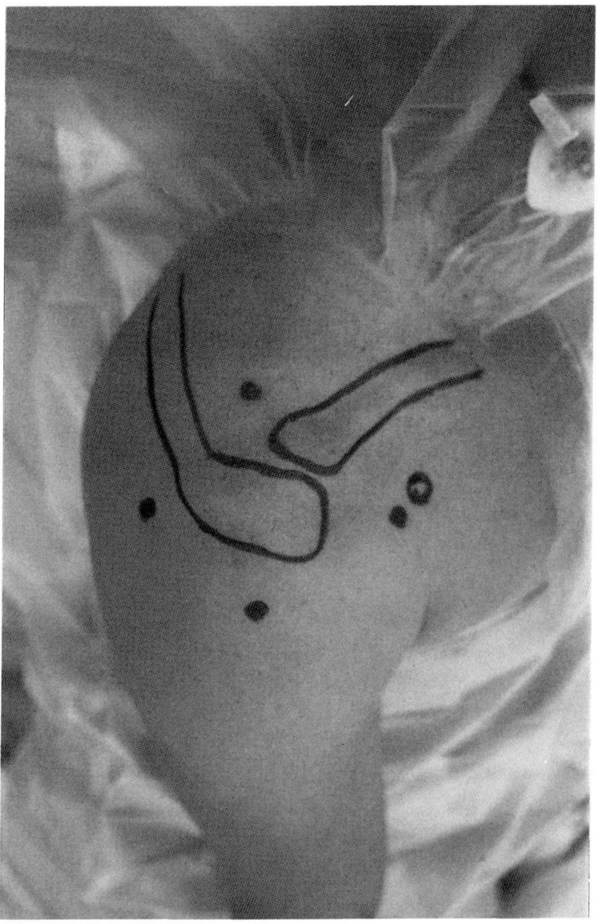

Figure 7-2. Surface landmarks drawn include the acromion and scapular spine, the clavicle, and the acromioclavicular articulation. The posterior, superior, lateral, and anterior arthroscopic portals and the tip of the coracoid (*circle*) are indicated.

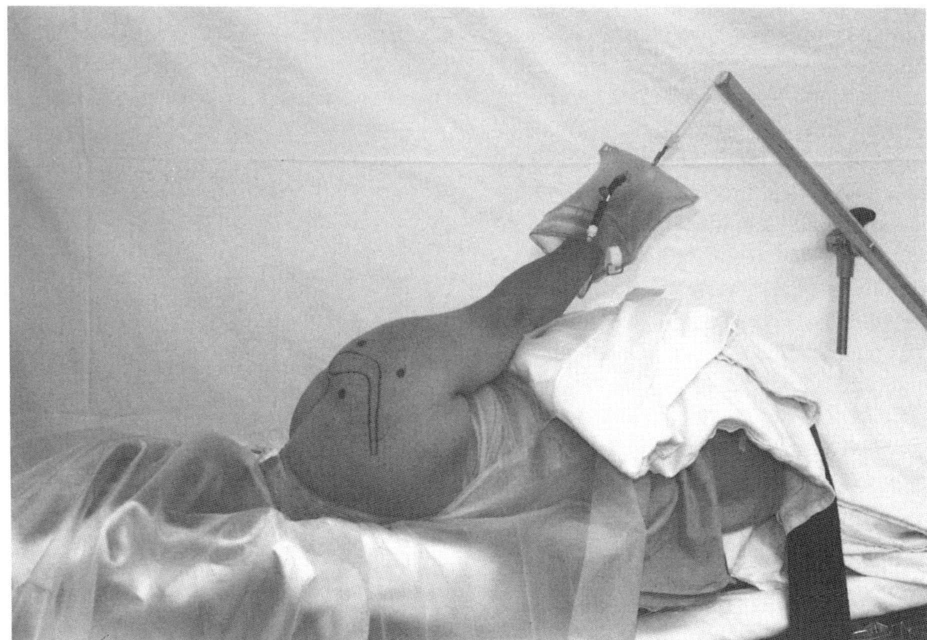

A

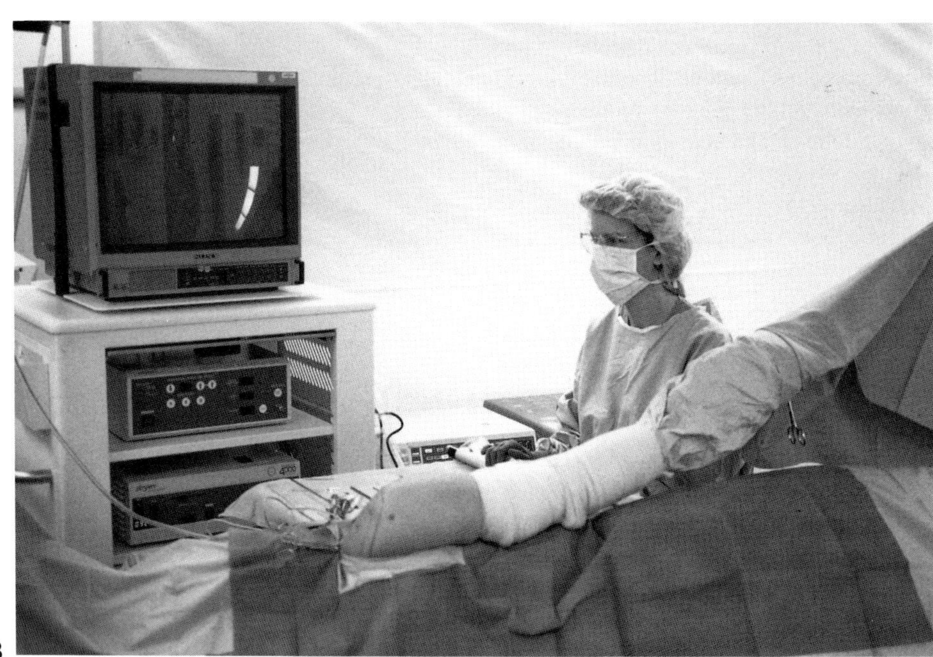

B

Figure 7-3. **(A)** The anatomy as seen in the lateral decubitus position. **(B)** The monitor and the nurse are positioned across the patient from the surgeon. The arthroscopic tools are placed on a stand in direct reach of the surgeon for easy access.

the posterior deltoid angled toward the coracoid process. The blunt tip of the trocar can be used to palpate the curve of the humeral head and the stepoff of the posterior glenoid, and thus the posterior joint line. Once the curve of the head and stepoff of the joint line have been identified, the changing rod is advanced between the humeral head and glenoid and passed through the capsule, feeling a slight pop. Then, the arthroscope cannula is passed over the changing rod and slid into the joint with a twisting motion. It is important to angle the cannula toward the superior aspect of the joint so that when the capsule is entered, the mouth of the cannula does not gouge the articular cartilage of the humeral head. We have not found preinfusion of the glenohumeral joint using a needle and syringe to be useful.

The posterior portal passes through the posterior deltoid, subdeltoid bursa, and infraspinatus or interval between the external rotators and then through the joint capsule.[7]

The suprascapular nerve enters the infraspinatus muscle 2 cm medial to the posterior edge of the glenoid and lies on the neck of the glenoid in that location. The axillary nerve passes through the quadrangular space inferior to the teres minor and innervates this muscle from below. Failure to establish the posterior portal precisely may place these nerves at risk. If needed, a second posterior portal can be made above or below the primary portal, keeping in mind the anatomic restraints of the acromion and axillary nerve.

Anterior Portal

The anterior approach is used mainly for anterior instrumentation and visual examination of the posterior portion of the joint as well as the posterior rotator cuff. Portal placement is performed under direct visualization through the posteriorly placed arthroscope. It is usually placed in the rotator interval, the space between the supraspinatus and subscapularis tendons. There are several ways of establishing this portal; the method used depends on the habitus of the patient and the desired use of this entry. The easiest method is to pass the arthroscope into the rotator interval bounded by the subscapularis tendon inferiorly, the biceps tendon and supraspinatus tendon superiorly, and the anterosuperior glenoid rim posteriorly. When this anterior approach is established, the only muscle pierced is the anterior deltoid. The arthroscope is advanced through the interval toward a point just lateral and slightly superior to the coracoid until resistance is met. The light of the arthroscope can usually be seen through the skin anteriorly, and this assists in placement of the portal. An 18-guage spinal needle is passed through the skin in the direction of the light as the arthroscope is slowly withdrawn to check the position of the needle. In larger patients, this transillumination technique is less reliable. Here, forward pressure is maintained on the arthroscope cannula, the arthroscope removed, and a double-ended changing rod or blunt-tipped Steinmann pin is passed into the cannula. It is advanced through the anterior structures until the skin is tented, and an incision is made to allow exit of the end of the rod through the front of the shoulder. The arthroscopic cannula is withdrawn slightly and the rod advanced carefully. The arthroscope is inserted posteriorly and the back end of the rod visualized within the joint. If the placement is satisfactory, the operative cannula is advanced over the rod from anterior until it enters the joint. Removal of the rod completes establishment of the portal.

This technique may not allow the desired flexibility in positioning, and individualized placement may be necessary. An alternative method useful in operative arthroscopy is to use a large spinal needle to enter the joint anteriorly in the desired location, making a skin incision and advancing the operative cannula with a long tapered blunt trocar into the joint under direct visualization. Because the trocar usually enters the joint with a pop, care should be taken to avoid hitting the arthroscope and damaging its optics. When entering more inferiorly as in the approach for arthroscopic repair of a Bankart lesion, the subscapularis muscle is also traversed with the portal. A second anterior portal for inflow may be placed superior to the long head of the biceps adjacent to the rotator interval portal and along a line between the coracoid process and the acromioclavicular joint, thus through the coracoacromial ligament. The inflow cannula will be kept out of the operative field by the biceps tendon. Care must be taken to always remain lateral to the coracoid when developing either the primary anterior or an accessory anterior portal. By staying lateral to the coracoid and thus lateral to the conjoined tendon, the musculocutaneous nerve that runs along the inferior surface of the conjoined tendon is protected. The brachial plexus is also medial to the conjoined tendon. Also, the axillary nerve lies along the inferior neck of the glenoid and may be put at risk with low anterior portals.

Superior Portal

A third, less commonly used portal is a superior portal through the supraspinatus muscle. This entry is most useful as an irrigation inflow but may also be used for visualization of a limited portion of the rotator cuff, the posterior glenoid labrum, and posterior portion of the humeral head. It may be useful in operative repair of SLAP lesions; however, the use of this portal in operative arthroscopy is limited because of the limitation of mobility caused by the osseous structures that surround it. The entry is bounded anteriorly by the clavicle, laterally by the acromion, and posteriorly by the base of the acromion and the scapular spine. It is bordered inferiorly by the posterosuperior rim of the glenoid.

The junction of the clavicle and the scapular spine with the acromion is palpated and the soft spot identified. A large spinal needle is introduced at a 40 degree angle to the skin, the object being to enter the joint posterior to the attachment of the long head of the biceps just above the posterosuperior glenoid rim.[13] The cannula with trocar is advanced through a skin incision along the same line. The cannula is thus placed behind the glenoid in the posterior joint recess so as not to interfere with visualization or manipulation through the other portals. The superior portal is relatively safe because the only major nerve in the area, the suprascapular nerve, is about 3 cm inferior to the path of entry in the suprascapular notch. The suprascapular nerve passes medial to the base of the coracoid, through the notch, and on to the supraspinatus fossa to innervate the supraspinatus muscle. The rotator cuff is not damaged by this approach as the instruments pass through the muscular portion of the supraspinatus. If a sharp trocar is used, care should be taken to avoid tearing the biceps tendon or its attachment along the posterosuperior glenoid labrum.

Subacromial Portals

Subacromial portals are used for examination of the superficial surface of the rotator cuff for partial- or full-thickness tears and for bursectomy and subacromial decompression. Usually the surgeon has performed an arthroscopic examination of the glenohumeral joint before approaching the subacromial space, so one or two posterior portals are already present at the start of the subacromial examination. The primary posterior portal is often satisfactory for entry of the arthroscope, and the secondary posterior portal can be used for inflow irrigation if the cannula does not interfere with manipulation of the arthroscope. Before the subacromial space is entered, the angle of the arm traction may need to be changed to maximize the acromiohumeral distance rather than the glenohumeral space. After adjustment of the traction, the shoulder should be somewhat subluxated inferiorly, and the gap between the posterior acromion and humeral head should be more easily palpable. The skin incision and deltoid perforation of the primary posterior portal are used to introduce the arthroscopic cannula and blunt trocar into the subacromial space. The angle of entry is changed, however, with the cannula being directed toward the central portion of undersurface of the acromion. Bone and periosteum of the acromion, as well as the coracoacromial ligament, should be palpable with the trocar. The cannula is swept from side to side to open up space and to break up adhesions. The space is then distended through this portal, and the arthroscope is introduced. A second portal for irrigation is sometimes necessary, because bleeding in the subacromial space can be profuse. The second portal should be superior and lateral to the primary posterior portal so that it lies 1 cm below and 1 cm anterior to the posterior angle of the acromion. This procedure is the same as for the primary portal. In some cases, the primary portal is too low and posterior to allow adequate visualization of the coracoacromial ligament and anterior acromion. In these cases, the arthroscope is interchanged with the inflow cannula. This usually improves the field of view significantly. The primary operative portal for the subacromial space is positioned 3 cm distal and lateral to the anterolateral corner of the acromion. This places the instrumentation parallel to the anterior acromion, nearly perpendicular to the fibers of the coracoacromial ligament, and allows for better operative control during subacromial decompression. As with all the shoulder portals, this entry should be maintained with a cannula to avoid excessive damage to the deltoid muscle as a result of instrument changes during the procedure. This, in turn, protects the axillary nerve, which lies along the undersurface of the deltoid, about 5 cm distal to the acromial origin of the deltoid.

Acromioclavicular Portal

The standard posterior portal used for glenohumeral and subacromial visualization lies in such a location that, with a 30 degree arthroscope, it is possible to look down the length of the acromioclavicular joint. The extent of the acromioclavicular joint can be visualized from posterior to anterior and from inferior to superior. The superior acromioclavicular ligaments can be seen after resection of the distal clavicle. If acromioclavicular arthroplasty is planned preoperatively, the surgeon has the option to slightly medialize the standard posterior portal to be in a more optimal position for visualization of the acromioclavicular joint. The standard anterior operative portal through the rotator interval will usually lie approximately 5 cm anterior and inferior to the acromioclavicular joint. This allows placement of arthroscopic equipment in an excellent position to perform resection of the distal clavicle. If a previous anterior portal has not been established, it is useful to place a spinal needle in a similar position, anterior and inferior to the acromioclavicular joint, such that it parallels the direction of the joint. Under direct visualization then, the portal can be established such that passage of instruments will be directly parallel to the acromioclavicular joint and allow good access to the posterior and superiormost aspects of the acromioclavicular joint.

ARTHROSCOPIC ANATOMY AND NORMAL ANATOMIC VARIANTS

It is important to develop a systematic approach to the arthroscopic examination of the shoulder. This results in a thorough examination with less chance of missing pathologic findings. The format outlined here allows for adequate examination with a minimum of wasted motion.

Glenohumeral Joint

The initial approach is made through the posterior portal, and an anterior outflow portal is developed as needed. Often, an 18-gauge needle placed anteriorly gives sufficient outflow to allow satisfactory diagnostic arthroscopy. The biceps tendon is identified and used as a reference throughout the examination. Fraying or partial avulsion of this tendon's insertion on the posterosuperior rim of the glenoid may be seen, particularly in a throwing athlete. Inflammation or wear of the tendon may be seen as it exits the joint at the bicipital groove. By withdrawing the arthroscope slightly, the articular surface of the humeral head is examined. Rotation of the arm and small superior-inferior panning motions allow most of the humeral head to be examined. In addition to nonspecific degenerative changes of the articular surface, a Hill-Sachs lesion may be identified in this manner. A normal finding posterolaterally is the "bare area," a sulcus found between the articular surface and the synovium. The normal bare area has vascular channels and a smooth surface. The pathologic Hill-Sachs lesion found in up to 80 percent of recurrent dislocators is a posterolateral lesion of the articular surface found medial to the bare area. This lesion has a raw cancellous surface distinguishing it from the smooth normal bare area.[1] Next, the glenoid and labrum are examined. Additional distraction is usually necessary for a complete examination. A view of the posterior glenoid and labrum from an anterior portal later in the procedure may be needed for complete visualization. The glenoid labrum should be smooth and have minimal mobility. Degenerative changes may be seen in the glenoid fossa, and lesions of the labrum can be identified. Labral fraying, bucket handle tears, and avulsion of the labrum from the glenoid (Bankart lesion) may be seen. In 35 percent of patients, the anterosuperior quarter of the glenoid labrum is not attached to the glenoid rim. This is not a Bankart lesion, but a normal anatomic variant called a sublabral foramen (Plate 7-1). True Bankart lesions occur below the equator of the glenoid (Plate 7-2). The labrum is variable, usually thinner superiorly and thicker inferiorly. The glenoid itself is then studied. A normal variant exists with a central bare area devoid of cartilage. Observations of the location of glenoid wear or effacement and labral tearing are important clues to the primary direction of pathologic instability and should be noted. The arthroscope is passed anteriorly between the biceps tendon and the humeral head. The subscapularis tendon and recess is visualized, and the superior, middle, and inferior glenohumeral ligaments are identified. Great variability is found in the glenohumeral ligaments, and sometimes it is impossible to distinguish three individual ligaments. The superior glenohumeral ligament appears as a confluence of the capsule at the inferior edge of the rotator interval, between the biceps tendon and the superior edge of the subscapularis tendon.

The middle glenohumeral ligament has wide attachments along the anterior glenoid labrum and may be difficult to distinguish as a discrete structure. It lies inferior to the subscapularis tendon and appears to form a sling along the tendon's deep surface. Of the glenohumeral ligaments, the middle is the most variable; it is not present in all patients.

The inferior glenohumeral ligament is the most important in traumatic anterior and inferior glenohumeral instability. It may be difficult to visualize without additional joint distraction and rotation, which tenses the ligament. The inferior ligament attaches along the anteroinferior edge of the labrum from about the 4- to 6-o'clock position on the face of the glenoid and inserts along the anteroinferior aspect of the anatomic neck of the humerus. The inferior glenohumeral ligament has three distinct portions. The superior band, which is absent in up to 25 percent of normal subjects, tightens to resist anterior translation at 45 to 90 degrees of abduction and resists external rotation with the arm adducted. The axillary recess and inferior portion, with progressive abduction and external rotation, wind up decreasing from the capacious volume in adduction to a tight fibrous band covering the humeral head in full external rotation and abduction.[15]

The biceps tendon is relocated and followed distally until it exits the joint in the bicipital groove. The rotator cuff insertion is now clearly seen with the subscapularis insertion being medial to the biceps and, in order, the supraspinatus, infraspinatus, and teres minor tendons inserting laterally. Rotator cuff tears usually begin in the impingement area, just lateral to the biceps tendon in the substance of the supraspinatus or infraspinatus tendon insertions on the greater tuberosity.[12]

If the posterior aspect of the joint was not well visualized through the posterior portal, the arthroscope is placed through the anterior portal with the inflow posterior. The posterior portions of the glenoid labrum can now be easily examined. Fraying or avulsion (a reverse Bankart lesion) may be seen in shoulders with posterior or multidirectional instability. The axillary recess and the subscapularis bursa must be well visualized as these are frequent locations for loose bodies.

After completing the examination of the glenohumeral joint, the shoulder is drained and the arthroscope is withdrawn. If the anterior portal has been established, it is usually maintained for later installation of 0.5 percent bupivacaine with epinephrine at the completion of the procedure. The arthroscope is introduced into the subacromial space as previously described. If the field is obscured by bleeding, it is sometimes necessary to develop a second portal for irrigation. Some patients have a distinct subacromial bursal space, but most subacromial spaces are filled with multiple loose areolar tissue layers that make visualization difficult. A simple sweeping motion of the arthroscope back and forth often breaks up some of these adhesions and allows for good visualization. If a simple diagnostic subacromial arthroscopy is being performed, the use of motorized instrumentation to resect the tissue is not recommended because the bleeding produced is often counterproductive. The anterior acromion can often be identified by palpating with the inflow cannula through a second anterolateral operative portal. It is sometimes difficult to differentiate the subdeltoid fascia and the undersurface acromion from the coracoacromial ligament, but the ligament should be readily identified by palpating with a blunt probe. The probe can also be used to identify the anterior subacromial hook of a type III acromion or spurs on the undersurface of the acromioclavicular joint. The coracoacromial ligament normally attaches to the undersurface of the anterior third of the acromion, but the attachment may extend laterally all the way around the anterolateral corner and medially onto the undersurface of the clavicle. The ligament is usually 2 to 3 cm wide at its acromial insertion. While looking at the anterior acromion, a simple rotation of the arthroscope 180 degrees permits examination of the superficial surface of the rotator cuff in the impingement area. If this is not well visualized, the arm can be brought up into 30 or 40 degrees of abduction by an assistant. To differentiate the rotator cuff from subacromial bursa, an assistant can take the arm through internal and external rotation maneuvers. Bursal tissue will remain more or less stationary, whereas the rotator cuff will move in synchrony with the humeral head. In this way, partial- or full-thickness rotator cuff tears can be identified. After completing the subacromial examination, the subacromial space is drained and 20 ml of 0.5 percent bupivacaine with epinephrine instilled, the cannula is removed, and all skin wounds are closed with 3-0 nylon.

OPERATIVE INDICATIONS AND PROCEDURES

Loose Body Removal

Although not as common as in the knee, osteochondral loose bodies can be a source of pain and clicking in the shoulder. They are most often found in patients who have sustained single or multiple dislocations in which there is a Hill-Sachs defect in the humeral head or a glenoid rim fracture. They also occur in shoulders with advanced arthritis, particularly that due to avascular necrosis in which portions of the crescent lesion have broken free. Loose bodies tend to be particularly difficult to appreciate by arthrography in the shoulder and may be better visualized by computed tomographic scan or arthroscopy. The operative approach is that for a diagnostic arthroscopy, and a thorough systematic examination is performed. Loose bodies in the shoulder are usually found in the inferior pouch below the glenoid, the posterior recess behind the glenoid, and the subscapularis recess. If the subscapularis recess is not readily viewed from the posterior portal, switching the arthroscope anteriorly may bring loose bodies trapped there into view. Loose bodies also have a predilection for the biceps tendon and can be found in synovial folds behind the biceps tendon insertion on the glenoid and in the area where the tendon exits from the joint at the bicipital groove. If loose bodies are found, their etiology is considered. If there is a Hill-Sachs lesions or glenoid fracture, glenohumeral instability must be ruled out as the patient's primary pathology.

Synovectomy and Biopsy

Diagnostic arthroscopy with synovial biopsy or operative arthroscopy for synovectomy can be performed satisfactorily in the shoulder. In the absence of a joint effusion, it can be difficult to perform aspiration and synovial biopsy of the glenohumeral joint, and specimens obtained may be inadequate for a diagnosis. The arthroscope can be used to sample the synovium selectively under direct vision, thus increasing the chance of a tissue diagnosis. Total synovectomy as an open procedure is difficult for the surgeon and debilitating for the patient. The arthroscopic approach, however, allows for near-total synovectomy without disrupting the deltoid or rotator cuff. The approach is the same as for operative arthroscopy. Again, adequate irrigation must be established early, because bleeding can be brisk. Once again, maintenance of hypotensive anesthesia and adequate irrigation pressure will allow for better visualization and a more thorough and accurate procedure. The motorized synovial resector is introduced anteriorly first, then exchanged with the arthroscope posteriorly. A full-radius tip works well. It may be necessary to establish additional anterior and posterior portals to complete the synovectomy.

Drainage and Debridement

In many cases, it is possible to perform a satisfactory debridement and drainage of the glenohumeral joint for pyarthrosis via arthroscopy. The procedure can be performed several times if necessary. When successful in controlling the infectious process, arthroscopy avoids the morbidity of an open procedure. You should always be prepared, however, to proceed with incisional drainage should it be needed. The arthroscope has advantages over repeated needle aspirations in that the surgeon can break up intra-articular loculations manually, direct irrigation and drainage throughout the joint, and debride necrotic tissue. Also, a drain can be placed directly through the arthroscopic cannula for suctioning.

Labral Tears

In the shoulder, symptomatic lesions of the glenoid labrum similar to those seen with the meniscus of the knee may be treated arthroscopically. All configurations seen in the knee can also be seen in the shoulder. The glenoid labrum, however, is very different anatomically from the meniscus. Its structure, composition, and function are continuing sources of debate. Mosely et al[10] described the labrum as primarily fibrous tissue, in contradistinction to the knee meniscus, which is fibrocartilage. There is a small fibrocartilaginous component within the labrum, confined to its attachment to the glenoid rim. The most important difference between the glenoid labrum and the knee meniscus is that, in the shoulder, the capsule and ligaments, including the biceps tendon, are attached to and become part of the glenoid labrum, which in turn attaches to the glenoid. Thus, lesions of the labrum suggest more significant pathology, such as glenohumeral instability. Aside from nonspecific fraying, the most common type of tear is a circumferential tear in which the labrum is pulled off the glenoid along its rim. Occasionally, a true bucket handle tear that can be dislocated into the joint is seen. These tears are often found in conjunction with a Bankart lesion, in which the labrum and attached ligaments are avulsed from the glenoid rim. This is diagnostic of glenohumeral instability. The Bankart lesion is usually found on the anteroinferior or posteroinferior glenoid rim. Detachment of the labrum between 12 and 3 o'clock on the anterior glenoid rim is a normal anatomic variant and need not be resected or repaired.

Circumferential tears are also seen along the anterosuperior and posterosuperior rim. The term *SLAP lesion,* which stands for superior labrum anteroposterior, has been coined for this problem.[14] The etiology of the lesion is unclear but may be due to excessive strain on the long head of the biceps caused by a rapid deceleration of the arm during the follow-through of the throwing motion. We believe, however, that forced abduction and external rotation brings the greater tuberosity to bear on the superior labrum-biceps complex, damaging these structures or pushing them off the glenoid rim.

Complex tears and transverse or parrot beak tears may be seen in conjunction with circumferential tears or as isolated entities. If the underlying problem is glenohumeral instability, then simple resection of the tear is unlikely to alleviate the symptoms completely. In many patients, however, resecting a torn labrum results in symptomatic relief. Only the loose or frayed portion should be removed because further resection can compromise the attachments of the glenohumeral ligaments and capsule and thus produce instability, while at the same time making future operative repair more difficult or impossible.

Biceps Tendon Lesions

Lesions at the biceps tendon within the glenohumeral joint occur in two locations: at the attachment of the tendon to the superior labrum and glenoid rim, and at the bicipital groove as the tendon exits the joint. Fraying and partial detachment of the tendon from the rim of the glenoid with or without accompanying labral pathology can be seen, particularly in the throwing athlete. This has been called the SLAP lesion. Some believe that debriding these lesions with a motorized instrument is beneficial, but why this should be the case is unclear at present. Repair of the lesions is a development procedure, and long-term results are not yet known. The lesions at the bicipital groove are suggestive of subacromial impingement syndrome and usually occur on the superior surface of the tendon. Biceps tendinitis as an isolated entity is rare. More commonly, irritation of the tendon is the result of impingement of the anterior acromion on the area of the greater tuberosity and the bicipital groove. This causes the tendon to become inflamed and erythematous and results in fraying if the process continues. Debridement of the ragged portion of the tendon may stimulate healing and give temporary relief. The underlying process of subacromial impingement syndrome, however, must be addressed, otherwise symptoms will recur.

Subacromial Decompression

Anterior acromioplasty and coracoacromial ligament resection for chronic subacromial impingement lesion as described by Neer[11] is simple and has an excellent success rate. It has one major drawback, which is also its major source of morbidity: detachment of the anterior deltoid. This delays active use of the shoulder for 4 to 6 weeks and may result in weakness and pain if the deltoid is not properly reattached or if avulsion of the repair occurs postoperatively. Arthroscopic decompression avoids this major source of complications because the deltoid is not detached.

In 1985, Morrison and Bigliani[8] showed that there is a direct correlation between the morphology of the acromion and rotator cuff tears. Most rotator cuff tears occur in patients with type III acromions that have a hook on the anteroinferior surface. The goal of arthroscopic subacromial decompression should therefore be to remove this hook, which will convert the type III or hooked acromion to a type I or flat acromion. As much bone can be removed arthroscopically as is removed through open techniques. A definite correlation exists between the amount of bone removed and the results of arthroscopic subacromial decompression. Arthroscopic decompression is indicated in patients with symptomatic chronic subacromial impingement syndrome of greater than 6 to 8 months' duration that has been unresponsive to aggressive conservative management. More than 70 percent of patients treated with an adequate conservative management protocol will obtain long-term symptomatic relief without surgery.[5] Contraindications to acromioplasty alone are the presence of a rotator cuff tear, symptomatic acromioclavicular joint arthritis, or calcific tendinitis. The use of combined procedures to address both impingement syndrome and these concurrent pathologies has proved safe and effective. Positioning and operative portals are described in the section on operative technique (Fig. 7-4). After establishing the arthroscopic portal and high-volume irrigation portal, the primary operative portal is developed. We use glycine as our irrigation fluid. The subacromial space is examined and the coracoacromial ligament is identified (Plate 7-3). It is sometimes difficult to distinguish the ligament from periosteum and bursa, but its acromial attachment can be delineated by placing needles at the anterior edge of the acromioclavicular joint and the anterolateral corner of the acromion. Coagulation current is used to divide the ligament between the two needles under direct visualization. A cautery may be used as necessary to control bleeding. The acromial branch of the thoracoacromial artery travels along the superior surface of the most medial portion of the ligament. Time should be taken to coagulate this artery because bleeding can be profuse. If adequate hypotensive anesthesia is present and if irrigation pressure is proper, often the artery can be seen pulsating before coagulation. After resecting the ligament, the undersurface of the acromion is attended to. Using the full-radius synovial resector, bursa and periosteum are removed from the anterior third. A large arthroplasty burr is used to perform the acromioplasty (Plate 7-4). The goal is to remove enough bone to flatten the slope of the anterior acromion. The full-radius resector is used to remove residual fragments of bone, periosteum, and bursa (Plate 7-1). The subacromial space is drained, 30 ml of local anesthetic with epinephrine instilled, and skin wounds closed with sutures. The lateral portal can be enlarged enough to admit the surgeon's fifth finger into the subacromial space (Fig. 7-5). The acromion and distal clavicle can then be palpated to determine the adequacy of the acromioplasty. If the acromion has not been flattened or if residual spurs are present, they can be removed under direct visualization. We recommend the use of this manual palpation for a surgeon's first 40 or 50 subacromial decompressions. In fact, some experienced shoulder arthroscopists use this palpation technique routinely on all their cases.

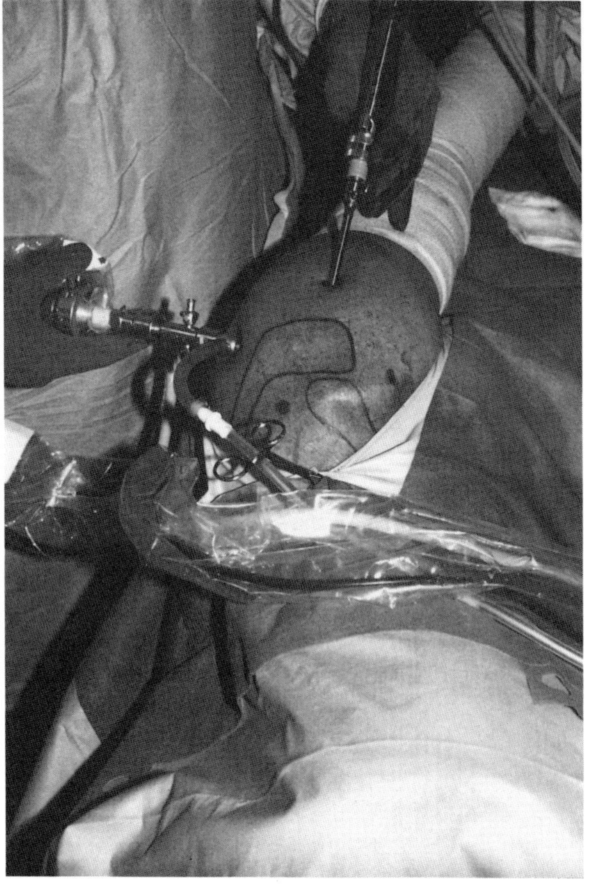

Figure 7-4. The arthroscope is in the posterior portal and the motorized tissue resector is in the lateral portal. Arthroscopic subacromial decompression can be performed using only these portals.

Any surgeon who has performed an arthroscopic subacromial decompression has encountered vigorous bleeding at some time during the procedure. If the coracoacromial artery is cut in a hypertensive patient, the massive bleeding can result in abandonment of the arthroscopic procedure and open coagulation. At other times, sinusoidal and bursal bleeding is so extensive that adequate visualization cannot be obtained even to perform the acromioplasty, and the procedure may have to be abandoned in favor of an open operation. To avoid these problems, we recommend the use of controlled blood pressure during any arthroscopic shoulder surgery. We recommend that systolic pressure be kept at about 95 mmHg and an irrigation pressure of at least 50 mmHg be used. This can be obtained either with gravity inflow, which is preferred, or with an arthroscopic pump. With control of the blood pressure and adequate inflow irrigation pressure, it is possible to cut the coracoacromial artery under direct visualization, observe the bleeding, and coagulate it without loss of clarity of the visual field. This would be impossible in a normotensive patient. An added benefit of controlling the blood pressure during the procedure is that irrigation pressures can be significantly lower, thus greatly decreasing the amount of fluid extravasation. Extravasation is not only unsightly and of concern to the patient but also significantly lowers the patient's core temperature, making the patient more uncomfortable and increasing the probability of anesthetic chills in the immediate postoperative period. With an expe-

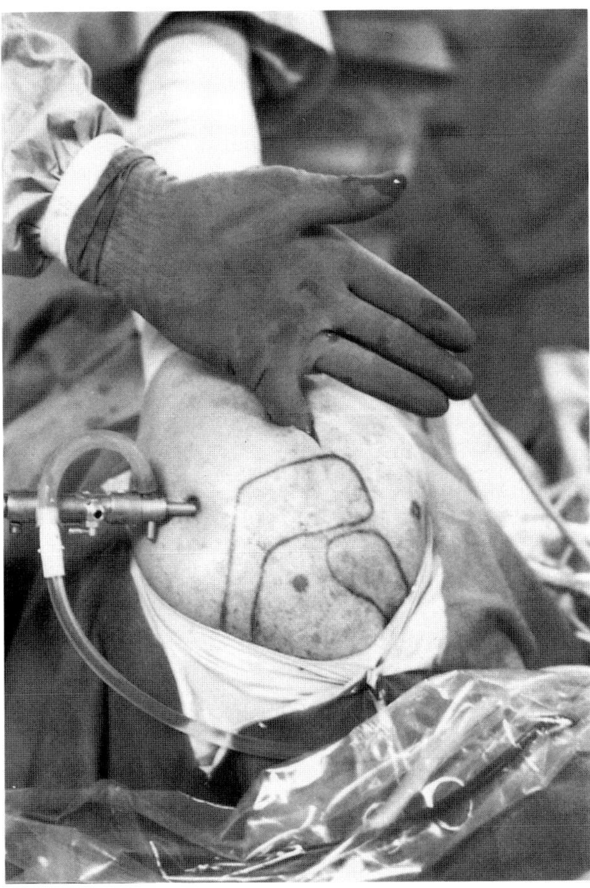

Figure 7-5. The small finger can be inserted through the extended lateral portal to check the adequacy of the subacromial decompression.

rienced anesthesiologist, it is unnecessary to use arterial lines to obtain blood pressures in the area required. We have performed more than 700 consecutive subacromial decompressions using these techniques with no complications whatsoever and believe that controlled blood pressure is the key to adequate visualization in shoulder arthroscopy.

After surgery, the arm is placed in a sling for comfort, but the patient is encouraged to use the arm for all light activities and to discard the sling as soon as possible. A standard rehabilitation program is undertaken. There are no restrictions to normal active use, although strenuous or repetitive overhead activities are discouraged for 3 to 6 weeks.

Rotator Cuff Tears

As with bicipital tendinitis, most rotator cuff tears are caused by chronic subacromial impingement. The exception is in the young athlete, in whom tears are usually partial thickness and related to trauma. The trauma may be a single violent episode but is more commonly repetitive in nature, such as throwing or competitive swimming. Tears are usually located near or at the insertion of the supraspinatus tendon on the greater tuberosity. For these lesions, subacromial decompression is usually unnecessary because the symptoms can be controlled by modifying the kinematics of the athlete's activity. There is some suggestion that recovery may be accelerated by arthroscopic debridement, which is believed to stimulate healing of the partial-thickness tears. Debridement of full-thickness rotator cuff tears without repair cannot be recommended. The preferred treatment of a full-thickness rotator cuff tear remains operative repair; debridement and decompression alone do not give satisfactory results. Attempts have been made to perform a true arthroscopic rotator cuff repair through the use of staples and other anchoring devices. Currently, these procedures remain developmental. The advantages of arthroscopic subacromial decompression is in the preservation of the deltoid origin. Open decompression and rotator cuff repair is not necessary in all patients. Instead, we have developed a technique for a limited open rotator cuff repair after arthroscopic subacromial decompression. The size of the rotator cuff tear can be very accurately diagnosed using magnetic resonance imaging with true sagittal images.[9] If a rotator cuff tear is less than 2 cm in diameter, it is possible to perform an arthroscopic subacromial decompression and then repair the rotator cuff through a limited deltoid splitting incision without detaching the anterior deltoid. This preserves the deltoid origin, allowing early mobilization, and is much less painful than a formal open rotator cuff repair. Often, the procedure can be performed on an outpatient basis. After completing arthroscopic subacromial decompression, we extend the anterolateral operative subacromial operative portal to the edge of the lateral acromion and distally to a total length of 3 to 4 cm. The deltoid is split in the line of its fibers, and a self-retaining retractor is used to expose the underlying rotator cuff (Fig. 7-6). The remaining bursa has a thick and gelatinous appearance because of the irrigation used during the arthroscopic procedure. It must be totally excised to allow adequate exposure of the cuff. Although the skin incision is small, it is inevitably directly over the rotator cuff tear, and excellent exposure of the full extent of the rotator cuff can be obtained by simple internal and external rotation of the humerus at the side. A trough is cut at the articular margin as in a more formal, open procedure. The tear is repaired using large nonabsorbable sutures, pulling the edge of the rotator cuff down into a trough in the bone, and obtaining fixation via a horizontal mattress technique with the ends of the sutures being brought out and tied over the lateral humerus. Often, a stout needle is sufficient to pass these sutures through

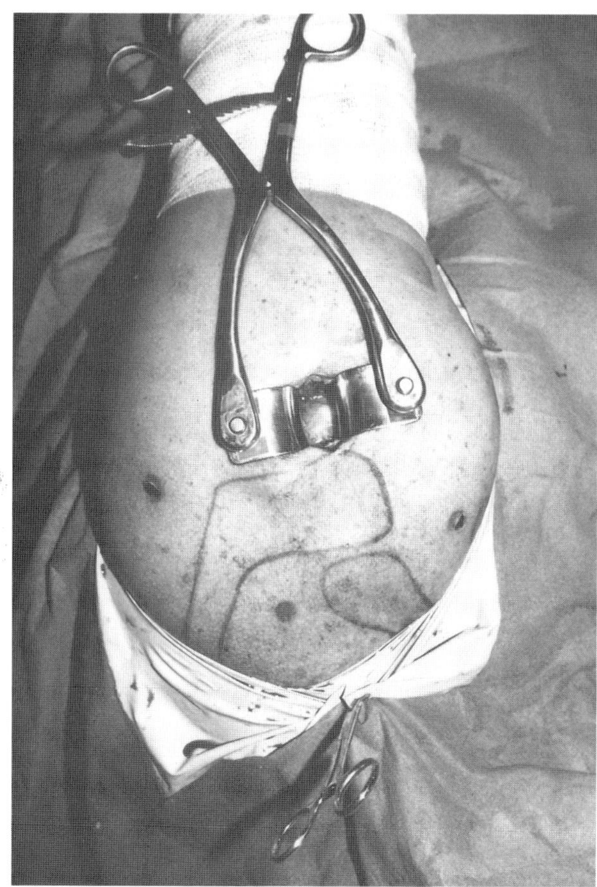

Figure 7-6. A modified Korbel retractor placed under the deltoid provides excellent visualization for the rotator cuff repair.

osteoporotic bone, but in younger patients, drill holes may be required. This is facilitated by abducting the arm, bringing the lateral humerus up into the wound to allow easy passage of the sutures, and then returning the arm to the side to pass the sutures through the rotator cuff. Multiple interrupted inverted figure of eight sutures are used for a solid repair. If the tear is larger than 2 or 3 cm in diameter or if it is very old, the standard technique of open rotator cuff repair can be added. If the tear is larger than expected, the limited procedure is abandoned and the incision is carried across the anterior acromion and 2 cm of anterior deltoid for greater exposure. This is usually unnecessary, however, if adequate preoperative planning and diagnostic imaging has been used. During arthroscopy of the glenohumeral joint, if a partial-thickness rotator cuff tear is seen or if there is some question as to whether the tear is full thickness, we use a marking suture passed directly through a spinal needle placed into the area of the tear. This suture is located on entering the subacromial space, and under direct vision, the area through which the suture passes is carefully inspected to determine whether the tear is partial thickness or full thickness. A probe is usually necessary for adequate evaluation of the cuff. The partial-thickness tear is inevitably located underneath the area of maximal impingement, and bony resection in that location should be reviewed to ensure that an adequate decompression has been obtained.

Staple Capsulorrhaphy

The first use of bone staples to reattach an avulsed inferior glenohumeral ligament was described in 1931 by Fouche.[1] Dutoit and Roux[4] also found this procedure to be successful. Modifications of the original procedure are still used today. The instrumentation is available to perform staple capsulorrhaphies arthroscopically. Even in the best of hands, this technically difficult procedure yields only an 80 to 85 percent satisfactory result. Because of this, many surgeons have abandoned this procedure in favor of alternative open or arthroscopic techniques. The best candidates for arthroscopic stabilization are those with a Bankart lesion and well-defined middle and inferior glenohumeral ligaments. In a shoulder with multiple dislocations, the glenohumeral ligaments may be shredded and torn away from the labrum rather than remaining attached to it as in a classic Bankart lesion. In this case, staple capsulorrhaphy is difficult and the repair tenuous. Likewise, patients with multidirectional instability are poor candidates for arthroscopic stabilization. Given the above limitations, the repair may be performed on patients with unidirectional anterior instability, although we do not recommend it in high-demand athletes. Staple capsulorrhaphy will likely be replaced with absorbable techniques or newer suturing techniques using anchors. Staple capsulorrhaphy needs to be mentioned for historic perspective and for cognizance of its potential complications.

The major complications encountered with this procedure relate to the placement of the staples. If the head of the staple is within the joint or the prongs penetrate the articular surface, devastating damage to the articular surface of the humeral head can result. Also, if the shoulder should redislocate, the prominent heads of the arthroscopic staples can gouge out large sections of humeral articular cartilage. Multiple modifications of this technique using bioabsorbable staples, screws, and tacks are being developed and look very promising. They all have the advantages of the staple technique but do not risk the multiple complications of metal devices. The general principle of the repair is to try to attach the thick healthy portion of ligament slightly more superior and medial than its original anatomic location and onto a bed of meticulously prepared, burred, bleeding bone. Enough fixation must be provided to maintain the tissue in that position until tissue healing is adequate. Most investigators agree that failure is caused by either poor tissue or an inadequate period of immobilization. It is difficult to evaluate the position of nonmetal devices because they are not seen on plain radiographs.

Capsulorrhaphy Using Suture Anchors

Suture anchors can be used arthroscopically to repair capsulolabral lesions. Anteroinferior, anterosuperior, and the standard posterior portals are necessary for adequate visualization. Initially, viewing can be from the anterosuperior portal with a 30 degree arthroscope or from posterior with a 70 degree arthroscope; later placement of the most proximal sutures and anchors is best viewed from posterior to avoid crowding of the anterosuperior portion of the joint.

After arthroscopic examination of the glenohumeral joint, a full-radius resector and periosteal elevator are used to trim and mobilize the inferior glenoid labrum ligamentous complex, which has often healed medially. Internal rotation of the arm relaxes the anterior capsular structures and allows for more mobilization and anatomic repair under less tension. Next, a full-radius resector and a motorized burr are used to decorticate the glenoid rim and scapular neck to bleeding bone to create a fibroblastic bed.

A large 8.5-mm threaded arthroscopic cannula is then placed in the anteroinferior portal for instrumentation. A Mitek guide and drill are inserted, and three holes are drilled, positioned as far superiorly and inferiorly as possible within the lesion and midway between the two. It is critical for the holes to be at the anterior border of the cartilage surface and not on the glenoid neck to accomplish anatomic repair of the labrum. The angle of the holes should be 15 to 20 degrees to the plane of the glenoid surface. A suture hook passes size 0 or 1 PDS suture through the ligament complex. With this technique, 0.5 to 1 cm of plication is possible and is determined by the amount of tissue grasped by the suture hook. A suture grasper retrieves through the cannula, the inner limb of the suture over which the suture anchor is then passed. The suture anchor is additionally secured to its inserter with a size 0 Dexon suture to avoid loss of the anchor within the joint. The anchor, once secured in its hole, allows sliding of the suture; a slipknot is tied outside the cannula and advanced and tightened with a knot pusher. In general, three sutures are sufficient, but some cases require individualized variations.

Postoperatively, 3 weeks of immobilization are followed by range of motion to tolerance and sling use at night, for a total of 6 weeks. At 6 weeks, active and passive range of motion are aggressively pursued. Wolf[17] reported on 50 cases of suture anchor capsulorrhaphy with no intraoperative complications and only one recurrence.

Suture Capsulorrhaphy

New techniques have been devised using suture material to repair Bankart lesions and stabilize the shoulder arthroscopically. At present, there are multiple proprietary techniques available, and no single procedure has been shown to be superior to others. Today's techniques will eventually be replaced by the absorbable technology previously discussed or by newer suture techniques. For this reason, we do not present a lengthy discussion of the technique of suture capsulorrhaphy. Rather, we would like to make some recommendations as how to avoid complications and improve results with the current techniques. The goal of any arthroscopic stabilization is to reattach the inferior glenohumeral ligament to the anterior glenoid rim. In the suture technique, drill holes are made in the anterior glenoid rim and sutures passed through the glenoid in a front-to-back fashion. These are then tied, either anteriorly or posteriorly, to reapproximate the labrum to the glenoid. The placement of the drill holes is the major source of error and complications in suture capsulorrhaphy. Anteriorly, the drill holes should be just at the interface between the articular cartilage and the subchondral bone or just below the subchondral bone. In this way, when the labrum is reapproximated to the glenoid, it will be pulled up on the articular margin and into its normal anatomic position. The major error here is to make the drill holes too far down on the glenoid neck, so that the reapproximated labrum is below the level of the articular surface and thus fails to reconstruct the cup-shaped interface between the labrum and articular cartilage complex. The step-off produced allows the humeral head to subluxate anteroinferiorly, resulting in wear and degenerative changes of the anteroinferior third of the glenoid, as well as the humeral head. This may occur even though gross dislocations have been corrected by the arthroscopic procedure.

Posteriorly, the suprascapular nerve, after winding around the spinoglenoid notch, passes approximately 1.5 cm medial to the articular surface of the glenoid. Drill holes for the suture technique that attempt to parallel the subchondral bone and exit the glenoid at its posterior neck must be extremely accurate. Slight angulations away from the articular cartilage place the nerve in jeopardy when the posterior cortex of the glenoid is exited. A safer and more accepted technique directs the drill more medially. This approach decreases risk to the neurovascular structures and also allows the sutures to be tied in a more proximal portion of the infraspinatus muscle belly, thus minimizing muscle damage secondary to necrosis. A small skin incision is made at the area where the drill exits the posterior scapula and splits the infraspinatus muscle in a line of the fibers, exposing the underlying body of the scapula, and the sutures are tied over the bone so as not to tether the infraspinatus muscle. Another major area of concern is the placement of the sutures through the labrum ligament complex. It is important to pass the sutures inferior enough on the avulsed labrum so that, when tied, the labrum ligament complex is advanced and secured to its anatomic position or just above. Failure to adequately advance these ligaments superiorly results in poor coaptation of the ligaments on the glenoid neck as well as a redundant inferior capsular pouch and thus persistence or recurrence of instability. Postoperatively, a period of immobilization followed by a therapy protocol similar to that used in the open techniques allows for healing before return to athletics.

Acromioclavicular Joint Arthroplasty

A partial acromioclavicular arthroplasty can be performed during arthroscopic decompression. Often, the inferior surface of the joint, due to its shape or presence of osteophytes, may contribute to impingement syndrome. In these cases, the supraspinatus outlet can be further decompressed by beveling the undersurface of the acromioclavicular joint. This often violates the capsule of the acromioclavicular joint, however, and may result in painful acromioclavicular joint postoperatively. When there is pain in the acromioclavicular joint preoperatively, a complete excisional arthroplasty of the joint should be considered. Physical therapy and increased activity after arthroscopic acromioplasty can exacerbate any pre-existing painful acromioclavicular arthritis and result in failure of an otherwise satisfactory procedure if subacromial decompression is performed in isolation. The acromioclavicular arthroplasty can be performed open or, as we prefer, arthroscopically. The arthroscopic procedure is performed through the same anterior rotator interval portal, which is located 3 cm below the anterior aspect of the acromioclavicular joint (Fig. 7-7). The portal placement is facilitated by use of a large spinal needle. The spinal needle is directed from anterior in such a position as it is parallel to the acromioclavicular joint. The portal is then made in this position. The arthroscopic burr is used to remove 5 mm of distal clavicle and 2 mm of the acromial articulation. We have found that 5 to 7 mm of bone removal is optimal; if more bone is removed, the incidence of unsatisfactory results increases. Care should be taken to preserve the superior acromioclavicular ligaments and joint capsule, as this will help maintain stability of the distal clavicle and prevent dimpling of the skin over the area of resection (Plate 7-5). Operative visualization is best obtained through the standard posterior portal. If an acromioclavicular joint resection is planned preoperatively, often the posterior portal can be medialized slightly to allow better visualization from posterior using a 30 degree arthroscope. An adequate amount of bone must be removed posteriorly and superiorly. These sections of the clavicle are somewhat more difficult to visualize, and failure to do so may result in inadequate resection.

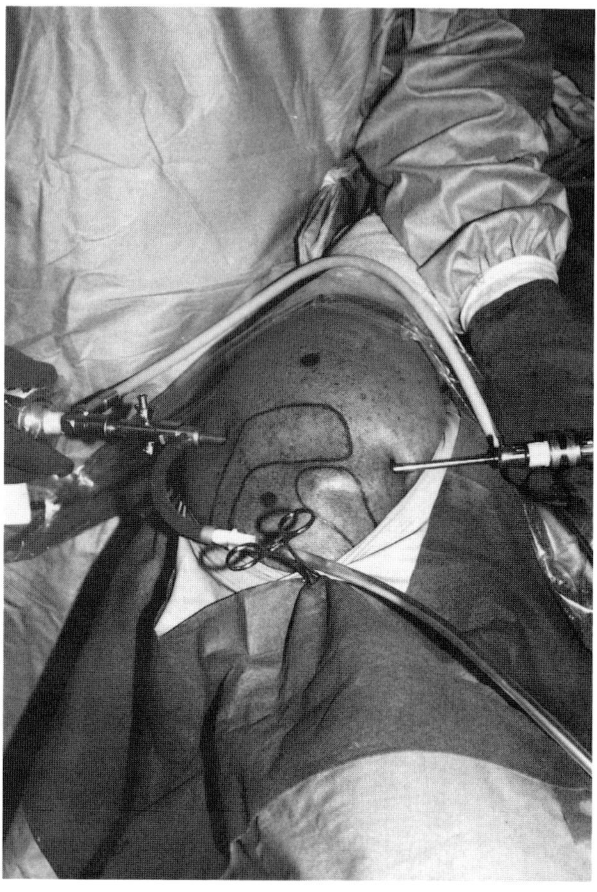

Figure 7-7. The motorized resector can be placed in the anterior portal parallel to the acromioclavicular joint for arthroscopic distal clavicular resection.

Degenerative Conditions

Arthritic conditions and rotator arthropathy present a special problem. Their correction requires major open surgery in the form of total shoulder replacement or massive rotator cuff repair. Unfortunately, these conditions occur most frequently in an elderly population in which such surgery may not be desirable. Shoulder arthroscopies have shown some promise in the partial control of these disorders without the significant morbidity of major open surgery. In degenerative arthritis, it is possible to remove loose bodies and portions of the osteophyte about the humeral head to allow increased motion and decreased pain. Also, there appears to be short-term decrease in pain simply by the irrigation during an arthroscopy. Gentle manipulation under anesthesia can also be performed at the time of shoulder arthroscopy and, when combined with an intra-articular debridement, will often give patients a significant short-term decrease in pain. It should be remembered, however, that the best treatment for patients with significant degenerative arthritis is replacement arthroplasty of the shoulder. Likewise, in patients with massive rotator cuff tears or early rotator cuff tear arthropathy, partial debridement may be in order. These patients may be told that no attempt is being made to improve their function, rather their goal is simply to decrease pain. An arthroscopic subacromial decompression in conjunction with a bursectomy and synovectomy is used in these patients; however, in our experience, increase in function is extremely unpredictable and should not be expected postoperatively. This debridement is considered only in patients with massive irreparable rotator cuff tears. In any patient in which the cuff can be mobilized, an open operative repair should be considered if medically feasible. The most predictable satisfactory results in terms of pain relief and function remain with open rotator cuff repair. Postoperatively, rehabilitation is begun as soon as possible to maintain and increase the range of motion and return patients to active use of the extremity.

CONCLUSION

Shoulder arthroscopy is well established. Knowledge of surface and underlying anatomy is critical to safely use this technology. Developmental procedures presented here are rapidly expanding the therapeutic indications of shoulder arthroscopy. We must use the new technologies with sound surgical judgment to minimize patient morbidity and maximize patient satisfaction.

REFERENCES

1. Altchek DW, Skyhar MJ, Warren RF: Shoulder arthroscopy for instability. Course Lect 38:187, 1989
2. Andren L, Lundberg BJ: Treatment of rigid shoulders by joint distention through arthrography. Acta Orthop Scand 36:45, 1965
3. Berman MS: Arthroscopy or the direct visualization of joints: an experimental cadaver study. J Bone Joint Surg 13:669, 1931
4. Dutoit GT, Roux D: Recurrent dislocation of the shoulder, a 24-year study of the Johannesburg stapling operation. J Bone Joint Surg [Am] 38:1, 1956
5. Frogameni AD, Morrison DS, Woodworth P: Conservative management for subacromial impingement syndrome. Presented at American Shoulder and Elbow Surgeons Specialty Day, American Academy of Orthopedic Surgeons, San Francisco, 1993
6. Klein AH, France JC, Mutschler TA, Fu FH: Measurement of brachial plexus strain in arthroscopy of the shoulder. Arthroscopy 3:45, 1987
7. Mathews LS, Terry G, Vetter WL: Shoulder anatomy for the arthroscopist. Arthroscopy 1:83, 1985
8. Morrison DS, Bigliani LU: Variations in shape and their relationships to subacromial impingement. Orthop Trans 1986
9. Morrison DS, Ofstein RA: The use of MRI in the diagnosis of rotator cuff tears. Orthopedics 13:633, 1990
10. Mosely HF, Overgaard B: The anterior capsular mechanism in recurrent anterior dislocation of the shoulder: morphological and clinical studies with special reference to the glenoid labrum and the glenoid ligaments. J Bone Joint Surg [Br] 44:913, 1962
11. Neer CS II: Anterior acromioplasty for the chronic impingement syndrome in the shoulder. J Bone Joint Surg [Am] 54:41, 1972
12. Neer CS II: Impingement lesions. Clin Orthop 173:70, 1983
13. Neviaser TJ: Arthroscopy of the shoulder. Orthop Clin North Am 18:361, 1987
14. Snyder SS, Karzel RP, DelPizzo et al: SLAP lesions of the shoulder. Arthroscopy 6:274, 1990
15. Turkel SJ, Panio MW, Marshall JL et al: Stabilizing mechanisms preventing anterior dislocation of the glenohumeral joint. J Bone Joint Surg [Am] 63:1208, 1981
16. Warner JJP: Shoulder arthroscopy in the beach chair position: basic setup. Tech Orthop 1:147, 1991
17. Wolf EM: Arthroscopic capsulolabral repair using suture anchors. Orthop Clin North Am 24:59, 1993

CHAPTER EIGHT

Rotator Cuff Disorders

Anthony Miniaci
Paul A. Dowdy

Codman[9–11] was the first to make a plea for the recognition of rotator cuff disorders. He made astute clinical observations of the patients he found had complete rupture of the supraspinatus tendon and stated that most of these patients were older than 40 years of age, were heavy laborers, and commonly had associated acromioclavicular and biceps tendon pathology. Our current understanding of rotator cuff disorders stems from the vast clinical experience of Dr. Charles Neer. Neer[45,46] has proposed a clinical staging system and treatment plan for patients with recalcitrant rotator cuff pathology.

Rotator cuff pathology is a common and disabling ailment affecting athletes who usually participate in overhead sports, most notably baseball, football, tennis, golf, and swimming.[19,31,32,35,36,38,39] Rotator cuff disorders can occur in athletes of all calibers. To manage these injuries optimally, it is essential to have an accurate approach and understanding of the rotator cuff.

ROTATOR CUFF FUNCTION

The rotator cuff forms an integral and essential part of the shoulder. It is generally agreed that the main functions of the rotator cuff are to provide dynamic stability to the glenohumeral joint, provide a fulcrum for flexion and abduction, provide strength in abduction and internal and external rotation, and perhaps provide a watertight seal to enhance cartilage nutrition.

The rotator cuff acts as a dynamic stabilizer preventing anteroposterior and superior-inferior glenohumeral translation during motion. In 1944, Inman and colleagues,[27] by inserting electrodes into the shoulder muscles, found that the rotator cuff (especially subscapularis, infraspinatus, teres minor) functions to depress the humeral head through the arch of flexion and abduction. Basmajian and Bazant,[1] in an electromyographic and morphologic study, found the supraspinatus was an important factor in preventing downward dislocation of the adducted shoulder. Similarly, Poppen and Walker,[60] in a cadaveric study, found that the supraspinatus, subscapularis, and infraspinatus compressed the humeral head into the center of the glenoid cavity throughout the arc of flexion and abduction. In a separate investigation, these authors found that the average glenohumeral excursion in the superior-inferior plane was less than 1.5 mm between each 30 degree arc of motion.[59] They attributed this to the rotator cuff tendons because patients with rotator cuff tears had greater excursion. D'Alessandro et al[13] found that the rotator cuff and deltoid muscle are important dynamic stabilizers of the glenohumeral joint. They performed an electromyographic analysis of 13 normal shoulders during a resisted apprehension test and found that, anteriorly, the pectoralis major and subscapularis were the most important dynamic stabilizers, whereas the infraspinatus and posterior deltoid were most important posteriorly. They concluded that this information should be used in designing rehabilitation protocols for patients with rotator cuff problems. Glousman et al[20] found that patients with anterior shoulder instability have overactivity of the supraspinatus and biceps but decreased activity of the subscapularis, pectoralis major, latissimus dorsi, and serratus anterior in a position of instability. They proposed that the supraspinatus and biceps were working to try to overcome the instability, while the lack of subscapularis activity was exacerbating the instability.

Saha[64] has shown that the supraspinatus initiates abduction, and this occurs only because of the fixed fulcrum provided by the rotator cuff as it depresses the humeral head against the glenoid so the deltoid can function efficiently. Burkhart[8] imaged 12 shoulders with known massive rotator cuff tears fluoroscopically. He found that patients with tears of the superior rotator cuff (supraspinatus and a portion of the infraspinatus) had stable fulcrum kinematics. The patients with tears of the superior and posterior rotator cuff (infraspinatus plus teres minor) subluxed anteriorly and posteriorly and could not establish a fulcrum. Patients with massive tears involving all four rotator cuff tendons had an acromial-humeral fulcrum.

The rotator cuff provides significant power to the shoulder. Colachis and Strohm[12] used selective axillary and suprascapular nerve blocks to show that the supraspinatus and infraspinatus muscles provide 45 percent of the abduction and 90 percent of the external rotation strength. Howell et al[25] found that the supraspinatus and deltoid muscles had equal torque in forward flexion and abduction.

Neer et al[47] has proposed that the rotator cuff may also function as a watertight seal. In massive tears of the rotator cuff, there is continuous leakage of synovial fluid under reduced pressure, leading to deterred diffusion of nutrients into articular cartilage. This is one of the proposed mechanisms for the development of rotator cuff arthropathy.

PATHOPHYSIOLOGY

Rotator cuff disorders are generally thought to be secondary to mechanical impingement, tendon degeneration associated with aging, or hypovascularity. In 1972, Neer[45] described impingement of the rotator cuff tendons under the anteroinferior surface of the acromion, not by the posterior or lateral surface as was previously believed. He described a surgical procedure (anterior acromioplasty) to correct this phenomenon. Neer[46] believed that 95 percent of rotator cuff tears were caused by mechanical impingement. He also thought that the reason tears develop in some people but not others can best be explained by variations in the shape and slope of the acromion. This mechanical impingement can lead to tendinitis, fibrosis, and then eventually bursal-sided partial tears and finally to full-thickness tears. Bigliani et al[4] later classified acromion morphology as type I, II, or III, based on their anatomic studies. Type I acromion has a flat undersurface, type II a smooth curved undersurface, and type III an anterior hook or beak (Fig. 8-1). These investigators later confirmed their findings in a clinical series. They found that 80 percent of the patients with rotator cuff tears had type III acromions.[42] Fukuda et al[18] performed a pathologic study of 12 bursal-sided partial cuff tears that supported Neer's hypothesis. In this study, the investigators noted at surgery that the site of the tear was impinged by the anteroinferior acromion with arm elevation in each case. The site of impingement showed degenerative changes histologically. These authors concluded that the changes were caused mainly by impingement and to a lesser extent by primary tendon degeneration and hypovascularity. The coracoacromial arch consists of the acromion, coracoacromial ligament, and the coracoid process. The subacromial bursa, rotator cuff tendons, and superior portion of the glenohumeral joint capsule occupy the space between the coracoacromial arch and the proximal humerus. Any process that decreases the volume of this space may lead to impingement.[5] Zuckerman et al,[69] in a cadaveric study, noted that specimens with rotator cuff tears had a significantly increased coracoacromial angle, increased posterior displacement of the superior acromial tip, and decreased acromial tilt. They concluded that coracoacromial arch stenosis may play an important etiologic role in rotator cuff tears.

Neer[46] has classified rotator cuff pathology according to clinical and radiologic presentation. In stage 1, there is edema and hemorrhage in the rotator cuff; in stage 2, there is tendinitis and fibrosis; and in stage 3, there are bone spurs and tendon rupture. This classification has helped orthopaedic surgeons identify and manage patients with

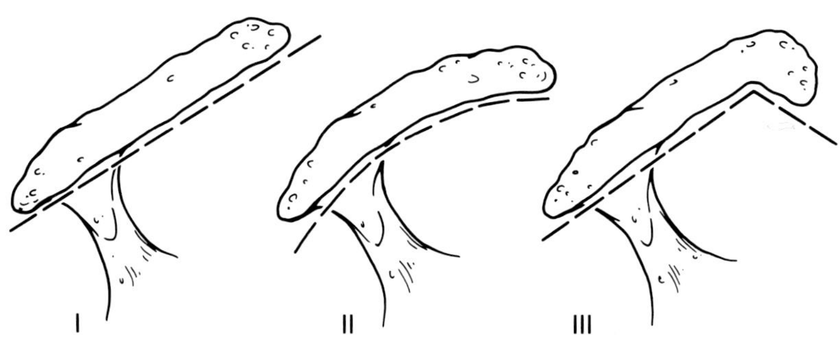

Figure 8-1. Acromion morphology. Type I, flat; type II, curved; type III, anterior hook.

rotator cuff pathology. Nirschl[52] has noted at surgery that the rotator cuff tendons appear gray, dull, edematous, and friable and that the abnormal sections can be grossly recognized from the surrounding normal tendon. Histologically, there are degenerative changes, mainly noted to be angiofibroblastic hyperplasia. There appeared to be a distinct lack of inflammatory cells, which is not unlike those changes seen in lateral epicondylosis of the elbow.[53] These histologic findings have been confirmed by Fukuda et al[18] in their pathologic analysis of bursal-sided partial rotator cuff tears obtained at the time of surgery. Thus, the later stages of rotator cuff pathology may be more appropriately called "rotator cuff tendinosis," because there is no active inflammation. Degenerative changes in the rotator cuff tendons have also been confirmed histologically in adolescents suffering rotator cuff tears.[29] No histologic samples of early rotator cuff lesions have been available, because this stage usually resolves with conservative treatment and is not subject to surgical intervention.

With further experience in the treatment of rotator cuff disorders, some investigators have been unable to find a direct mechanical cuase of impingement in a significant proportion of patients operated on for "impingement syndrome" and thus do not agree that mechanical impingement is the primary problem in the development of rotator cuff disorders but think that intrinsic tendon degeneration may be the inciting event. Nirschl[52] has determined that only 10 percent of his patients operated on with rotator cuff tendinitis have distinct acromial beaks. Another 18 percent of those patients had coracoacromial arch stenosis without obvious acromial pathology. He concluded that most rotator cuff tendinitis was caused by tendon degeneration, likely secondary to repeated eccentric tensile overloading of the rotator cuff tendons. Anatomic studies have supported this belief. Ogata and Uhthoff,[56] in a radiologic and histologic study of the coracoacromial arch, found articular side partial tears in 34 of 36 specimens in which a partial rotator cuff tear was present. They also found significant acromial and rotator cuff degeneration in the absence of bony spurs on the anteroinferior acromion. They concluded that most rotator cuff tears are initiated not by impingement but by a primary degenerative tendinopathy. Ozaki et al[58] analyzed 200 shoulders in 100 cadavers morphologically and histologically, trying to correlate pathologic changes in the acromion with rotator cuff tears. They found degenerative lesions of the coracoacromial ligament and anterior third of the undersurface of the acromion in each case in which a bursal-sided partial-thickness rotator cuff tear or full-thickness tear was present. By contrast, if an articular-sided partial-thickness tear was present, the acromion appeared normal morphologically and histologically. They concluded from their findings that most tears of the rotator cuff are degenerative lesions associated with increased age and that the acromial changes were secondary. Certainly, in athletes, degenerative rotator cuff tendinitis and primary mechanical impingement are usually seen in those 35 years of age or older.[3,32]

Decreased vascularity of the rotator cuff has also been implicated as an important factor in the development of rotator cuff disorders. Codman[9] described the "critical zone" in the supraspinatus as the distal 1 cm involved in all rotator cuff ruptures. Moseley and Goldie[44] noted that after injection of 72 cadaveric shoulders with micropaque, the critical zone corresponded to an area of anastomosis between tendinous and osseous vessels to the rotator cuff. Rathbun and MacNab[61] analyzed the blood supply to the rotator cuff grossly in cadaveric specimens. They found an area of avascularity in the supraspinatus tendon, corresponding to the critical zone where rotator cuff pathology occurs. This avascular area was dependent on arm position. Withe the arm abducted, there was complete filling of all vessels in the supraspinatus tendon. However, with the arm at the side, the distal portion of the supraspinatus tendon became avascular. This phenomenon could be produced in the other rotator cuff tendons as well as at the biceps tendon insertion. The authors concluded that the anatomic disposition of the rotator cuff tendons makes them subject to constant pressure from the humeral head, which wrings out the blood supply and leads to degenerative changes. Lohr and Uhthoff,[37] in another anatomic study in which the arms were abducted 45 to 50 degrees, noted that the articular side of the supraspinatus tendon is completely avascular. They concluded that the tenuous blood supply of the supraspinatus was an important etiologic factor in the production of rotator cuff pathology. Brooks et al[7] performed a quantitative histologic study of the vascularity of the rotator cuff tendons. They found that both the supraspinatus and infraspinatus tendons were hypovascular in their distal 15 mm. They did not mention a difference in vascularity between the articular and bursal sides of the tendons. Hypovascularity most likely plays an integral role in the development of rotator cuff pathology. The decreased vascularity can lead to tendon degeneration with aging, or it may exacerbate the wear and tear associated with mechanical impingement.

Jarvholm and colleagues[30] found that the supra- and infraspinatus muscle pressures were high compared with the trapezius and deltoid muscles in an abducted arm position. They postulated that with arm abduction, the increased pressure could result in ischemia to these muscles with subsequent degeneration of their tendons.

It is unlikely that one specific etiologic factor is responsible for rotator cuff disorders in most cases. More likely, it is a combination of the above factors working synergistically to produce these problems. Whatever the etiology, the believed pathophysiology of rotator cuff disorders goes through the same basic sequence (Fig. 8-2). Tendonitis leads to tendinopathy with subsequent partial and then

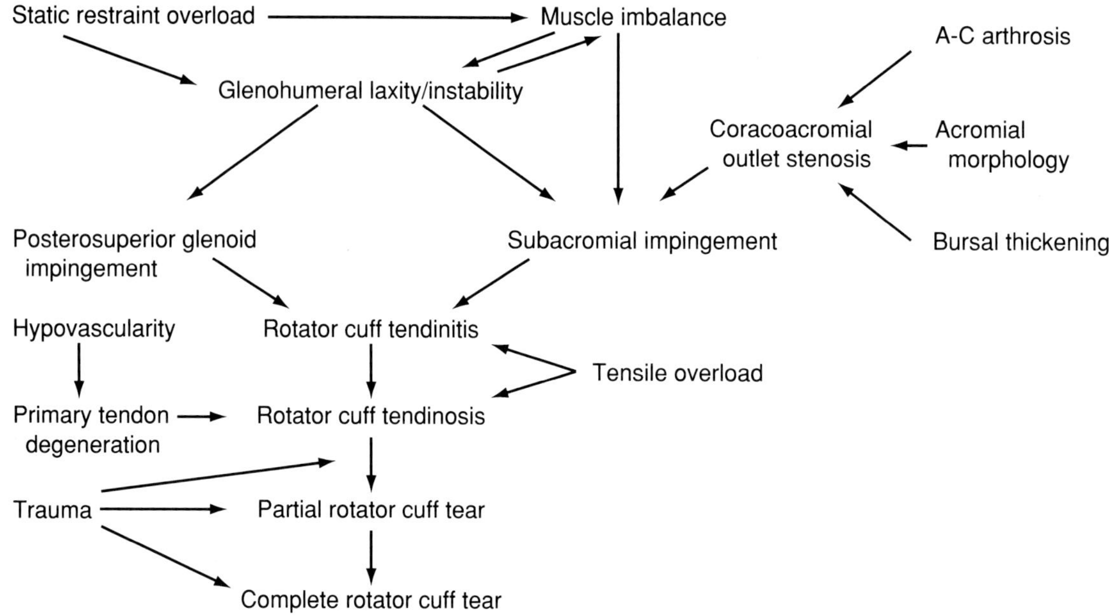

Figure 8-2. Pathophysiologic sequence of most rotator cuff tears.

complete tearing of the rotator cuff. Rotator cuff tears can also be iatrogenic and secondary to inaccurate placement of trocars during arthroscopy or improper intramedullary nail insertion in the surgical management of humeral shaft fractures.[55]

Neer[46] stated that rotator cuff tears do not occur in normal tendon. He thought that "acute" rotator cuff tears represented an acute extension of an incomplete-thickness tear. Hawkins and Kennedy[24] stated that a complete-thickness rotator cuff tear is always preceded by a long history of shoulder problems. Bassett and Cofield[2] found that most of the acute rotator cuff tears that they operated on had an area of pre-existing degeneration. Norwood et al[54] thought that the most common cause of a complete tear of the rotator cuff was an acute traumatic episode superimposed on a chronic degenerative process. This was based on the fact that the patients in their study who had a full-thickness tear had a high incidence of associated orthopaedic conditions (degenerative) and orthopaedic surgical procedures. Pre-existing degenerative cuff lesions explain the finding of rotator cuff rupture in those suffering a primary dislocation at an age older than 40 years. All clinical evidence suggests that normal rotator cuff tendons do not tear.

In athletes involved in overhead activities such as throwing, swimming, volleyball, and racquet sports, rotator cuff tendonitis is not frequently associated with primary impingement from mechanical tightness of the subacromial space. Most of the impingement that occurs in young athletes is secondary to another underlying primary problem, such as instability, muscle imbalance, os acromiale, or malunited fractures. However, most tendonitis in young athletes is not related to either primary or secondary impingement. Most young athletes develop rotator cuff tendonitis secondary to overuse. This overuse can be related to such factors as practice regimen or intensity, faulty technique, or faulty equipment. As the rotator cuff fatigues due to overuse, its ability to perform the functions of stabilization and control of the humeral head diminishes. Sometimes, the end result of this process is a secondary impingement as the humeral head displaces superiorly because of the lost depressor effect of the cuff. In some cases, however, the athlete suffers from rotator cuff irritation and dysfunction without impingement. Most commonly, this is seen in throwers who develop rotator cuff tendonitis of the infraspinatus due to eccentric overload as the cuff repeatedly works to decelerate the arm during the follow-through phase of the throwing motion.

In the shoulder joint, there is a fine line between stability, laxity, and instability. The static stabilizers are composed of the glenohumeral ligaments, joint capsule, and secondarily, the glenoid labrum. The dynamic stabilizers are the rotator cuff musculature and the scapular rotators. As mentioned, the rotator cuff functions to depress the humeral head within the glenoid cavity, whereas the scapular rotators position the glenoid in the proper plane for stability with arm motion. With repeated supra physiology loads, as in the throwing athlete, there are repetitive stresses on the static stabilizers. In overhead sports, the arm is in the abducted and externally rotated position, placing the anterior structures, especially the inferior glenohumeral ligament, under stress.[66] Eventually, these structures fatigue, which may lead to minor subluxation. With laxity, the dynamic restraints work harder to keep the glenohumeral joint located. Eventually, the rotator cuff can fatigue, and this may result in subluxation of the glenohumeral joint. With anterior subluxation, the rotator cuff tendons may be impinged under the acromion (Fig. 8-3). Alternatively, the anterior humeral translation causes the undersurface of the supraspinatus and infraspinatus tendons to become impinged on the posterosuperior surface of the glenoid rim.[33–35,67] This secondary impingement leads to rotator cuff tendonitis and potential tearing of the rotator cuff. Jobe and Kvitne[32] have called this the ''instability complex.'' They have classified these pathologies and clinical syndromes as a spectrum ranging from pure impingement to pure instability.

Superior labral anteroposterior (SLAP) lesions, as defined by Snyder et al,[65] may also cause instability and subsequent rotator cuff pathology. In a recent biomechanical study in which a superior labral lesion was created in the biceps tendon, there was an increase in glenohumeral instability.[17,63] Secondary impingement can also result from muscular imbalance. Fowler[16] has noted fatigue and weakness of the rotator cuff musculature and scapular rotators in swimmers with rotator cuff tendonitis.

Clinical Evaluation

The importance of an accurate history and physical examination in the assessment of rotator cuff disorders has been recognized.[23,40,57] Athletes with rotator cuff problems usually present with shoulder pain and occasionally with dysfunction. The nature and location of the pain is important. The onset of the pain and its occurrence with activities should be determined accurately. Athletes participating in overhead sports will commonly experience anterior or posterior shoulder pain with their arm in the abducted/externally rotated position. In this position, the humeral head may be subluxing anteriorly, causing secondary impingement of the rotator cuff tendons. Alternatively, the athlete may present with a history of shoulder pain and the feeling that their shoulder is ''coming out of joint.'' Also, complaints such as inability to elevate their arm and night and rest pain are significant and may represent a rotator cuff tear, whereas activity-related pain may signify tendonitis alone.[19,32,35]

Examination may reveal wasting of the supraspinatus or infraspinatus muscles with prominence of the scapular spine. There may be loss of the normal contour above or below the scapular spine, with wasting of the supraspinatus or infraspinatus muscles, respectively. The supraspinatus test may be decreased. In this test, the patient actively abducts their arm against the examiner with the patient's arm abducted 90 degrees, forward flexed 30 degrees, and internally rotated. Range of motion should be determined. The impingement sign may be positive. Whether instability coexists with the impingement is of paramount importance. This is evaluated with the anterior apprehension sign and relocation test. Patients that are grossly apprehensive during the anterior apprehension test usually have recurrent anterior dislocations. In these cases, the diagnosis is usually clear. In the patient who is not grossly apprehensive, the presence of shoulder pain in the 90 degree abducted and externally rotated position, relieved by applying a posteriorly directed force on the humeral head (relocation test), may signify anterior glenohumeral subluxation. Translation tests of the glenohumeral joint may be increased in patients with underlying instability. Throwing athletes may have a tight posterior capsule giving obligate anterior glenohumeral translation with forward elevation or external

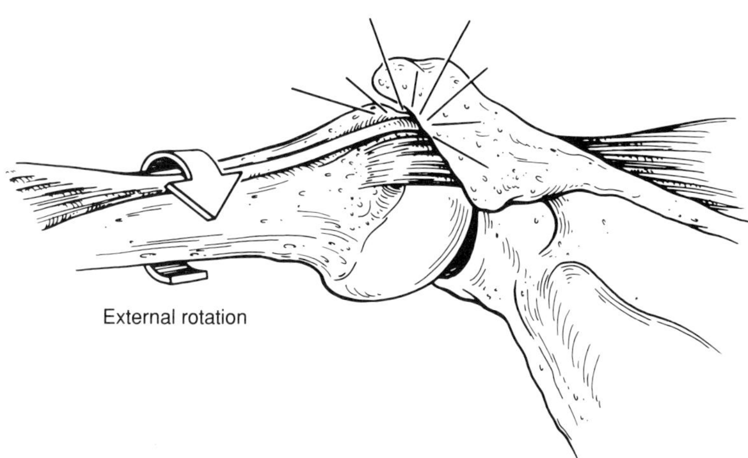

Figure 8-3. During anterior subluxation of the abducted and externally rotated humerus, secondary impingement may occur.

rotation.[21] They may also have associated loss of internal rotation.

Radiology

Routine anteroposterior, lateral, and axillary view radiographs are examined for stigmata of instability or rotator cuff disease (sclerosis, cysts, and irregularity of the greater tuberosity/sclerosis and spur formation of the anteroinferior acromion/narrowing of the acromiohumeral gap). Supraspinatus outlet views are obtained to assess acromial morphology[48] (Fig. 8-4). On routine anteroposterior shoulder radiographs, Weiner and MacNab[68] have shown that if the acromiohumeral distance is 5 mm or less (Fig. 8-5), a rotator cuff tear is likely present.

If significant rotator cuff tear is suspected clinically, an arthrogram or magnetic resonance imaging (MRI) scan is usually ordered. MRI has been shown to be very sensitive in the evaluation of full-thickness rotator cuff tears[14,26] (Fig. 8-6). The authors caution on the routine use of MRI in the evaluation of these patients because abnormal signals are present even in normal shoulders.[41]

Norwood and colleagues[54] have found that patients with multiple rotator cuff tendons torn are older, have decreased range of motion, and are less active. These patients more often have radiologic indicators of rotator cuff disease and more often suffer an acute injury.

Treatment: Acute Rotator Cuff Injuries

In Neer's[46] stages of rotator cuff impingment, acute injuries to the cuff typically occurred early and at a younger age. Acute cuff injury/contusion occurs with initial tensile overloading from eccentric muscle contraction.[51] Unless treated appropriately, the acute cuff contusion may proceed to tendonitis and fibrosis and then possibly to tearing. Bassett and Cofield[2] analyzed the results of repair of acute rotator cuff tears. They found the tears were caused by either a direct fall, a strong eccentric or concentric muscular contraction, or a motor vehicular accident. Bigliani et al[3] noted that 11 of 23 tennis players they had operated on for rotator cuff tears suffered a definite traumatic episode. Norwood and colleagues[54] noted that a high percentage of patients with full-thickness rotator cuff tears could remember a distinct traumatic episode beginning their symptomatology, especially those with tearing of multiple rotator cuff tendons. Several authors have noted that primary anterior dislocation in the older patient is often associated with rotator cuff tears. Hawkins et al[22] found that rotator cuff

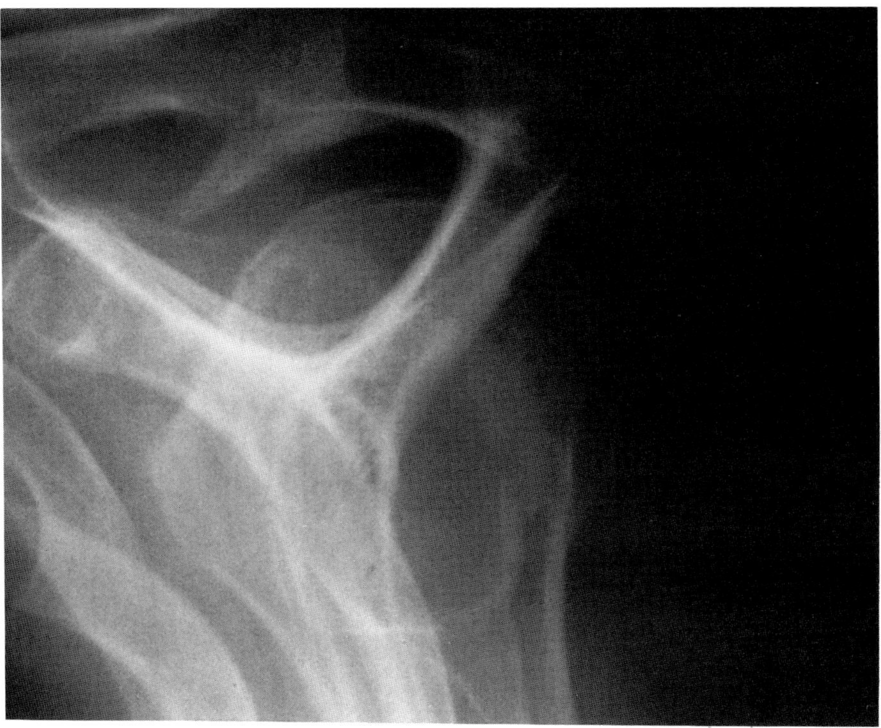

Figure 8-4. The supraspinatus outlet view reveals the acromion morphology. In this case, a large spur projects from the anterior acromion.

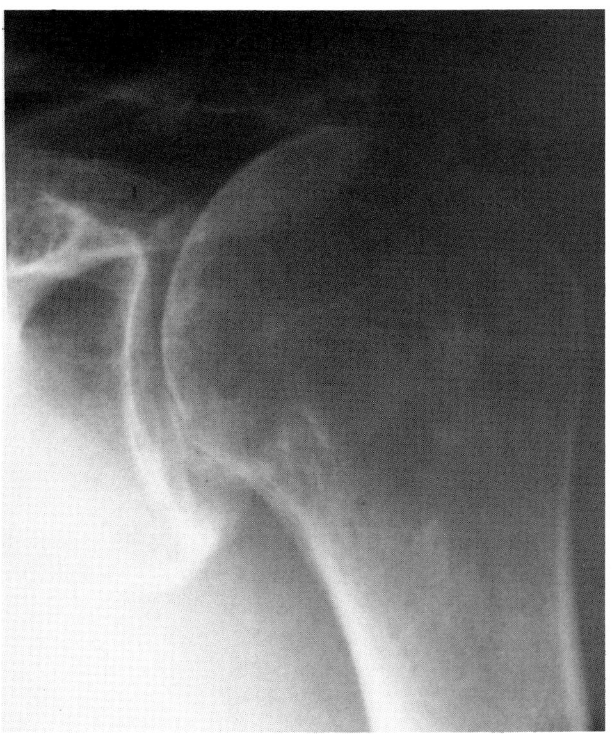

Figure 8-5. The acromiohumeral distance is demonstrated on an anteroposterior radiograph. In this case, a distance of less than 5 mm indicates the likely presence of a large cuff tear.

tears were present in most of the 61 shoulders in patients 40 years of age or older that had suffered an initial anterior shoulder dislocation. Neviaser et al[50] have treated 37 patients older than 40 years of age for rotator cuff rupture after sustaining primary anterior shoulder dislocations. In each case, there was rupture of the subscapularis and anterior capsule from the lesser tuberosity. These authors cautioned of the strong association between first-time anterior dislocation at an age older than 40 years and rotator cuff rupture. A displaced fracture of the greater tuberosity of the proximal humerus is, by definition, a rotator cuff rupture.[15,49]

Acute rotator cuff tendonitis is best managed conservatively. Rest, ice, and anti-inflammatory medication are used initially. After the acute pain has subsided (1 to 2 weeks maximum), physiotherapy is started to regain motion and increase rotator cuff flexibility and strength.

The management of acute rotator cuff tears remains controversial. The natural history of acute rotator cuff tears is not known. Many authors believe that most acute tears become relatively asymptomatic with conservative management.[6,28] Bassett and Cofield[2] analyzed the results of rotator cuff repair in 37 patients within 3 months of injury. The patients were divided into three groups: those operated on within 3 weeks of injury, those operated on between 3 to 6 weeks after injury, and those operated on between 6 weeks and 3 months of injury. The patients that were operated on within 3 weeks of initial injury had significantly better active shoulder abduction and better muscle strength than those operated on more than 3 weeks after their injury. These authors proposed that if a patient has a full-thickness rotator cuff tear and has significant compromise of shoulder function, then the patient should have that tear repaired within 3 weeks of injury for optimal results. We currently offer early surgery to patients suffering acute rotator tears, especially young athletes. Patients with significantly displaced fractures of the greater tuberosity and patients who have rotator cuff rupture after anterior shoulder dislocation and continue to have shoulder dysfunction despite conservative treatment are offered surgery.

Chronic Rotator Cuff Injuries

The mainstay of treatment in rotator cuff disorders, whether they are degenerative in nature or secondary to glenohumeral instability, is conservative. Neer[45] noted that most of his patients with impingement responded favorably

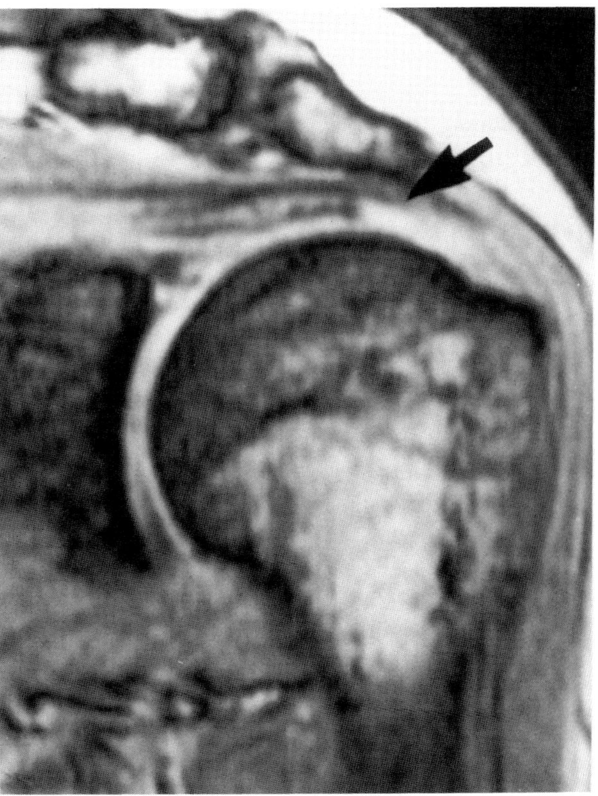

Figure 8-6. Magnetic resonance imaging scan showing a complete tear of the rotator cuff (*arrow*) at the supraspinatus tendon tear.

to a rehabilitation program. Rockwood and Lyons[62] noted that a large percentage of the patients referred to them for surgery responded to a rehabilitation program. Morrison et al[43] followed 616 patients with isolated subacromial impingement syndrome and found that 67 percent responded to a directed rehabilitation protocol. Bokor et al[6] followed 53 patients with full-thickness rotator cuff tears treated conservatively for an average 7.6 years. They found that 76 percent of the patients had substantial improvement in pain. They had slightly less improvement in function and range of motion. There was a tendency toward better results with longer follow-up. The patients who presented less than 6 months from the onset of their shoulder symptoms fared significantly better than those presenting more than 6 months from the onset of their problems. These authors concluded that conservative management of rotator cuff tears is an effective method to relieve pain, especially if the treatment was started early.

Activity modification is an important factor in conservative care. For the athlete, this means no overhead activity. Nonsteroidal anti-inflammatory medications can be used to control inflammation and pain. A physiotherapy program is prescribed. This entails the achievement of flexibility and synchronous power of the rotator cuff muscles, scapular stabilizers, trapezius, deltoid, and pectoralis major muscles. During rehabilitation of a patient with glenohumeral instability/laxity, any positions that produced symptoms or subluxation are avoided. Judicious use of corticosteroid injections into the subacromial space are used (maximum, three).

Indications for surgery must be individualized. Before considering surgery, the patient must have a normal range of motion. Patients who have undergone at least 6 months of an *appropriate* rehabilitation program directed at their underlying pathology are considered for surgery. Itoi and Tabata[28] have noted that the results of conservative treatment of rotator cuff tears tend to deteriorate with time and that the natural history of conservatively treated rotator cuff tears in the high demand population is uncertain. Athletes with a full-thickness rotator cuff tear are offered surgery, with the thought that greater motion and better function may be obtained if the patients are operated on early.[2]

Overuse Tendonosis in Athletes

Because overuse tendonosis in most young athletes is not associated with impingement, surgery to enlarge the subacromial space is usually fraught with failure. Treatment must be directed toward alleviating the cause for the overuse problem. In most cases, rehabilitation exercises to improve the strength, endurance, and coordination of the rotator cuff muscles are effective. Also, adjustment of the athlete's practice regimen or technique if often necessary. In some cases, athletes develop overuse tendonosis simply because they are trying to exceed their own physical capabilities. In those cases, education of the athletes to recognize their own physical limitations is necessary. In nearly all cases, treatment by conservative means is successful.

SUMMARY

Rotator cuff disorders are a very important shoulder ailment affecting adults of all ages. The etiology is controversial but most likely a combination of mechanical impingement, intrinsic tendinopathy, and hypovascularity. In overhead athletes, underlying laxity or instability must be suspected. The treatment of these disorders is, by and large, conservative. The indications for surgery in acute rotator cuff tears remains controversial. Surgery in chronic cases is reserved for patients who do not respond to an appropriate rehabilitation program directed at the underlying pathology.

REFERENCES

1. Basmajian JV, Bazant FJ: Factors preventing downward dislocation of the adducted shoulder joint. J Bone Joint Surg [Am] 41:1182, 1959
2. Bassett RW, Cofield RH: Acute tears of the rotator cuff: the timing of surgical repair. Clin Orthop 175:18, 1983
3. Bigliani LU, Kimmel J, McCann PD, Wolfe I: Repair of rotator cuff tears in tennis players. Am J Sports Med 20:112, 1992
4. Bigliani LU, Morrison DS, April EW: The morphology of the acromion and its relationship to rotator cuff tears. Orthop Trans 10:216, 1986
5. Bigliani LU, Ticker JB, Flatow EL et al: The relationship of acromial architecture to rotator cuff disease. Clin Sports Med 10:823, 1991
6. Bokor DJ, Hawkins RJ, Huckell GH et al: Results of nonoperative management of full-thickness tears of the rotator cuff. Clin Orthop 294:103, 1993
7. Brooks CH, Revell WJ, Heatley FW: A quantitative histological study of the vascularity of the rotator cuff tendon. J Bone Joint Surg [Br] 74:151, 1992
8. Burkhart SS: Fluoroscopic comparison of kinematic patterns in massive rotator cuff tears: a suspension bridge model. Clin Orthop 284:144, 1992
9. Codman EA: The Shoulder. Thomas Todd, Boston, 1934
10. Codman EA: Rupture of the supraspinatus—1834–1934. J Bone Joint Surg 19:643, 1937
11. Codman EA: Rupture of the supraspinatus. Am J Surg 42:603, 1938
12. Colachis SC, Strohm BR: Effect of suprascapular and axillary nerve blocks on muscle force in upper extremity. Arch Phys Med Rehabil 52:22, 1971
13. D'Alessandro DF, Jobe FW, Perry J et al: Dynamic stabilizers

of the glenohumeral joint: an anatomic and electromyographic analysis. Orthop Trans 14:260, 1990
14. Farley TE, Neumann CH, Steinbach LS et al: Full-thickness tears of the rotator cuff of the shoulder: Diagnosis with MR imaging. AJR 158:347, 1992
15. Flatow EL, Cuomo F, Maday MG et al: Open reduction and internal fixation of two-part displaced fractures of the greater tuberosity of the proximal part of the humerus. J Bone Joint Surg [Am] 73:1213, 1991
16. Fowler PJ: Swimming injuries to the rotator cuff. American Academy of Orthopaedic Surgeons 52nd Annual Meeting, Las Vegas, 1985
17. Fu FH, Harner CD, Klein AH: Shoulder impingement syndrome. A critical review. Clin Orthop 269:162, 1991
18. Fukuda H, Hamada K, Yamanaka K: Pathology and pathogenesis of bursal-side rotator cuff tears viewed from en bloc histologic sections. Clin Orthop 254:75, 1990
19. Glousman RE: Instability versus impingement syndrome in the throwing athlete. Orthop Clin North Am 24:89, 1993
20. Glousman RE, Jobe FW, Tibone J et al: Dynamic electromyographic analysis of the throwing shoulder with glenohumeral instability. J Bone Joint Surg [Am] 70:220, 1988
21. Harryman DT II, Sidles JA, Clark JM et al: Translation of the humeral head on the glenoid with passive glenohumeral motion. J Bone Joint Surg [Am] 72:1334, 1990
22. Hawkins RJ, Bell RH, Hawkins RH, Koppert GJ: Anterior dislocation of the shoulder in the older patient. Clin Orthop 206:192, 1986
23. Hawkins RJ, Chris T, Bokor D, Kiefer G: Failed anterior acromioplasty. A review of 51 cases. Clin Orthop 243: 106, 1989
24. Hawkins RJ, Kennedy JC: Impingement syndrome in athletes. Am J Sports Med 8:151, 1980
25. Howell SM, Imobersteg AM, Seger DH, Marone PJ: Clarification of the role of the supraspinatus muscle in shoulder function. J Bone Joint Surg [Am] 68:398, 1986
26. Iannotti JP, Zlatkin MB, Esterhai JL et al: Magnetic resonance imaging of the shoulder: sensitivity, specificity, and predictive value. J Bone Joint Surg [Am] 73:17, 1991
27. Inman VT, Saunders JBM, Abbott LC: Observations of the function of the shoulder joint. J Bone Joint Surg 26:1, 1944
28. Itoi E, Tabata S: Conservative treatment of rotator cuff tears. Clin Orthop 275:165, 1992
29. Itoi E, Tabata S: Rotator cuff tears in the adolescent. Orthopedics 16:78, 1993
30. Jarvholm U, Palmerud G, Karlsson D et al: Intramuscular pressure and electromyography in four shoulder muscles. J Orthop Res 9:609, 1991
31. Jarvinen M: Epidemiology of tendon injuries in sports. Clin Sports Med 11:493, 1992
32. Jobe FW, Kvitne RS: Shoulder pain in the overhand or throwing athlete. The relationship of anterior instability and rotator cuff impingement. Orthop Rev 18:963, 1989
33. Jobe CM, Sidles J: Evidence for a superior glenoid impingement upon the rotator cuff. Presented at the Fifth International Conference on Surgery of the Shoulder, Paris, 1992
34. Jobe CM, Walch G, Sidles J: Evidence for a superior glenoid impingement upon the rotator cuff. Anatomic, kinesiologic, MRI and arthroscopic findings. Orthop Trans 16:763, 1992
35. Kvitne RS, Jobe FW: The diagnosis and treatment of anterior instability in the throwing athlete. Clin Orthop 291:107, 1993
36. Lehman RC: Shoulder pain in the competitive tennis player. Clin Sports Med 7:309, 1988
37. Lohr JF, Uhthoff HK: The microvascular pattern of the supraspinatus tendon. Clin Orthop 254:35, 1990
38. Maylack FH: Epidemiology of tennis, squash, and racquetball injuries. Clin Sports Med 7:233, 1988
39. McMaster WC, Troup J: A survey of interfering shoulder pain in United States competitive swimmers. Am J Sports Med 21:67, 1993
40. Miniaci A, Dowdy PA, Fowler PJ: Clinical assessment of shoulder injuries. In Chan KM (ed): Sports Injuries of the Hand and Upper Limb. Churchill Livingstone, London, 1994
41. Miniaci A, Dowdy PA, Willits K, Vellet AD: Magnetic resonance imaging evaluation of the asymptomatic shoulder. Am J Sports Med, in press
42. Morrison DS, Bigliani LU: The clinical significance of variations in acromial morphology. Orthop Trans 11:234, 1987
43. Morrison DS, Frogameni A, Woodworth P: Conservative management for subacromial impingement of the shoulder. Presented at the American Shoulder and Elbow Surgeons Ninth Open Meeting, San Francisco, 1993
44. Moseley HF, Goldie I: The arterial pattern of the rotator cuff of the shoulder. J Bone Joint Surg [Br] 45:780, 1963
45. Neer CS II: Anterior acromioplasty for the chronic impingment syndrome in the shoulder: a preliminary report. J Bone Joint Surg [Am] 54:41, 1972
46. Neer CS II: Impingement lesions. Clin Orthop 173:70, 1983
47. Neer CS II, Craig EV, Fukuda H: Cuff-tear arthropathy. J Bone Joint Surg [Am] 65:1232, 1983
48. Neer CS II, Poppen NK: Supraspinatus outlet. Orthop Trans 11:234, 1987
49. Neviaser RJ, Neviaser TJ: Observations on impingement. Clin Orthop 254:60, 1990
50. Neviaser RJ, Neviaser TJ, Neviaser JS: Anterior dislocation of the shoulder and rotator cuff rupture. Clin Orthop 291:103, 1993
51. Nirschl RP: Rotator cuff surgery. Instr Course Lect 38, 1989
52. Nirschl RP: Rotator cuff tendinitis: basic concepts of pathoetiology. Instr Course Lect 38, 1989
53. Nirschl RP, Pettrone FA: Tennis elbow: the surgical treatment of lateral epicondylitis. J Bone Joint Surg [Am] 61:832, 1979
54. Norwood LA, Barrack R, Jacobson KE: Clinical presentation of complete tears of the rotator cuff. J Bone Joint Surg [Am] 71:499, 1989
55. Norwood LA, Fowler HL: Rotator cuff tears: a shoulder arthroscopy complication. Am J Sports Med 17:837, 1989
56. Ogata S, Uhthoff HK: Acromial enthesopathy and rotator cuff tear. A radiologic and histolgic postmortem investigation of the coracoacromial arch. Clin Orthop 254:39, 1990
57. Ogilvie-Harris DJ, Wiley AM, Sattarian J: Failed acromioplasty for impingement syndrome. J Bone Joint Surg [Br] 72:1070, 1990
58. Ozaki J, Fujimoto S, Nakagawa Y et al: Tears of the rotator cuff of the shoulder associated with pathological changes in the acromion. J Bone Joint Surg [Am] 70:1224, 1988
59. Poppen NK, Walker PS: Normal and abnormal motion of the shoulder. J Bone Joint Surg [Am] 58:195, 1976

60. Poppen NK, Walker PS: Forces at the glenohumeral joint in abduction. Clin Orthop 135:165, 1978
61. Rathbun JB, MacNab I: The microvascular pattern of the rotator cuff. J Bone Joint Surg [Br] 52:540, 1970
62. Rockwood CA, Lyons FR: Shoulder impingement syndrome: diagnosis, radiographic evaluation, and treatment with a modified Neer acromioplasty. J Bone Joint Surg [Am] 75:409, 1993
63. Rodsky MW, Rudert MJ, Harner CD et al: Significance of a superior labral lesion of the shoulder: a biomechanical study. Trans Orthop Res Soc 15:276, 1990
64. Saha AK: Dynamic stability of the glenohumeal joint. Acta Orthop Scand 42:491, 1971
65. Snyder SJ, Karzel RP, Del Pizzo W et al: SLAP lesions of the shoulder. Arthroscopy 6:274, 1990
66. Turkel SJ, Panio MW, Marshall JL, Girgis FG: Stabilizing mechanisms preventing anterior dislocation of the glenohumeral joint. J Bone Joint Surg [Am] 63:1208, 1981
67. Walch G, Liotard JP, Boileau P, Noel E: Postero-superior impingement in the throwing athlete. Presented at the Fifth International Conference on Surgery of the Shoulder, Paris, 1992
68. Weiner DS, MacNab I: Superior migration of the humeral head: a radiological aid in the diagnosis of tears of the rotator cuff. J Bone Joint Surg [Br] 52:524, 1970
69. Zuckerman JD, Kummer FJ, Cuomo F et al: The influence of coracoacromial arch anatomy on rotator cuff tears. J Shoulder Elbow Surg 1:4, 1992

CHAPTER NINE

Open Surgery for Rotator Cuff Repair

Sanford Kunkel

This chapter discusses open surgery for rotator cuff disorders. Previous chapters have discussed the role of arthroscopy for rotator cuff tendinitis and tears. At times, arthroscopic evaluation of the rotator cuff for partial-thickness tears and small full-thickness tears is advocated. This chapter discusses the open approach to partial- and full-thickness rotator cuff tears.

INDICATIONS

Treatment of the athlete with rotator cuff symptoms usually includes nonsteroidal anti-inflammatory medications, preoperative rehabilitation for rotator cuff and scapular strengthening, and occasionally a few subacromial injections. As Neer[6] has suggested, most patients with stage I or II rotator cuff disease should be treated for a minimum of 12 months nonoperatively. In dealing with an athletic population in which the use of the athlete's upper extremity is important to his or her profession or livelihood, the nonoperative period of treatment may be shortened. With a high-caliber or professional athlete who has failed to show significant improvement with nonoperative treatment for 6 months, surgical intervention is often recommended. An arthrogram or magnetic resonance imaging (MRI) may be used to evaluate the extent of rotator cuff disease and aid in preoperative planning and consultation. In those patients who show clinical signs of partial- or full-thickness rotator cuff tearing and radiographic studies that confirm a rotator cuff tear, surgical intervention should be considered. In the younger athlete, partial- or full-thickness cuff tears may be difficult to diagnose clinically, and the classic symptoms of night pain, weakness to external rotation and abduction, and muscle atrophy will often be absent. MRI plays a particularly helpful role in evaluating the young well-muscled athlete for rotator cuff pathology. The decision regarding open rotator cuff surgery involves consideration of the recovery time, which is discussed later in this chapter. This decision will have a different effect on the collegiate or professional athlete than it does on the middle-aged recreational athlete.

As a general guideline, any patient with a documented rotator cuff tear and clinical findings and complaints consistent with rotator cuff pathology should be considered a surgical candidate. The decision for surgery should be based on the patient's individual demands and symptomatology. The decision and timing of rotator cuff surgery need to be individualized for each particular patient. Often, the middle-aged recreational athlete will chose to modify his or her activity or give up the sport altogether until surgery is convenient, whereas the higher-profile athlete may choose to proceed with surgery immediately to begin the rehabilitation process and return to his or her sport as quickly as possible.

Once a decision to proceed with open rotator cuff repair has been made, every effort should be made to achieve a secure repair of the rotator cuff to a trough in bone or side-to-side watertight closure. Adequate decompression and a secure tendon repair afford the patient the most reliable results.[3–5] Currently, no studies demonstrate that decompression alone for a rotator cuff tear is as effective as decompression and rotator cuff repair.

SURGICAL TECHNIQUE

Patients are placed on the operating room table or on a beach chair positioner in the supine position, and general anesthesia, a scalene block, or both are administered to the involved upper extremity. The patient is then placed in a semisitting position in which diagnostic arthroscopy may be performed. If clinical evaluation or radiographic studies indicate partial- or full-thickness rotator cuff tear, the surgeon may wish to proceed to open surgery without arthroscopy. For the open procedure, the patient is positioned in approximately 30 degrees of flexion, with padding behind the knees and heels (Fig. 9-1). The shoulder and upper extremity are prepared and draped free for positioning and exposure of the rotator cuff. A sand bag or inflatable bladder may be placed under the ipsilateral scapula to bring the shoulder into a more advantageous position. A skin incision is made from just proximal to the anterior acromion, approximately 5 to 7 cm in length, in line with the fibers of the deltoid (Fig. 9-2). The skin and subcutaneous layer are incised, and self-retaining retractors are placed in the wound. The anterior deltoid is reflected off the anterior acromion in a fiber-splitting approach, peeling the white aponeurotic insertion of the deltoid from the acromion and following this distally to a raphe in the deltoid, which often exists at the junction of the middle and anterior thirds of the deltoid (Fig. 9-3). By splitting the deltoid in the direction of its fibers over the acromion, a subsequent side-to-side repair can be performed. The deltoid can safely be split up to 5 cm from the lateral edge of the acromion, at which point the axillary nerve courses on the undersurface of the deltoid. A stay suture is used in the distal deltoid split to prevent damage to the nerve (Fig. 9-4).

An anterior acromioplasty is then performed using a power saw or osteotome, removing the anteroinferior aspect of the acromion (Fig. 9-5). With the patient positioned in approximately 30 degrees of incline, the osteotome or saw may be directed to the apex of the undersurface of the acromion. The undersurface of the acromion can be smoothed with a power burr and smeared with bone wax to prevent further bleeding and future bony overgrowth. The undersurface of the acromioclavicular joint is evaluated, and degenerative spurs are debrided with a rongeur or burr. Electrocautery is often necessary due to the abundant blood supply in the fat surrounding the acromioclavicular joint. If the acromioclavicular joint is noted to be degenerative and painful to palpation during physical examination, distal clavicle resection may be performed. I perform a distal clavicle resection approximately 10 percent of the time with a rotator cuff repair. The coracoacromial ligament is often released with the anterior acromioplasty; if the ligament remains after the acromioplasty, it should be released with cutting cautery. Care should be taken to cauterize the acromial branch of the thoracoacromial artery.

The subacromial bursa is then inspected, and if significant scarring or thickening is noted, this should be excised. Uhtoff et al[10] have demonstrated that the bursa provides

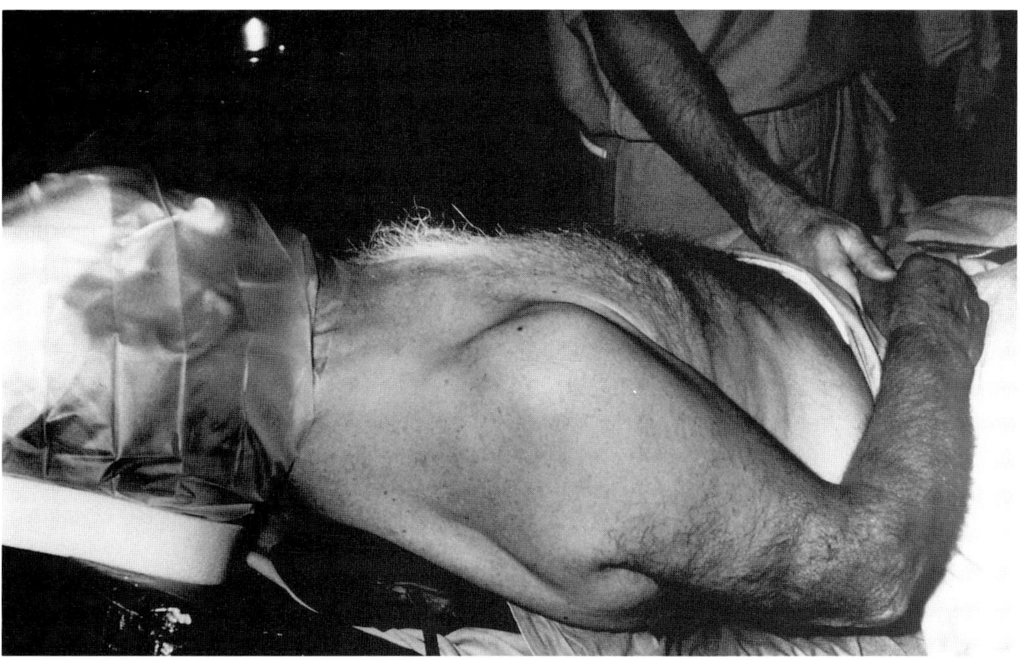

Figure 9-1. Patient positioned in semisitting position for open rotator cuff surgery.

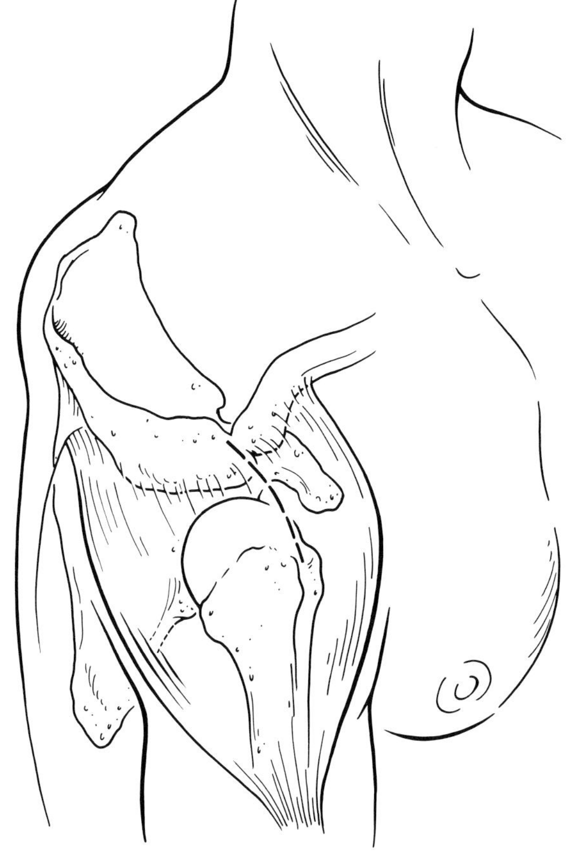

Figure 9-2. Deltoid-splitting incision for open rotator cuff repair.

an important source of blood supply and potential healing for the rotator cuff. Overzealous resection of the bursa should be avoided. With deep retraction of the deltoid, the rotator cuff tear is exposed and evaluated for size and condition. Often, cuff tears appear small on the bursal surface, but further evaluation of the undersurface shows lamination of the rotator cuff layers or retraction of the undersurface of the rotator cuff, making these cuff tears functionally much larger than they appear on the bursal surface (Fig. 9-6). If lamination and retraction of the undersurface of the cuff are present, the undersurface layer should be evaluated for elasticity. If this layer can be reapproximated to a trough in bone near the greater tuberosity, then the bursal layer of the rotator cuff should be trimmed back to the level of the tear of the undersurface layer (Fig. 9-7A). If the undersurface layer of the laminated tear lacks the flexibility to allow reapproximation of this layer to the trough-in-bone repair, then the undersurface layer may be sewn to the bursal surface layer in a vertical mattress fashion to prevent further retraction after repair (Fig. 9-7B). The free edge of the cuff tear is trimmed with a #15 blade scalpel to a viable tendon margin. Excessive trimming of the rotator cuff edge should be avoided. For laminated tears, I have recently used SCOI technique suture placement in the free edge of the tear to prevent cutting out of the suture between the tear layers (Fig. 9-8). If there is no lamination of the rotator cuff edge, then a simple horizontal mattress suture or Kessler-type grasping suture with size 2 nonabsorbable suture or a 1-mm braided Dacron

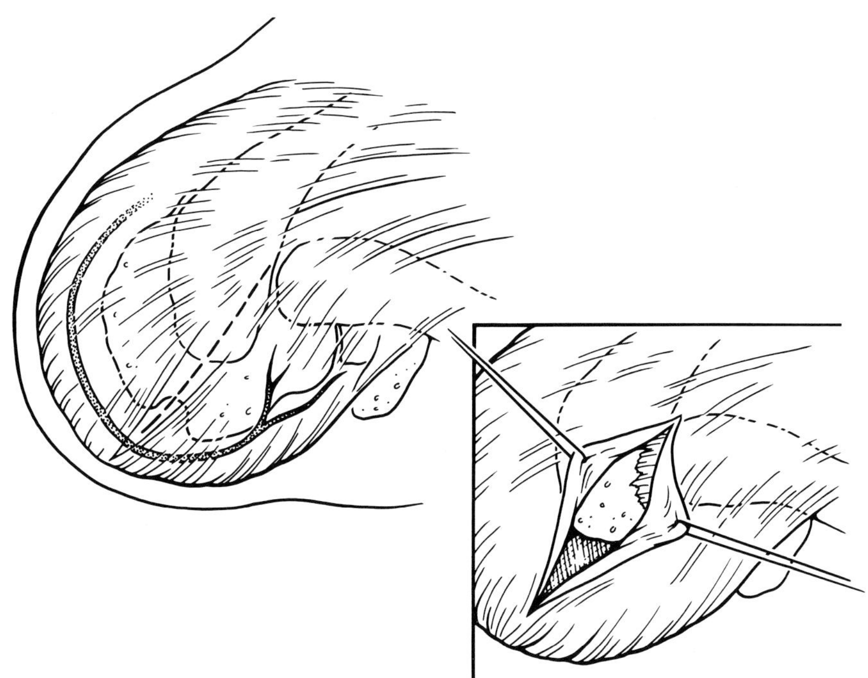

Figure 9-3. Deltoid fascia and muscle are split in line with its fibers.

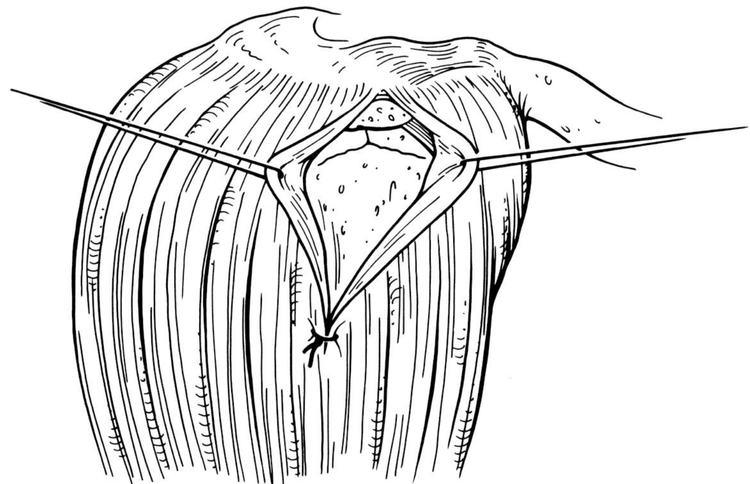

Figure 9-4. Stay suture in apex of deltoid split to prevent injury to axillary nerve.

suture. Once the sutures are placed in the free edge of the cuff tear, the tissue can be evaluated for elasticity and determination of the placement for the trough in bone. If possible, the trough should be made at the junction of the anatomic neck and greater tuberosity. Reapproximation of the cuff near the greater tuberosity helps to restore the normal biomechanics of the rotator cuff. If the tear is retracted and scarred with poor elasticity or is large in size, it may be reapproximated to a trough in bone that is placed slightly more medial onto the articular surface of the humeral head. The placement of the trough should be determined by the tension created in the rotator cuff during the reapproximation. For massive tears that appear chronic and have limited mobility and elasticity, the cuff is mobilized with stay sutures and release of adhesions on the bursal side of the cuff and subdeltoid bursa. The cuff may be mobilized with blunt dissection intra-articularly, including the undersurface of the teres minor, infraspinatus, supraspinatus, and subscapularis. A Cobb elevator can be used to strip the capsule from the glenoid neck outside of the labrum to mobilize the subscapularis. Dissection is limited medially to the spinoglenoid notch to prevent injury to the

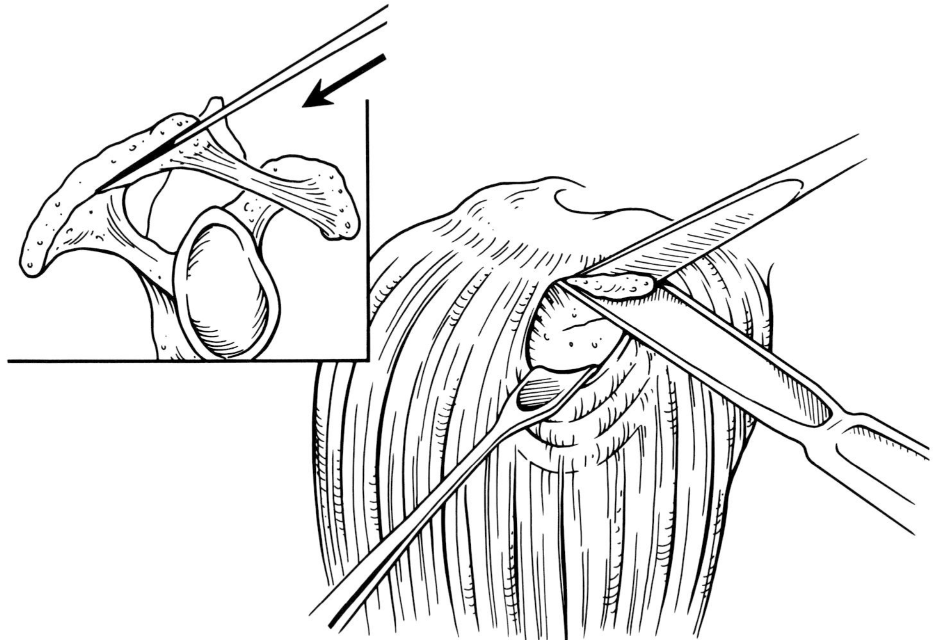

Figure 9-5. Anterior acromioplasty performed from an anterior (open) approach.

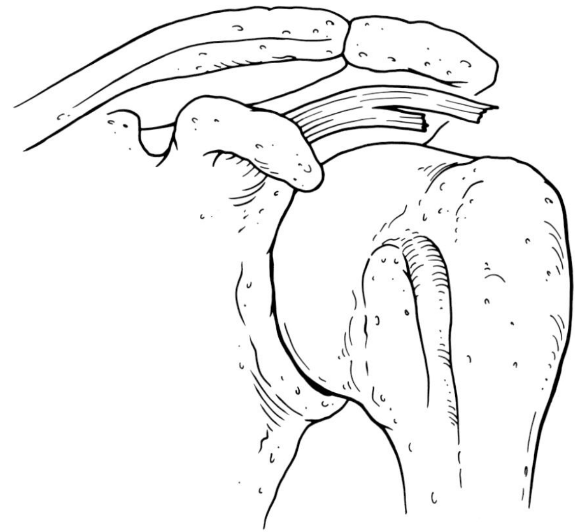

Figure 9-6. Rotator cuff tear with a layered and laminated appearance.

suprascapular nerve. Release of the coracohumeral ligament from the base of the coracoid will improve subscapularis mobility.

The trough in bone is made using a 1-in.-wide osteotome or power burr. For most tears, this trough will be 8 to 10 mm in width and should span the distance of the cuff tear itself (Fig. 9-9). My preference is to use drill holes in the base of the trough and a tenaculum to complete the bony tunnel from medial to lateral. A large bone bridge (1 cm or more in size) will lessen the likelihood of fracturing the bony bridge. We prefer to pass the sutures from medial to lateral, tying the sutures laterally (Fig. 9-10). Passing a pull suture with the suture for repair allows the suture to be pulled through, avoiding the need to pass the needle from the trough outward, which can be difficult. This allows the surgeon to draw the free edge of the tear into the trough. I have also performed cuff repair by tying the sutures over the free edge of the cuff in the trough itself, and this is also satisfactory.[5] Once the free edge of the tear has been reapproximated to the trough, the arm should be taken through a full range of motion to determine if there is any undue tension on the repair. If there is retraction of the tendon edge from the trough, particularly during adduction or with the arm at the side, an abduction pillow should be used for 6 weeks postoperatively.

If after decompression the bursal surface of the cuff is intact, finger palpation is used to feel for a defect or thinning of the cuff. My experience is that most rotator cuff tears begin on the articular surface, and significant partial-thickness tears may exist on the articular side of the cuff, with a normal-appearing bursal surface. If there is a question about the location or the thickness of the undersurface tear, an intraoperative arthrogram is performed using methylene dye or diluted Betadine. The dye is injected with an 18-gauge spinal needle into the shoulder joint at a distance from the area of the potential rotator cuff tear. The dye

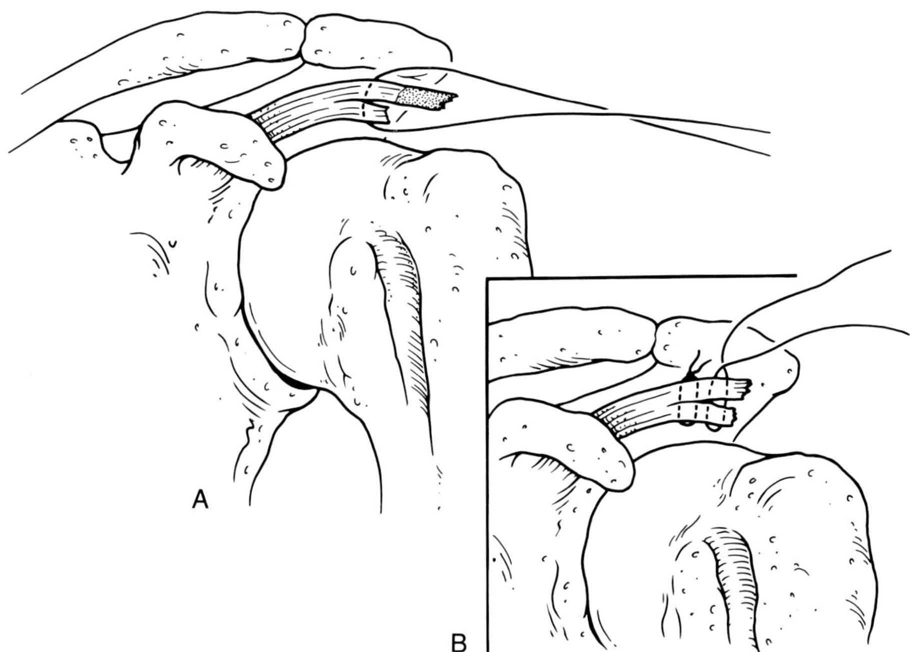

Figure 9-7. **(A)** Laminated tears are trimmed back to the undersurface layer. **(B)** Laminated tears with poor elasticity are repaired in situ.

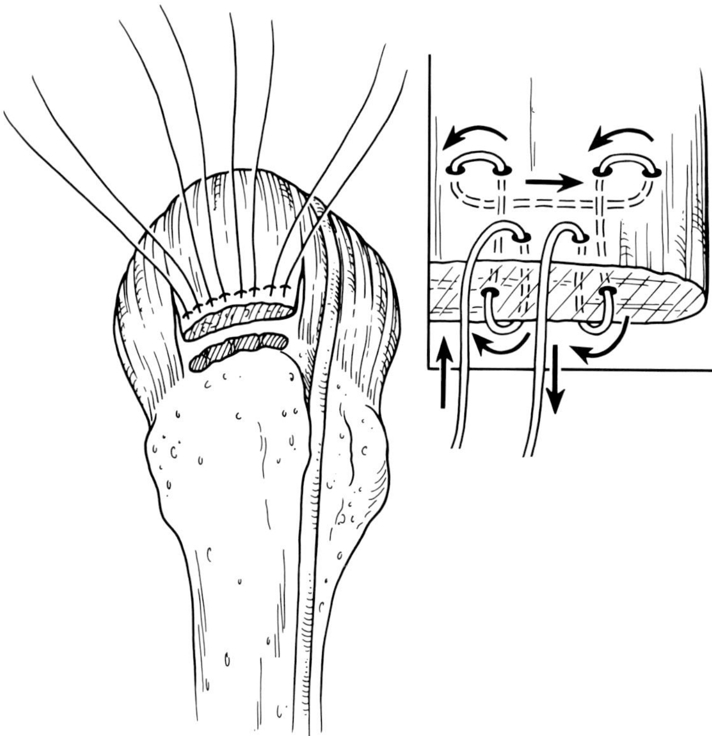

Figure 9-8. SCOI suture technique for rotator cuff repair. (Courtesy of Linvatec Corp., Largo, FL.)

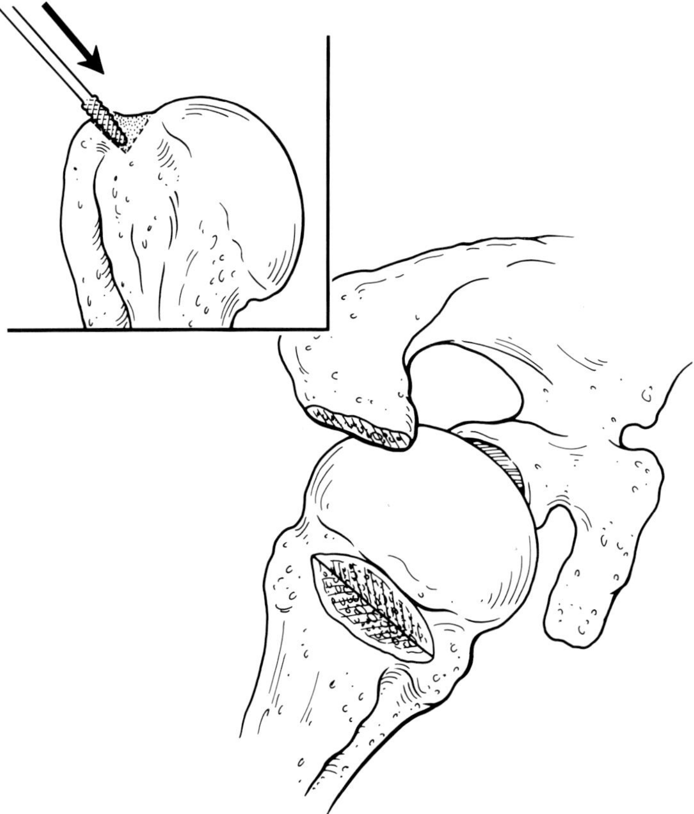

Figure 9-9. Trough in bone is made at the junction of the anatomic neck and greater tuberosity.

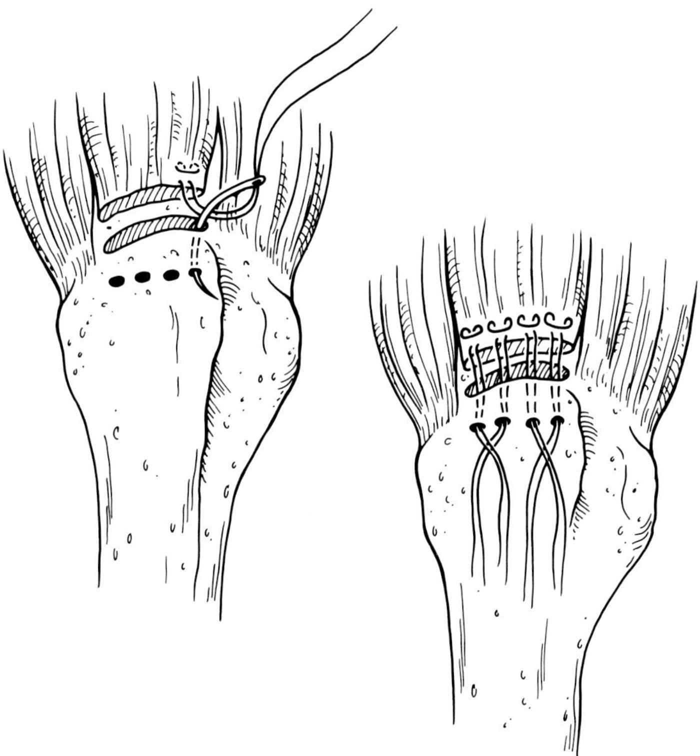

Figure 9-10. Sutures are passed through the greater tuberosity with a 1.5-in cutting needle or suture passer.

will be visible through the cuff if significant thinning has occurred. Small pinhole full-thickness tears demonstrate leakage of dye through the tear, leading the surgeon to the tear in the cuff. This is most often in the area of the supraspinatus insertion at the greater tuberosity. Once the location of cuff disease is localized, the cuff is split in line with the fibers for a distance of 1 to 2 cm. The undersurface of the cuff often has a "crabmeat" appearance, and we make every effort to excise this diseased tissue. The cuff may be repaired in a side-to-side fashion with size 2 nonabsorbable suture or 1-mm braided Dacron, although one always feels more secure with a trough-in-bone repair if significant resection of the cuff is required or there is tension on the side-to-side repair.

If diagnostic arthroscopy is performed and a partial-thickness cuff tear is diagnosed, an evaluation of the extent of the cuff tear is critical. I feel that partical-thickness tears involving more than 50 percent thickness of the cuff should be excised and repaired either side to side or preferably to a trough in bone. I feel that a tear of more than 50 percent thickness will most likely progress to a full-thickness tear over time.

If preoperative diagnostic studies or diagnostic arthroscopy demonstrates a partial-thickness or small full-thickness tear, an arthroscopic acromioplasty combined with a mini-incision approach can be used for rotator cuff repair. After the arthroscopic acromioplasty, a 3 to 5-in incision is used at the anterolateral corner of the acromion, often extending the anterolateral stab wound used for the acromioplasty and extended distally in line with the fibers of the deltoid (Fig. 9-11). The deltoid is split in line with its fibers from the lateral edge of the acromion up to 5 cm in line with the fibers of the deltoid. A deep self-retaining retractor is then used to expose the underlying bursa and rotator cuff. A limited bursectomy is performed, and the rotator cuff is evaluated. If a small full-thickness tear is noted, a side-to-side repair or a repair to a trough in bone is used, depending on the extent of the tear. If a partial-thickness tear is noted with the bursal side intact, an intraoperative arthrogram is used. Location of partial-thickness cuff tear can also be marked during arthroscopy, with a suture passed through an 18-gauge spinal needle. This will help the surgeon determine the site of rotator cuff pathology during the deltoid-splitting exposure. The trough-in-bone repair should be used when possible and that this may be technically difficult with the limited exposure of a mini-incision approach. For medium and large tears, the mini-incision does not allow the surgeon to perform adequate lysis of adhesions and mobilization of the cuff. The acromioclavicular joint cannot be evaluated through the mini-incision approach. If a mini-incision is used, a suture anchor device is of great benefit in repairing the tendon to a trough in bone due to the limited exposure. I have found particularly with the deltoid that with adequate closure of

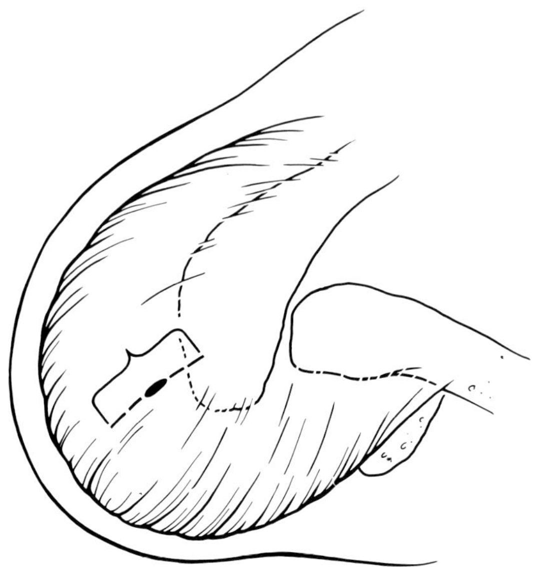

Figure 9-11. Mini-incision for small full-thickness rotator cuff repairs.

the deltoid over the anterior acromion, the mini-incision approach has limited benefits to formal open rotator cuff surgery.

Of critical importance to the success of open rotator cuff repair is the reattachment of the deltoid to the anterior acromion. If the deltoid has been detached (*deltoid off*), two drill holes are made in the anterior acromion approximately 5 to 7 mm posterior to the anterior edge of the acromion. Care must be taken that these holes are not to close to the anterior acromion to avoid fracture. The anterior deltoid is then reapproximated to the acromion with size 2 nonabsorbable suture in a vertical mattress or interrupted simple fashion (Fig. 9-12). If the deltoid fascia allows, a side-to-side repair of the deltoid may be performed with size 2 nonabsorbable sutures without the need for drill holes. This is my preferred method of handling the deltoid (*deltoid on*). The split in the deltoid is then reapproximated with size 1 absorbable suture (Fig. 9 13).

The subcutaneous layer is closed with interrupted absorbable size 2-0 sutures, and the skin is reapproximated with running size 3-0 subcuticular sutures. Routine postoperative dressings are applied, and the patient is placed in a sling or abduction pillow, depending on the tension of the repair.

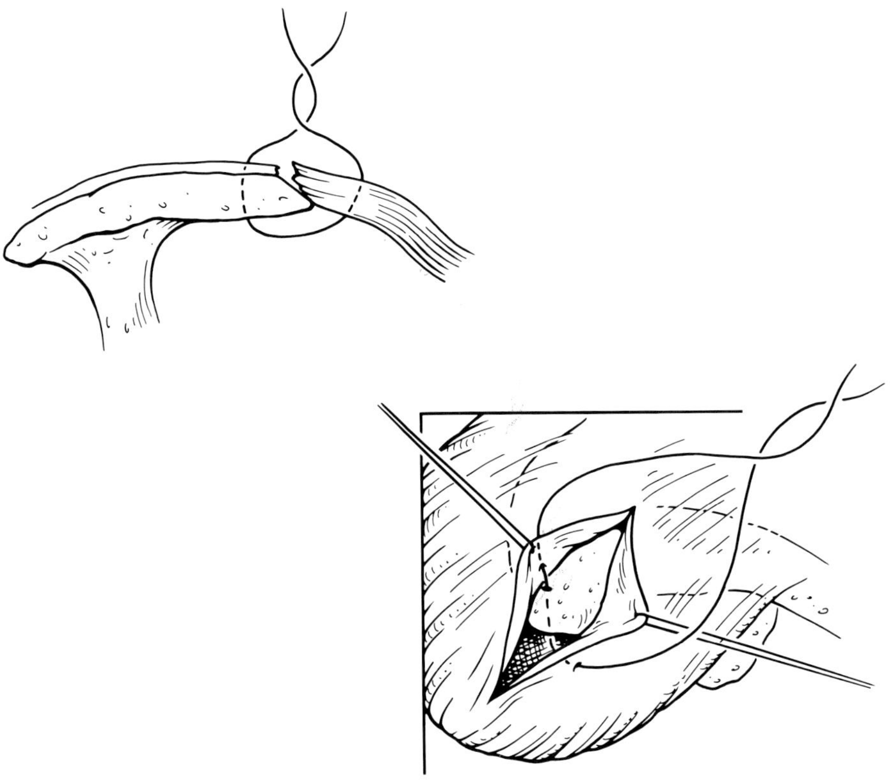

Figure 9-12. Deltoid fascia reapproximated to the anterior acromion using drill holes in acromion and vertical mattress suture technique.

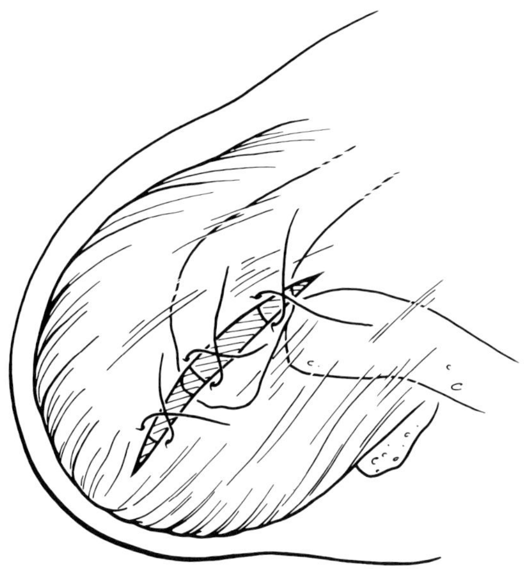

Figure 9-13. Side-to-side repair of deltoid splitting (deltoid on) incision.

POSTOPERATIVE REHABILITATION

Most patients are managed in a sling postoperatively except for those with tears that are massive and repaired under tension requiring an abduction pillow. Ice is applied to the operative shoulder for the first 72 hours for 15 to 20 minutes every hour while awake or continuously with a coolant system.

Phase I

Passive range of motion exercises in external rotation, forward elevation, and pendulum exercises begin the first postoperative day; two to four sets a day with 10 repetitions of each exercise are recommended. There is a tremendous variability in the patient's ability to obtain passive range of motion in the first 6 weeks, but I emphasize that all patients have full passive motion in the first 6 weeks if possible. Passive internal rotation is delayed for 3 weeks after surgery.

If the mini-open surgical approach has been used for repair of small full- or partial-thickness tears, the patients may experience less postoperative pain. The splitting of the deltoid lessens the possibility of deltoid detachment during postoperative rehabilitation. However, I think that the weak link in rotator cuff surgery is the repair of the rotator cuff either in a side-to-side or trough-in-bone fashion. Therefore, all patients undergoing open surgery for rotator cuff repair must be protected from active exercises for the first 6 weeks postoperatively. For large and massive tears, passive motion should be continued for 8 weeks.

Phase II

Active motion with terminal stretching begins at postoperative week 7 for most patients but can be delayed up to 8 or more weeks if there is a large or massive tear. During phase II, patients are educated to begin active assisted and subsequently active exercises in external rotation, internal rotation, and forward elevation. This is followed by gentle terminal stretching. Pendulum exercises are also maintained during this phase. For large tears, resumption of the supine position to begin phase II allows success. Many patients require two weeks to actively elevate in the upright position when beginning phase II.

Phase III

Phase III generally begins about the third postoperative month but again may be delayed, depending on the size of the tear. This phase involves active motion with terminal stretching (i.e., phase II) and a resistance program with resistance tubing. Active motion with terminal stretching is maintained as performed in phase II. Resistance exercises are performed in external rotation, internal rotation, forward flexion, and overhead punch press fashion. These are performed in two to three sets a day for 10 to 15 repetitions. It is beneficial to begin all phases of the rehabilitation program in the supine position to allow gravity to work in favor of the patient. The patient can then progress to sitting and then to a standing position.

RESULTS

Few articles in the orthopaedic literature have reported on the results of rotator cuff surgery in athletes.[1,9] Hawkins and Misamore[4] have reported 86 percent relief of pain in patients with rotator cuff tear that was repaired to a trough in bone. Most of the patients in this study were of the nonathletic population. Other authors have reported good or excellent relief of pain in 58 to 85 percent of their patients in dealing with the general population.[2,7,8]

Tibone et al[9] have reported on 45 athletes with a partial- or full-thickness rotator cuff tear treated with an anterior acromioplasty and repair of the rotator cuff. Eight-seven percent of their patients stated that they were improved compared with their preoperative status, although only 34 patients (76 percent) thought that they had a significant reduction in pain postoperatively. Objectively, only 56 percent of the patients were rated as having a good result that allowed them to return to their former competitive level without significant pain. Forty-one percent of the 29 athletes who had been involved in pitching and throwing returned to their former competitive status. In their experience, a repair of the rotator cuff combined with an acromioplasty in the young athletic population provided satisfactory relief of pain but did not guarantee that the athlete would be able to return to his or her former competitive status in all sports.

Bigliani et al[1] have reported on 23 tennis players with symptomatic full-thickness rotator cuff tears having undergone anterior acromioplasty and rotator cuff repair. Eighty-three percent of their patients achieved a good result, signified by being pain-free, and were able to play tennis at their presymptomatic competitive level.

My experience is that full-thickness rotator cuff tears rarely occur and are less symptomatic in the young athletic population compared with the average patient. With the advent and increased use of MRI, it may be possible to detect partial-thickness rotator cuff tears that were previously diagnosed as rotator cuff tendinitis. Full-thickness rotator cuff tears tend to occur in the athletic population at an age similar to that of the nonathletic population. The average age for patients in Bigliani's study was 58 years of age, whereas the average age in the Tibone study was 29 years. Bigliani's patients all had full-thickness rotator cuff tears. The Tibone group included 65 percent who had partial-thickness rotator cuff tears and perhaps had an element of underlying instability due to their predilection for overhead throwing activities.

As a general rule, a secure repair of the rotator cuff to a trough in bone should be strived for in all patients undergoing rotator cuff repair. The ability of an athlete to return to his or her presurgical level of competition probably relates more to the upper extremity requirements of the particular sport.

Diagnosis and surgical treatment of rotator cuff pathology in the athlete are both challenging and demanding. Preoperative education, a secure repair of the rotator cuff and repair of the deltoid, and a comprehensive postoperative rehabilitation program offer patients a predictable and successful outcome.

REFERENCES

1. Bigiliani LU, Kimmel J, McCann PD: Repair of rotator cuff tears in tennis players. Am J Sports Med 20, 1992
2. Debeyre J, Patte D, Elmelik E: Repair of ruptures of the rotator cuff of the shoulder with a note on advancement of the supraspinatus muscle. J Bone Joint Surg [Br] 47:436, 1949
3. Hawkins RJ, Kunkel SS: Rotator cuff repair utilizing a trough in bone. p. 149–154. In Paulos LE, Tibone JE (eds): Operative Techniques in Shoulder Surgery. Aspen Publishers, Gaithersburg, MD, 1992
4. Hawkins RJ, Misamore MD, Hobeika PE: Surgery for full thickness rotator cuff tears. J Bone Joint Surg [Am] 67: 1349–55, 1985
5. Kunkel SS, Hawkins RJ: Rotator cuff repair utilizing a trough in bone. Techniques Orthop 3:51–57, 1989
6. Neer CS II: Anterior acromioplasty for chronic impingement syndrome in the shoulder: a preliminary report. J Bone Joint Surg [Am] 54:41–50, 1972
7. Peterson C: Long term results of rotator cuff repair. In Bailey JI, Kessel L (eds): Shoulder Surgery. Springer, Berlin, 1982
8. Samilson RL, Binder WF: Symptomatic full thickness tears of the rotator cuff: an analysis of 292 shoulders in 276 patients. Orthop Clin North Am 6:449, 1975
9. Tibone JE, Elrod B, Jobe FW et al: Surgical treatment of tears of the rotator cuff in athletes. J Bone Joint Surg [Am] 68:877–89, 1986
10. Uhthoff H, Sarkar K: Repair in rotator cuff tendons. p. 216–9. In Surgery of the Shoulder. CV Mosby, St. Louis, 1990

CHAPTER TEN

Arthroscopy for Rotator Cuff Disorders

James R. Andrews
Timothy B. Sutherland

Rotator cuff disorders in the athlete's shoulder remain a diagnostic and therapeutic challenge for the sports medicine physician. Timely and accurate diagnosis, coupled with appropriate treatment, allows expedient return to preinjury status. Shoulder arthroscopy has become a valuable tool for diagnostic and therapeutic treatment of both professional and recreational athletes.

The most crucial diagnostic tools in the evaluation of the athletic rotator cuff injury remain a complete and accurate history and physical examination.[18] The athlete's history, in addition to the traditional questions regarding pain location, onset, quality, severity, and timing, must include athlete and sports-specific questions. For the throwing athlete, these include the sport and level of competition (recreational, collegiate, professional), the position played, the exact activity and motion that reproduced the patient's disability, and the phase of throwing affected (windup, cocking, acceleration, deceleration, and follow-through). The thrower's control, velocity, and endurance (both pitch count and innings pitched) should also be carefully scrutinized to obtain subtle hints as to the underlying pathology. The collision athlete should be carefully questioned regarding the location and position of the injured extremity at impact, the presence of any neurologic symptoms, and current functional disability. The player's protective equipment (padding) should be carefully assessed for its role in both preventing injury and allowing early return to competition. Competitive and highly trained athletes are often able to precisely pinpoint the location and exacerbating activities of their shoulder injury, thus greatly assisting in diagnosis.

A complete physical examination is essential. Observation of the athlete at rest, disrobing, and reproducing athletic motions can provide subtle information regarding muscular atrophy and abnormal motion patterns. Game films of the athlete, if available, can be reviewed to evaluate both the initial mechanism of injury and current postinjury status. Gentle palpation can reveal specific areas of tenderness and should include the sternoclavicular joint, the acromioclavicular joint, rotator cuff insertion, and the anterior and posterior glenohumeral joint. Strength testing with manual muscle testing and carefully documented active and passive range of motion should be performed for both shoulders. Range of motion testing should be performed in both the sitting and supine positions. Specific tests for impingement, stability, and labral pathology are then performed.

After a complete history and physical examination, ancillary tests are ordered as necessary. A standard set of plain radiographs is obtained on most athletes. This evaluation includes anteroposterior views in internal rotation and external rotation, a West Point axillary view, and a Stryker notch view. With suspected rotator cuff injury, additional views (the suprasinatus outlet view[16] and the acromial profile view[3]) are used to fully define the anatomy of the acromion and the coracoacromial arch. Additional radiographic studies including magnetic resonance imaging (MRI) scans, contrast enhanced MRI scans, and arthrograms are ordered on a case-by-case basis if necessary to make therapeutic decisions. Isokinetic muscle testing can be used to document and diagnose subtle motor deficiencies. Electrodiagnostic testing (electromyograms and nerve conduction velocity studies) is occasionally used if suspicion of primary nerve lesion is present.

Rotator cuff disease can be classified by both mechanism of injury and morphology. The four major categories of rotator cuff injury in the athlete are primary compressive cuff disease, secondary compressive cuff disease, tensile failure of the cuff, and acute traumatic rotator cuff tears. The overhead athlete most commonly presents with some manifestation of overuse cuff failure, whereas acute traumatic rotator cuff tears are seen more commonly in collision sports and high-energy injuries.

Primary compressive cuff disease is essentially the classic impingement lesion described by Neer.[15] Extrinsic compression on the rotator cuff from the coracoacromial arch combined with age-related degenerative changes within the tendon itself lead to primary compressive disease. Clinically, these patients present with insidious onset of shoulder pain, radiation to the deltoid muscle, nocturnal pain, and exacerbation of symptoms with overhead activities. Examination generally reveals a positive impingement sign (pain with internal rotation and forward flexion)[13] in a painful arc from 80 to 120 degrees. The impingement test, or relief of symptoms with injection of local anesthetic into the subacromial space, generally confirms the diagnosis. Primary compressive disease is found most commonly in athletes older than 40 years of age, most often involved in overhead sports. The pain can often be temporally localized to the follow-through stages in both throwing and racquet sports when the internally rotated arm enters the painful arc from 80 to 120 degrees. Variable amounts of weakness can be present secondary to either pain or actual rotator cuff involvement (tendonitis, partial-thickness rotator cuff tearing, or full-thickness rotator cuff tearing).

Weakness should be evaluated with external rotation strength at 0 degrees and 90 degrees abduction, empty can test, and internal rotation at 0 degrees abduction. Weakness secondary to pain is often completely alleviated with subacromial injection of local anesthetic (the impingement test). Primary compressive disease is uncommon in young athletes younger than 35 years of age. These young patients with true primary compressive cuff disease will generally demonstrate bony abnormalities of the coracoacromial arch, either a congenitally hooked (or type III) acromion[9,10] or the presence of an os acromionale.[11] Most commonly, athletes younger than 35 years of age with impingement symptoms have underlying anterior instability. History and physical examination will reveal evidence of this instability and should be carefully sought in the young athlete.[11]

Anterior instability often presents as secondary compressive cuff disease in these young athletes.[14] Failure of the glenohumeral ligament capsule complex, the static stabilizers of the shoulder, leads to fatigue of the dynamic stabilizers of the shoulder, the rotator cuff muscles. This fatigue allows abnormal translation of the humeral head with impingement under the coracoacromial arch. This abnormal translation can also lead to impingement of the posterosuperior rotator cuff on the glenoid in the cocking position of abduction with maximal external rotation.[19] Distinguishing secondary from primary compressive disease is critical, as treatment approaches are radically different.

Tensile lesions are most commonly seen in overhead athletes and usually occur as undersurface rotator cuff tears or lesions of the biceps labral complex.[1,2,6] This tensile failure is due to microtrauma with eccentric overload of the rotator cuff during the deceleration phase of throwing as the cuff resists horizontal adduction, internal rotation, anterior translation, and distraction forces. Partial tears secondary to repetitive microtrauma are usually seen in the undersurface of the supraspinatus and posterior cuff tendons.[4] Tensile lesions can also be secondary to anterior laxity, with increased forces placed on the posterior cuff musculature. On physical examination, the patients often have minimal weakness, with pain primarily over the supraspinatus and infraspinatus tendons and posterior capsule. Advanced imaging with computed tomographic arthrogram or contrast MRI may reveal partial undersurface tearing.

Acute traumatic rotator cuff tears are uncommon in the athlete's shoulder and are most commonly seen in the collision sports or as a sequelae of high-energy trauma. The usual mechanism of injury is forced adduction or active abduction against resistance. These athletes present with a single well-defined traumatic episode. Examination reveals variable degrees of discomfort with significant weakness of the rotator cuff musculature. Expedient diagnosis and early treatment with rotator cuff repair seems to offer these athletes the best functional result.

Except for the acute traumatic tear, the initial treatment of most rotator cuff injuries is conservative. This conservative treatment involves a supervised rehabilitation program that emphasizes protection of healing tissues with progression to complete return of motion and strength. All patients enter a carefully supervised interval return to sports program that is activity- and sport-specific and tailored to each athlete's underlying pathology.

The arthroscope is a secondary tool used for the diagnosis of elusive shoulder disorders and for the treatment of many common athletic rotator cuff injuries that prove recalcitrant to conservative treatment.

Diagnostic arthroscopy of the shoulder allows enhancement of the clinical assessment of the rotator cuff pathology, verification of the suspected clinical lesion, and precise delineation of the location and degree of the underlying shoulder pathology. The arthroscope can also be used for appropriate decompression and debridement as indicated by the patient's clinical and arthroscopic examination and presentation.

Surgical arthroscopy of the shoulder begins with the preoperative education and preparation of the athlete. Careful explanation of the proposed procedure to the athlete greatly facilitates postoperative rehabilitation. Both the goals for surgery and the limitations of surgery should be reviewed with the athlete; the postoperative rehabilitation regimen should be outlined and its importance emphasized to ensure compliance.

As intraoperative hemostasis is critical in achieving visualization of the subacromial space, preoperative evaluation should include assessment of any bleeding tendencies or coagulopathies. All nonsteroidal anti-inflammatories and other prostaglandin inhibitors should be discontinued 7 to 10 days before surgery. If any question of bleeding disorder exists, appropriate laboratory studies (including prothrombin time, partial thromboplastin time, and bleeding times) should be checked.

Supraspinatus outlet views and acromial profile views should be reviewed before surgery to assess size of the acromial hook and acromial thickness. This allows estimation of the amount of bone to be resected anteriorly as well as the total amount of bone that can be removed without increasing the risk of acromial fracture postoperatively. This acromions (less than 8 mm in thickness on outlet view) should be decompressed carefully to avoid overthinning and fracture. Preoperative muscle strength and ancillary studies (MRI scan, arthrograms if available) should be reviewed to allow for planning of rotator cuff repair if clinically indicated.

After appropriate preoperative preparation, the patient is taken to the operating suite. We generally use general anesthesia for our routine shoulder arthroscopy unless contraindicated by the patient's overall medical health. A careful examination under general anesthesia is then performed on both shoulders. Translation anteriorly, posteriorly, and inferiorly is assessed in neutral, internal, and external rotation and is documented. The patient is then carefully positioned in the lateral decubitus position and is supported by a beanbag or kidney rest. All bony prominences are carefully padded, and an axillary roll is used if necessary. The arm is then suspended from the overhead pulley system in about 60 to 70 degrees of adduction and 15 degrees of forward flexion. The suspension rope is secured to a free-hanging weight of 10 to 20 lb. The lightest weight that will adequately suspend the arm without exerting undue traction is used. The operating room table is then rotated to allow access to both the anterior and posterior aspect of the shoulder. After the shoulder is sterilely prepared and draped, the bony anatomic landmarks are marked with a sterile marking pen—the anterolateral and posterolateral corners of the acromion, the acromioclavicular joint, and the coracoid process.[5]

We routinely add epinephrine to our arthroscopic fluid (one ampule of 1 : 1,000 epinephrine per 3-liter bag of fluid). At this point, we also check the patient's blood pressure and request that the patient's blood pressure be decreased to a systolic pressure of 90 mmHg or less (if the overall cardiovascular condition of the athlete permits). These two maneuvers help obtain hemostasis in the bursal space and ensure adequate visualization for diagnostic and therapeutic arthroscopy.

The acromioclavicular joint is then palpated, and an 18-gauge spinal needle is inserted into the joint. This assists in localizing the acromioclavicular joint when in the subacromial space and is most easily accomplished before insertion of the arthroscope with possible distension of the soft tissues. The posterior portal is established first, and its location is identified by palpating the posterior "soft spot" over the glenohumeral joint. This point is approximately 2 to 3 cm inferior and 1 cm medial to the posterolateral corner of the acromion and represents the interval between the infraspinatus and the teres minor. Gentle internal and external rotation of the arm can assist in the location of this interval. Care should be taken to avoid being too close to the posterior acromion, as this can make visualization of the anterior acromion and acromioclavicular joint difficult. An 18-gauge spinal needle is then inserted in the soft spot and advanced toward the coracoid process anteriorly. A gentle pop is felt as the needle penetrates the posterior capsule. The glenohumeral joint is then distended with 40 to 50 ml of saline, and free backflow from the needle ensures proper placement. As the joint reaches maximal distension, the arm will also be observed to gently rotate. The spinal needle is then removed, and a small stab incision is made in the skin with a #11 blade. The arthroscopic cannula and dull trocar are then advanced to the glenohumeral joint. Only dull trocars are used, and the sharp trocars may be removed from the operative field to avoid inadvertant use. The tip of the dull trocar is used to palpate the posterior rim of the glenoid, and the arthroscopic cannula is inserted just lateral to the posterior rim. The arthroscope is then inserted, and an initial assessment of the glenohumeral joint is performed. The biceps tendon is used for orientation and is carefully examined for any degenerative change or detachment of the biceps labral anchor. The anterior capsulolabral complex is then carefully evaluated for evidence of a traumatic Bankart lesion, with detachment of the anteroinferior labrum from bone, or the presence of capsular laxity. If the arthroscope can be advanced without difficulty anteroinferiorly between the humeral head and glenoid, this is considered evidence of abnormal capsular laxity. The articular surfaces of the humeral head and glenoid are then examined for evidence of chondral damage. The posterior and anterior humeral heads are evaluated for the presence of Hill-Sachs or reverse Hill-Sachs lesions consistent with pathologic laxity. The rotator cuff is then carefully visualized, the subscapularis is checked, and the superior cuff is checked for any evidence of undersurface tearing (Plate 10-1). Fraying of the undersurfaces of the supraspinatus and the posterior cuff is seen with tensile failure of the cuff in overhead athletes and is commonly seen in veteran pitchers at the professional level[2] (Plate 10-2).

To allow complete visualization of the joint and the use of operating instruments, an anterior portal is established. This portal is established halfway between the coracoid process and the anterolateral corner of the acromion. A spinal needle is passed from this location into the joint and visualized with the arthroscope. The needle should pass just below the biceps tendon, through the rotator interval when viewed intra-articularly. If the initial examination revealed a traumatic Bankart lesion and consideration is being given to arthroscopic stabilization, the position of the anterior portal may be altered. In this situation, the portal may be moved superiorly to just below the anterolateral corner of the acromion. Again, the intra-articular position should be confirmed with spinal needle placement. The needle is then removed, a small skin incision is made, and the arthroscopic cannula and dull trochar are introduced into the joint under direct visualization. The arthroscope is then inserted into the anterior portal, and diagnostic arthroscopy of the shoulder is completed. The anterior capsuloligamentous structures are evaluated, and the posterior cuff and labrum are evaluated for undersurface tearing or degenerative change. Undersurface tears of the cuff can then be debrided sequentially using the anterior and posterior portals using a 4.2-mm motorized debrider. Any degenerative labral tears are then carefully debrided, taking care to prevent destabilization of the shoulder joint.[8,17] An additional anterior portal may be established adjacent to and inferior to the original anterior portal if necessary for additional instrumentation.

Large partial-thickness tears should be carefully palpated to avoid missing a full-thickness tear. Internal and external rotation of the arm assist in visualizing the entire undersurface of the rotator cuff.

After glenohumeral arthroscopy is completed, subacromial bursoscopy is performed. Before beginning the bursoscopy, the athlete's blood pressure is once again checked to ensure adequate hypotension has been maintained. The arthroscope and cannula are then removed from the glenohumeral joint. The arthroscopic cannula and dull trocar are taken through the posterior skin incision. The posterior acromion is palpated, and the cannula and trocar are advanced into the bursa. The coracoacromial ligament can often be palpated anteriorly with the tip of the trocar. Before inserting the arthroscope, the general position of the cannula is checked by lining up a second cannula of identical length on the superior aspect of the shoulder. Care is taken that the tip of the cannula is under the anterior aspect of the acromion and not medially under the acromioclavicular joint or laterally into the deltoid muscle. The arthroscope is then inserted into the subacromial space. Even with the presence of bursal adhesions and scarring, a bursal space should be identifiable (Plate 10-3). If not, often the posterior bursal curtain has not been penetrated, and the arthroscope should be removed, the dull trocar replaced, and the cannula advanced more anteriorly (Plate 10-4).

The subacromial space is then carefully evaluated. The coracoacromial ligament, undersurface of the acromion, superior surface of the rotator cuff, and the acromioclavicular joint are identified (Plate 10-5). Subacromial adhesions and scarring often make visualization difficult, and a lateral portal must be established. A spinal needle is inserted approximately 1 cm posterior and 3 cm distal to the anterolateral corner of the acromion. This needle is then visualized in the bursal space. The needle should be roughly parallel to the undersurface of the acromion. If the needle must be angled too far caudal or cephalad to be identified in the subacromial space, then manipulation of instruments in the lateral portal will be difficult. A small skin incision is then made, and the cannula with dull trocar is advanced into the bursa. Debridement of the subacromial adhesions is then accomplished with a motorized debrider. After careful debridement, the subacromial space is carefully evaluated for any evidence of impingement or rotator cuff tearing. The undersurface of the acromion and the coracoacromial ligament are examined for areas of abrasion or wear (Plate 10-6). The bursa over the rotator cuff is carefully debrided, and the cuff is assessed for any evidence of abrasion or superficial partial-thickness rotator cuff tears (Plate 10-7). The arm is gently internally and externally rotated to facilitate complete visualization of the cuff. The lateral portal may be used to complete visualization of the cuff if this cannot be performed through the posterior portal.

Visualization in the subacromial space can be problematic secondary to bleeding, and strict attention must be paid to hemostasis. Electrocautery is used liberally to coagulate areas of bleeding (Plate 10-8). Instrumentation of the subacromial space often causes an increase in the patient's blood pressure, and as previously noted, bleeding is reduced with a systolic blood pressure below 90 mmHg. We routinely use an arthroscopic pump system (3M), and in the bursa we will increase the pump pressure from 30 mmHg (used for glenohumeral arthroscopy) to 50 to 60 mmHg in the subacromial space.

If evidence of impingement is present or a full-thickness rotator cuff tear is identified, we proceed with arthroscopic subacromial decompression. With the arthroscope in the posterior portal, a motorized debrider from the lateral portal is used to debride all soft tissues off the undersurface of the acromion. The acromioclavicular joint is then visualized. Localization of the acromioclavicular joint is assisted by the previously placed 18-gauge spinal needle. Electrocautery is used liberally in this stage, as the soft tissues below the acromion and surrounding the acromioclavicular joint are quite vascular. The electrocautery is then used to divide and elevate the coracoacromial ligament off the anterior aspect of the acromion. At this point, the anterior hook of the acromion can be identified, and the acromion appears to be longer in its posterior-to-anterior dimension (secondary to the anterior hook) (Plate 10-9). An oval motorized burr is then inserted through the lateral portal, and the anterior edge of the acromion is removed. Difficulty in removing the anterior acromion often indicates that osteophytes are present on the lateral acromion, and these must be removed before removing the anterior acromion. As the anterior acromion is removed, the anterior acromioclavicular joint and the distal clavicle will be identified. The remainder of the acromion is then flattened using the motorized burr. Care must be taken to avoid taking too much bone from the center of the acromion and creating a concavity or "soup bowl" on the undersurface of the acromion. This occurs most commonly in individuals with soft cancellous bone or very hard cortical bone. The acromion is flattened posteriorly approximately 2 to 3 cm, and this drop-off point can be visualized by withdrawing the arthroscope slightly in the posterior portal.

The depth and adequacy of the acromioplasty is then assessed. The periosteal sleeve anteriorly is used to estimate the amount of bone removed. This layer is easily identifiable, and its depth can be estimated by the outside diameter of the burr cannula (Plate 10-10). We typically excise 8 to 10 mm from the anterior acromion. The thickness of the acromion and the size of the anterior hook may alter the amount of bone resected. The distal clavicle is then visualized, and the anterior resection is checked by the depth of exposed distal clavicle. Depending on the presence of preoperative infraclavicular osteophytes, this should also measure approximately 8 mm. If any spurs are present on the undersurface of the clavicle, they are resected with the motorized burr at this point. Finally, the overall configuration of the acromion is examined. After adequate acromioplasty, the long diameter visualized should not run in a medial-to-lateral direction secondary to excision of the anterior spur.

If preoperative examination revealed significant acromioclavicular joint pain, we then proceed with arthroscopic distal clavicle excision.[12] An anterior portal is established just anterior to the acromioclavicular joint by using an 18-gauge spinal needle. A small skin incision is made, and the soft tissues are debrided. Hemostasis is obtained, and a large motorized burr is used to excise the lateral 1 to 1.5 cm of the distal clavicle. Care must be taken to adequately resect the superior and posterior clavicle. Visualization can be improved with the use of the 70 degree arthroscope.

Full-thickness tears of the rotator cuff are evaluated arthroscopically from both the glenohumeral joint and the subacromial space (Plate 10-11). Nonviable tissue is carefully debrided using a motorized debrider. In young athletes, we proceed with arthroscopic subacromion decompression and then prefer a "mini-open" repair of the rotator cuff. Arthroscopic evaluation and subacromial decompression must be performed expediently in this situation to avoid excessive fluid extravasation into the soft tissues, which can make mini-open repair difficult.

Arthroscopic debridement of the full-thickness tear can be considered in some situations (Plate 10-12). Debridement is usually considered in the older patient who presents with a chief complaint of pain without weakness. Physical examination should reveal no significant weakness of the cuff. Arthroscopic debridement alone can be considered in this situation, although the patient should be carefully counseled that an additional procedure may be necessary. If there is a question as to the functional significance of a tear and it is reparable, we will proceed to a mini-open repair of the rotator cuff. Arthroscopic debridement may also be considered in the massive irreparable rotator cuff deficit. In these patients, usually elderly, decompression and debridement often provide significant pain relief and surprising improvement in function. Postoperative rehabilitation emphasizes the anterior and middle deltoids to compensate for the absent rotator cuff. Care should be taken in debridement of these patients with massive cuff defects to avoid destabilization of the coracoacromial arch. For this reason, minimal bone resection is performed with the acromioplasty, and the coracoacromial ligament is not excised.

Partial-thickness tears of the rotator cuff are debrided as described above.[2] Debridement alone is performed with undersurface tears as if no evidence of impingement exists in the subacromial space. Superior (bursal surface) partial-thickness tears are debrided and combined with an arthroscopic subacromial decompression.

Appropriate diagnosis and treatment of rotator cuff injuries in athletes allow safe and early return to sports participation. Shoulder arthroscopy provides an additional diagnostic and therapeutic modality with the athlete fails to respond to conservative treatment. Surgical arthroscopy combined with a well-supervised rehabilitation program returns many of those athletes to their preinjury status.[20]

REFERENCES

1. Andrews JR, Angelo RL: Shoulder arthroscopy for the throwing athlete. In Paulos LE, Tibone JE (eds): Operative Techniques in Shoulder Surgery. Aspen Publishers, Gaithersburg, MD, 1991
2. Andrews JR, Brousard TS, Carson WG: Arthroscopy of the shoulder in the management of partial tears of the rotator cuff: a preliminary report. Arthroscopy 1:117, 1985
3. Andrews JR, Byrd JWT, Kupferman SP, Angelo RL: The profile view of the acromion. Clin Orthop 263:142, 1991

4. Andrews JR, Carson WG, McLeod WD: Glenoid labral tears related to the long head of the biceps. Am J Sports Med 13:337, 1985
5. Andrews JR, Carson WG, Ortega K: Arthroscopy of the shoulder: technique and normal anatomy. Am J Sports Med 12:1, 1984
6. Andrews JR, Gidumal RH: Shoulder arthroscopy in the throwing athlete. Perspectives and prognosis. Arthroscopy 6:374, 1990
7. Andrews JR, Gillogly S: Physical examination of the shoulder in throwing athletes. In Zarins B, Andrews JR, Carson WG (eds): Injuries to the Throwing Arm. WB Saunders, Philadelphia, 1985
8. Andrews JR, Kupferman SP, Dillman CJ: Labral tears in throwing and racquet sports. Clin Sports Med 10:901, 1991
10. Bigliani LU, Morrison D, April EW: The morphology of the acromion and its relationship to rotator cuff tears. Orthop Trans 10:228, 1986
11. Bigliani LU, Norris RT, Fischer J: The relationship between the unfused acromial epiphysis and subacromial impingement lesions. Orthop Trans 7:138, 1983
12. Gartsman GM, Combs AH, Davis PF, Tullos HS: Arthroscopic acromioclavicular joint resection: an anatomical study. Am J Sports Med 19:2, 1991
13. Hawkins RJ, Kennedy JD: Impingement syndrome in athletes. Am J Sports Med 8:151, 1980
14. Jobe FW, Glousman RE: Rotator cuff dysfunction and associated glenohumeral instability in the throwing athlete. In Paulos LE, Tibone JE (eds): Operative Techniques in Shoulder Surgery. Aspen Publishers, Gaithersburg, MD, 1991
15. Neer CS: Anterior acromioplasty for the chronic impingement syndrome in the shoulder. J Bone Joint Surg [Am] 54:41, 1972
16. Neer CS, Poppen NK: Supraspinatus outlet. Orthop Trans 11:234, 1987
17. Pappas AM, Goss TP, Kleinman PK: Symptomatic shoulder instability due to lesions of the glenoid labrum. Am J Sports Med 11:279, 1983
18. Scarpinato DF, Bramhall JP, Andrews JR: Arthroscopic management of the throwing athlete's shoulder. Clin Sports Med 10:913, 1991
19. Walch G, Boileau P, Noel E, Donell ST: Impingement of the deep surface of the supraspinatus tendon on the posterosuperior glenoid rim, an arthroscopic study. J Shoulder Elbow Surg 1:238, 1992
20. Wilk KE, Arrigo C, Courson R: Preventive and Rehabilitative Exercises for the Shoulder and Elbow. 3rd Ed. American Sports Medicine Institute, Birmingham, AL, 1991

CHAPTER ELEVEN

Overview of Glenohumeral Instability

Richard J. Hawkins
Gary W. Misamore

Interest in glenohumeral instability has increased in the past few years, due in part to the vast number of basic research publications that have recently appeared in the peer review literature. The current concepts of shoulder instability, however, remain confusing and challenging. This chapter presents an overview of glenohumeral instability, with particular emphasis on basic concepts and their impact on the clinical aspects of glenohumeral instability.

In past years, our appreciation of instability in the athlete focused on the individual who sustained significant trauma, resulting in an acute dislocation that was reduced and often progressed to recurrent instability, and who eventually had an operation with a reasonably good outcome. However, there is now much more to an appreciation of instability, with other more confusing areas involving multidirectional instability,[39] posterior instability,[20] and the more subtle forms of anterior instability, particularly in the overhead athlete such as in the thrower, tennis player, or swimmer.[12,27,28,30] We also now have the overlap disorder secondary to instability, such as impingement tendinitis, both intrinsically and extrinsically. This overlap of rotator cuff and capsuloligamentous control presents a new and unique challenge to the treating physician.[30]

Considerable research has focused on the static constraints of ligaments and capsule and how they control the glenohumeral joint.[2,3,9,40,41,50,51,53,54] Patients' tissues vary significantly, and variations in collagen production and architecture may play a role in stability. The rotator cuff, as a dynamic stabilizer of the shoulder, has received significant interest.[3,5,6,9,12,19,29,32,45,47] The scapula, long neglected in the past, is now appreciated as an integral part of shoulder mechanics, and its coordinated action plays a vital role in stabilizing the glenohumeral joint.[30,47]

Problems unique to the overhead athlete commence with overuse, progress to eccentric overload, leading to dynamic and static failure, and eventually resulting in instability. This tissue breakdown and altered biomechanics with scapular dysfunction and secondary impingement are particularly prevalent in the throwing athlete with its more subtle form of anterior instability. The issue of sorting out these various problems in athletes poses a challenge[4,12,27,28,30,39] (Fig. 11-1).

CLASSIFICATION

To communicate clearly and have an appreciation of prognosis and treatment, there needs to be an agreed-on classification of glenohumeral instability. In general, we consider direction, degree, onset, timing, and volition as components of a classification system.

Historically, *direction* of instability has been a key ingredient, consisting of anterior, posterior, and now multidirectional. Inferior instability, previously classified as unidirectional, is almost always associated with multidirectional instability. The *degree* of instability has been described as subluxation or dislocation. It is now understood that there are more subtle forms of subluxation, particularly in the overhead athlete. The *onset* of instability may be traumatic

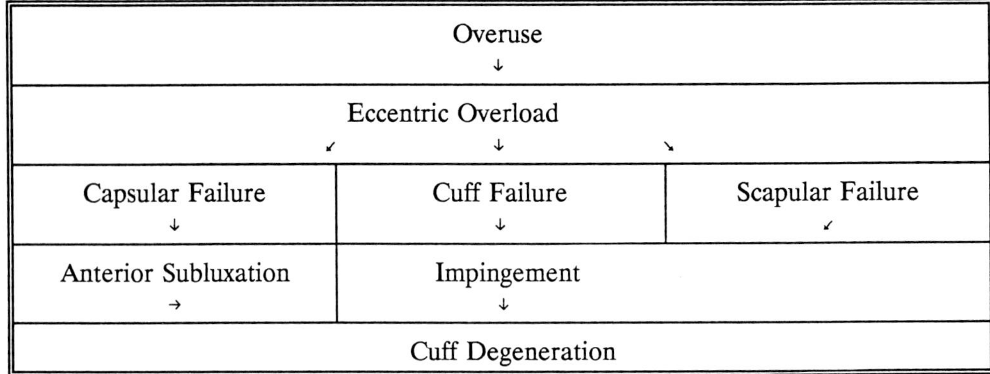

Figure 11-1. Common sequence of events leading to shoulder dysfunction.

or atraumatic. If atraumatic, it may have overuse superimposed on a predisposed tissue deficiency that leads to instability. There can also be traumatic instability superimposed on previously existing ligamentous laxity, which may or may not have been symptomatic before the traumatic onset. *Volition* is sometimes present in patients with posterior instability, produced either by muscular contraction or arm position, or both. It may occasionally be seen in patients who have multidirectional or anterior instability. The final component of a classification system considers an instability pattern as being *acute* or *chronic* (recurrent) in nature.

Matsen has provided a mnemonic to understand and classify instability at the extreme ends of the spectrum: TUBS and AMBRI, now referred to as AMBRII (Table 11-1). The TUBS variety of instability is *t*raumatic in onset *u*nidirectional (anterior) in direction with a *B*ankart lesion, and generally responding to *s*urgery. At the opposite end of the spectrum is the *AMBRII* type of patient, whose problem is *a*traumatic in onset, usually *m*ultidirectional in nature, typically with *b*ilateral shoulder laxity noted on examination, and usually responding to a *r*ehabilitation program, and if an operation is to be performed, it is an *i*nferior capsular shift with reconstruction of the *i*nterval lesion. An understanding of these two ends of the spectrum should help us with the difficult challenges of diagnosing and treating these problems. Unfortunately, there are many gradations between these extremes, such as an AMBRI type of patient who has a Bankart lesion, and thus, diagnosis, classification, and selection of the best treatment for each patient still often remain a challenge. Many athletes who function overhead have an instability pattern not incorporated in these mnemonics, in that they have more subtle forms of instability.

Table 11-1. Classification Mnemonic for Shoulder Instability

*T*raumatic	*A*traumatic
*U*nidirectional (anterior)	*M*ultidirectional
Bankart	*B*ilateral
*S*urgery	*R*ehabilitation
	*I*nferior capsular shift
	*I*nterval closure

There is an overlap between instability and impingement, and Jobe et al[30] have helped us appreciate this overlap by classifying patients into type I (pure impingement), type II (anterior subluxation with labral damage), type III (anterior instability with loose ligaments), and type IV (pure instability). Although not well standardized, this classification helps provide an understanding of this overlap.

COLLAGEN CHARACTERISTICS

Tissue characteristics play a role in instability. There are patients who have normal tissue subjected to trauma. There are patients who have abnormal tissues subjected to sometimes normal or minimal force, leading to instability. Finally, there are patients who have abnormal tissue subjected to significant trauma. The interaction of these tissue characteristics and the degree and nature of the trauma to which patients are subjected may lead to different instability patterns.

The football lineman who is arm tackling and undergoes a violent wrench with the arm thrust into extension in the externally rotated and abducted position will likely sustain a traumatic anterior dislocation of the shoulder with a Bankart lesion. The baseball pitcher who continually overuses the shoulder, subjecting it to eccentric overload, will eventually undergo capsuloligamentous failure, resulting in more subtle forms of anterior instability, often presenting as pain, without a subjective feeling of instability. There is also the patient who has symptomatic and lax tissue, whose shoulder is subjected to overuse, resulting in a loose shoulder that becomes symptomatic.

Recent work suggests that there is an excessive rate of production of collagen or an excessive turnover of collagen in patients who have multidirectional instability.[18] There are many ways to analyze increased joint laxity, which is frequently present in patients who have loose shoulders or classical multidirectional instability. Features such as thumb-to-forearm hyperextension of the fingers, hyperextension of the elbows, hypermobile patellae, or an ability to touch the palms to the floor with the knees straight are all manifestations of increased laxity or flexibility. Collagen abnormalities may also manifest as spreading of a scar in a patient whose surgical operation for instability failed, perhaps indicating that the collagen of the capsule may well have stretched in the same manner as the collagen of the skin.

STABILIZING FACTORS

Several components are important to glenohumeral stability:

1. Ligamentous restraints (Plate 11-1)
2. The rotator cuff and larger muscles of the shoulder providing dynamic control
3. Glenohumeral orientation such as glenoid version and proximal humeral torsion
4. Aspects of the tissues related to collagen (as already discussed)
5. Concavity compression
6. Intra-articular negative pressure

Ligamentous Restraints

Important ligamentous constraints to stability consist of the inferior glenohumeral ligament anterior and posterior bands, the middle glenohumeral ligament, the superior glenohumeral ligament, and probably the coracohumeral ligament.

The original static experimental work was performed by Turkel et al[51] in 1981, using a cadaveric model to demonstrate that the anterorinferior glenohumeral ligament provided stability to the glenohumeral joint with the arm externally rotated and abducted.

Additional cutting experiments demonstrated that to achieve an anterior dislocation in a cadaveric model, the anterior ''middle and inferior'' glenohumeral ligament (anterior and posterior bands), as well as subscapularis, needed to be incised.[54] The corollary of that, however, in trying to achieve a posterior dislocation was not the same. When the posterior infraspinatus and posterior ligamentous structures, including the inferior glenohumeral ligament (posterior and anterior bands), were incised, a posterior dislocation could not be achieved. In fact, a posterior dislocation could not be achieved until the middle and superior anterior glenohumeral ligaments had been incised. O'Brien et al[40] showed a hammock effect of the pouch, with the anterior and posterior bands controlling stability in different positions of external and internal rotation.

Further selective cutting experiments performed by Warner et al[53] demonstrated that with the arm at the side in 0 degrees of abduction, the ''superior'' glenohumeral ligamentous complex provided stability against inferior translation. At 45 degrees of abduction, both bands of the inferior glenohumeral ligament provided stability. At 90 degrees of abduction, the inferior glenohumeral ligament, particularly the posterior band, provided stability, preventing inferior translation. This aids in an understanding of stability in different positions and helps us appreciate the role of superior reconstruction for inferior instability with the arm at the side in the neutral position.

The ''coracohumeral'' ligamentous structure has been reported on by Harryman et al,[14] as well as in the Japanese literature, which indicates that when the coracohumeral ligament is released, there is an increase in external rotation and an increase in an ability to translate the humeral head in the glenoid (Fig. 11-2). When the coracohumeral ligament is imbricated through surgical reconstruction, there is a loss of external rotation and a diminution in the amount of posterior and inferior translation. Many of these studies relate to the ''circle'' concept of ligamentous control of the glenohumeral joint.

The circle concept of the shoulder suggests that if there is excessive translation in one direction, there is likely excessive translation in another direction[22] (Fig. 11-3). For example, we appreciate in patients who have multidirectional instability that they have excessive translation often in three directions.[39] Similarly, patients who have recurrent anterior dislocations also have excessive inferior or posterior translation of the shoulder in addition to the expected excessive anterior translation.

Muscle Function

Recently, there has been a focus on the muscles of the shoulder and their role in stability. Recent work by Blasier et al[4] has shown that the force required to translate the humeral head is much greater with the greater degrees of muscle pull of the cuff into glenoid. This is in a cadaveric model but does relate to the critical role of the rotator cuff muscles in stablizing the shoulder.

Fine-wire electromyographic analysis of the shoulder has looked at various stabilizing muscles in a concentric and eccentric mode.[5,12,19,29] It is now well appreciated that the rotator cuff muscles are the fine-tuners of the shoulder, probably functioning more effective eccentrically to stabilize rather than provide power to the shoulder. Based on cross-sectional analyses, the subscapularis supplies 53 percent of the cuff moment, undergoing significant eccentric contraction when the throwing arm is brought into external

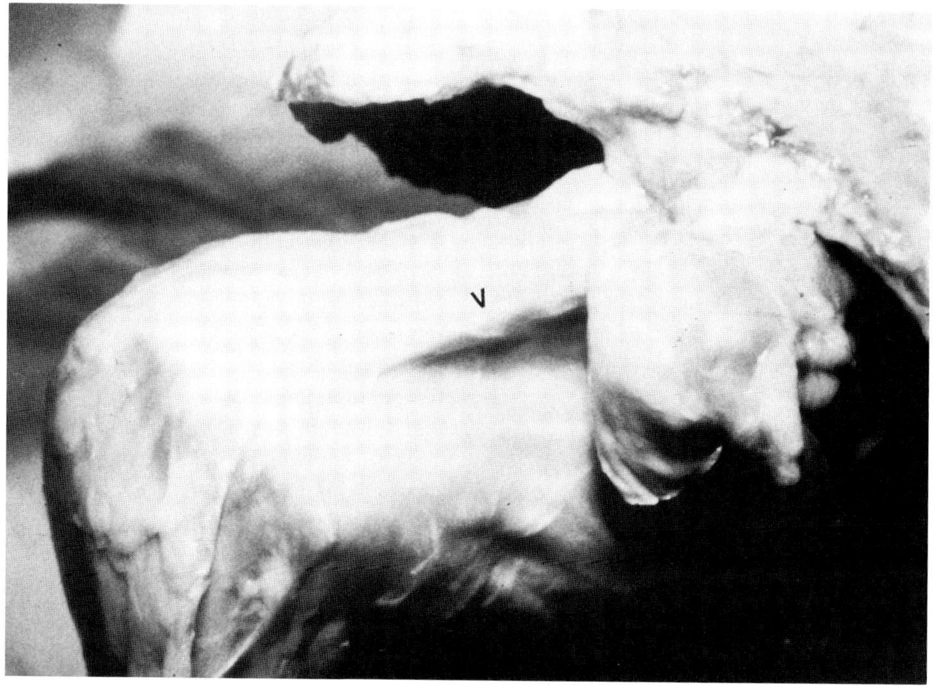

Figure 11-2. Coracohumeral ligament (*arrowhead*).

rotation and abduction.[32] This is probably as a stabilizing maneuver to maintain the humeral head in the socket, and probably opposing forces such as the infraspinatus on the opposite side play a similar role.

There has been considerable focus on rehabilitation of the rotator cuff to establish eccentric control and develop the larger muscles (e.g., pectoralis and deltoid) of the shoulder for concentric power.[6,7,9,30,32,36,55] In terms of overhead activities, we throw from the ground up, with the shoulder muscles providing only a small amount of the overall energy involved in generating the velocity of an overhead activity (perhaps 20 percent). Obviously, the effect of the kinetic chain from the ground up provides most of the energy for power.

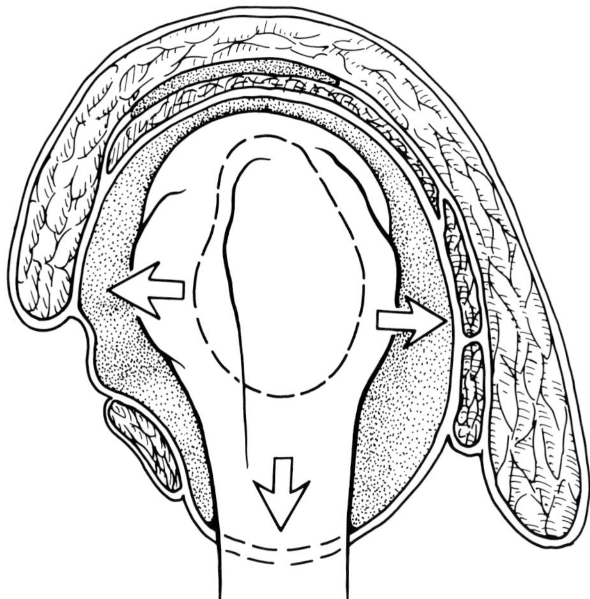

Figure 11-3. Circle concept of shoulder instability.

Version of the Glenohumeral Joint

In the literature, abnormalities of version of the glenoid or torsion of the proximal humerus have not been shown to relate to instability.[43] Rarely, they may be present and, if so can contribute to instability. Diagnosis of abnormal version is based on computed tomography or magnetic resonance imaging. Glenoid version often is easy to determine but seldom does it contribute to instability. It is more difficult to establish influence of abnormal torsion of the proximal humerus because of the difficulties in measurement, but it plays the same role as glenoid version.[47] Likewise, during scapular protraction, the scapula follows the movement of the humerus, reducing the stresses on the anterior aspect of the joint. Inability of the scapular muscles to stabilize the scapula effectively decreases the efficiency of the rotator muscles because a stable base is not provided for this glenohumeral relationship.

Concavity Compression

Concavity compression is provided by the concave contour of the glenoid, which is deepened by the labrum and related to the forces by which the muscles centralize the humeral head in the socket.[23,24] As glenoid depth is increased and with appropriate muscle forces centralizing the humeral head into the glenoid fossa, there is less possible translation of the humeral head in the socket[3,35] (Fig. 11-4).

It is not only the amount of muscular force by which the humeral head is pulled into the socket but also the direction of that force. An eccentric force might relate to an instability problem, whereas a balanced concentric force might provide stability. The rotator cuff and larger muscles of the shoulder obviously play an important functional role in this area.

A flat glenoid allows significant translation.[23] A concave glenoid provides stability with less translation. The muscular forces, if directed appropriately, stabilize the shoulder; if directed inappropriately, they may contribute to instability.[4]

Negative Pressure

In 1858, Humphrey[24] stated that the weight of the limbs is borne entirely by atmospheric pressure. When a needle is inserted into the joint, there is a pressure differential such that air rushes into the joint.[11,33] In this circumstance, there is excessive passive translation, up to 50 percent greater than when the pressure is not normalized. The role of this capsular venting phenomenon in a clinical setting of instability is uncertain. When experimental biomechanical work is performed, one must consider venting of the joint in these translation studies relating to static constraints of the shoulder.[2,3,11,14,25,33,40,45,50,51,53,54]

Appreciating that decreased force is required to translate the humeral head in a vented situation, one might consider this important in the presence of a lax capsule. For example, does the presence of a lax capsule increase joint volume and are translational forces apt to create an instability pattern? Also, the presence of synovial fluid within the joint can affect stability to a small degree because it contributes to cohesion between the articular surfaces.

ASSESSING SHOULDER LAXITY

During physical examination of the shoulder, we perform translational testing, noting the amount that the humeral head moves within the glenoid fossa, both in a sitting and supine position, awake and under anesthesia, and with the arm in different positions[4] (Fig. 11-5). Anterior and posterior translation can be described as a ''load-and shift test.'' The principle is to load the humeral head into the socket to be sure it is centered and then to stress anteriorly and posteriorly, documenting the amount of translation. There is no standard classification to document translation, but we might suggest descriptive terms:

Grade 0: the humeral head moves not at all

Grade I: the humeral head moves up the glenoid face 0 to 1 cm

Grade II: the humeral head rides up the glenoid face to the rim 1 to 2 cm

Grade III: the humeral head rides up and over the glenoid rim greater than 2 cm (this may remain dislocated when the stress is released but still constitutes grade III)

Similarly, a sulcus sign is an inferior translation test performed by applying longitudinal traction on the arm with the arm at the side. This may also be performed by levering inferiorly with the arm in the abducted position. It is difficult to feel the relationship of the humeral head in the glenoid with this testing, so it is best to describe the centimeters of displacement inferiorly with the arm at the side. This represents the measurement between the undersurface of the acromion and the superior aspect of the humeral head, which is crude at best. This might be described as

Grade 0: none

Grade I: less than 1 cm

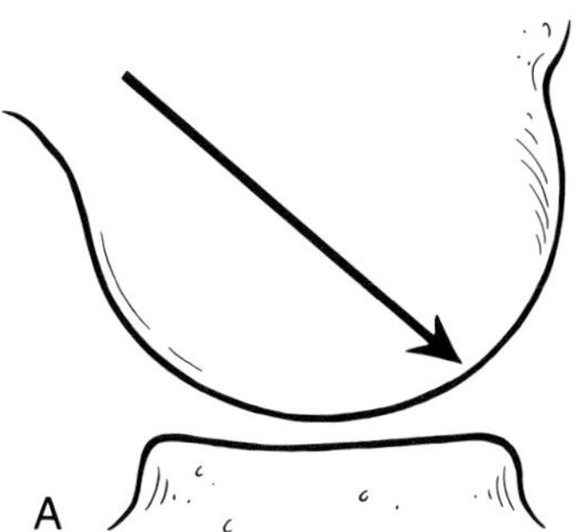

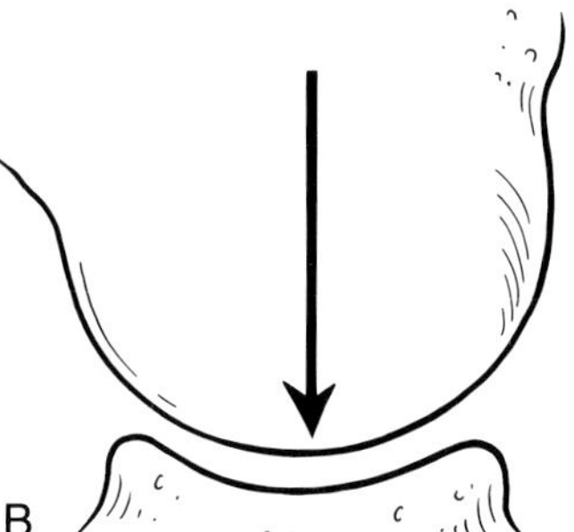

Figure 11-4. (**A**) Flat glenoid with asymetric muscle action, increasing tendency to translation. (**B**) Concave glenoid with centralizing muscle action, diminishing translation.

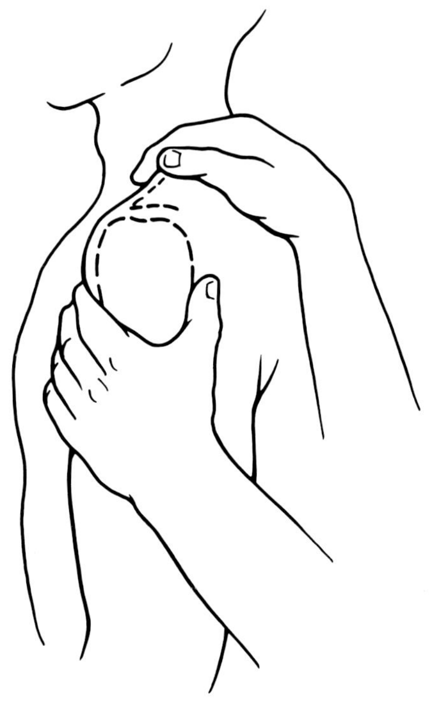

Figure 11-5 Physical examination to determine translation.

Grade II: 1 to 2 cm

Grade III: greater than 2 cm

Most patients with multidirectional instability would have grade III anteroposterior excursion and greater than 2 cm of inferior excursion on translation testing in the relaxed state or under anesthesia.

Recent studies of in vivo quantification of stability have suggested that anterior, posterior, and sulcus drawering in a group of normal patients approximates close to 1 cm in each direction, and the following conclusions were made:

1. Even in normal shoulders, substantial translation can occur.
2. These translations were reproducible
3. There was marked intersubject variability.[15]

Therefore, we must be careful in our interpretation of translation of the humeral head in the glenoid socket and not attribute it to instability simply because there is significant translation. Side-to-side differences may be the most meaningful; therefore, comparison is critical.

It is also prudent to examine the arm in different positions. For example, if a patient has an incompetent inferior glenohumeral ligament, then excess translation compared with the opposite extremity should be present with the arm externally rotated and abducted in the provocative position. When performing these translation tests, it is very helpful to ask the patient if this reproduces his or her symptom complex. For example, if a patient has posterior instability when the examiner translates the head posteriorly, the patient may say that is his or her problem, reproducing the symptoms of instability. The meaning of translation under anesthesia can be confusing. Some believe it is very meaningful, whereas others think it is worthless. It is only a part of the assessment related to a diagnosis of instability.

Laxity, or excessive translation, does not equal instability.[15] Stability is least important in the midranges of motions, from a functional point of view, but may be important in the AMBRI type of instability. Stability, related to static constraints, is important at the extremes of motion, particularly external rotation and abduction, as in the TUBS variety of instability or in the throwing athlete with subtle anterior capsule failure.

ANALYSIS OF THE ATHLETE'S SHOULDER

Much can be learned about instability in the shoulder from analyzing the athlete's shoulder. Athletes often present with a painful shoulder, and the diagnosis of underlying instability can be difficult. Further, there is the frequent presence of an overlap between instability and impingement.

Physical Examination

The physical examination features in the athlete's shoulder frequently consist of limitation of internal rotation and crossed-arm adduction, scapular dysfunction, excessive anterior translation with positive relocation testing, weakness of external rotation, and frequently, the presence of impingement signs.

The aspect of a painful shoulder in an athlete having loss of internal rotation associated with limitation of crossed-arm adduction is supported in the laboratory by the work of Harryman et al.[15] They demonstrated an obligate anterior translation with forward elevation of the arm. With suturing of the posterior structures, there was a greater degree of anterior translation. This coincides in the athlete's shoulder that has posterior capsular tightness, pushing the humeral head forward in a subluxed position, and because of this architectural arrangement, results in an impingement pattern. The concept of a tight posterior capsule pushing the humeral head forward, resulting in impingement, is likened to a yo-yo effect.

The scapular dysfunction of athletes often consists of diminution of scapular protraction with some form of scapular dyskinesia, often with winging (Plate 11-2). This feature can also contribute to proximal migration of the humeral head, with secondary impingement.[27,28,30]

Certain physical signs are very reliable in providing a

diagnosis in the shoulder; others are not. Speer et al[49] have shown that the apprehension sign, when present, is highly sensitive, specific, and accurate for anterior instability of the shoulder. The "relocation test" consists of stressing the shoulder in external rotation and abduction, resulting in pain. By pushing the upper arm posteriorly, one can gain greater external rotation in the abducted position with less pain, which is suggested to relate to anterior instability. They have shown this test was 50 percent accurate, in that other pathologies such as a rotator cuff tear had a positive relocation test. Although the degree of translation is important, perhaps even more important is the symptomatic reproduction of the patient's complex with translational testing. This is particularly so with posterior and multidirectional instability. Other aspects of clunks and grinds in the shoulder are occasionally meaningful, suggesting labral pathology that may be present with instability.

BICEPS AND SUPERIOR LABRAL COMPLEX

The biceps complex probably plays a role in anterior stability.[36,45] The biceps attaches to the superior labrum, and there are lesions that occur in this area. Biceps and superior labral lesions, now called SLAP (superior labral, anterior and posterior) lesions, were originally attributed by Andrews to eccentric overload, resulting in avulsion of the superior labral complex. We now appreciate this as being commonly a shear phenomenon related to instability. Rodosky et al[44] have performed experiments creating this SLAP lesion in the shoulder joint. In the presence of a SLAP lesion, there was significant strain on the anteroinferior glenohumeral ligament. With repair of the SLAP lesion, this strain was dramatically reduced. A recent report by Altchek et al[1] has indicated that patients who have SLAP lesions have slightly greater anterior translation. Repair eliminated this translation.

INTRINSIC IMPINGEMENT

Recent work by Walsh et al[52] and Jobe[26] has indicated that with the arm in external rotation and abduction, an area of intrinsic impingement is located above the superior glenoid labrum where the superior glenoid impinges against the undersurface of the rotator cuff. The relationship of this intrinsic impingement to instability is unclear.

PATHOLOGY IN INSTABILITY

The pathology seen in anterior unidirectional instability of the shoulder may consist of the following: (1) Hill-Sachs lesion, (2) Bankart lesion, (3) capsular stripping, (4) capsular laxity, anterior and inferior, (5) combinations of these (e.g., a very small Bankart lesion with excessive capsular laxity), and (6) mild anterior labral fraying and subtle capsular laxity, as in a thrower.

One can appreciate the wide variation and pathology that may be present, ranging from a little instability with little pathology to a large instability with a large amount of pathology.

In the past, the pathology of instability has been classically thought to be a Bankart lesion. This relates to the TUBS kind of anterior instability. With subtle forms of instability, there are more subtle forms of anterior capsular lesions. Sometimes patients have only mild labral fraying anteriorly with a redundant pouch. Bigliani et al[3] have shown in a cadaveric model that the capsule is stretched at the same time a Bankart lesion is created. Then comes the questions of what needs to be corrected and what is the best way to correct this lesion. Some patients have capsular redundancy with no labral pathology. This can be anterior, inferior, or a combination of these.

Some forms of pathology in the unstable shoulder present with lax pouches inferiorly, eventually predisposing to multidirectional instability. These patients often have minimal visible pathology in the shoulder other than a lax pouch, which is difficult to document.[39] Patients with posterior instability frequently only have lax capsules posteriorly. It is unusual to have a posterior Bankart lesion requiring correction.[31]

MANAGEMENT OF INSTABILITY PROBLEMS

An appreciation of basic research concepts that have added to our knowledge of shoulder instability will aid in the managing of these problems. Obviously, it is critical to diagnose the type of instability and correct the underlying biomechanical problems. A nonoperative approach is preferred whenever possible. This may not be very successful in the presence of a patient with a large Bankart lesion and recurrent anterior instability, but it is often very successful in the overhead athlete with subtle anterior instability or in the athlete with posterior or multidirectional instability. The thrust of a rehabilitation program is based on eccentric control of the shoulder rotators, provision of a stable and efficient scapular platform, along with biceps and latissimus control. The latissimus aids in protecting the supraspinatus as deceleration occurs in the follow-through in overhead activities. Stretching the posterior capsule is critical. If surgery is to be entertained, it must be carefully tempered with an accurate diagnosis and appropriate correction of the pathology. It seems in recent years that less surgery is providing a more functional outcome.[30] Earlier aggressive rehabilitation after surgery does not seem to compromise the outcome. We have learned that we should violate the tissues as little as possible, perhaps now leaning toward splitting the subscapularis and doing some form of Bankart repair. We also have applied the principles of capsular mobilization to correct redundancies, tailoring it to the instability, and this is particularly applicable to the athletic population. The functional demands of the athlete can be much greater and, as such, require a specialized approach.

Complications can occur with surgery, and one pitfall to avoid is making the shoulder too tight.[16,17,37] The present policy of management in these athletes is to obtain stability and provide painless mobility. The further functional challenge in the athlete is to restore the athlete to as normal a shoulder as possible, with the appropriate amount of translation or ''slop'' remaining in the shoulder.

It is important, in approaching surgical stabilization of the athlete's unstable shoulder, to consider whether the athlete is a pitcher, second baseman, quarterback, lineman, or soccer player. It is also important to consider the level of participation, whether recreational, high school, college, or professional. It may be inappropriate to apply the same stabilizing procedure to the football lineman with a large Bankart lesion and to the professional baseball pitcher with subtle anterior labral and capsular stretching.

Historically, procedures such as Magnuson-Stack, Putti-Platt, and Bristow have not stood the test of time, particularly for the functional demands of the overhead athlete. They have stood the test of time in athletes who do not participate overhead.

The classical Bankart procedure, performed for many years by Carter Rowe, M.D., has been the most successful. We have now modified that procedure to violate the subscapularis less, to do less of a capsular repair, and to be vigorous with our postoperative rehabilitation.[30,46]

The recent introduction of the capsulolabral reconstruction by Jobe et al[30,46] has greatly advanced our ability to surgically stabilize the shoulder and achieve a better outcome for our overhead athletes.

The concept of arthroscopic stabilization of the shoulder is new and exciting, yet still developing. We are not yet in the position in which we can achieve the gold standard results as we can for an overhead athlete with an open repair. There are situations in which an arthroscopic stabilization would be appropriate for an overhead athlete. For example, in the patient with subtle instability who has a small Bankart lesion, we may wish only to put that Bankart lesion back down to the glenoid. This might achieve as good a result as we can achieve any other way. It is difficult arthroscopically to do the fine-tuning demanded, but as we get better with instrumentation and techniques, that will be achieved.

The eventual goal arthroscopically is to be able to restore the capsule or labrum to the anterior glenoid, suturing it down as we now do with a Bankart type of operation with secure sutures, thus allowing early range of motion. Once achieved, we may stabilize many of these athletes arthroscopically. At the present time, an open procedure remains the gold standard for our shoulder athletes.

REFERENCES

1. Altchek D, Pagnani MJ, Speer KP et al: Arthroscopic fixation of shoulder labral lesion. J Shoulder Elbow Surg 3:S68, 1994
2. Belle RM, Hawkins RJ: Collagen typing and production in multidirectional instability of the shoulder. Orthop Trans 15:188, 1991
3. Bigliani L, Pollock R, Soslowsky L et al: Tensile properties of the inferior glenohumeral ligament. J Orthop Res 10:187–97, 1992
4. Blasier RB, Guldberg RE, Rothman ED: Anterior shoulder stability: contributions of rotator cuff forces and the capsule ligaments in a cadaver model. J Shoulder Elbow Surg 1:140–50, 1992
5. Boublik M, Hawkins RJ: Clinical examination of the shoulder complex. J Orthop Sports Phys Ther 18:379–85, 1993
6. Bradley JP, Tibone JE: EMG analyses of muscle action about the shoulder. Clin Sports Med 10:789–809, 1991
7. Brown LP Niehuess SSL, Harrah A et al: Upper extremity range of motion and isokinetic strength of the internal and external rotator in major league baseball pitchers. Am J Sports Med 16:577–85, 1988
8. Chinn JC, Priest JD, Kent BE: Upper extremity range of motion, grip strength and girth in highly skilled tennis players. Phys Ther 54:474–82, 1988
9. Cleland FRC: Notes on raising the arm. J Anat Physiol 18:275–8, 1984
10. Dillman CJ, Fleisig GS, Werner SL, Andrews JR: Biomechanics of the shoulder in sports: throwing activities. In Postgraduate Advances in Sports Medicine. Independent Study Course, Chapters IV-IX. Forum Medicum Inc., 1991
11. Gainor BJ, Piotrowski G, Puhl J et al: The throw: Biomechanics and acute injury. Am J Sports Med 8:114–8. 1980
12. Gibb T, Sidles J, Harryman D et al: The effect of capsular venting on glenohumeral laxity. Clin Orthop 268:120–7, 1991
13. Glousman R, Jobe FW, Tibone JE et al: Dynamic electromyographic analysis of the throwing shoulder with glenohumeral instability. J Bone Joint Surg [Am] 70:220–6, 1988
14. Harryman DT II: Role of the coracohumeral ligament in passive motion and stability of the shoulder. Orthop Trans 4:595, 1990
15. Harryman DT II, Sidles JA, Clark JM et al: Translation of the humeral head on the glenoid with passive glenohumeral motion. J Bone Joint Surg [Am] 72:1334–43, 1990
16. Harryman DT II, Sidles JA, Scott LH, Matsen FA: Laxity of the normal glenohumeral joint: a quantitative in vivo assessment. J Shoulder Elbow Surg 1:66–76, 1992
17. Hawkins RH, Hawkins RJ: Failed anterior reconstruction for shoulder instability. J Bone Joint Surg [Br] 67:709–14, 1985
18. Hawkins RJ, Angelo RL: Glenohumeral osteoarthrosis: a late

complication of the Putti-Platt repair. J Bone Joint Surg [Am] 72:1193–6, 1990
19. Hawkins RJ, Belle RM: Dynamic electromyographic analysis of the shoulder muscles during rotational and scapular strengthening exercises. pp. 32–5. In Post M, Morrey BF, Hawkins RJ (eds): Surgery of the Shoulder. CV Mosby, St. Louis, 1990
20. Hawkins RJ, Koppert G, Johnston G: Recurrent posterior instability (subluxation) of the shoulder. J Bone Joint Surg [Am] 66:169–74, 1984
21. Hawkins RJ, Murnaghan JP: The shoulder. In Cruess RL, Rennie WR (eds): Adult Orthopaedics. Vol. 2. Churchill Livingstone, New York, 1984
22. Hawkins RJ, Schutte JP: The assessment of glenohumeral translation using manual and fluoroscopic techniques. Orthop Trans 12:727, 1988
23. Howell SM, Galint BJ: The glenoid-labral socket: a constrained articular surface. Clin Orthop 243:122–5, 1989
24. Humphrey GM: A treatise on the Human Skeleton (Including the Joints). Macmillan, London, 1858
25. Itoi E, Motzin NE, Morrey BF, An KN: Scapular inclination and inferior stability of the shoulder. J Shoulder Elbow Surg 1:131–9, 1992
26. Jobe CM: Evidence for a superior glenoid impingement upon the rotator cuff. J Shoulder Elbow Surg 2:S19, 1993
27. Jobe FW, Bradley JB: Rotator cuff injuries in baseball: preventions and rehabilitation. Sports Med 6:377, 1988
28. Jobe FW, Bradley JB: The diagnosis and nonoperative treatment of shoulder injuries in athletes. Clin Sports Med 8:419, 1989
29. Jobe FW, Moynes DR, Tibone JE, Perry J: An EMG analysis of the shoulder in pitching: a second report. Am J Sports Med 12:218–20, 1984
30. Jobe FW, Tibone JE, Jobe CM, Kvitne RS: The shoulder in sports. p. 961–90. In Rockwood CA, Matsen FA III (eds): The Shoulder. WB Saunders, Philadelphia, 1990
31. Johnston GH, Hawkins RJ, Fowler PJ, Haddad R: A complication of posterior glenoid osteotomy for recurrent posterior shoulder instability. Clin Orthop 187:147–9, 1984
32. Keatin JF, Waterworth P, Shaw-Dunn J, Crossan J: The relative strengths of the rotator cuff muscles. J Bone Joint Surg [Br] 75:137, 1993
33. Kumar VP, Balasubramaniam P: The role of atmospheric pressure in stabilizing the shoulder: an experimental study. J Bone Joint Surg [Br] 67:719–21, 1985
34. Lippitt SB, Harryman DT, Sidles JA, Matsen FA: Diagnosis and management of AMBRI syndrome. Techniques Orthop 6:61–73, 1991
35. Lippitt SB, Vanderhook JE, Scott HL et al: Glenohumeral stability from concavity-compression: a quantitative analysis. J Shoulder Elbow Surg 2:27–35, 1993
36. Litchfield RB, Hawkins RJ, Dillman CJ et al: Rehabilitation for the overhead athlete. J Orthop Sports Phys Ther 18:433–441, 1993
37. MacDonald PB, Hawkins RJ, Fowler PJ, Miniachi A: Subscapularis release for internal rotation contracture after anterior instability shoulder repair. Orthop Trans 16:767, 1992
38. Moseley JB, Jobe FW, Pink M et al: EMG analysis of the scapular muscles during a shoulder rehabilitation program. Am J Sports Med 20:128–34, 1992
39. Neer CS II, Foster CR: Inferior capsular shift for involuntary inferior and multidirectional instability of the shoulder: a preliminary report. J Bone Joint Surg [Am] 62:897–908, 1980
40. O'Brien SJ, Arnoczky SP, Warren RF et al: The anatomy and histology of the inferior glenohumeral ligament complex of the shoulder. Am J Sports Med 18:449, 1990
41. O'Connell P, Nuber G, Mileski R: The contribution of the glenohumeral ligaments to anterior stability of the shoulder joint. Am J Sports Med 18:579–84, 1989
42. Pappas AM, Goss TP, Kleinman PK: Symptomatic shoulder instability due to lesions of the glenoid labrum. Am J Sports Med 11:279, 1983
43. Randelli M, Gombioli PL: Glenohumeral osteometry by computed tomography in normal and unstable shoulder. Clin Orthop 280:151–6, 1986
44. Rodosky MW, Harner CD, Fu FH: The role of the long head of the biceps muscle and superior glenoid labrum in anterior stability of the shoulder. Am J Sports Medicine 22:121–30, 1994
45. Rodosky MW, Rudert MJ, Harner CD, Fu FH: The long head of the biceps: a biomechanical study of its contribution to shoulder stability. Trans Orthop Res Soc 15:276, 1990
46. Rubinstein DL, Jobe FW, Glousman RE et al: Anterior capsulolabral reconstruction of the shoulder in athletes. JSES 1:229, 1992
47. Saha AK: Dynamic stability of the glenohumeral joint. Acute Orthop Scand 42:491–505, 1971
48. Snyder SJ, Kaszel RP, DelPizzo W et al: SLAP lesions of the shoulder. Arthroscopy 6:274–9, 1990
49. Speer KP, Hannafin JA, Altchek DW, Warren RF: An evaluation of the shoulder relocation test. Am J Sports Med 22:177–83, 1994
50. Terry GC: The stabilizing function of passive shoulder restraints. Am J Sports Med 19:26–34, 1991
51. Turkel SJ, Panio MW, Marshall JL, Girgis FG: Stabilizing mechanisms preventing anterior dislocation of glenohumeral joint. J Bone Joint Surg [Am] 63:1208–17, 1981
52. Walch G, Boileau P, Noel E, Donell ST: Impingement of the deep surface of the supraspinatus tendon on the posterosuperior glenoid rim: an arthroscopic study. J Shoulder Elbow Surg 1:238–45, 1992
53. Warner JJP, Deng H, Warren RF et al: Static capsuloligamentous restraints to superior-inferior translation of the glenohumeral joint. Trans Orthop Res Soc 17:497, 1991
54. Warren RF, Korndlatt IB, Marehand R: Static factors effecting posterior shoulder stability. Orthop Trans 8:89, 1984
55. Wilk KE, Arrigo CA, Andrews JR: Standardized isokinetic testing protocol of the throwing shoulder: the throwers' series. Isokinetics Exerc Sci 1:63–71, 1991

CHAPTER TWELVE

Natural History of Shoulder Instability—Options for Treatment

Nick Mohtadi

NATURAL HISTORY

The natural history of any disease can be looked at from an epidemiologic standpoint as having different stages. The disease starts with the *biologic onset* and ends with an *outcome.*[34] Prevention would logically occur before the biologic onset. The clinical manifestations of any disease are the hallmark of the *clinical onset.* With many diseases, it is plausible to make an early diagnosis before the clinical onset and therefore introduce screening or early detection. With respect to traumatic instability of the shoulder, the onset is at the time of injury. Screening is not a viable option, and prevention, although possible, involves a careful evaluation of risk factors including the mechanism of injury and the role of environmental conditions. This chapter focuses on the *clinical course*[34] or natural history of traumatic anterior dislocation of the shoulder after the initial injury. Minimal reference is made to other types of instability, such as multidirectional instability or posterior instability, as appropriate.

Acute Anterior Instability

The clinical course of acute anterior dislocation of the shoulder has been documented since the time of Hippocrates.[32] He outlined management principles including techniques of reduction, initial immobilization with protection, and rehabilitation with massage. He was concerned about the long-term prognosis as it related to recurrence of instability and the effect of repeated dislocations on work and athletic function. The recommended treatment at that time was cauterization of the shoulder from the axilla. With the advent of more formal surgical intervention, the focus of the problem was defining the essential lesion responsible for recurrent instability. Bankart[3] in 1923 brought a new understanding to the problem with his description of the lesion that bears his name. Up to that time, the main theories applying to instability were related to capsular laxity and muscular weakness. More recently, the understanding of glenohumeral instability has been aided by cadaveric,[28,37,38] clinical,[10] and arthroscopic correlations.[8]

There have been several specific attempts to address the natural history of anterior instability of the shoulder.[1,16–22,24,25,33,35] The main concern has been the problem of recurrent instability. The main factor accounting for recurrence is clearly the age of the patient at the time of the first traumatic episode of instability. The risk of recurrence has been calculated in these studies and is summarized in Table 12-1. The true natural history of any disease must reflect the situation in which no treatment has been offered. Furthermore, to compare the recurrence rates, the patient populations must be similar, their risks of reinjury the same, and the pathology at initial dislocation the same. It is impossible to compare all the studies on all potential confounding variables. Nevertheless, the evi-

Table 12-1. Age As a Factor in Rate of Recurrence of Anterior Instability

Study	Age <20 yr (%)	Age 20–29 yr (%)	Age >30 yr (%)
Hoelen et al	64 (<30 yr)		8
Kiviluoto et al	56	26	6
Kazar & Relovszky	46	31	5
Hovelius	64 (<23 yr)	48 (23–29 yr)	19
Henry & Genung	88 (<32 yr)		NA
Aronen & Regan	25 (18–22 yr)		NA
Rowe	83	63 (20–40 yr)	16 (>40 yr)
McLaughlin & Cavallaro	94	78	9
Simonet & Cofield	66	40 (20–40 yr)	0 (>40 yr)
Marans et al	100 (<17 yr)	NA	NA

Abbreviation: NA, not available.

dence is abundantly clear that the younger the patient with an acute traumatic anterior dislocation, the greater the likelihood of recurrence of instability.[22]

Other factors implicated in a higher recurrence rate or poorer prognosis are male sex, lesser degree of trauma, humeral head defect (Hill-Sachs or Hermodsson lesion), athletic participation or manual labor, and length of time of immobilization and rehabilitation.

The poorer prognosis with respect to being male[35] and the activity level[18,19,21,24,25,35] may be confounding variables or at least reflect a multifactorial nature to the higher rate of recurrence. The amount of trauma accounting for the initial episode is also related to recurrence. The greater the trauma, the less the recurrence rate.[18,19,21,24,25,33] This is also reflected in patients with associated greater tuberosity fractures and in those with associated nerve lesions as complications of the dislocation.[21,24,25,33] In situations in which a humeral head defect was present after the initial episode, the recurrence rate is higher.[18,19,33] The effects of immobilization and rehabilitation are discussed under the category of treatment.

With respect to traumatic anterior subluxation, the natural history is believed to be similar to the traumatic dislocation.[7] The mechanism of injury is usually the same; however, the signs and symptoms are not always evident.[11] Subluxation is also likely to occur due to the repetitive stress of an overhead activity.[27] The pathology associated with this mechanism may be quite different. As a result of differing mechanisms of injury, symptoms, and physical findings, it is more difficult to confirm the diagnosis of anterior subluxation. Without a clear way of defining the clinical onset, there are no true natural history studies from which to base an understanding.

Posterior Instability

The natural history of posterior instability of the shoulder is not known. This is in part due to the uncommon nature of the problem and mostly because the problem is not well recognized and documented.[14] The acute posterior dislocation is unlikely to result in recurrence of instability,[14] although one report suggests that 6 of 10 resulted in further problems.[33] There are reports on the management of recurrent instability,[13,36] but true inferences on natural history cannot be made.

Multidirectional Instability

The natural history of multidirectional instability is only made from inference in those individuals who have been treated for "uncontrollable and involuntary inferior subluxation or dislocation."[29] Many patients present with pain as the primary symptom due to an overuse traumatic etiology.[12] The true natural history of this condition is not known.

OPTIONS FOR TREATMENT

Treatment of the athlete's shoulder with primary traumatic anterior instability remains a controversial area.[15] There are two options for treatment. The first involves a nonoperative approach. This would combine the period of time of immobilization with rehabilitation.[1] The second option is that of early surgical repair[4] for primary instability.[5]

The evidence for the use of prolonged immobilization with or without rehabilitation is conflicting.[1,5,15–17,19–21,24,35,40] Aronen and Regan[1] showed excellent results with an aggressive rehabilitation program. In this series, a 3-week period of immobilization was followed by a strengthening program and restriction of provocative activities until the goals of rehabilitation had been achieved. A recurrence rate of 25 percent was achieved. In a similar series of young athletes with a first-time dislocation, a recurrence rate of 17.3 percent was reported. The treatment protocol included strict immobilization for 5 weeks, followed by 6 weeks of limited abduction with graduated exercises.[40] In a prospective randomized trial, length of time of immobilization showed no difference in recurrence rate.[18,19] Other reports have a variety of recurrence rates irrespective of time of immobilization.[5,16,21,24,33] It is very difficult to resolve this dilemma based on the literature. In a review of this controversy, Hawkins and Mohtadi[15] suggested that the issue of immobilization should be resolved on the basis of the healing response in the tissues involved. After the dislocation, hemorrhage, hemostasis, and inflammation occur in the damaged area.[9,23] Once the inflammatory phase has subsided, the pain diminishes. At this point, the reparative phase is in full gear with a fibroblastic healing response.[9,23] The recommended approach is to immobilize the shoulder until the symptoms of pain are under control. Rehabilitative exercises are instituted, avoiding the provocative position of abduction and external rotation.[15] This more pragmatic approach considers the clinical evidence and has a theoretical grounding in the basic science of healing.

The suggestion of early surgical repair is one that has been referred to by several authors,[2,4,18,24,39] going back to as early as 1942.[30] In a prospective but nonrandomized study of cadets with an initial episode of anterior dislocation, standard treatment was compared with early arthroscopic intervention.[39] There was a recurrence rate of 92 percent in the standard treatment group versus 22 percent in the patients treated with arthroscopy. Bokor[5] presented preliminary results on nine patients younger than 25 years of age. There were no recurrences reported, with a minimum follow-up at 6 months. This preliminary information shows a dramatic difference between operative and nonoperative treatment. These results should be interpreted with cautious optimism because the selection of patients and arthroscopic technique was not standardized.

In the recurrent situation, the use of exercise has been shown to have poor results in those patients with an etiology of traumatic instability.[7,27] It is apparent that the role of nonoperative treatment in recurrent shoulder instability has been only minimally represented in the literature. Very few articles are devoted to this method of treatment. This is likely because the experience of most surgeons is unfavorable, and surgical treatment has excellent results.[27] Here again, the evidence is conflicting,[6] although in this series the patients had muscular weakness documented before the treatment with the training program. In the series of Burkhead and Rockwood, those patients with atraumatic subluxation did well with nonoperative treatment, and in the series of Brostrom et al, the failures were primarily in individuals with generalized joint laxity. It is difficult to make strong conclusions based on the evidence of nonoperative treatment in the chronic recurrent situations. Patient selection, lack of randomization, and different outcomes are confounding variables in determining the value of this treatment. A great deal of empirical evidence that has not been reported suggests that surgical treatment of recurrent traumatic anterior dislocations is the treatment of choice. The key element in this treatment is to fix the pathologic lesion.[3,15,26,31] The current trend is to avoid restriction of motion and allow for best possible functional return.[27]

SUMMARY

The natural history of many orthopaedic problems is not well known. Acute traumatic anterior dislocation of the shoulder has a reasonably well-defined natural history, particularly in the active individual younger than 20 years of age. This is the high-risk group for recurrent instability. The evidence is consistent and makes biologic sense. The reported recurrence rates range from 25 to 94 percent. It is clear what needs to be done in situations in which nonoperative treatment fails; however, a case can be made for early operative stabilization. Nevertheless, stronger evidence is required to suggest that surgery is the treatment of choice for the first-time dislocator.

REFERENCES

1. Aronen JG, Regan K: Decreasing the incidence of recurrence of first time anterior dislocations with rehabilitation. Am J Sports Med 12:283, 1984
2. Baker CL, Uribe JW, Whitman C: Arthroscopic evaluation of acute initial anterior shoulder dislocations. Am J Sport Med 18:25, 1990
3. Bankart ASB: Recurrent or habitual dislocation of the shoulder joint. BMJ 2:1132, 1923
4. Benedetto KP, Glotzer W: Arthroscopic Bankart procedure by suture technique. Arthroscopy 8:111, 1992
5. Bokor DJ: Management of acute first-time anterior shoulder instability, abstracted. J Shoulder Elbow Surg 2(suppl. 1):S50, 1993
6. Brostrom LA, Kronberg M, Nemeth G, Oxelback U: The effect of shoulder muscle training in patients with recurrent shoulder dislocations. Scand J Rehabil Med 24:11, 1992
7. Burkhead WZ, Rockwood CA: Treatment of instability of

the shoulder with an exercise program. J Bone Joint Surg [Am] 74:890, 1992

8. Caspari R, Geissler W: Arthroscopic manifestations of shoulder subluxation and dislocation. Clin Orthop 291:54, 1993
9. Clayton ML, Weir GJ: Experimental investigations of ligamentous healing. Am J Surg 98:373, 1959
10. Cofield R, Nessler J, Weinstabl R: Diagnosis of shoulder instability by examination under anesthesia. Clin Orthop 291:45, 1993
11. Garth WP, Allman FL, Armstrong WS: Occult anterior subluxations of the shoulder in noncontact sports. Am J Sports Med 15:579, 1987
12. Hawkins RJ, Bell RH: Shoulder instability—diagnosis and management. Can J Sport Sci 12:67, 1987
13. Hawkins RJ, Koppert G, Johnston G: Recurrent posterior instability (subluxation) of the shoulder. J Bone Joint Surg [Am] 66:169, 1984
14. Hawkins RJ, McCormack RG: Posterior shoulder instability. Orthopaedics 11:101, 1988
15. Hawkins RJ, Mohtadi NGH: Controversy in anterior shoulder instability. Clin Orthop 272:152, 1991
16. Henry JH, Genung JA: Natural history of glenohumeral dislocation—revisited. Am J Sport Med 10:135, 1982
17. Hoelen MA, Burgers AMJ, Rozing PM: Prognosis of primary anterior shoulder dislocation in young adults. Arch Orthop Trauma Surg 110:51, 1990
18. Hovelius L: Anterior dislocation of the shoulder in teenagers and young adults. J Bone Joint Surg [Am] 69:393, 1987
19. Hovelius L, Eriksson K, Fredin HEA: Recurrences after initial dislocation of the shoulder. J Bone Joint Surg [Am] 65:343, 1983
20. Kazar B, Relovszky E: Prognosis of primary dislocation of the shoulder. Acta Orthop Scand 40:216, 1969
21. Kiviluoto O, Pasila M, Sundholm J, Sundholm A: Immobilization after primary dislocation of the shoulder. Acta Orthop Scand 51:915, 1980
22. Marans JJ, Angel KR, Schemitsch EH, Wedge JH: The fate of traumatic anterior dislocation of the shoulder in children. J Bone Joint Surg [Am] 74:1242, 1992
23. Mason ML, Allen MS: Rate of healing of tendons. Ann Surg 113:424, 1941
24. McLaughlin HL, Cavallaro WU: Primary anterior dislocation of the shoulder. Am J Surg 80:615, 1950
25. McLaughlin HL, Maclellan DI: Recurrent anterior dislocation of the shoulder. II. A comparative study. J Trauma 7:191, 1967
26. Mohtadi NGH: Advances in the understanding of anterior shoulder instability. Clin Sports Med 10:863, 1991
27. Montgomery WH, Jobe FW: Functional outcomes in athletes after modified anterior capsulolabral reconstruction. Am J Sports Med 22:352, 1994
28. Moseley H, Overgaard B: The anterior capsular mechanism in recurrent anterior dislocation of the shoulder. J Bone Joint Surg [Br] 44:913, 1962
29. Neer CS, Foster CR: Inferior capsular shift for involuntary inferior and multidirectional instability of the shoulder. J Bone Joint Surg [Am] 62:897, 1980
30. Nicola T: Anterior dislocation of the shoulder: the role of the articular capsule. J Bone Joint Surg [Am] 24:614, 1942
31. O'Brien SJ, Warren RF, Schwartz E: Anterior shoulder instability. Orthop Clin North Am 18:395, 1987
32. Papachristou G: The classic: injuries of the shoulder: dislocations (Hippocrates). Clin Orthop 246:4, 1989
33. Rowe CR: Prognosis in dislocations of the shoulder. J Bone Joint Surg [Am] 38:957, 1956
34. Sackett D, Haynes R, Guyatt G, Tugwell P: Clinical Epidemiology. A Basis Science for Clinical Medicine. 2nd Ed. Little, Brown, Boston, 1991
35. Simonet WT, Cofield RH: Prognosis in anterior shoulder dislocation. Am J Sports Med 12:19, 1984
36. Tibone JE, Prietto C, Jobe FWEA: Staple capsulorrhaphy for recurrent posterior shoulder dislocation. Am J Sports Med 9:135, 1981
37. Turkel S, Panio M, Marshall J, Girgis F: Stabilizing mechanisms preventing anterior dislocation of the glenohumeral joint. J Bone Joint Surg [Am] 63:1208, 1981
38. Warner J, Deng XH, Warren RF, Torzilli P: Static capsuloligamentous restraints to superior inferior translation of the glenohumeral joint. Am J Sports Med 20:675, 1992
39. Wheeler JH, Ryan JB, Arciero RA, Molinari RN: Arthroscopic versus nonoperative treatment of acute shoulder dislocations in young athletes. Arthroscopy 5:213, 1989
40. Yoneda B, Webb RP, MacIntosh DL: Conservative treatment of shoulder dislocation in young males. J Bone Joint Surg [Br] 64:254, 1982

CHAPTER THIRTEEN

Surgery for Anterior Instability

Jeffrey S. Abrams
Peter MacDonald

The young athlete who sustains an anterior shoulder dislocation faces the prospect of a high rate of recurrence, especially if he or she plans to remain active in sports.[11,19,22,30] Recurrence rates after initial dislocations are high, but disability may be variable. The rate of recurrence of instability range from Rowe's[19] 94 percent redislocation rate in patients younger than 20 years of age to the 64 percent of Hovelius[11] in patients younger than 22 years. Disability may be greater when you include athletes with apprehension.

In young patients, it remains controversial whether the natural history is altered by conservative treatment. Nonoperative management includes immobilization, rehabilitative exercises, and refraining from provocative activities. Immobilization after an acute dislocation for 3 to 4 weeks did not alter the long-term results according to Hovelius,[11] nor Simonet and Cofield.[22] Aronen and Regan[3] and Yoneda et al[30] reported a decreased rate of recurrence after strict adherence to a rehabilitative program. The greatest issue may be avoidance of provocative activities, which is difficult to adhere to in the athletic population. If subsequent instability cannot be managed nonoperatively, then surgical reconstruction can be considered.

Surgical candidates are those disabled by pain, recurrent instability, or apprehension. The lifestyle of the patient may be an important factor in determining whether a patient needs to be operated on for traumatic instability. Patients who choose to remain active in overhead athletics will often be unhappy with recurrences of subluxation and dislocations.

An athlete who is apprehensive and thinks that maximum external rotation and extension must be avoided may not be able to return to the previous level in overhead or contact athletics. A patient who chooses a less aggressive lifestyle might find an occasional dislocation with a relatively asymptomatic interval to be an acceptable alternative.

In certain circumstances, a first-time dislocation patient may be a candidate for surgical repair. Some overhead or contact athletes may choose to lessen the risk of recurrence. Recurrence rates after initial dislocation are high in this age group, and nonoperative measures may not alter the natural history of recurrent instability. These athletes may choose early surgical intervention at a convenient time rather than risk a recurrence at an inconvenient time. Some athletes, after an initial episode of instability, will choose a 3- to 6-month trial of supervised goal-directed rehabilitation before determining the degree of disability. Those who remain disabled because of apprehension or recurrent episodes of instability may wish to proceed to surgery.

Many repairs have been used for anterior instability. Historically, some repairs have attempted to obtain stability with little regard for maintaining motion and subsequent function. The Putti-Platt repair can create excessive loss of external rotation. In some cases, this has led to the development of osteoarthrosis.[10] It has been postulated that the joint contact forces have been altered with the abnormal biomechanics of the contracture. Shoulder reconstructions that use large metal implants such as staples and screws have been associated with complications as a result of metal breakage, loosening, or impingement[31] (Fig. 13-1).

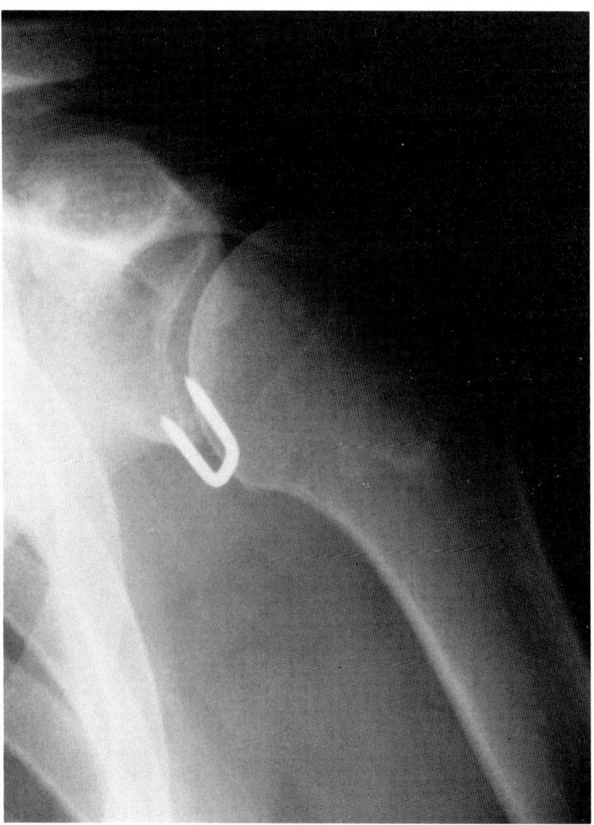

Figure 13-1. Malpositioned staple presents significant risk for articular damage.

Patients with prior shoulder stabilization resulting in significant loss of external rotation or loose hardware may require additional surgery.

A classification of instability is helpful to direct treatment. Traditionally, instability has been classified according to direction (anterior, posterior, inferior, or multidirectional), etiology (traumatic versus atraumatic), degree (dislocation, subluxation, apprehension), frequency (acute, recurrent, chronic), and volition (voluntary versus involuntary). Lippitt et al[14] and Thomas and Matsen[26] have introduced acronyms to help direct management, *t*raumatic *u*nidirectional instability with a *B*ankart lesion best responds to *s*urgery (TUBS). At the other end of the spectrum is *a*traumatic *m*ultidirectional instability that is often *b*ilateral and best treated by *r*ehabilitation (AMBRI). In cases that fail to respond to nonoperative treatment, an *i*nferior capsule shift and correction of the rotator cuff interval lesion is recommended. The clinician may be faced with patients who fall between the two ends of this spectrum. Many athletes with occult shoulder instability have shoulder pain as a result of repetitive microtrauma. These patients might not have an initial traumatic event that precipitated instability. Athletes can develop an incompetent and stretched capsule labral system that allows excessive glenohumeral translation. For difficult cases, examination under anesthesia combined with diagnostic and arthroscopy can improve accuracy in making the diagnosis.[9]

As a result of past experience and current understanding of the pathophysiology of traumatic anterior instability, certain basic principles are used in the selection of the type or repair used:

1. *Address the pathology:* It makes sense to use a repair that is aimed at the underlying problem. A Bankart repair, for example, is best applied to anterior instability in which a labral detachment or capsular stripping is the underlying cause. Surgery can be performed either arthroscopically or via arthrotomy (Fig. 13-2). If anterior instability exists with no significant labral detachment, then anterior capsular tightening is recommended. Although an arthroscopic capsule repair is technically possible, it is not recommended for the casual arthroscopic surgeon. If the pathology is multidirectional capsular laxity, then rehabilitation is the primary treatment. Failing a rehabilitation program, an inferior capsular shift may be considered. The classical inferior shift, as described by Neer and Foster,[16] both obliterates the axillary pouch as well as reinforces the rotator cuff interval superiorly.

   Turkel and co-workers, in 1981,[28] found that the inferior glenohumeral ligament was the predominant restraint while the shoulder was in the position of 90 degrees of abduction and 90 degrees of external rotation. This work was supported by the in vitro model created by Terry et al[25] and O'Brien et al.[17] Bigliani et al[6] have studied the mechanical properties of the inferior glenohumeral ligament and noted elongation before failure. Several authors therefore suggest addressing the capsule in addition to the Bankart lesion. The anterior capsulolabral reconstruction has been popularized by Jobe et al[13] (Fig. 13-3). This procedure repairs a Bankart lesion if present and simultaneously shifts the capsule. The resultant capsule is shifted on the glenoid side of the joint through the inferior and middle glenohumeral ligament. The middle glenohumeral ligament often escapes scrutiny when discussing pathology of instability but has an important role in restricting anterior translation in the position of 45 degrees of abduction.[28,29] The advantage of procedures directed at the intra-articular pathology is to minimize loss of external rotation, which is important in throwers and other overhead athletes.
2. *Avoid the use of large metallic implants in or around the joint:* Many reports are in the literature of complications regarding hardware in and around the shoulder joint.[31] The use of large metallic objects such as screws or staples to secure the subscapularis or labrum may be hazardous. Modern repair techniques have included the development of buried suture anchors or tags that allow relatively easy repair of a Bankart lesion. The pull-out strength of several implants has recently been tested and shown to be comparable with the strength of many sutures that are used to reattach soft tissue to bone.[5] Biodegradable suture anchors are currently under investigation and might provide additional benefit as the implant is reabsorbed.
3. *Maintain range of motion:* Loss of motion, particularly external rotation, is detrimental to function and significantly increases the risk of osteoarthrosis. A repair that preserves almost complete external rotation is desirable. Some loss of external

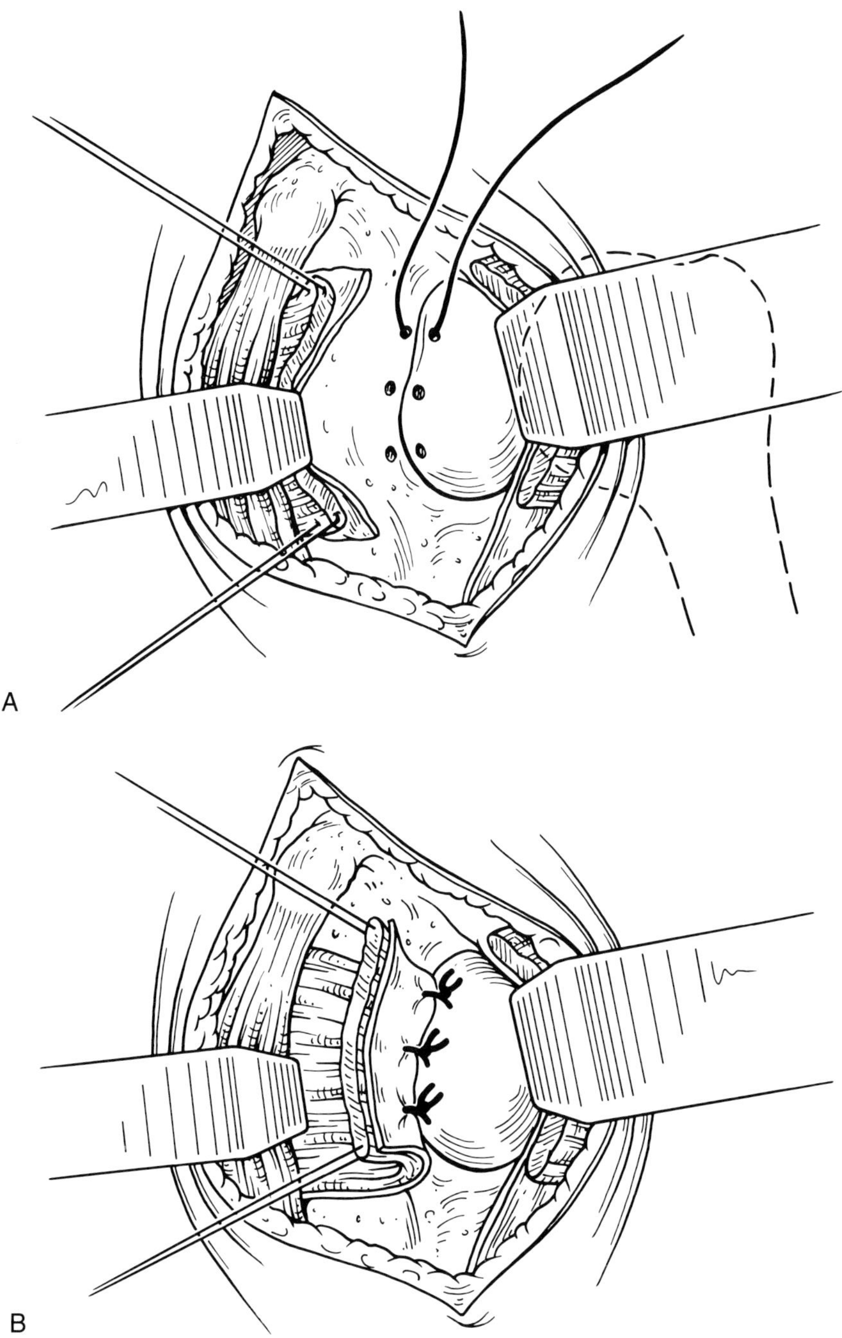

Figure 13-2. Bankart repair. **(A)** Subscapularis and capsule are released laterally and reflected to expose the anterior glenoid rim. Drill holes are placed and sutures passed through the glenoid rim. **(B)** Sutures are passed through the avulsed labrum and capsule. As the sutures are tied, the Bankart lesion is repaired.

rotation may be unavoidable if capsular redundancy is corrected. However, repairs such as the Putti-Platt and Magnuson-Stack depend on external rotation loss to control instability.[18] Anatomically directed procedures as in the Bankart and capsulolabral reconstruction minimize loss of rotation.[4,13,21] Incising and spreading rather than detaching the subscapularis may maximize external rotation.

4. *Aim for early rehabilitation:* The postoperative management and therapy of shoulders that have undergone anterior stabilization are based on the surgeon's interpretation of tissue quality, security of the repair, intraoperative examination after the repair, and the patient's ultimate desired range of motion of the shoulder. Some arthroscopic shoulder stabilization procedures have the disadvantage of requiring a period of immobilization

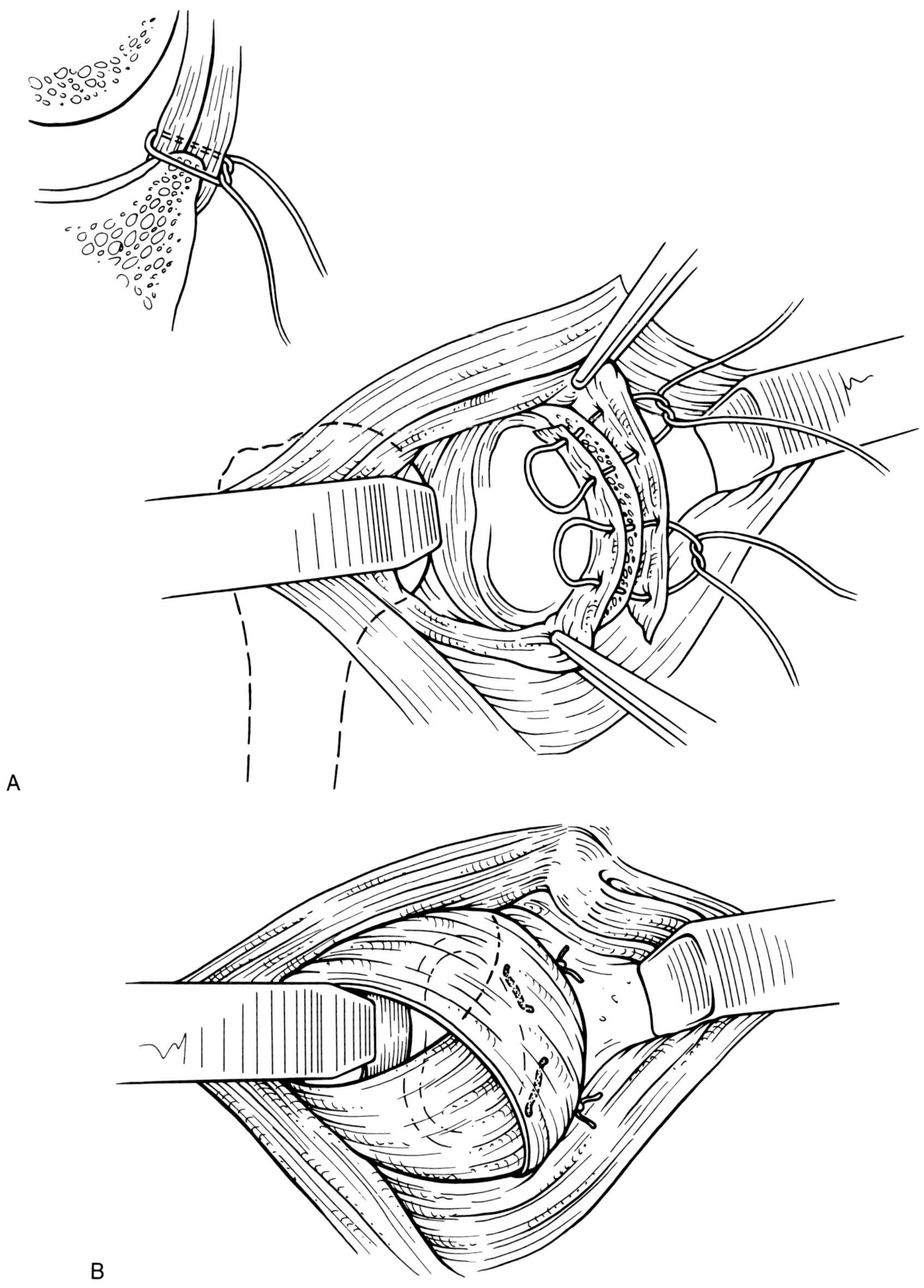

Figure 13-3. Anterior capsulolabral repair. **(A)** The anterior capsule is exposed by splitting the subscapularis in the line of the muscle fibers. A transverse incision is made through the capsule. Sutures are placed along the glenoid rim and passed through the inferior leaf of capsule, resulting in superior and medial advancement. **(B)** The superior leaf is advanced over the repaired inferior leaf. (*Figure continues.*)

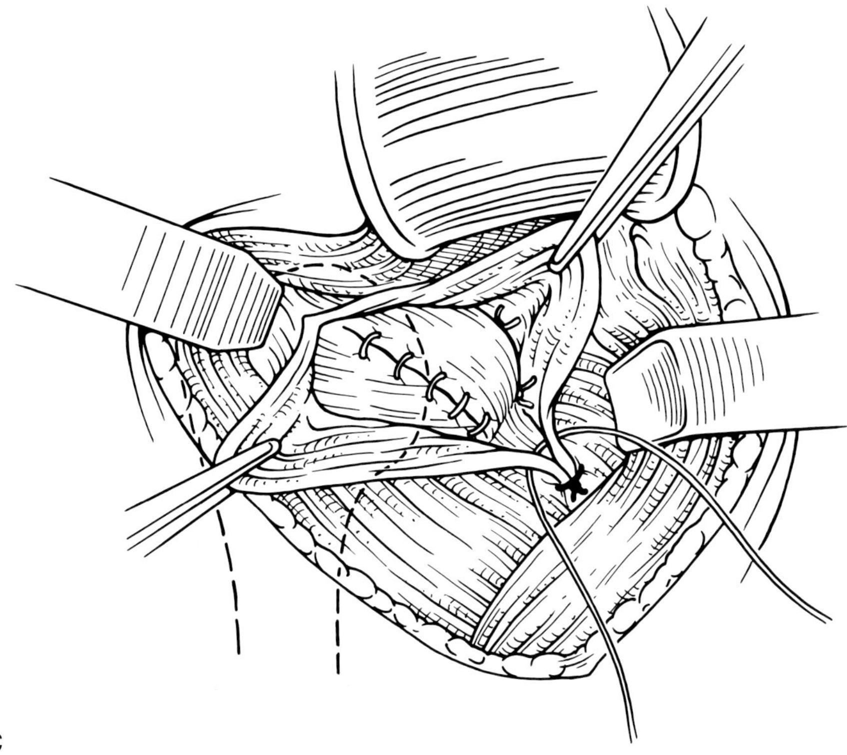

Figure 13-3 (*Continued*). **(C)** The transverse incision is closed to complete the repair.

to protect the repair. In any repair, the goal is to provide enough stability to allow early passive range of motion exercises. One advantage of the anterior capsulolabral reconstruction is the preservation of the subscapularis muscle insertion, which in theory allows early active exercises. Return to sport is often delayed until the shoulder has a pain-free range of motion, loss of apprehension, and muscle strength to actively protect the internal repair.

Patient selection is an important feature that may define success and failure. Repairs performed arthroscopically may create less scar tissue, cause less restriction of motion, and be anatomically precise. Patients who might require a stronger repair may be best treated by an arthrotomy and surgical reconstruction. For most surgeons, an open procedure is preferred for athletes. In the near future, we may see this change. Improved arthroscopic techniques are being used to obtain a secure repair, allowing early motion and low recurrence. The surgeon's experience, the patient's compliance in the postoperative period, noted pathology, quality of the tissue, and the expectations of the athlete are important considerations when choosing between open or arthroscopic procedures.

Surgery begins with examination under anesthesia. A load and shift maneuver is helpful to identify increased translation, clicks due to incompetent labrum, and obvious dislocation and reduction.[9] Range of motion, specifically rotation, is recorded in both shoulders.

BANKART REPAIR

Bankart repair is familiar to most orthopaedic surgeons.[4] With this technique, the subscapularis muscle is divided 1 cm medial to the lesser tuberosity and sharply dissected from the underlying capsule. The arm is externally rotated, and the capsule is opened by a vertical incision 0.5 cm lateral to the anterior glenoid rim. The lateral capsular flap is sutured to the anterior glenoid neck with the arm in external rotation. Rowe and Zarins[20] have modified the procedure by overlapping the medial and lateral parts of the anterior capsule for reinforcement of the repair. Many modifications have been made to the original description allowing for improved exposure, improved anatomic fixation, and early rehabilitation. The surgeon should "customize" a surgical approach to address the precise pathology and direct appropriate rehabilitation to obtain the result. The surgical repairs in this chapter are our preferred approaches, although others are reasonable alternatives. The surgeon should be familiar with the multiple pathologies that may be discovered and be able to alter the repair as required.

The approach uses the supine position with slight flexion of the hips and knees and the shoulder at the edge of the table resting on an arm board. The examination under anesthesia should precede preparing and draping to avoid any restrictions due to adhesive drapes. A longitudinal deltopectoral approach is used with the skin incision within

Langer's lines. A more inferior skin incision within the axillae may result in a more satisfactory cosmetic result, especially desired in women. Undermining the skin to palpate the coracoid process from beneath provides exposure of the anterior and anteroinferior portion of the shoulder. The cephalic vein is retracted laterally with the deltoid and the pectoralis medially, allowing for the exposure of the subscapularis tendon on the lesser tuberosity. A small nick in the superior portion of the conjoined tendon fascia allows for careful medial retraction of coracobrachialis and short head of the biceps, along with the pectoralis. Techniques that take off the coracoid process or divide the conjoined tendon are usually unnecessary. When left intact, these structures can serve to protect the musculocutaneous nerve from overzealous retraction. The cluster of vessels at the inferior margin of the subscapularis is identified and cauterized. A vertical incision through the subscapularis and capsule is made 1.5 cm medial and parallel to the palpable biceps tendon. Through this anterior window, the surgeon can confirm the presence of a Bankart lesion by pushing the humeral head posteriorly with a blunt instrument. Transverse divergent incisions at the upper and lower edges of the subscapularis and capsule allow entrance of a humeral head retractor that pushes the head posteriorly, allowing excellent exposure of the glenoid. The absence of a Bankart lesion may change the procedure of choice to one that addresses the capsule alone. In this case, the subscapularis can be separated from the underlying capsule to expose the latter for a cruciate capsulorrhaphy (see next section). Another option may be to create a Bankart lesion and perform a reconstruction.

The anterior glenoid can be exposed by retracting the humeral head posteriorly and an using anterior glenoid neck retractor medially deep to the separated labrum anteriorly. The anterior neck of the glenoid is decorticated to a bleeding surface with either curettes or a high-speed burr. Sutures can be passed through drill holes, or suture anchors can be placed along the anterior edge of the articular surface to allow for anatomic restoration of the labrum. Depending on the size of the Bankart lesion, multiple sutures or suture anchors are used. The typical Bankart lesion can be repaired with anchors at approximately the 2, 4, and 6 o'clock position (right shoulder). Drill holes can be developed with a high-speed burr and completed with a towel clip. Larger lesions may require additional anchoring sutures. Nonabsorbable sutures (Ethibond #2) and suture anchors are used for the repair, although longer-acting absorbable sutures can be used.

The sutures are, in turn, passed through the anterior labrum and capsule as the subscapularis and capsule are pulled upward. Sutures are placed adjacent to the glenoid articular surface. Care must be taken not to take too large a bite in the capsule, which could result in subsequent limitation to external rotation. The sutures through the anterior labrum and its capsular attachment are secured (Fig. 13-2). The subscapularis tendon unit and capsule are then reattached anatomically to their original position adjacent to the lesser tuberosity. The shoulder should be examined for range of motion and stability. If the shoulder remains unstable, further tensioning of the subscapularis tendon and underlying capsular can be made laterally by advancing this flap. In general, at least 30 degrees of external rotation should be demonstrated at this time. The superior border of the subscapularis is reinforced laterally to secure the rotator cuff interval.

The deltopectoral interval may be closed with absorbable sutures. Subcutaneous and skin closure is by surgeon's choice. Postoperatively, a sling is used for comfort. Patients are instructed on local hygiene to the axillae until the wound has healed.

ANTERIOR CAPSULOLABRAL RECONSTRUCTION

Many surgeons perform a classical Bankart procedure separating subscapularis and capsule. It may be preferable to correct the pathology with minimal disruption of the remaining shoulder anatomy. Jobe et al[13] have described a modification of the Bankart repair that approaches the shoulder joint through a split in the subscapularis tendon. In theory, this technique may be advantageous in overhead athletes and throwers and may allow for a more aggressive rehabilitation program. Early abduction and external rotation will not jeopardize the subscapularis attachment to the lesser tuberosity. The repair may address a Bankart lesion if present and also repairs capsular laxity by shifting the capsule in an inferior-superior direction avoiding any medial-lateral shortening that may limit external rotation. In throwers, labral pathology often coexists with capsular pathology. Repairs that significantly limit external rotation in this population are unacceptable.

The anterior capsulolabral reconstruction is a technically demanding procedure. Specially designed retractors by Jobe facilitate the repair. A right angle Gelpi retractor, a special glenoid spike, and humeral head retractor and retractors to expose the deltopectoral interval are important. In muscular athletes, it may be particularly difficult to obtain adequate exposure, and additional assistants are recommended.

A standard deltopectoral approach as in the Bankart repair is followed by a transverse incision along the middle and distal thirds of the subscapularis tendon and fascia, exposing the underlying capsule. Meticulous dissection beginning medially can further develop the interval between the capsule and the undersurface of the subscapularis (Fig. 13-3). Separating the subscapularis laterally from the underlying capsule is difficult. Retaining sutures along the cut edge of the subscapularis allow a sharp periosteal elevator or knife to be used to free the tendon from the underlying capsule. Special retractors designed by Jobe greatly enhance exposure. An extensive separation of the subscapularis from the capsule is advisable. Self-retaining Gelpi retractors to hold the subscapularis apart are helpful.

The capsule is horizontally split from lateral to medial, extending medially over the glenoid neck. Usually, three suture anchors are placed in the anterior glenoid rim. Any labral detachments can be anatomically reapproximated as the sutures are passed through the labrum. If the labrum is intact, the anchors are placed just medial to the edge of the articular surface. The inferior flap is advanced superiorly, and the superior flap is advanced inferiorly, with the sutures coming through both flaps and tied in a mattress fashion. The subscapularis is allowed to fall together and sutured edge to edge (Fig. 13-3).

A sling or abduction brace is used during the early postoperative period. Return to sports is based on the athlete's range of motion, scapular muscular strength, and appropriate rehabilitation to the dominant muscle groups about the shoulder. Throwing is generally delayed 6 to 12 months. The advantages of this technique include splitting rather than dividing the subscapularis, inferior-superior reconstruction of capsule, aggressive early rehabilitation, and abduction brace to reduce contractures.

ANTERIOR CRUCIATE CAPSULAR REPAIR

The anterior cruciate capsule repair may be used for anterior instability where the labrum is intact and anterior capsular redundancy is present. This can also be used to treat a Bankart lesion associated with a stretched-out capsule. Usually, when one suspects an intact labrum, the subscapularis can be separated from the underlying capsule. A medial retractor can then be placed to retract the subscapularis medially.

A horizontal incision is made through the midcapsule to the glenoid rim. If a previous lateral capsular division was made, the edges of the capsule should have traction sutures placed for reference. An inferior and superior flap can then be developed and overlapped in a south-north repair. A vertical T may not be necessary in most cases. The stretched-out capsule can be obliterated by superiorly advancing the inferior flap (Fig. 13-4). If the labrum is intact, sutures can be placed along the medial capsular edge and reattached to the labrum after an oblique shift in a superior direction. Overlapping the capsular edges medially removes any remaining capsular redundancy. If present, the lateral capsule incision is anatomically closed. The subscapularis muscle tendon unit is returned and repaired to its origin without lateral advancement. The postoperative program is similar to the Bankart (see Postoperative Program).

CONSIDERATIONS FOR ARTHROSCOPIC SHOULDER STABILIZATION VERSUS OPEN REPAIR

Arthroscopic techniques to repair traumatic anterior shoulder instability continue to be developed and refined. The goal of arthroscopy is to reproduce the same objectives as those performed with open surgery. These objectives are

1. A procedure performed anteriorly where the major pathology is located
2. Repair labrum to the glenoid to deepen "the socket"
3. Create appropriate tension in the capsule that will limit excessive translation without limiting external rotation
4. Improved techniques of tissue fixation allowing early rehabilitation and minimizing immobilization

The surgeon may select arthroscopic stabilization based on the pathology, the surgeon's experience, and the ability of the patient to cooperate with the postoperative regimen. As in open procedures, the surgeon must adapt his or her surgery to address the discovered pathology. Decreased success rates can be expected if this is not accomplished. Correction of the pathology by similar technique of tissue reattachment should have results similar to open procedures.[2,24]

Arthroscopic stabilization is a preoperative decision based on the patient's history of trauma, physical findings, and preoperative discussions regarding the patient's expectations. If poor visualization or difficulty with obtaining appropriate capsular tension occurs, surgeons may convert to an open procedure.

POSTOPERATIVE PROGRAM

The duration of immobilization after surgical repair remains controversial. Arthroscopic stabilization techniques have, in general, been followed by 3 weeks immobilization with a sling before rehabilitation. Open techniques have popularized earlier and more aggressive rehabilitation, but some continue to recommend a sling for the early postoperative period. This appears to be a contradiction of open versus arthroscopic techniques performed in other joints. The goal of arthroscopic surgery is to allow early motion similar to an open repair. As of now, arthroscopic techniques continue to necessitate immobilization during the initial 3 weeks and a more gradual stretching program especially in external rotation. A period of immobilization should be based on

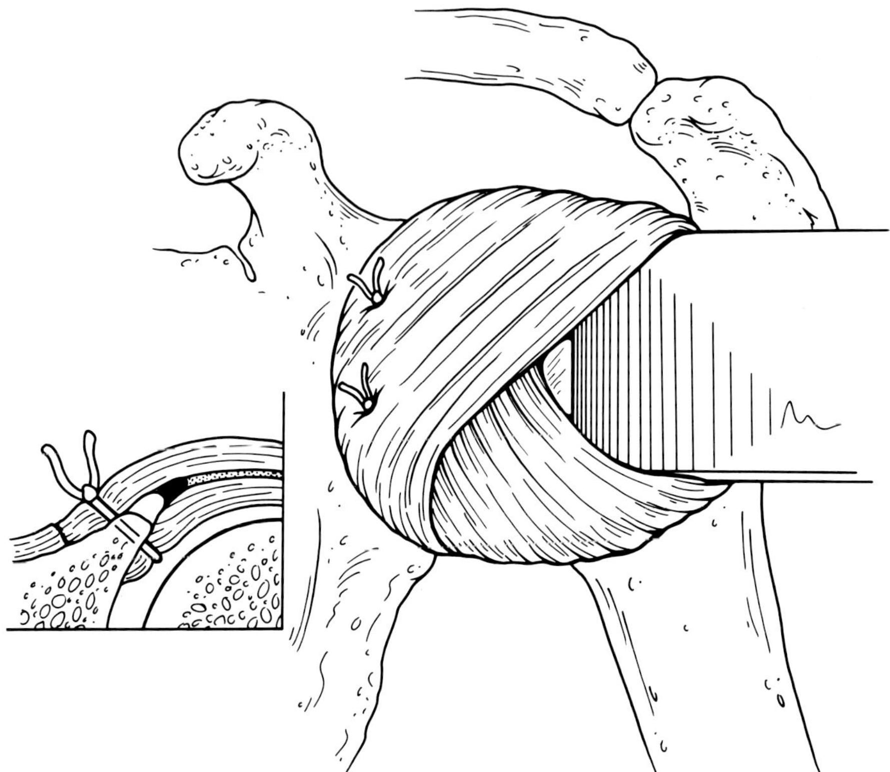

Figure 13-4. Anterior cruciate capsular repair. Capsular flaps are created by incisions transversely from the humerus to the glenoid and vertically along the glenoid. The inferior flap is advanced superior and medial, and the superior flap is advanced inferior and medial. The inset illustration is a cross section through the anterior glenoid rim showing placement of suture and overlap of capsular flaps.

1. Security of the repair
2. Tissue quality
3. Additional augmentation or implants used
4. Demonstrable range of motion on the operative table at the completion of surgey, before stretching the repair. If Bankart repair is performed arthroscopically, the surgeon may visualize the repair during rotation.
5. Expectations of the patient

Securing a thick portion of labrum and ligament with excellent glenoid fixation allows early motion whether open or arthroscopic. Patients who can obtain 30 degrees of external rotation without stressing the repair at the completion of the operation can often begin early rehabilitation with close monitoring.[2,21] In general, thin capsular repairs and reconstruction are restricted for a longer period, whereas labral repairs can be moved early.

The goals of rehabilitation include a stable shoulder with a painless full range of motion, normal strength, endurance, and a return to normal activities. This can be accomplished through four stages of rehabilitation: (1) early protected mobilization; (2) progressive strengthening; (3) sport-specific re-education and neuromuscular proprioceptive training; and (4) a maintenance program. Early phases of rehabilitation are designed to allow assisted motion using the healthy arm. Pendulum exercises can be used to warm up. Forward flexion as tolerated and external rotation to 30 degrees can be allowed during the first 2 weeks. This program can be used after both open and arthroscopic techniques. In cases in which the fixation is more tenuous, 2 to 3 weeks of immobilization before beginning rehabilitation is recommended. Lateral abduction can be started early and may be helpful in patients returning to overhead athletics. Further external rotation stretching is closely monitored and progressed based on expectations and security of the repair. Active exercises can usually be started at 2 weeks, and gentle resistive exercises are generally started 4 to 8 weeks postoperatively, depending on the technique used.

Most arthroscopic and open procedures aim to obtain the majority of rotation with the elbow at the side by 6 to 8 weeks after surgery. External rotation should be compared pre- and postoperatively to the normal side. Examination under anesthesia on the unstable shoulder might reveal an external rotation deficit due to chronic capsular or medialization of the capsule and labrum. Delays in obtaining motion can postoperatively result in capsule contractures, posterior subluxation, and loss of full elevation. Combined abduction and external rotation can gradually be pursued if maximal external rotation is desired, as in pitching. Athletes attempting more than 90 degrees of external rotation in 90 degrees of abduction before 3 months can stretch their repair, possibly inviting recurrent subluxation.

Crossed chest and internal rotation stretching is helpful after initial labral healing at 4 to 6 weeks. In cases in which posterior capsule tightness is present, the humeral head can ride anteriorly, putting pressure along the labral repair. Preoperative stretching of the posterior capsule structures might be helpful in the postoperative course.

Isometric shoulder strengthening can be started early. Resistive strengthening of the elbow and forearm, along with general body conditioning, can begin immediately. Once motion is significantly recovered, rotator cuff, deltoid, and scapular strengthening is pursued. The rotator cuff can be concentrically and eccentrically strengthened with rubber tubing or hand-held weights. By externally rotating to 45 degrees and slowly releasing, an eccentric emphasis is made on the posterior and superior rotator cuff. Scapular strengthening including trapezius, rhomboid, pectoralis, and serratus anterior is important in protecting the repair by maintaining the glenoid in an acceptable position to complement the humeral head and reduce shearing forces. Standing shrugs, bent over and standing rows, and push-ups (narrow grip) are important. The latissimus helps control deceleration of the arm, which may diminish eccentric overload of the supraspinatus.[7] More advanced strengthening can begin in 8 to 10 weeks. Plyometric or explosive movement training is usually started after 12 to 16 weeks postoperatively.

Sport-specific exercises to improve glenohumeral and scapulothoracic synchronization are important to regain specific functions. Swimming and tennis can usually be started by 4 months. Contact sports are best judged on protective internal rotation strength and may require 6 months or more to allow for adequate healing. Throwing may be started when sport-specific rehabilitation has progressed. This generally takes 4 to 6 months before starting the interval training program. A strength maintenance program for at least 1 year is suggested.

PROGNOSIS WITH SURGERY

With careful selection of patients, good results from a Bankart repair can be obtained.[20] Hovelius et al[12] found only a 2 percent recurrence after Bankart repair, compared with 36 percent after Putti-Platt repair. Likewise, the success of anterior capsulolabral reconstruction has been noted in professional athletes including pitchers.[21] In a series of 75 athletes with a follow-up averaging 39 months, 92 percent excellent or good results were reported, with 75 percent of the professional baseball players returning to their sport. Range of motion was reported as full in 79 percent of the athletes. Patients can often return to overhead and contact sports after anterior stabilization. Improved understanding of the pathology and the desire to maintain maximum external rotation have produced results with minimal restriction. Return to throwing in a highly skilled pitcher may be difficult to achieve. Other factors including rotator cuff damage and changes in scapular thoracic rhythm might interfere with return to pitching.

Although the successful results of arthroscopic stabilization have not been as consistent as open techniques, these results can be expected to improve with better refinement of instruments and skills. Recent data using a biodegradable tack for all cases of anterior instability in which a Bankart lesion exists found a redislocation rate of 14 percent.[24] This population included contact athletes who in others series were found to have high redislocation rate. In 35 patients stabilized by a transglenoid technique, recurrent subluxation or dislocation occurred in 12 percent.[1] The loss of external rotation ranged from 0 to 15 degrees and averaged less than 5 degrees. More recently, a review of 25 patients with suture anchors placed arthroscopically found 4 percent recurrent instability.[2] Arthroscopic stabilization represents multiple types of procedures and may be technique-dependent, with the best results limited to surgeons who have a large experience in this area. One must remain critical when comparing arthroscopic stabilization with the commonly performed open techniques.

A common denominator in all reports of failed stabilization for shoulder instability include an incorrect diagnosis of the direction of instability and a failure to correct the pathologic lesions with an appropriate surgical procedure.[8] It is therefore important that shoulder surgeons develop their own approach to shoulder instability based on sound principles and using procedures with which they are most familiar. This begins preoperatively in obtaining a careful history and performing a precise physical examination. Multidirectional instability will generally yield poor results with the techniques mentioned above and therefore requires special consideration.

FAILED SURGERY

Failures include recurrence of instability, repairs made too tight, or other complications relating to surgery. One must identify the reason for failure before planning correction. The initial principles are still critical to this success: (1) making the proper diagnosis, which includes direction(s); (2) addressing the pathology including correcting capsule tension and labral reattachment to the articular edge; (3) the avoidance of hardware or implants that cannot be adequately secured in bone; and (4) compliance with rehabilitation.

Repeat shoulder surgery can be challenging. Shoulders made too tight with significant loss of external rotation may lead to osteoarthritis with or without posterior subluxation.[10,15] An anterior Z-plasty with release of the capsule is necessary to avoid serious arthrosis (Fig. 13-5). Occasionally, an early release should be considered if external rotation does not exceed 0 degrees (i.e., 4 to 6 months). As an alternative, this release can be performed arthroscopically.

Recurrence of instability because of not correcting the pathology can be diagnosed arthroscopically and corrected by either open or arthroscopic techniques. Labral integrity should be confirmed as well as identification of capsular redundancy. After previous surgical failure, most surgeons would recommend open surgical techniques to provide additional security of repair. Longer periods of immobilization might be recommended as well. This decision might be altered if you had performed the index surgery and had not adequately addressed the capsule tension at that time. The amount of trauma necessary for the recurrence is helpful in formulating a plan.

Revision of previous extra-articular procedures (i.e., Bristow, duToit) can be difficult if recurrence occurs. The arthroscope posteriorly may identify persistence of intra-articular pathology. Anterior portal placement might be hazardous due to the transferred structures. Patients with persistence Bankart lesion are best approached by an arthrotomy with careful elevation of the subscapularis and capsule as a unit, just medial to the biceps. Tissue reattachment to their anatomic location is the objective.

Painful hardware may require removal. The transferred coracoid process is traditionally fixed with a screw to the anterior glenoid in a Bristow procedure. Anterior-placed staples are used to secure the subscapularis in the duToit or Magnuson-Stack procedures. If these forms of fixation become symptomatic (i.e., loosening or impingement), they should be removed. If asymptomatic, they are best left alone. The soft tissue or the coracoid might require additional suturing if the hardware is removed.

Multidirectional instability remains a frequent cause of failure of unidirectional surgery.[10] Excessive tightness can push the head posteriorly. Inadequate attention to the inferior sulcus allows the head to remain unstable despite capsular plication anteriorly. The superior structures adjacent to the rotator cuff interval play a role in preventing inferior instability.[29] The inferior glenohumeral ligament is not effective in preventing anterior and posterior translation

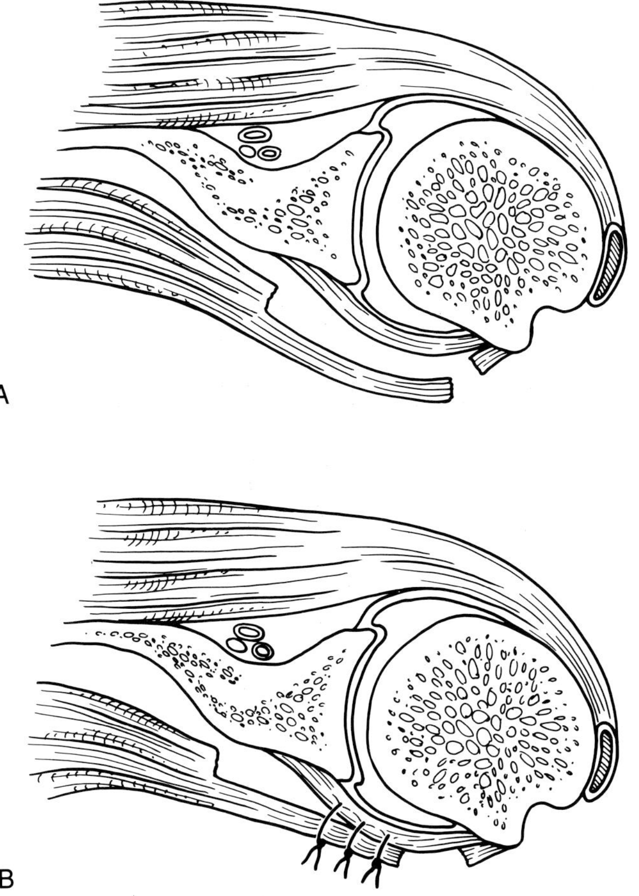

Figure 13-5. (A & B) Anterior release for internal rotation contracture.

when this redundancy is present. Multidirectional instability is best treated by nonoperative measures. Physical therapy may gradually stretch out tight repairs, and rotator cuff strengthening might prove sufficient to salvage surgical failure. Surgical restoration of the rotator cuff interval and a balanced inferior capsule shift are essential for surgical correction.

CONCLUSION

Young athletes with traumatic anterior instability of the glenohumeral joint can be treated surgically, achieving a high rate of success. Surgery is best applied to those patients disabled by recurrent dislocation or subluxation or who remain apprehensive. First-time dislocators who are disabled by persistent pain or apprehension after a rehabilitation program should be considered as well.

Selected athletes may consider immediate surgical repair. This may avoid the complication and disability found in high-risk activities, especially in the young age group. After surgery, the risk of recurrence is significantly reduced; yet not all athletes are disabled by shoulder instability. These considerations need to be judged on an individual basis.

A patient's history defines the etiology and degree of force sustained to create initial or recurrent shoulder instability. Physical examination may identify apprehension and suspected directions(s) of instability. Examination under anesthesia is helpful to demonstrate labral pathology and record external rotation in both shoulders. Arthroscopy may be helpful in identifying "the essential lesion." Operative reconstruction is often best managed by some modification of the Bankart procedure, especially in overhead athletes.

Patient selection and experience of the surgeon should identify which procedure is most beneficial and successful to correct the pathology. The surgical goal is to re-establish the glenoid labrum and proper capsule tension, specially the inferior and middle glenohumeral ligaments. The delicate balance of mobility and restored stability may return athletes to a high functional level. The rehabilitation program needs to be individualized to meet these demands. Failures of surgery due to loose hardware, arthrosis, or capsular tightness with posterior subluxation require early surgery for salvage before severe arthrosis. Patients with multidirectional instability should begin with an appropriately designed rehabilitation program. If problems persist, however, an appropriate surgical procedure needs to be used.

Rehabilitation and protective activities are important to the successful outcome. Young athletes need to be reminded of the importance of complying to achieve the best end result. Long-term experience is available for many procedures performed via open surgery. As arthroscopic surgical techniques mature, the procedures should share similar success. Surgeons need to remain equipped with a series of operations that are directed at correcting the pathology.

REFERENCES

1. Abrams JS: Arthroscopic shoulder stabilization for recurrent subluxation and dislocation. J Shoulder Elbow Surg, suppl. 2, 1:S25, 1993
2. Abrams JS: Arthroscopic capsulolabral anchor. Presented at the Fourth Annual Steadman-Hawkins SportsMedicine Foundation Meeting, Vail, CO, 1993
3. Aronen JG, Regan K: Decreasing the incidence of recurrence of first time anterior shoulder dislocations with rehabilitation. Am J Sports Med 12:283, 1984
4. Bankart ASB: The pathology and treatment of recurrent dislocations of the shoulder joint. Br J Surg 26:23, 1938
5. Barber FA, Cawley P, Prudich JF: Suture anchor failure strength—an in vivo study. Arthroscopy 9:647, 1993
6. Bigliani LU, Pollock RG, Soglowsky LJ et al: Tensile properties of the inferior glenohumeral ligament. J Orthop Res 10:187, 1992
7. Dillman CJ, Fleisig GS, Werner SL, Andrews JR: Biomechanics of the shoulder in sports: throwing activities. In Matsen FA, Fu FH, Hawkins RJ (eds): The Shoulder: A Balance of Mobility and Stability. American Academy Orthopaedic Surgeons, Rosemont, IL, 1993
8. Hawkins RH, Hawkins RJ: Failed anterior reconstruction for shoulder instability. J Bone Joint Surg [Br] 67:709, 1985
9. Hawkins RJ, Abrams JS, Schutte JP: Multidirectional instability of the shoulder: an approach to diagnosis. Orthop Trans 11:246, 1987
10. Hawkins RJ, Angelo RL: Glenohumeral osteoarthritis: a late complication of the Putti-Platt repair. J Bone Joint Surg [Am] 72:1193, 1990
11. Hovelius L: Anterior dislocation of the shoulder in teenagers and young adults: five years prognosis. J Bone Joint Surg [Am] 69:393, 1987
12. Hovelius L, Thorling J, Fredin H: Recurrent anterior dislocation of the shoulder: results after the Bankart and Putti-Platt operations. J Bone Joint Surg [Am] 61:566, 1979
13. Jobe FW, Giangarra CE, Kvitne RS, Glousman RE: Anterior capsulolabral reconstruction of the shoulder in athletes in overhand sports. Am J Sports Med 19:428, 1991
14. Lippitt SB, Harryman DT, Sidles JA, Matsen FA: Diagnosis and management of AMBRI syndrome. Techniques Orthop 6:61, 1991
15. MacDonald PB, Hawkins RJ, Fowler PJ, Miniaci A: Release of the subscapularis for internal rotation contracture and pain after anterior repair for recurrent anterior dislocation of the shoulder. J Bone Joint Surg [Am] 74:734, 1992
16. Neer CS, Foster CR: Inferior capsular shift for involuntary inferior and multidirectional instability of the shoulder: a preliminary report. J Bone Joint Surg [Am] 62:897, 1980

17. O'Brien SJ, Neves MC, Arnoczky SP et al: Anatomy and histology of the inferior glenohumeral ligament complex of the shoulder. Am J Sports Med 18:449, 1990
18. Regan WD, Webster-Bogaert S, Hawkins RJ, Fowler PJ: Comparative functional analysis of the Bristow, Magnuson-Stack and Putti-Platt procedures for recurrent dislocation of the shoulder. Am J Sport Med 17:42, 1989
19. Rowe CR: Prognosis in dislocations of the shoulder. J Bone Joint Surg [Am] 38:957, 1956
20. Rowe CR, Zarins B: Recurrent transient subluxation of the shoulder. J Bone Joint Surg [Am] 63:863, 1981
21. Rubenstein DL, Jobe FW, Glousman RE et al: Anterior capsulolabral reconstruction of the shoulder in athletes. J Shoulder Elbow Surg 1:229, 1992
22. Simonet WT, Cofield RH: Prognosis in anterior shoulder dislocation. Am J Sports Med 12:19, 1984
23. Snyder SJ, Strafford BB: Arthroscopic management of instability of the shoulder. Orthopedics 16:993, 1993
24. Speer KP, Pagnani M, Warren RF: Arthroscopic anterior shoulder stabilization, two to five year followup using a biodegradable tac. Presented at the American Shoulder and Elbow Surgeons Specialty Day, New Orleans, 1993
25. Terry GC, Hammon D, France P, Norwood LA: The stabilizing function of passive shoulder restraints. Am J Sports Med 19:26, 1991
26. Thomas SC, Matsen FA: An approach to the repair of avulsion of the glenohumeral ligaments in the management of traumatic anterior glenohumeral instability. J Bone Joint Surg [Am] 71:506, 1989
27. Tsai L, Wredmark T, Johansson C et al: Shoulder function in patients with unoperated anterior shoulder instability. Am J Sports Med 19:469, 1991
28. Turkel SJ, Panio MW, Marshall JL, Girgis FG: Stabilizing mechanisms preventing anterior dislocation of the glenohumeral joint. J Bone Joint Surg [Am] 63:1208, 1981
29. Warner JJP, Caborn DNM, Berger R et al: Dynamic capsuloligamentous anatomy of the glenohumeral joint. J Shoulder Elbow Surg 2:115, 1993
30. Yoneda B, Welsh RP, MacIntosh DL: Conservative treatment of shoulder dislocation in young males. J Bone Joint Surg [Br] 64:254, 1982
31. Zuckerman JD, Matsen FA: Complications about the glenohumeral joint related to the use of screws and staples. J Bone Joint Surg [Am] 66:175, 1984

CHAPTER FOURTEEN

Arthroscopy for Anterior Instability

James D. Cash
Jeffrey S. Abrams

Arthroscopy of the shoulder has profoundly affected our knowledge regarding many aspects of the treatment of the unstable shoulder. The development of a multitude of arthroscopic techniques over the past 10 years in an attempt to recreate previously described open surgical procedures has offered the orthopaedic surgeon a variety of methods for surgical stabilization. Unfortunately, description of a technique does not guarantee good results, and one must be careful to analyze the anatomic basis for the procedure described and the results obtained. Because long-term studies of the outcomes of these procedures are not yet possible, decisions based on preliminary results have to be sufficient for now.

The standard to which these arthroscopic stabilization procedures should be compared is open anterior shoulder reconstruction. More than 150 different open surgical procedures have been described with varying degrees of success. The goals of any stabilization procedure about the shoulder are to have a low recurrence and complication rate, to maintain motion with no traumatic arthritis, to allow joint inspection, and to treat the pathologic condition with a procedure that is not too technically difficult.[10] Long-term reports of open surgical stabilization show recurrence rates for instability from 2 to 13 percent, depending on the series reviewed.[38] The standard open Bankart repair is thought by many to be the most anatomically correct open procedure, as it restores stability by repairing the lateral capsular flap directly to the anterior glenoid rim. The procedure as described by Rowe[37] is associated with a recurrence rate of less than 5 percent. Despite these glowing results with the Bankart and other open repairs, complication related to the use of hardware near the joint,[52] loss of motion,[19] and failure to return to the desired level of athletics[25] have led to the use of the arthroscopic techniques as an alternative to open stabilization.

ARTHROSCOPIC ADVANTAGES

With the multitude of techniques available for stabilizing the shoulder, the most attractive one should be the easiest to perform with the best results and least trauma for the patient. Watson-Jones[45] reflected the feelings of many surgeons in regard to open shoulder reconstruction by noting that "the only factor common to the many operative procedures is a bloody dissection in an anterior approach." The technical aspects of the Bankart procedure can be particularly demanding and require skilled, knowledgeable, and attentive assistants for adequate retraction and visualization. Arthroscopic stabilization permits a single surgeon to perform the procedure, with the same assistance needed for a regular arthroscopic procedure. Both loss of motion and failure to return to the desired level of sporting activity have been described with open surgical stabilization. In describing the results of the Bristow procedure, Hill et al[20] reported an average of 12 percent loss of external rotation, and only 6 of 41 throwers returned to their preinjury level of activity. Despite regaining complete elevation and external rotation in 69 percent of the patients who had a Bankart repair, Rowe[37] found that only 10 of 30 patients who engaged in throwing sports were able to return to their preinjury throwing level. Hawkins[18] described a 22 degree loss of external rotation in his patients who had a Putti-Platt procedure, with none of eight throwers returning to the preinjury athletic level. In Rowe's series,[37] the return of maximum external rotation was associated with an increase rather than decrease in stability. Rowe found that any restriction of external rotation could be a handicap in athletes needing complete elevation and external rotation in overhead activities such as that performed when serving in tennis, pitching a baseball, throwing a football, making a lay-up in basketball, swimming, and particularly in gymnastics. Some types of work, such as plastering, painting, and paper hanging, also require full shoulder rotation. Arthroscopic stabilization, by addressing only the labrum-ligamentous complex and by decreasing the anterior shoulder scar formation, may provide a means of limiting postoperative loss of motion.

Thorough visualization of the glenohumeral joint, rotator cuff, and subacromial bursa is a routine part of diagnostic arthroscopy. In review of 45 shoulders examined arthroscopically after acute initial anterior dislocation, Baker et al[4] found five rotator cuff tears (12 percent), osteochondral fragments in four shoulders (9 percent), free-floating attached labrum in three shoulders (9 percent), and two other shoulders with glenoid avulsion fractures (4 percent). Twenty-eight of 45 (62 percent shoulders in this series were found to be grossly unstable with complete capsular labral detachment. Although the recurrent shoulder dislocation with radiographic confirmation is easy to diagnose, a subset of patients exists, particularly those with subluxation, in whom symptoms and office examination cannot prove instability.[3] When these patients fail rehabilitation and have persistent symptoms, examination under anesthesia and arthroscopy may be indicated. A posterolateral Hill-Sachs lesion, tear of the labrum-ligamentous complex, redundant patulous anterior capsule, and anterior glenoid rim fracture are all signs of glenohumeral instability. Matthews et al[30] have reported that open surgery is contraindicated immediately after shoulder arthroscopy because of the fluid extravasation and soft tissue swelling that invariably accompany an arthroscopic procedure. When diagnostic arthroscopy uncovers a lesion of instability, the ability to stabilize the shoulder arthroscopically in the same surgical setting may preclude the associated surgical and anesthetic risks of a second procedure.

ARTHROSCOPIC STABILIZATION TECHNIQUES

The common denominator underlying all arthroscopic stabilization procedures for anterior instability is reestablishment of a functional inferior glenohumeral ligament complex. This can be achieved by reattaching the avulsed labrum with the ligament in continuity or by reattaching the ligament directly to the glenoid neck. Anatomic dissection and arthroscopic visualization of acute dislocations have shown capsular tears with stretching and subsequent capsular laxity to be another frequent cause of anterior instability. This must often be addressed at the time of reconstruction along with Bankart lesion repair to prevent recurrence of instability. The arthroscopic techniques to be described are all a variation of an open stabilization procedure and can be divided in three main categories depending on the type of fixation device used (i.e., metal devices such as staples or screws, suture-based repairs, and absorbable devices).

Metallic Staples and Screws

Capsular stapling was first performed by Perthes in 1906[34] and was later popularized by duToit and Roux.[12] In August 1982, Johnson[23] performed the first arthroscopic stabilization (on an orthopaedic surgeon) and in 1983 described the arthroscopic procedure for capsulorrhaphy using a modified metal staple and cannula system. In this technique, a 4-mm staple is introduced through an anterior arthroscopic portal on a specially designed staple holder through a staple cannula (Fig. 14-1). The glenoid labrum with its attached capsular ligaments is engaged with the staple and advanced superiorly. The staple is then impacted into the anterior glenoid neck. Staple insertion technique is critical.[11] The staple must be inserted at the correct angle and must be positioned away from the glenoid articular surface. The tines must not disrupt the glenoid articular surface or enter the joint. To prevent skiving of the staple, the handle of the staple driver must frequently be angled forcefully toward the axilla to insert the staple at the correct angle. Counterpressure stabilizes the scapula and aids insertion. To test the security of the insertion, the surgeon palpates the posterior scapula as the staple driver is angulated posteriorly and inferiorly. If the staple is secure, the motion of the staple driver is translated to the posterior scapula. Radiographs are routinely obtained immediately after the operation to confirm correct position of the staple.[11]

Johnson[23] began using the staple capsulorrhapy technique in 1982 and continues to use a similar technique. The results for patients operated on early (1982 to 1984) in his series with a minimum 2-year follow-up revealed a 21 percent redislocation rate. Those patients that were operated on from 1985 to 1987 with a minimum 2-year follow-up had a 13 percent redislocation rate (L. Johnson, personal communication, 1990). Johnson believes the discrepancy is due to the shorter postoperative immobilization time used in the earlier operations. He currently recommends shoulder immobilization in a sling for 3 to 4 weeks after surgery, with pendulum exercises at 1 to 4 weeks,

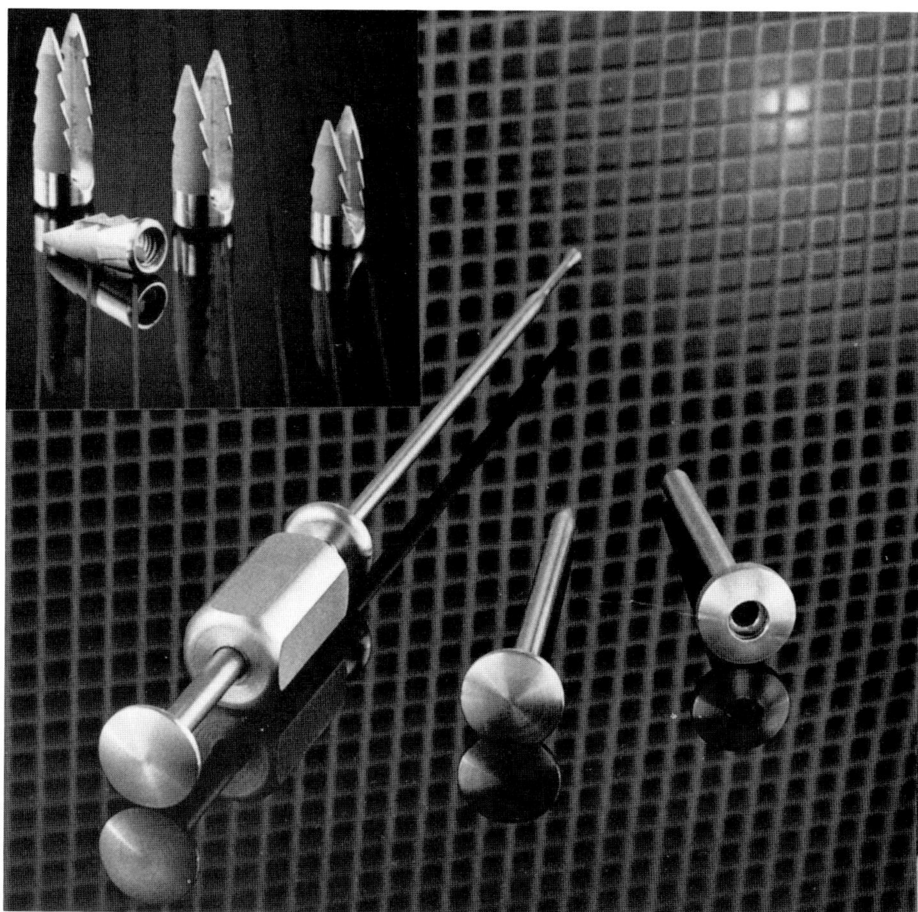

Figure 14-1. Arthroscopic staple system. (Courtesy of Instrument Makar, Inc., Okemas, MI.)

isometric and tubing exercises at 6 weeks, and holding athletes out of competition for 6 months.[11]

Matthews[29] reported on the first 25 consecutive patients undergoing staple capsulorrhaphy. Five patients required reoperation: three for recurrent anterior instability, one for posterior instability, and one for pain alone. The results were good or excellent in 67 percent of the patients, fair in 8 percent, and poor in 24 percent. Gross[17] used a similar stapling procedure but devised his own tools. He reported on 12 patients with a 44.8-month follow-up. Six patients had excellent results, two had good results, two had fair results, and two had poor results. The poor results were redislocations, giving a 17 percent (2 of 12) rate of redislocation.

Maki[26] reported the results of 21 patients undergoing staple capsulorrhaphy with a follow-up of 34 months. Five of 21 patients (21 percent) experienced recurrent instability. Maki recommended avoiding this procedure in patients returning to athletic activities. Lane and co-workers[24] reported that 18 to 54 patients (33 percent) who underwent staple capsulorrhaphy for anterior instability experienced at least one espisode of postoperative instability. Eighteen percent (10 of 54) required further open stabilization.

Wiley[48] devised a threaded collared pin with a beveled shank of various lengths (Fig. 14-2) that could be driven into the glenoid neck with the shank located just under the skin so it could be removed at a later date (Fig. 14-2). Curettes were used to debride the anterior glenoid rim. The rivet was used to impale the loose labrum and was driven inward until the flange rested on the glenoid margin. Four weeks later, with the patient under local or general anesthesia, the device was removed by incising the skin over it, slipping the special duct on to the beveled shank, and extracting the rivet. With a follow-up period of 6 months to more than 2 years, Wiley reported that the operation succeeded in 9 of 10 patients.

Wolf[49] and Snyder and Strafford[41] had devised a method for arthroscopic reattachment of torn ligaments to bone using a cannulated bone screw with attached washer (Dyonics, Inc., Andover, MA). After preparation of the glenoid, a guide pin is introduced through a cannula, used to pierce the labrum and capsule, and advanced on to the bone of the anterior glenoid. A cannulated drill is then passed over the guide pin and is used to create a drill hole in the anterior glenoid. The guide pin is left in place as the drill is removed. The cannulated screw is then placed over the pin, the screw

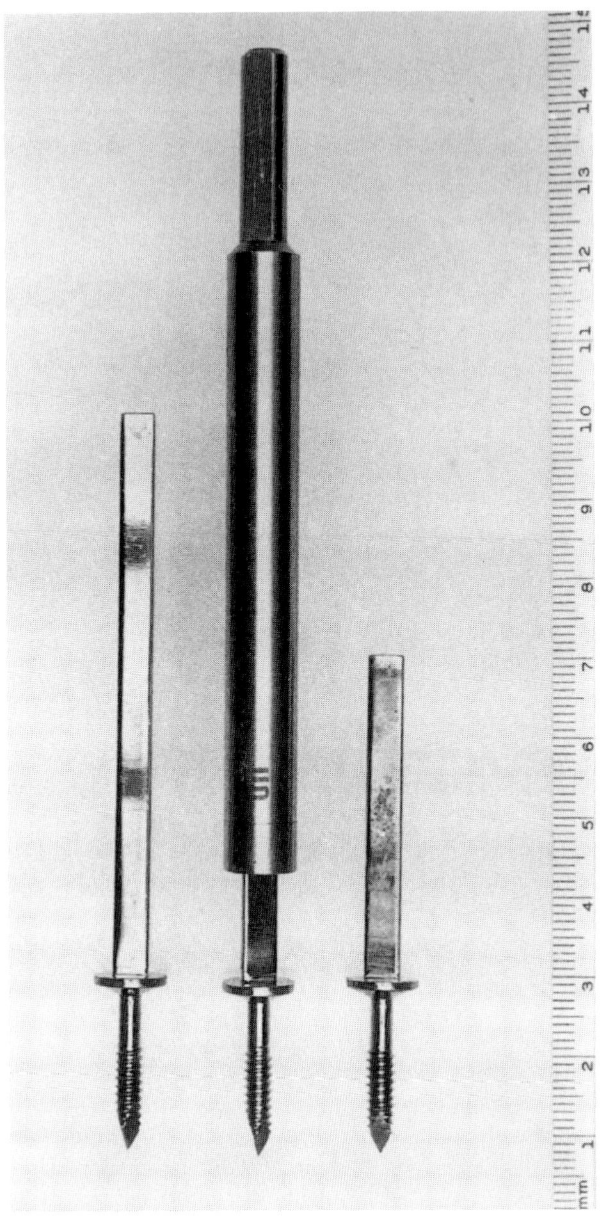

Figure 14-2. The removable rivet. (Courtesy of Xomed/Treace, Division of Bristol Myers Squibb, Jacksonville, FL.)

is tightened, and the labrum and capsule are drawn to the anterior neck of the glenoid (Fig. 14-3). The guide pin is then removed, completing the repair.[51]

Snyder and Strafford[41] reconstructed 36 shoulders using the Dyonics cannulated screw and washer and had a 14-month average follow-up (range, 3 to 40). Fifty percent of the patients had excellent results with complete recovery of range of motion and full activity. Twenty percent (7 of 36) of the patients had elimination of their instability and required arthroscopic screw removal due to persistent pain and irritation. Thirty percent of the patients experienced failures with recurrent instability. Gartsman used a Dyonics screw in 17 patients with anterior instability (G.M. Gartsman, personal communication, 1992). After a minimum 3-year follow-up, six patients (28 percent) had experienced recurrent instability, and four of them underwent repeat surgery. At that time, two of the Bankart lesions had failed to heal. None of the patients experienced screw-related complications. Wolf[49] used the OSI cannulated screw in 31 patients between 1984 and 1987. He found a 15 percent recurrence rate, which was also associated with some degree of trauma. He noted that six additional patients had their screws removed to relieve minor irritation symptoms resulting from the head of the screw. He has since abandoned the use of the screw because he thinks it does not address the ligament laxity that often results from anterior instability.

Suture Capsulorrhaphy

Attachment of the anterior labrum-ligamentous complex with sutures through an open approach has been well described with good success.[35] Classically, three holes are made in the anterior rim of the glenoid using specialized instruments. Sutures are passed through the holes and then through the edge of the lateral capsular flap and are tied to hold the lateral flap securely against the freshened glenoid rim. The remaining limbs of the sutures are then passed through the medial flap of the capsule and tied to one another.[5]

Although the efficacy of the Bankart repair in patients with anterior instability of the shoulder is widely accepted, the technical difficulty of reattaching the anterior part of the shoulder capsule to the lip of the glenoid fossa has limited its popularity.[5,21,35] One problematic part of the procedure is to reattach the torn anterior capsule and labrum to the bony rim. This can be technically difficult because the operative field is small and the glenoid rim is often blunted, both of which make it difficult to fashion the bony tunnels necessary to accept the sutures for capsular or labral repair.[35] Reider and Inglis[35] developed a technique using modified polypropylene (Prolene) pull-out sutures to perform the same function as the Bankart procedure more simply and efficiently. Size 1 Prolene sutures are passed through the glenoid in an anterior-to-posterior direction over Keith needles placed through the cut lateral edge of the capsule. The sutures are retrieved posteriorly and tied snugly over buttons padded with surgical felt on the back of the shoulder. Reider and Inglis[35] reported on 31 patients with an average 4-year 3-month follow-up with no recurrence of instability.

Morgan and Bodenstab[32] described an arthroscopic trans-

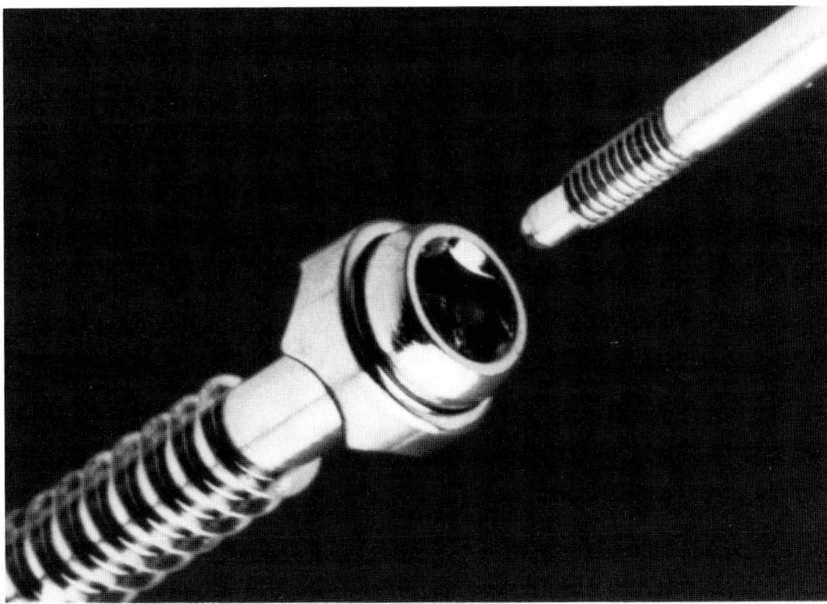

Figure 14-3. Cannulated screw and washer. (Courtesy of Smith & Nephew Dyonics, Inc., Andover, MA.)

glenoid absorbable suture technique based on the open technique described previously by Reider and Inglis.[35] Suture material is delivered through the separated soft tissue of the Bankart lesion and glenoid bone from anterior to posterior in a transglenoid fashion by using a modified Beath pin. Two separate passes of the pin (one superior and one inferior) are required to create a single large anterior horizontal mattress suture with transglenoid suture tails that exit the scapular neck and skin posteriorly through two separate posteroinferior skin portals (Fig. 14-4). The sutures are then brought out through the same posterior portal and tied over the thick fascia of the posterior one-third of the deltoid. All the 25 patients in their series (with 17-month average follow-up) were rated as excellent, with full active range of motion, and all were able to return to their preinjury level of activity, including contact and throwing sports. Grana et al[16] used this technique in 27 patients and reported discouraging results after an average 36-month follow-up. Ten patients were not compliant with the 3-week postoperative immobilization and had an 80 percent redislocation rate (8 of 10). The 17 remaining patients had four recurrences, a 23 percent redislocation rate. Failures were associated with younger patients, shorter immobilization periods after surgery, and patients with recurrent dislocations or who participated in contact sports.

Caspari et al[9] have devised a suture punch (Concept, Inc., Clearwater, FL), which is a standard basket forceps handle and shaft with modified jaws (Fig. 14-5). The inferior jaw consists of a cannulated needle, which passes back through the shaft of the punch and exits at the superior margin of the back handle. A feeder wheel is also located on the back of the handle, which facilitates the passing of the suture down the shaft and out the end of the needle. The upper jaw of the punch has a hole drilled through it so the end of the needle fits into the hole. The device is used by punching the labrum-ligamentous complex in the desired location for placing the suture. The needle passes through the labrum and into the hole in the upper jaw. The

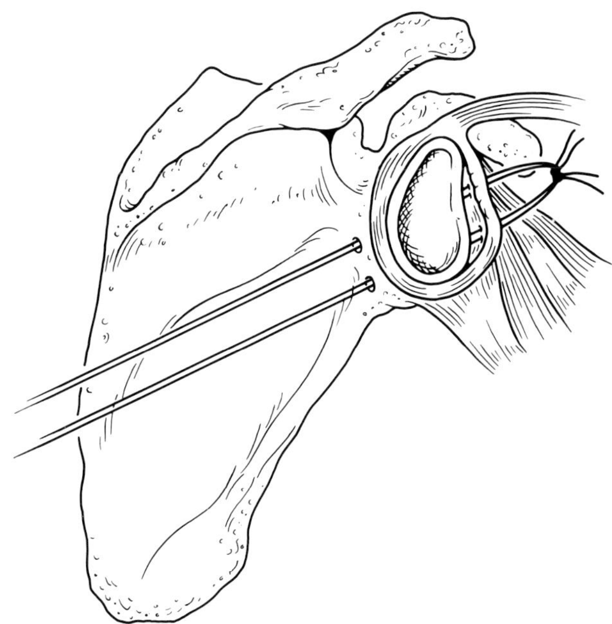

Figure 14-4. Arthroscopic transglenoid suture technique. (From Morgan and Bodenstab,[31] with permission.)

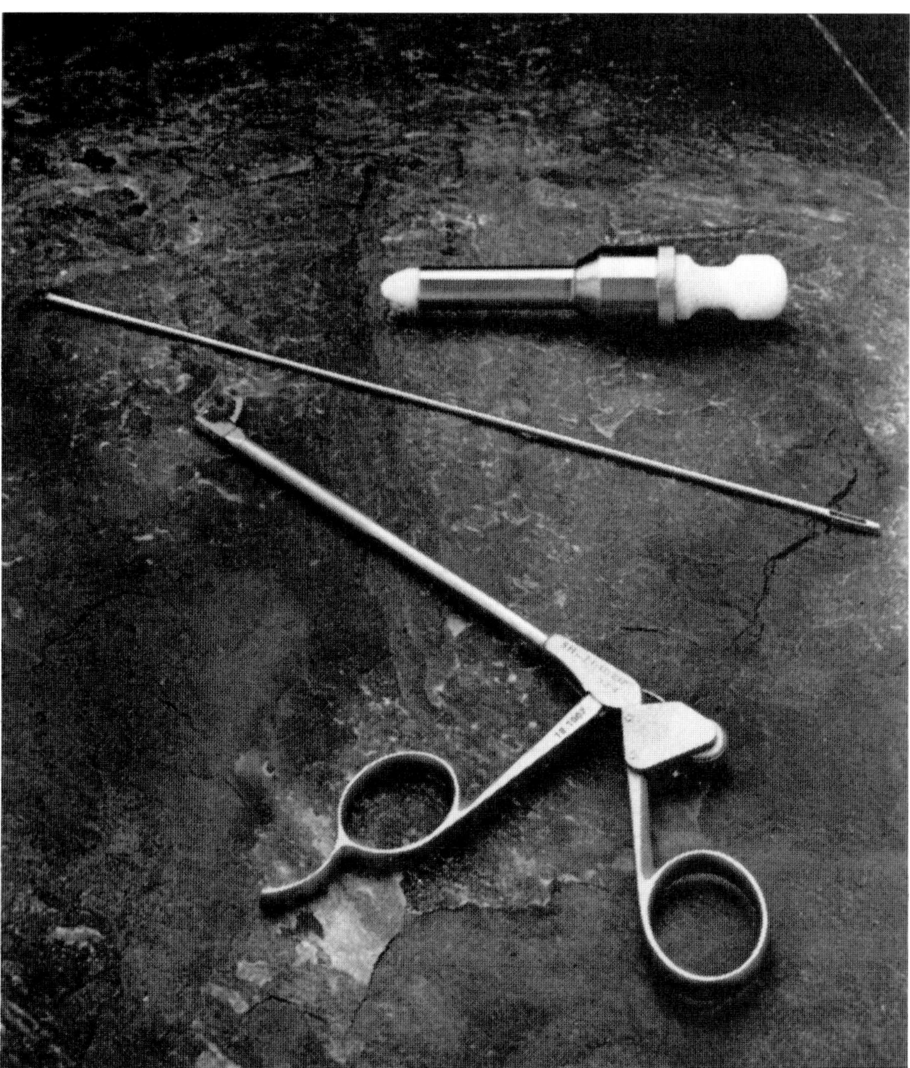

Figure 14-5. Suture punch system. (Courtesy of Concept, Inc., Clearwater, FL.)

feeder wheel is then used to pass the suture through the punch, out the end of the needle, and through the hole in the upper jaw. The punch is then opened, disengaging the needle from the labrum, and the entire punch is removed from the joint through the cannula, pulling both ends of the suture with it. The suture is thus passed through the labrum, and both ends of the suture can be tagged anteriorly on the outside of the joint. Once a sufficient number are passed, usually four to six sutures, a drill guide is placed on the edge of the glenoid, and a modified Beath pin is passed from anterior to posterior at a 45 degree angle to the flat surface of the glenoid. With the drill guide placed at the 2-o'clock position on the glenoid (for a right shoulder), the pin should be directed toward the 7:30 position on the posterior aspect of the glenoid (Fig. 14-6). This ensures a proper exit in the infraspinatus fossa both medial and inferior to the main trunk of the suprascapular nerve, which should arborize well lateral to the exit hole[6] (Fig. 14-7). Morgan and Bodenstab[32] disagree with this placement and recommend the angle of the pin should be approximately 30 degrees inferior to a perpendicular line in reference to the long axis of the glenoid articular surface and either parallel to, less than, or equal to 15-degrees medial to the glenoid articular surface in an anterior-to-posterior direction. Their dissection showed this angle to permit pins to exit the scapular neck posteriorly greater than 1 cm lateral to and greater than 0.5 to 2 cm inferior to the main trunk of the suprascapular nerve[32] (Fig. 14-8). Neither of these surgeons has reported suprascapular nerve complications in their present series. Caspari et al[9] reported on 49 shoulders on which this technique was used with an average follow-up of 33 months. There was a 4 percent redislocation rate (2 of 49) and a 4 percent resubluxation rate (2 of 49). Goldberg et al[15] used the Caspari transglenoid suture

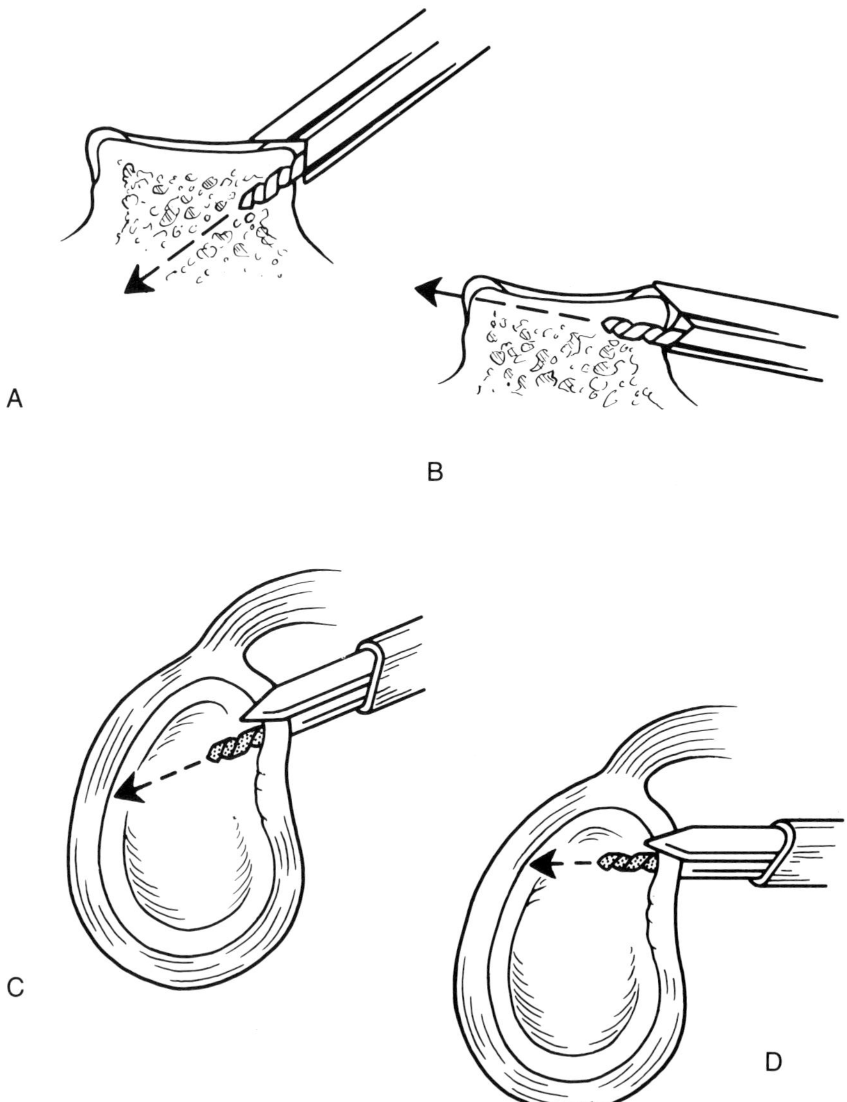

Figure 14-6. Positioning of guide pin through glenoid. (**A**) Correct positioning. (**B**) Incorrect positioning. (**C**) Correct positioning. Surgeon should aim for posteroinferior quadrant. (**D**) Incorrect positioning. (From Caspari RB, Cash JD, Meyers JF et al: Arthroscopic Bankart reconstruction. Presented at the AAOS annual meeting, New Orleans, 1990.)

technique on 38 shoulders for anterior capsulolabral repair and had a mean duration of follow-up of 36 months (24 to 54 months). There were no redislocations, but four shoulders (10 percent) had recurrence of instability. These authors found that return to contact sports did not result in an increase in recurrence and concluded that the technique showed great promise in appropriately selected patients. Weber[46] compared his results of the Caspari technique with those of open Bankart repairs. At a minimum 2-year follow-up, 3 of 11 of the arthroscopically repaired patients had sustained a recurrence of instability and none of the 24 open repairs had. At reoperation, the failures were all found to have recurrent Bankart lesions. The arthroscopically treated group had significantly greater external rotation, required less hospitalization and less pain medication, and were pain-free sooner than the open repair group.

One of the problems inherent to the techniques in which sutures are pulled through the glenoid and sutured over the fascia of the infraspinatus is the possible damage to the suprascapular nerve and other complications that can arise from drilling pins through the glenoid.[39] Maki[27] has described a technique that attempts to reduce the risk of damage to posterior neurovascular structures. A tissue grasper is used to secure the detached anteroinferior glenohumeral ligament with sutures. After passing at least two pins with sutures across the glenoid neck, the sutures are knotted posteriorly with multiple knots called Mulberry knots. The sutures are then drawn anteriorly back across

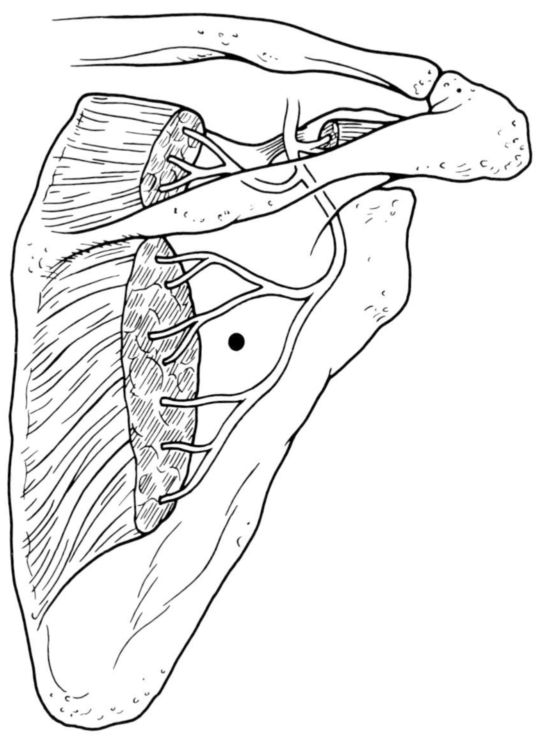

Figure 14-7. Arborization of suprascapular nerve with location of ideal exit hole well medial to main.

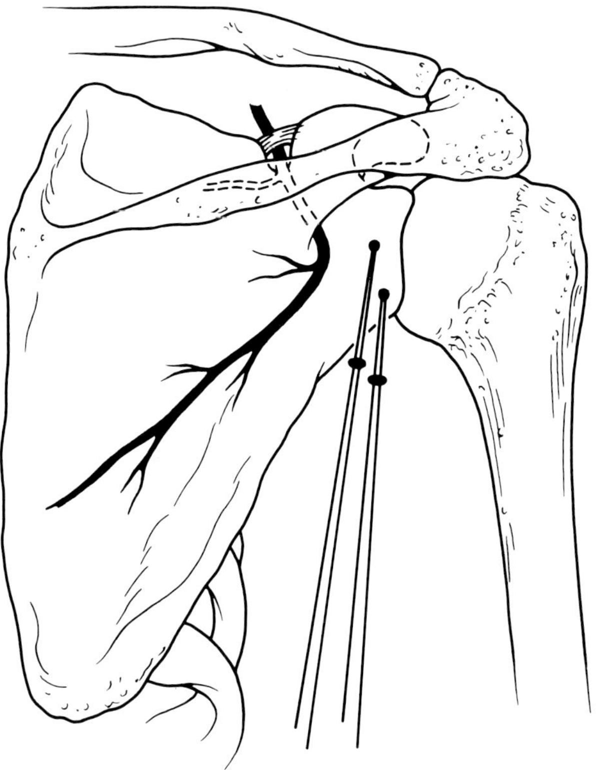

Figure 14-8. Posterior exit holes lateral to main trunk of suprascapular nerve. (From Morgan and Bodenstab,[31] with permission.)

the glenoid neck to secure the knots against the posterior glenoid. This provides support fixation to sutures tied over soft tissue and avoids entrapping muscles or nerves posteriorly. The suture can then be tied anteriorly through a cannula using a knot pusher (Fig. 14-9). An alternative method involves passage of the sutures back across the glenoid in an M-shaped fashion followed by tying the final knots posteriorly along the glenoid neck. Maki[28] reported on 15 patients who underwent this procedure and noted one failure. All the successful patients (93 percent) were able to resume their previous activity levels. Morgan[31] reported on 175 shoulders on patients who underwent this repair with a 1-to-7-year follow-up and noted 95 percent excellent results and a 5 percent failure rate with recurrent instability. Eighty-seven percent of his patients achieved full range of motion, and 13 percent lacked 5 to 10 degrees of terminal external rotation. He also discovered that most failures occurred in collision athletes, and when this group was analyzed separately, they had a 16.6 percent recurrence rate versus 1.5 percent rate in throwers and noncollision athletes.

In an effort to more closely mimic the desirable characteristics of the open Bankart repair, without the theoretical dangers of transglenoid drilling, anterior suturing methods have been developed.[41] Wolf[49] and Feldman and coworkers[14] have described techniques for arthroscopic reattachment of capsular and ligamentous tissue to bone using the Mitek suture anchor system (Mitek, Inc., Norwood, MA). The first-generation device consisted of a small wire arc made of nickel titanium alloy attached to a titanium body. Recently, a second-generation suture anchor has been developed that uses a double-armed device with even stronger fixation strength than the original anchor (Fig. 14-10). Wolf's[49] technique involves arthroscopically drilling three holes, each spaced as far as possible from each other, on the anterior glenoid rim. It is critical that the holes are made at the anterior border of the cartilaginous surface and not medial on the scapular neck. The angle of the drill bit should be approximately 15 to 20 degrees to the plane of the glenoid surface. This drill hole placement permits that surgeon to bring the inferior glenohumeral labrum-ligamentous complex onto the glenoid rim and create a buttress anteriorly.[49] A suture hook (Concept Corp., Largo, FL) is placed through the most inferior portion of the detached glenohumeral labrum-ligamentous complex. This suturing technique permits approximately 0.5 to 1.0 cm of soft tissue plication, which compensates for any labrum-ligamentous injury or redundancy that may exist. A suture anchor is then slid down the inside limb of the suture to enter the first drill hole. The GII Mitek anchor lets a size 0 or 1 PDS suture slide with the anchor and within its drill hole. The loop is closed using a slipknot that is tied outside the cannula, tightened outside the cannula, and slid down the cannula with a knot pusher (Arthrex Corp., Naples, FL).

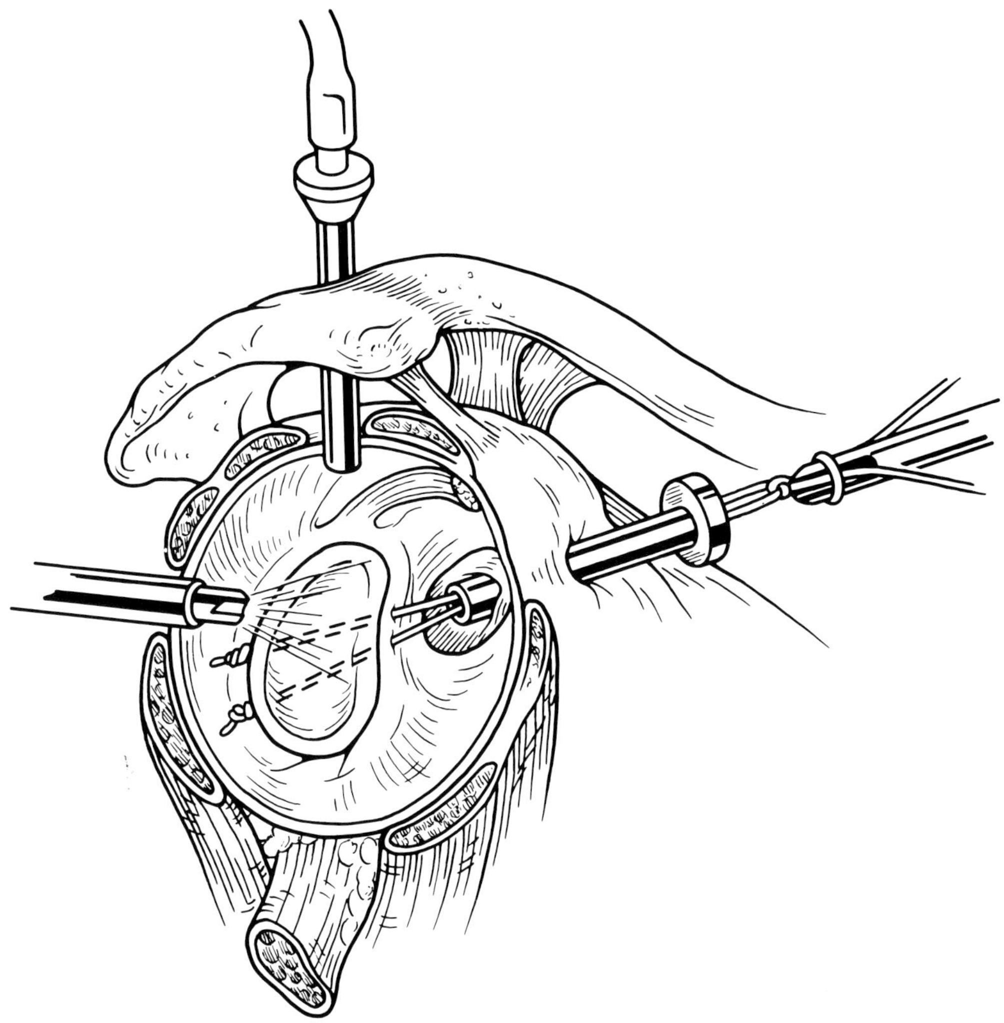

Figure 14-9. Mulberry knot technique. Knot pusher securing avulsed anterior labrum. (From Maki N: Scientific exhibit. Presented at the AAOS annual meeting, New Orleans, 1990.)

This closes the loop and approximates the inferior glenohumeral labrumligamentous complex to the anterior glenoid rim (Fig. 14-11). In general, three anchors are inserted, but two may be sufficient in some procedures. An immobilizer is worn for 3 weeks, at which time motion exercises are begun. Preliminary results in 50 patients since September 1989 have shown no complications and only one recurrence.[49] Feldman et al,[14] using a similar procedure in a multicenter study reported in 24 patients with an average follow-up of 10 months, had no recurrences, with a mean Bankart score of 93. Snyder and Strafford[41] described a similar procedure using a suture passing device called a shuttle relay (Linvatec Corp., Largo, FL). Several companies are developing absorbable suture anchors that are embedded into the bone in the same fashion as a Mitek metal anchor, yet avoid permanent metallic bony implants along with their concomitant disadvantages.

Bioabsorbable Implants

The use of metallic implants around the shoulder joint has been associated with loosening, migration, and breakage of the implant. Zuckerman and Matsen[52] analyzed a series of 37 patients with complications related to the use of these implants. It is thought that along with incorrect positioning or fixation of the implant at the time of the operation, the great mobility of the glenohumeral joint jeopardizes these implants and predisposes them to fatigue, failure, loosening, and migration.[42]

Bioabsorbable implants have therefore been developed as an attempt to alleviate its well-known possible complication of metallic shoulder implants. Speer and Warren[42] have described the use of a cannulated tack (Suretac, Acufex Microsurgical, Mansfield, MA) that is molded from a synthetic copolymer (polyglyconate) that is identical to that

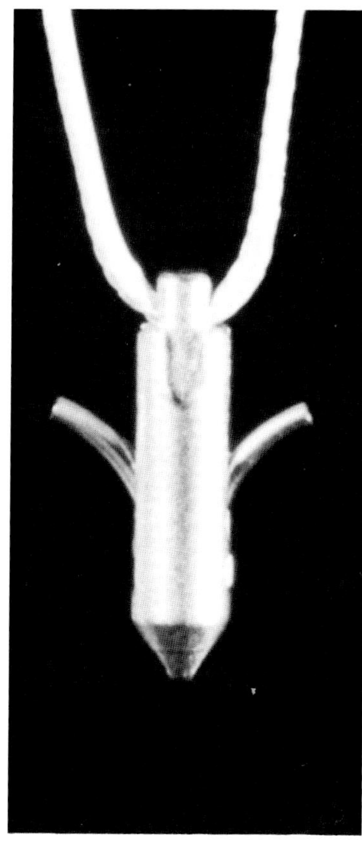

Figure 14-10. Mitek GII anchor. (Courtesy of Mitek, Norwood, MA.)

used in Maxon sutures (Davis and Geck, Danbury, CT). Ribs on the shaft of the tack increase its pull-out strength, and a broad flat head allows the tack to capture soft tissue and hold it to bone while the implant is being inserted (Fig. 14-12). The device is degraded by hydrolysis alone, and studies by the manufacturer show mean side-bending strength (kg) was 23.6 at insertion, 11.6 at 2 weeks, 1.2 at 3 weeks, and 0.0 at 4 weeks with implant in vivo strength loss of 4.13 kg/week. Histologic evaluation showed a very benign response within the bone tunnel environment and no evidence of a foreign body response.

This bioabsorbable implant has been assessed in two clinical trials in which it was used arthroscopically to repair a Bankart lesion in the shoulder. After glenoid bony rim abrasion, a cannulated drill placed through the labral lesion to be advanced creates the bone tunnel into which the implant is to be inserted. A wire fits through this drill to allow the wire to remain in bone when the drill is withdrawn. The bioabsorbable tack is implanted over the wire by means of a cannulated impactor, forcing the soft tissue against the abraded anterior glenoid bony rim (Fig. 14-13). Resch et al[36] reported on 18 patients who were treated with arthroscopic Bankart repair with this implant. An essential precondition for his application of this technique was that the labrum had not fully degenerated, which allowed refixation of the capsule by the labrum itself. His follow-up average was only 11 months (range, 4 to 18), but only 1 of the 18 patients (5.6 percent) had experienced

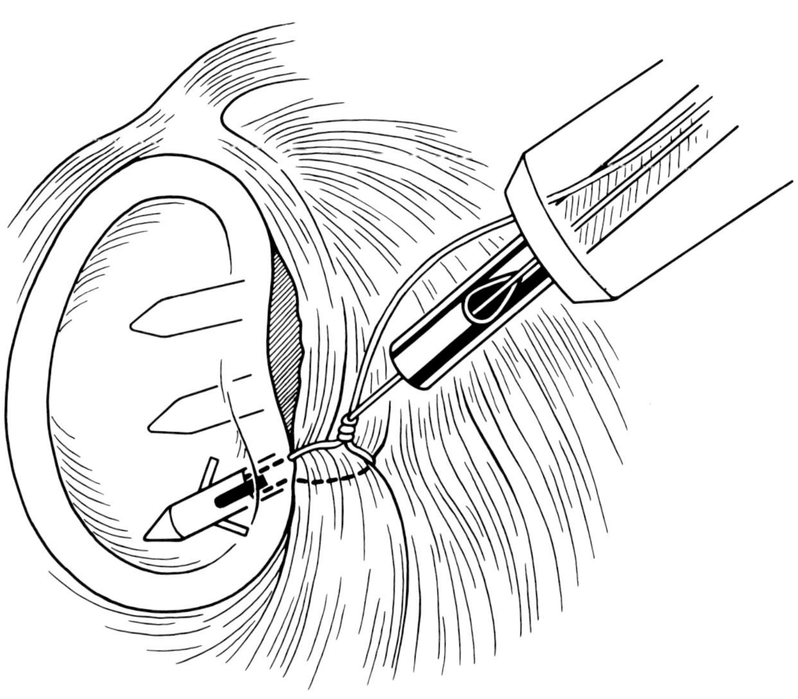

Figure 14-11. Knot pusher tightening noose around the ligament labral complex and reapproximating it to the glenoid cavity.

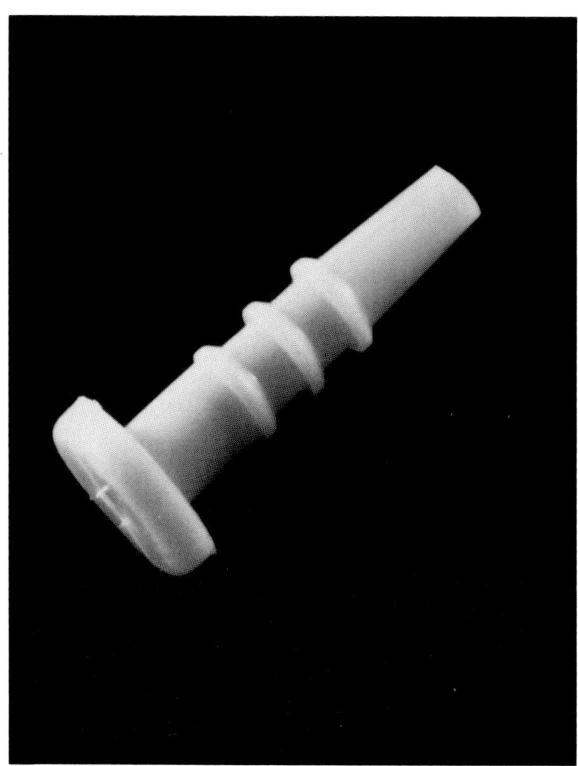

Figure 14-12. Suretac (Acufex Microsurgical, Mansfield, MA).

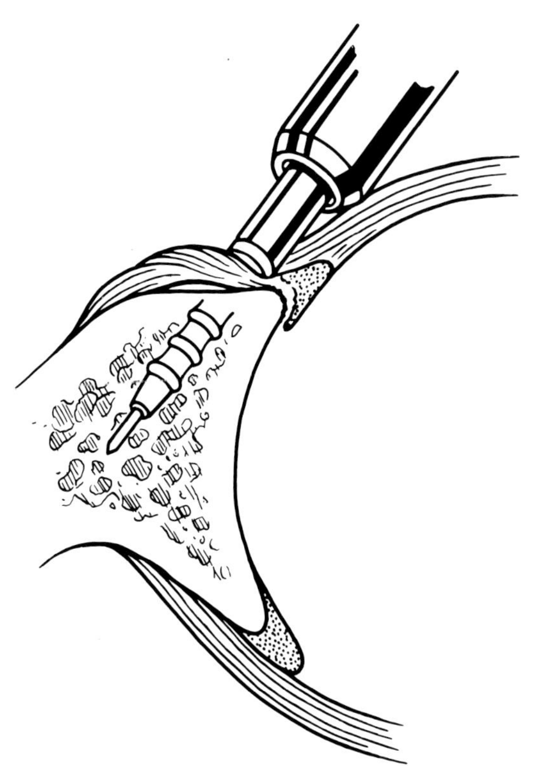

Figure 14-13. Suretac (Acufex Microsurgical, Mansfield, MA) impacting labral ligamentous complex to anterior glenoid rim.

resubluxation or redislocation. Fourteen of the 18 patients had regained full motion. Warner et al[44] have reported on their first 20 patients who were treated with arthroscopic Bankart repair with this implant. These patients had a minimum of 2 years follow-up examination. Postoperative care mandated shoulder immobilization in a sling for 4 weeks. With a mean 32-month follow-up, the recurrence rate was 10 percent (2 of 20). Both recurrences were subluxations that occurred primarily with throwing activities in the only two patients in the series not to have a true Bankart lesion noted at the time of arthroscopy. The mean loss of external rotation in the 10 patients in which it was measured at the time of last follow-up was 3 degrees (0 to 10 degrees) with the arm in full adduction and 7 degrees (range, 0 to 10 degrees) with the arm elevated to 90 degrees in the scapular plane. No complications were associated with the surgery.[44]

Altchek[2] reported a 13 percent recurrence rate in his first 50 patients with the use of the bioabsorbable tack. He further limited indications for the procedure to include only those with discrete labral detachments and a well-defined glenohumeral ligament lateral to the labrum. A subsequent group of 100 patients showed a recurrence rate of 7 percent.

My (JSA) Preferred Technique

As in open repair, surgery begins with examination under anesthesia. After examination of the supine patient, the lateral decubitus position uses an axillary roll and beanbag support. The sitting beach chair position with shoulder over the edge of the table is an alternative. With the patient lying sideways, additional tape is used to maintain the torso in a slightly posterior tilted position so that the glenoid is level with the floor. The shoulder is abducted less than 20 degrees and is often supported with minimum traction (i.e., 5 lb). An additional lateral sling or an assistant can provide a lateral distraction force during the surgical procedure.

Diagnostic arthroscopy identifies the pathology. Labral detachments, gross capsular tears and redundancy, and a Hill-Sach's lesion may confirm the diagnosis. Confusing cases of suspected occult instability and impingement need additional examination of the subacromial bursa. Intraoperative demonstration of excessive translation along with labral changes should precede capsular stabilization.

The most common pathology identified is a large labral detachment with intact capsular ligament as described by Bankart. There may be smaller labral detachments with increased capsular stretching and tears or an intact blunted labrum with chronic evidence of capsular stretching and redundancy. Rarely, a lateral capsular injury is noted just superior to the subscapularis. The anterior labrum may reattach to the glenoid in a more medial position reducing its ability to buttress the head.[33] Satisfactory stabilization needs to address whatever pathologies are encountered to minimize the recurrence rate.[1]

As previously discussed, there are multiple arthroscopic techniques to reattach the capsule and labrum to the glenoid rim. Surgeons may use suture or absorbable implants (tacks or staples). Caspari[7] introduced a technique to grasp labrum and capsular ligaments with a suture punch (Linvatec, Largo, FL) and pass transglenoid sutures to tie over infraspinatus fascia. Morgan[31] used a transglenoid technique to create a mattress suture over the anterior labrum. Wolf et al[49] popularized a technique using Mitek GII suture anchors to restore the labrum without transglenoid suture passage. Snyder and Strafford[41] have introduced a shuttle relay (Linvatec, Largo, FL), which allows multifilament nonabsorbable sutures to be used instead of monofilament absorbable sutures. Many new instruments are becoming available to pass sutures precisely through the detached Bankart lesion to anatomically correct it. We prefer suture anchors to anatomically restore the shoulder and avoid infraspinatus and possibly suprascapular nerve injury. Nonabsorbable sutures may prove advantageous to allow for prolonged support during early rehabilitation.

Capsular tensioning remains the most challenging aspect to restore anatomy.[1] While visualizing from a posterior portal, two anterior portals lateral to the coracoid and through the rotator cuff interval can be developed. The more inferior portal is adjacent to the superior edge of the subscapularis. The more superior portal is within the rotator cuff interval adjacent to the long head of the biceps entering inferior and lateral to the acromioclavicular joint. The glenoid is abraded and decorticated along the anterior neck (Fig. 14-14). A secure stitch in the superior border at the inferior glenohumeral ligament and labrum allows for superior mobilization and protection throughout the procedure.

Drill holes adjacent to the articular surface can be filled with buried suture anchors containing nonabsorbable sutures (Ethibond or Tevdek #2). Currently, mini-Revo screws (Linvatec, Largo, FL) and Mitek GII anchors (Norwood, MA) are used. The sutures are passed through the labrum and capsule using the shuttle relay or blitz suture retriever (Linvatec, Largo, FL) (Figs. 14-15 and 14-16). After placement of sutures through the labrum and capsule (Fig. 14-16), a knot teaser or loop handle knot pusher (Linvatec, Largo, FL) is used to place five throws of the suture to create secure knots so that the labrum and capsule are reapproximated to the bone (Figs. 14-17 and 14-18). In the future, absorbable implants combined with sutures might have a role in anchoring the labrum and avoiding the risk of a permanent implant near the joint. As the traction is reduced and the sutures are tied, the humeral head reduction and decreased joint volume can be arthroscopically visualized. Once the sutures are tied, the repair is probed and tested for security. The traction is released, and the shoulder is externally rotated 30 degrees while visualizing from the anterior portal. The postoperative program can be adjusted based on the security of the repair.

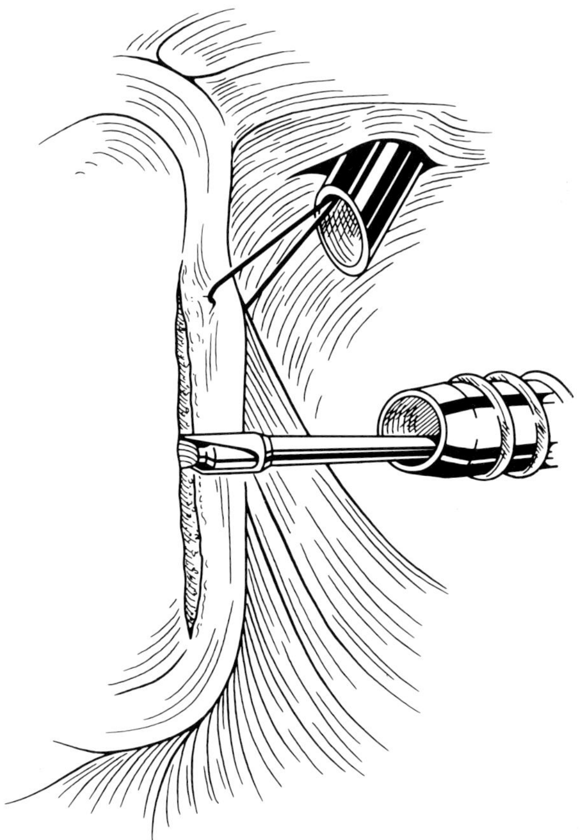

Figure 14-14. With the arthroscope visualizing from the posterior portal, two anterior portals are developed within the rotator interval. A suture placed through the labrum and superior edge of the inferior glenohumeral ligament places upward traction through the anterosuperior portal adjacent to the biceps tendon. A burr decorticates the anterior glenoid surface through the anteroinferior portal.

REHABILITATION

Regardless of which arthroscopic anterior shoulder stabilization technique is used, the arm should be placed to the side and internally rotated when the anterior labrum-ligamentous complex is fixed to the anterior glenoid. Once the fixation is completed, care should be taken to keep the arm in this position with the use of an arm sling or immoblizer to prevent loss of fixation of any repaired tissue. It would be distressing to see a patient awake from one of these procedures in a postanesthetic haze and place the arm in an abducted and externally rotated position.[6]

Most postoperative protocols stress the need to hold the arm in this adducted and internally rotated position for 3

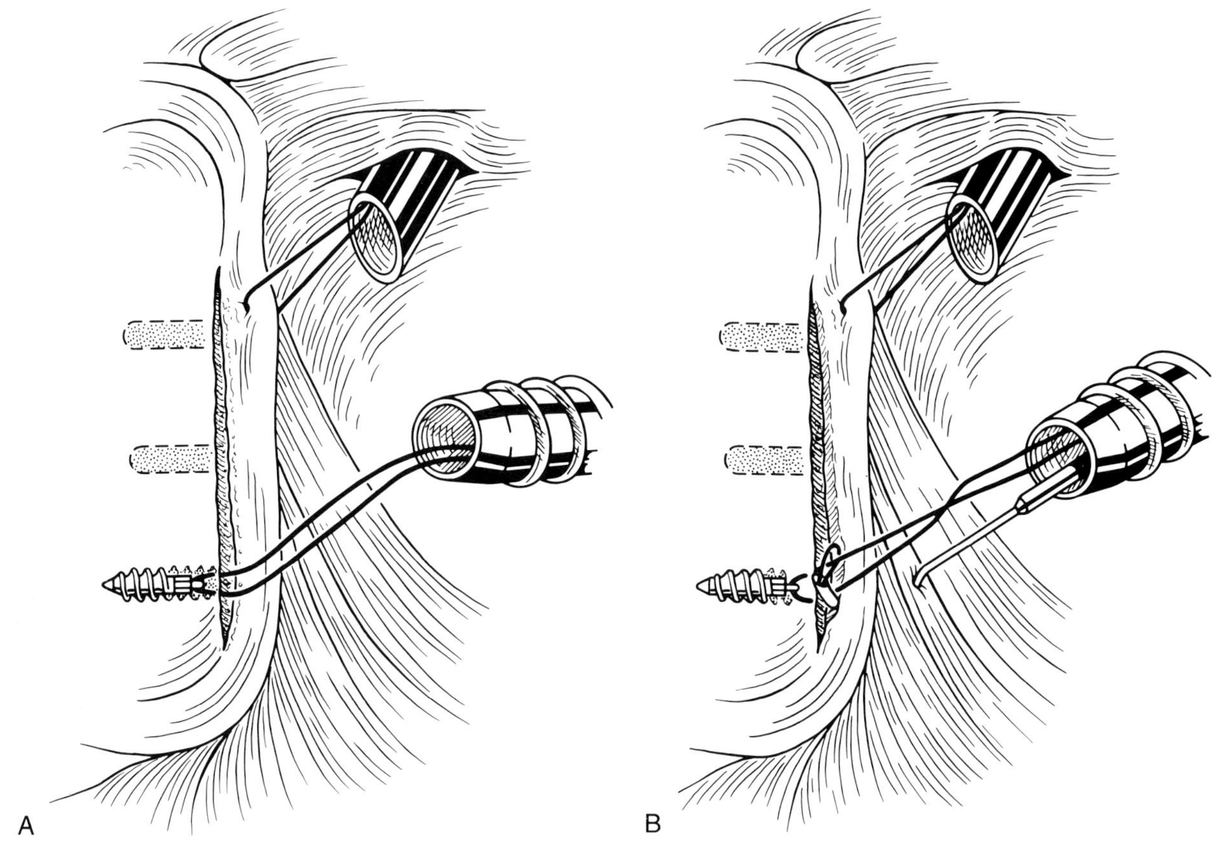

Figure 14-15. (**A**) A mini-Revo screw (Linvatec) with size 2 nonabsorbable suture is placed in a previously drilled hole at the inferior edge of the detached labrum. (**B**) While retracting the superior stitch, the anchor sutures are retrieved through the labrum and capsule with a blitz (Linvatec).

to 4 weeks in a sling or immobilizer.[3,13,16,24] In his first 24 months of stapling glenohumeral ligaments for traumatic dislocations, Johnson experienced one repeat dislocation among 19 patients. After April 1984, he reduced the immobilization time from 3 to 2 weeks to decrease morbidity and accelerate the return of range of motion. In the next 8 months, he saw seven repeat dislocations. He subsequently returned to a 3.5- to 4.5-week postoperative immobilization time and reports improved results (L. Johnson, personal communication, 1990). Of the 10 patients in Grana's study, who admitted removal of the immobilizer after 1 week, 8 rated as failed.[6]

Some think that the key to arthroscopic stabilization is not initial firm fixation of the soft tissue to bone but approximation of abraded tissues (apposing anterior glenoid neck and labrum) for enough time to allow soft tissue adherence to the glenoid. Eisenberg et al[13] reported on a series of 40 patients (18 recurrent dislocators, 17 recurrent subluxers, and 5 with one time dislocations that prompted chronic subluxations) in whom he debrided the capsuloligamentous complex down to bleeding tissue and decorticated the neck of the scapula, allowing the soft tissue and bone to heal against each other without initial fixation. The authors prescribed strict immobilization in a sling for 4 weeks, and on follow-up evaluation at 6 months to 5 years, 34 of 40 rated in the excellent range on the Rowe scale, with 2 good, 3 fair, and 1 poor. The average Rowe score for all patients was 93 of a possible 100. These findings certainly point out the possibility that the most important aspects to obtaining good results with these arthroscopic stabilization procedures may be both in the preparation/debridement and in the immobilization phase of the rehabilitation. Thus, the first phase of rehabilitation requires the operated shoulder be placed at least 3, preferably 4, weeks in an arm sling. Elbow and wrist range of motion as well as isometric internal and external rotation exercises can be instituted in the early postoperative period and should be performed with the arm to the side and internally rotated against the body.

The other important goal of the operation other than stabilization is return to function. A good or excellent result requires near-normal motion and strength. The second phase of rehabilitation should progress first through a passive, then active assisted, then active range of motion pro-

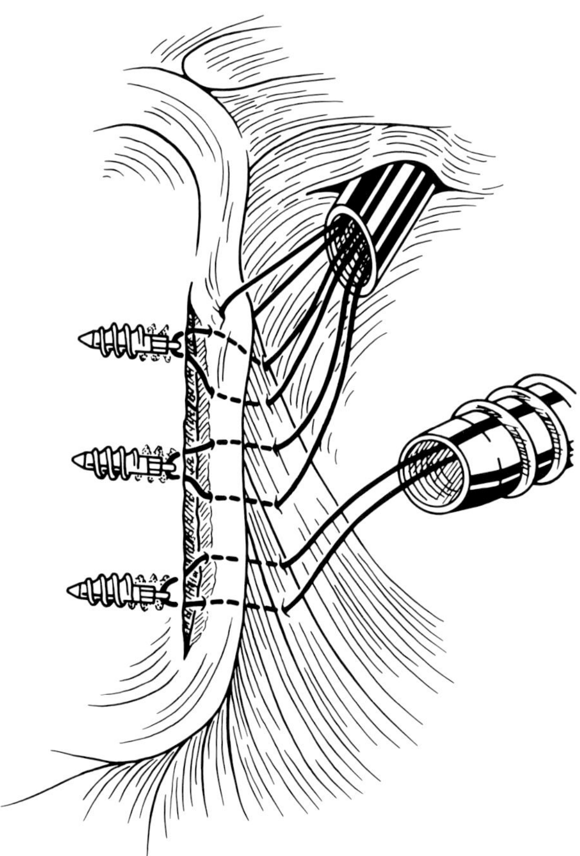

Figure 14-16. Suture anchors are placed along the anterior edge with the sutures drawn through the labrum and capsule ligaments.

gram to achieve near-normal range of motion at the 6- to 8-week postoperative time. We have found that it is especially helpful to start the range of motion passively in the supine position, thus negating the effects of gravity. Once near full passive motion is achieved supine, the patient can be moved to a reclining position and then to an upright position. Once upright full passive motion is achieved, active motion is instituted, again starting in a supine position and advancing as previously described to the upright position.[6]

The third phase of rehabilitation involves strengthening and stretching. Strengthening is usually performed with resistance exercises starting at approximately 6 weeks postoperatively, with terminal stretching following soon after in an attempt to obtain maximum motion. Sport-specific training begins when near-normal strength and motion are obtained. Four to six months are usually required for patients to start any gradual build-up to overhead sporting activities, and 6 to 9 months are required for consideration to return to unrestricted activity or contact sports.[3,15,29]

ARTHROSCOPY FOR ACUTE INITIAL DISLOCATIONS

Currently, arthroscopic reconstruction of the shoulder is most commonly used in the orthopaedic community for recurrent anterior shoulder dislocation. Acute initial dislocations are usually treated with closed reduction and either immobilization or early strengthening programs. There is, however, a high rate of redislocation of the glenohumeral joint after initial dislocations, especially in young patients.[19] Rowe[37] reported a 94 percent recurrence rate in patients younger than the age of 20 years at the time of initial dislocation and a 74 percent rate in a 20- to 40-year-old age group with follow-up of 1 to 10 years. Hovelius et al[22] reported no recurrences in 32 patients who had a greater tuberosity fracture in association with a dislocation, but there was a 50 percent instance of recurrence in those patients 22 years of age or younger. Baker and associates[4] performed arthroscopy on 45 shoulders after acute initial anterior dislocations and found three distinct types of lesions. Group 1 (six shoulders) had capsular tears with no labral lesions. These shoulders were stable under anesthesia. Group 2 (11 shoulders) had capsular tears and partial labral detachments. These shoulders were mildly unstable. Group 3 (28 shoulders) had capsular tears with complete labral detachments and were grossly unstable during examination under anesthesia. Hovelius et al[22] reported a 55 percent rate of radiologic impression fractures in the posterior part of the humeral head with initial anterior dislocations.

Although age is thought to be the principal factor in the development of a chronic instability, it appears that athletic participation also plays a significant if not predominant role. Simonet and Cofield,[40] in comparing two groups, noted an 82 percent recurrence rate among athletes and 30 percent recurrence rate among nonathletes after an initial anterior dislocation of the shoulder. At the U.S. Military Academy, Wheeler et al[47] compared conventional nonoperative treatment with early arthroscopic intervention. At arthroscopy, either staple fixation or anterior glenoid abrasion was performed. Except for the surgery, both groups were managed in a similar fashion. Recurrent dislocation in those treated with immobilization and rehabilitation was 92 percent versus 22 percent in those who underwent arthroscopic surgery before their immobilization and rehabilitation. Uribe and Hechtman[42] carried out arthroscopic stabilization of acute initial traumatic anterior dislocations in 11 young athletes using the Caspari[9] suture technique. Follow-up averaged 24.5 months (range, 18 to 38). There were nine excellent and two good results, with one patient having a transient episode of instability associated with trauma but no further sequelae. They point out that the secondary changes seen in recurrent dislocations including stretching of the anterior capsular structures, erosion of the

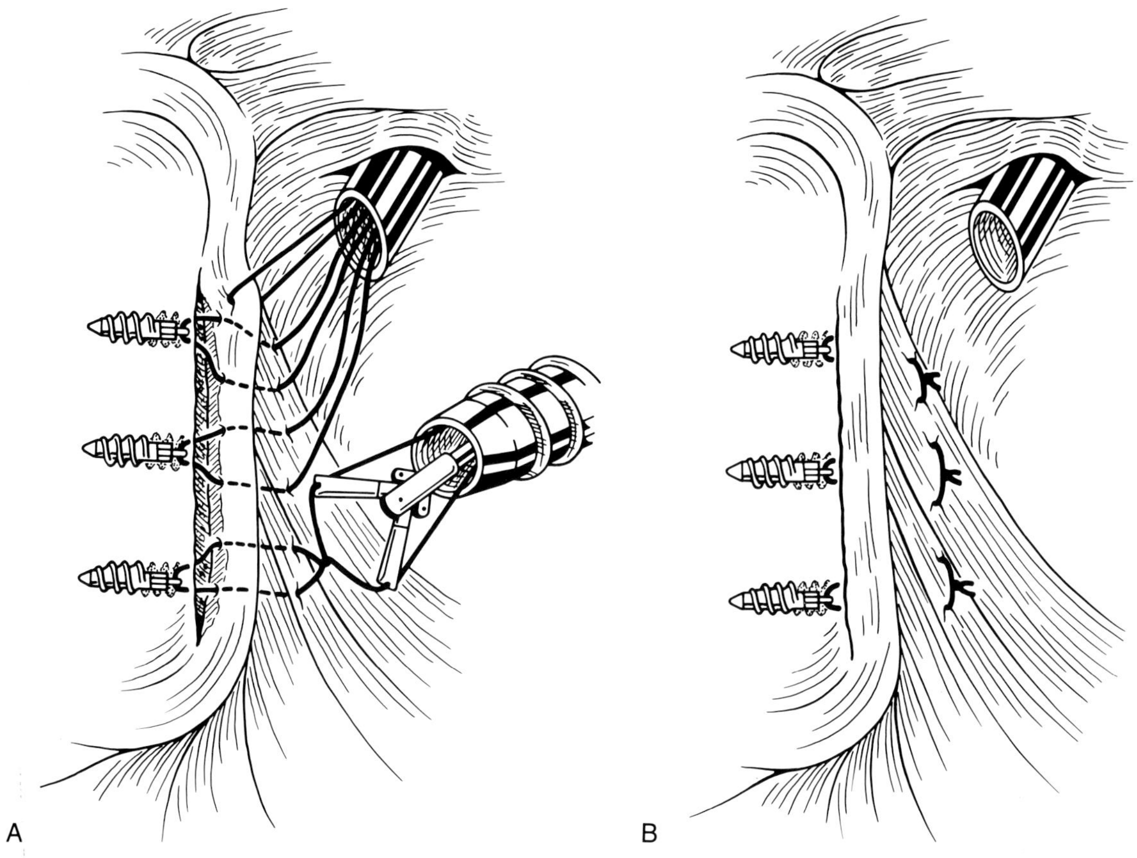

Figure 14-17. (**A**) Mattress sutures are tied with a "suture teaser" (Linvatec). (**B**) Four throws secure the capsule and labrum to the glenoid. The superior traction stitch is removed once proper tension has been established.

anterior glenoid rim, and enlargement of the posterolateral humeral head defect are not seen. No additional time is lost from athletic participation after repair, when compared with those who were managed in the traditional nonoperative manner. There appears to be a subgroup of patients in whom an initial episode of shoulder dislocation should be treated just like an initial episode of knee dislocation, with an offer being made for surgical stabilization if a lower rate of redislocation is desired. Certainly, more studies need to be performed before it can become common practice to offer surgical stabilization for initial anterior dislocation of the glenohumeral joint. However, from the currently available literature, the most appropriate candidate would be an athlete younger than 20 years of age who is found to be markedly unstable under anesthesia and to have a complete labral detachment on arthroscopic evaluation.

SUMMARY

The goal of surgical stabilization of the unstable glenohumeral joint is to produce a stable yet mobile joint that can return to preinjury function. Open surgical procedures (in particular, the Bankart procedure) have evolved to a point at which stability and mobility are being attained with a low complication rate, but the rate of return to preinjury function, particularly overhead athletes, has not been ideal. Arthroscopic stabilization is an attractive alternative to open procedures, particularly in those patients who have a history of traumatic and unidirectional recurrent dislocation with a labral detachment. A variety of techniques for reattaching a detached labrum-ligamentous complex has been described. Longer follow-up is needed to assess the efficacy of these procedures fully, particularly in the light of the good results now being obtained with the open Bankart procedure. Longer-term studies have shown a higher rate of recurrence of dislocation with the arthroscopic technique[15,26,42] than with the open technique.[22,38]

There appears to be no universal procedure that will allow the surgeon to best treat all anterior shoulder instabilities the same way. The systematic approach based on the best techniques and studies currently available might produce the following guidelines: (1) arthroscopic stabilization for anterior shoulder instability has the best chance

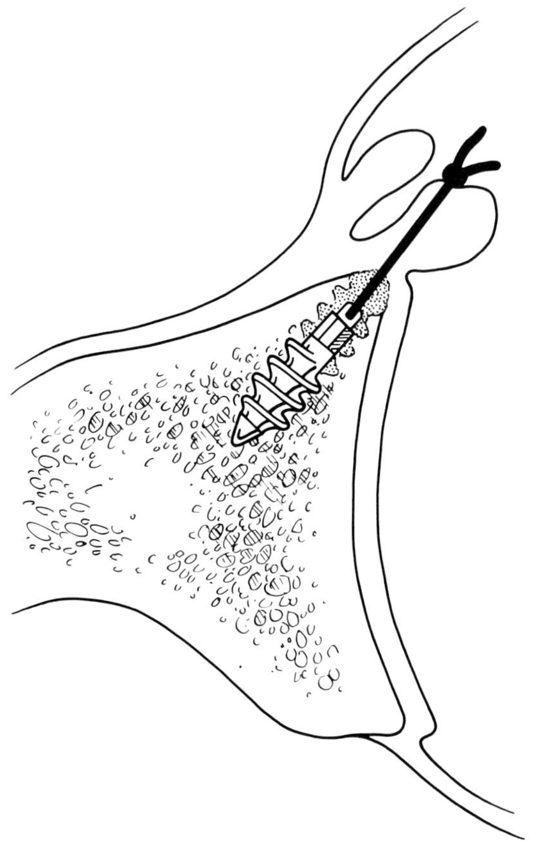

Figure 14-18. Profile of the entrance angle of the mini-Revo anchor and suture at the articular edge of the glenoid.

for success in traumatic unidirectional instability; (2) the surgeon should be prepared to perform a variety of stabilization procedures depending on the type of anterior capsular lesion seen at the time of surgery. The bioabsorbable tack and suture anchor methods have the best chance for success when a Bankart lesion with capsule attached to the labrum is present. When chronic interstitial tearing of the anterior structures, a patulous anterior capsule, or bucket handle labral tears exist, a pull-through suture technique or suture anchor capsulorrhaphy may afford the best results of the arthroscopic methods[9,32]; (3) if inadequate capsular plication to the glenoid is seen at the time of surgery, then conversion to an open technique can and should be considered; (4) adequate debridement of fibrotic soft tissue and abrasion of the anterior glenoid neck is essential for success with any of these techniques described; (5) 3 to 4 weeks of postoperative immobilization may improve results; and (6) young athletes with initial traumatic anterior dislocation are at an extremely high risk for recurrence of dislocation. With this knowledge, a better informed decision can be made regarding advisability of an arthroscopic repair of these acute injuries.

Arthroscopic stabilization offers the potential advantages of shorter hospitalization, less traumatic treatment of the soft tissues, more thorough examination of the glenohumeral joint and subacromial bursa, and greater cosmesis compared with open procedures. It could also provide a means by which selective stabilization of those initial anterior dislocations that might be prone to recurrence could be performed. Long-term follow-up and randomized studies comparing open and arthroscopic techniques are needed to further define the best role of arthroscopic shoulder stabilization and to determine which of the several techniques described provides the best results with the fewest complications.

REFERENCES

1. Abrams JS: Arthroscopic shoulder stabilization for recurrent subluxation and dislocation. J Shoulder Elbow Surg 2:25, 1993
2. Altchek DW: Presented at AANA Meeting, Palm Desert, CA, 1993
3. Altchek DW, Skyhar MJ, Warren RF: Shoulder arthroscopy for shoulder instability. p. 187. Course Lec 38, 1989
4. Baker CL, Uribe JW, Whitman L: Arthroscopic evaluation of acute initial anterior shoulder dislocations. Am J Sports Med 18:25, 1990
5. Berg EE, Ellison AE: The inside-out Bankart procedure. Am J Sports Med 18:129, 1990
6. Cash JD: Recent advances and perspectives on arthroscopic stabilization of the shoulder Clin Sports Med 10:871, 1991
7. Caspari RB: Arthroscopic stabilization for shoulder instability. p. 57. In Durr L (ed): Operative Techniques in Shoulder Surgery. Aspen Publishers, Gaithersburg, MD, 1991
8. Caspari RB, Cash JD, Meyers JF et al: Arthroscopic Bankart reconstruction. Presented at the AAOS annual meeting, New Orleans, 1990
9. Caspari RB, Savoie FH, Myers JP et al: Arthroscopic management of the unstable shoulder. Presented to the Annual Meeting of the American Academy of Orthopaedic Surgeons, Las Vegas, 1988
10. Cofield RH, Kavanagh BF, Frassica FJ: Anterior shoulder instability. p. 210. Course Lec 34, 1985
11. Detrisac DA, Johnson LL: Arthroscopic shoulder capsulorrhaphy using metal staples. Orthop Clin North Am 24:71, 1993
12. duToit GT, Roux D: Recurrent dislocations of the shoulder: a 24-year study of the Johannesburg stapling operation. J Bone Joint Surg [Am] 38:1, 1956
13. Eisenberg JH, Redler MR, Belkin SC: Arthroscopic stabilization of the shoulder without internal hardware. Presented to the Arthroscopy Association of North American Annual meeting, Palm Desert, CA, 1993
14. Feldman A, Harner C, Fu FH: Arthroscopic repair of glenoid capsular labral tears using the Mitek anchor. Presented to the Annual Meeting of the Academy of Orthopaedic Surgeons, New Orleans, 1990
15. Goldberg BJ, Nirschl RP, McConnell JP, Pettrone FA: Ar-

throscopic transglenoid suture capsulolabral repairs: preliminary results. Am J Sport Med 21:656, 1993
16. Grana WA, Buckley PD, Yates CK: Arthroscopic Bankart suture repair. Am J Sports Med 21:348, 1993
17. Gross RM: Arthroscopic shoulder capsulorrhaphy: does it work? Am J Sports Med 17:495, 1989
18. Hawkins RJ: Arthroscopic staple repair for shoulder instability—a retrospective study of 50 cases. Arthroscopy 5:122, 1989
19. Henry JH, Genung JA: Natural history of glenohumeral dislocation—revisited. Am J Sports Med 10:135, 1982
20. Hill JA, Lombardo SJ, Kerlan RK et al: The modified Bristow-Helfet procedure for recurrent anterior subluxation and dislocation. Am J Sports Med 9:283, 1981
21. Hovelius L, Eriksson K, Fredin H et al: Recurrences after initial dislocation of the shoulder: results of a prospective study of treatment. J Bone Joint Surg [Am] 65:343, 1983
22. Hovelius L, Thorling GJ, Fredin H: Recurrent anterior dislocation of the shoulder: results after the Bankart and Putti-Platt operations. J Bone Joint Surg [Am] 61:566 1979
23. Johnson L: Instrument Maker's educational film. Instrument Maker Co., Okemos, MI
24. Lane JC, Sachs RA, Riehl B: Arthroscopic staple capsulorrhaphy: a long term followup. Arthroscopy 9:190, 1993
25. Lombardo SJ, Kerlan RK, Jobe FW et al: The modified Bristow procedure for recurrent dislocation of the shoulder. J Bone Joint Surg [Am] 58:256, 1976
26. Maki NJ: Arthroscopic stabilization for recurrent shoulder instability. Presented at the Annual Meeting of the Academy of Orthopaedic Surgeons, Las Vegas, 1989
27. Maki NJ: Bankart repair: an arthroscopic technique. Presented to the Annual Meeting of the American Academy of Orthopaedic Surgeons, New Orleans, 1990
28. Maki NJ: Arthroscopic stabilization: suture technique. Operative Tech Orthop 1:180, 1991
29. Matthews LS: Results of arthroscopic capsulorrhaphy of the shoulder. Presented at the Arthroscopy Association of North American Annual Meeting, San Francisco, 1986
30. Matthews LS, Vetter WL, Oweida SJ et al: Arthroscopic staple capsulorrhaphy for recurrent anterior shoulder instability. Arthroscopy 1:106, 1988
31. Morgan CD: Arthroscopic transglenoid Bankart suture repair. Operative Tech Orthop 1:171, 1991
32. Morgan CD, Bodenstab AB: Arthroscopic Bankart suture repair: technique and early results. Arthroscopy 3:111, 1987
33. Neviaser TJ: The anterior labroligamentous periosteal sleeve avulsion lesion: a cause of anterior instability of the shoulder. Arthroscopy 9:17, 1993
34. Perthes G: Uber operationen bei habituellar schulterluxation. Dsch Zischr Chl 85:199, 1906
35. Reider B, Inglis AE: The Bankart procedure modified by the use of Prolene pull-out sutures. J Bone Joint Surg [Am] 64:682, 1982
36. Resch H, Golser K, Sperner G: Die arthroscopische labrumrefixation mit resorbierbaren staples. Arthroskopie 5:89, 1992
37. Rowe CR: Acute and recurrent anterior dislocations of the shoulder. Orthop Clin North Am 11:253, 1980
38. Rowe CR, Patel D, Southmayd WW: The Bankart procedure: a long-term end-result study. J Bone Joint Surg [Am] 60:1, 1978
39. Shea KP, O'Keefe RM, Fulkerson JP: Comparison of initial pull-out strength of arthroscopic suture and staple Bankart repair techniques. Arthroscopy 8:179, 1992
40. Simonet WT, Cofield RH: Prognosis in anterior shoulder dislocation. Am J Sports Med 12:19, 1984
41. Snyder SJ, Strafford BB: Arthroscopic management of instability of the shoulder. Orthopedics 16:993, 1993
42. Speer KP, Warren RF: Arthroscopic shoulder stabilization: a role for biodegradable materials. Clin Orthop 291:67, 1993
43. Uribe JW, Hechtman KS: Arthroscopically assisted repair of acute Bankart lesion. Orthopaedics 16:1019, 1993
44. Warner J, Pagnani M, Warren RF et al: Absorbable Bankart repair utilizing a cannulated absorbable fixation device. Orthop Trans 15:761, 1991
45. Watson-Jones R: Fractures and Joint Injuries. Vol. 11, Ed. 4. Livingston Ltd., Edinburgh, 1960
46. Weber SC: A prospective evaluation comparing open and arthroscopic treatment of recurent anterior glenohumeral dislocation. Presented at the American Academy of Orthopaedic Surgeons Annual Meeting, Anaheim, CA 1991
47. Wheeler JH, Ryan JB, Arciero RA, Molinari RN: Arthroscopic versus nonoperative treatment of acute shoulder dislocations in young athletes. Arthroscopy 5:213, 1989
48. Wiley AM: Arthroscopy for shoulder instability and a technique for arthroscopic repair. Arthroscopy 4:25, 1988
49. Wolf EM: Arthroscopic capsulolabral repair using suture anchors. Orthop Clin North Am 24:59, 1993
50. Wolf EM, Wilk RM, Richmond JC: Arthroscopic Bankart repair using suture anchors. Operative Tech Orthop 1:184, 1991.
51. Yahiro MA, Matthews LS: Arthroscopic stabilization procedures for recurrent anterior shoulder instability. Orthop Rev 18:1161, 1989
52. Zuckerman JD, Matsen FA: Complications about the glenohumeral joint related to the use of screws and staples. J Bone Joint Surg [Am] 66:175, 1984

CHAPTER FIFTEEN

Surgery for Posterior Instability

Jeffrey S. Noble
William Morin

Posterior glenohumeral instability remains a poorly understood pathologic entity that is not infrequently seen in an athletic population. The true incidence of posterior shoulder instability is uncertain but has been reported to represent 2 to 4 percent of those patients who present with shoulder instability.[5,35] Treatment of this variant of shoulder instability remains controversial. Diagnostic and therapeutic difficulty arises in part due to the confusion in terminology. Confusion also exists between posterior subluxation and dislocation. True posterior dislocation is an acute traumatic entity that is rare and most commonly associated with a low incidence of recurrence. Most commonly, an acute posterior dislocation presents with an impression defect as described by McLaughlin and requires careful treatment based on the size of the defect and duration of the dislocation.[21,26] Recurrent posterior subluxation is a distinct and separate entity, often not associated with trauma and troublesome related to its therapeutic implications.

Historically, early reports in the literature failed to distinguish recurrent posterior dislocation from subluxation and involved small, poorly defined patient populations. Reported surgical options for recurrent posterior instability have included glenoid[5,9,13,19,24,31,40,45] and humeral osteotomies,[7,24] posterior bone blocks,[1,11,12,28] posterior Bankart repairs,[22] posteroinferior capsular shifts,[4,15,18,20,25] staple capsulorrhaphy,[43,44] and posterior capsular plication with infraspinatus advancement[8,16,32,41] or biceps tendon transfers.[5] With locked posterior dislocation, using an anterior approach, procedures of subscapularis or tuberosity transfer as well as arthroplasty have been described.[21]

Historically, operative procedures were devised to address several presumed etiologies, including capsular laxity, excessive retroversion or hypoplasia of the glenoid, and posterior labral detachment.

In 1967, Scott[40] reported on three cases using a posterior glenoid osteotomy to diminish glenoid retroversion in patients with recurrent posterior instability. One shoulder was actually dislocated in the recovery room. Subsequent authors have reported variable results with his procedure.[3,11,28] Associated complications are worrisome and include joint contracture,[19] subcoracoid impingement,[13] intra-articular fracture,[23] and eventual development of glenohumeral arthritis,[23] particularly with violation of the joint surface.

Posterior stabilization procedures using bone blocks were aimed at extending the posterior bony glenoid rim. In 1949, Fried[11] reported satisfactory results in a small series of patients using an extracapsular bone block for "habitual posterior dislocation of the shoulder joint." More recently, Mowery and associates[28] reported excellent results in four of five patients using an intra-articular posterior bone block from the posterior iliac crest.

Although a reverse Bankart lesion is a rare pathologic entity, direct reattachment of the detached posterior labrum may be an effective surgical technique. Hindenach,[22] as well as Rowe,[35] authored case reports using "Bankart's method of repair" for recurrent posterior dislocation of the shoulder. Both papers reported favorable outcome after posterior capsular reattachment through drill holes in the posterior glenoid rim.

Procedures aimed at reducing excessive capsular redundancy include the posteroinferior modification of the inferior capsule shift as described by Neer and Foster.[29] Satisfactory long-term results have been reported by Bigliani et al[4] and in the series by Goss and Costello.[15]

Tibone and Ting[44] reported less than satisfactory results with posterior staple capsulorrhaphy in 20 athletes. Although stability was reasonably well restored, only one patient returned to his preoperative throwing level.

Fronek and associates[12] reported a success rate of 91 percent using posterior capsulorrhaphy for posterior subluxation of the glenohumeral joint. Despite the low recurrence rate, 70 percent of these athletes participated at a diminished level of competition or were forced to change to a less demanding situation.

Soft tissue posterior reconstruction involving capsular plication and infraspinatus advancement (i.e., "reverse" Putti-Platt procedure) has also been reported. In 1953, Severin[41] reported a technique in which the infraspinatus tendon was divided obliquely and advanced laterally over a double-breasted capsular plication. Hawkins and associates,[19] as well as Bell and Noble,[2] have reported satisfactory results without recurrence of instability using a modification of this procedure.

PATHOANATOMY

Stability of the glenohumeral joint can be divided into static and dynamic components. Static stability is divided into that provided by the capsuloligamentous structures and the congruence of the articular surfaces. Dynamic stability of the glenohumeral joint is related to the complex interaction of the glenohumeral ligaments, rotator cuff musculature, and the large muscles of the shoulder, such as the deltoid.

The static stabilizers, which control posterior translation, have been studied by capsular cutting experiments on cadaveric specimens.[38,39,46,47] Using such experiments, Warren et al[46] evaluated the stability of the shoulder to posterior displacement in two positions: (1) the neutral position, and (2) the classic position for posterior dislocation—that of flexion, adduction, and internal rotation. They noted that no posterior subluxation or dislocation occurred in the classic position after incising the infraspinatus, teres minor, and the entire posterior capsule from the 12- to 6-o'clock positions. Also, no posterior dislocation occurred with simply incising the anterior inferior and middle capsule from the 6- to 3-o'clock position. It was only after incising the anterior superior capsule from the 3- to 12-o'clock position that posterior dislocation occurred.

Schwartz et al[38] evaluated specimens positioned at 90 degrees of abduction or adduction and neutral humeral rotation. Variation of horizontal abduction was then used to simulate clinical examination. Through these studies, they concluded that the posterior inferior capsule provided the primary posterior restraint to posterior dislocation. Also, the anterior superior capsule and superior glenohumeral ligaments provided secondary restraints to posterior dislocation.

Recently, Harryman et al[17] evaluated the role of the rotator interval in instability of the shoulder using selective cutting studies and concluded that a major component in resisting posterior and inferior glenohumeral displacement was provided by an intact rotator interval capsule. Their studies revealed that sectioning of the rotator interval capsule increased and imbrication of these structures decreased, the translation seen on sulcus and posterior drawer tests. Furthermore, dislocation of the glenohumeral joint occurred both inferiorly and posteriorly when the interval capsule had been sectioned. Clinically, Nobuhara and Ikeda,[30] in characterizing lesions of the rotator cuff interval, noted in their experience that symptomatic posteroinferior instability of the glenohumeral joint substantially decreased after closing and reinforcement of the rotator cuff interval capsule.

In addition to stability offered by capsuloligamentous and bony structures, Gibb et al[14] evaluated the concept of stability due to a limited joint volume. Such a limited joint volume is able to resist translational forces when applied to the glenohumeral joint by creating a relative vacuum intra-articularly. Clinical testing, using anterior and posterior load-and-shift maneuvers and sulcus testing, was used both in the intact shoulder and after capsular venting. Simple capsular venting was shown to reduce the force necessary to translate the humeral head posteriorly by 10.8 N (43 percent).

The importance of dynamic stability has been theorized to aid in glenohumeral stability, either by pulling the head of the humerus posteriorly during external rotation or by compressing the humeral head congruently into the glenoid. Currently, several investigators are attempting to quantify and identify the crucial role dynamic stability plays in both posterior and overall glenohumeral stability. It is apparent that many questions about posterior instability remain unsolved. Future emphasis will undoubtedly center around dynamic shoulder modeling to better delineate the restraints to posterior displacement

CLASSIFICATION

The classification of posterior instability is presented in Table 15-1. Categories include traumatic versus atraumatic and subluxation versus dislocation. Traumatic posterior

Table 15-1. Classification of Posterior Instability

Acute posterior dislocation
Without impression defect
With impression defect
Chronic posterior dislocation
Locked (missed) with impression defect
Recurrent posterior subluxation
Voluntary
Habitual (willful)
Muscular control (not willful)
Involuntary
Positional (demonstrable)
Nonpositional (not demonstrable)

instability is further subdivided into acute posterior dislocation without an impression defect (rare) or acute posterior dislocation with an impression defect. When a traumatic posterior dislocation with an impression defect remains locked and undiagnosed, it then becomes a "missed" chronic posterior dislocation.

Atraumatic recurrent posterior subluxation is subdivided into voluntary and involuntary, with four subtypes emerging: voluntary habitual (emotionally disturbed), voluntary—not willful (muscular control), involuntary positional (demonstrable by the patient with arm position), and involuntary (not demonstrable by the patient by arm position or muscular contraction). Direction of instability may be described as unidirectional (posterior), which is the subject of this chapter. However, one must also be aware of the variants of multidirectional (posteroinferior), as well as global instability that must be considered when evaluating an athlete with presumed posterior instability.

The habitual subluxor was described by Rowe and associates in 1973.[36] The classic patient is a female adolescent with a psychiatric or personality disorder. Also described as "willful subluxors," these patients will not be helped by surgery and often require psychiatric evaluation. Although rare, it is important to distinguish this subset of patients in that they possess a subconscious desire to frustrate attempts at treatment and should not be considered surgical candidates.

Voluntary muscular and involuntary positional subluxors should not be confused with the previously habitual subluxor. Although these patients can demonstrate their instability, they do not have a willful desire to do so and exhibit no underlying psychiatric or personality disorder. Most often, these patients have a component of involuntary instability with certain movements or activities. The instability is termed *voluntary muscular* if demonstrable by muscular contractions and *involuntary* if posterior subluxation occurs with arm positioning. Some patients are both voluntary and involuntary.

The final subset of recurrent posterior subluxors is termed *involuntary* but is not demonstrable by the patient. Confirmation of this entity is difficult. As a diagnostic aid, "symptomatic translation" is useful in establishing the diagnosis clinically. During the load-and-shift maneuver, posterior translation of the proximal humerus on the glenoid rim may reproduce the patient's symptoms, strongly suggesting the diagnosis of posterior instability.

Acute Traumatic Posterior Dislocation

Acute posterior dislocation of the glenohumeral joint without an impression defect is extremely rare.[33,35] The subgroup of a locked posterior subluxation with an impression defect, sometimes termed a *dislocation* is discussed in the next section.

History

The history of an acute posterior dislocation without an impression defect is that of either indirect violent trauma including seizures, electrical shock, motor vehicle accident, or more commonly, a blow pushing posteriorly on the forward outstretched extremity with the arm in a position of flexion, adduction, and internal rotation. This may occur in a football lineman with posteriorly directed force. Most commonly, the humeral head subluxes posteriorly and reduces spontaneously. Occasionally, an actual dislocation may occur and remain temporarily locked out of the joint.

Physical Examination

In most circumstances, the acute posterior subluxation spontaneously reduces, as does the acute posterior dislocation, thus making it difficult to distinguish the two. With acute posterior dislocation presenting to the emergency department, the arm is in a fixed position and painful, with no motion and with the arm adducted and internally rotated. The patient is unable to externally rotate actively or passively. The humeral head may be palpable posteriorly, with a corresponding "empty" glenoid fossa anteriorly.

Radiographic Examination

Appropriate radiographic examination is critical in diagnosing this entity. In all patients, a standard trauma series should be obtained, consisting of a true anteroposterior view of the shoulder at a right angle to the scapula, a transcapular lateral taken parallel to the scapula, and an axillary view. The axillary view provides the most accurate roentgenographic evidence of dislocation. It also identifies an impression defect should it be present,[20] which is a different subset (i.e., locked posterior subluxation). Axial plane computed tomography may be helpful in assessing glenoid version, glenoid rim changes, impression defects in the humeral head, and associated glenoid fractures.

Treatment

Closed treatment is usually effective in the acute setting. After initial clinical and radiographic evaluation, reduction is facilitated by appropriate analgesia and muscular relaxants. The reduction is performed by flexion and adduction with longitudinal and lateral traction on the shoulder. Direct pressure may be applied to the humeral head from the posterior aspect of the shoulder to facilitate reduction. After successful reduction, stability of the shoulder should be assessed. If stable, the arm might be immobilized with the shoulder in mild extension and slight external rotation for 4 weeks. In fact, immobilization may be unnecessary. If unstable, the extremity should be immobilized in slight extension of the humerus and slight external rotation of the forearm for 6 weeks. After immobilization, physiotherapy emphasizes rotational strengthening. Although accurate epidemiologic data are lacking, recurrent instability seems to be uncommon after an acute posterior dislocation if immediately diagnosed and appropriately managed. This fact is unknown in that acute posterior dislocations without impression defects diagnosed and reduced are rare.

Chronic Posterior Dislocation (Locked/Missed Posterior Dislocation)

A locked posterior dislocation of the shoulder results when an acute posterior dislocation exists in the presence of an impression defect and the humeral head remains in actual fact subluxed posteriorly. If diagnosed immediately, the term is a *locked posterior subluxation.* If the diagnosis becomes delayed, some refer to this as a missed posterior subluxation. Although the term *dislocation* has been applied, this entity actually represents a subluxation with some of the humeral head outside the joint and some inside the joint. Unfortunately, if left untreated, progressive destruction of the humeral head may occur, and glenoid changes may result, altering the prognosis and treatment.

History

The initial mechanism of injury may be related to multiple trauma, a seizure disorder, or an alcohol-related incident. When patients present acutely, they are very painful with limited motion, and appropriate roentgenographic investigation (particularly an axillary view) confirms the diagnosis. At late presentation, pain is diminished and patients complain of a functional deficit. The chief complaint is that of inability to externally rotate the arm (i.e., an internal rotation deformity). These patients have difficulty

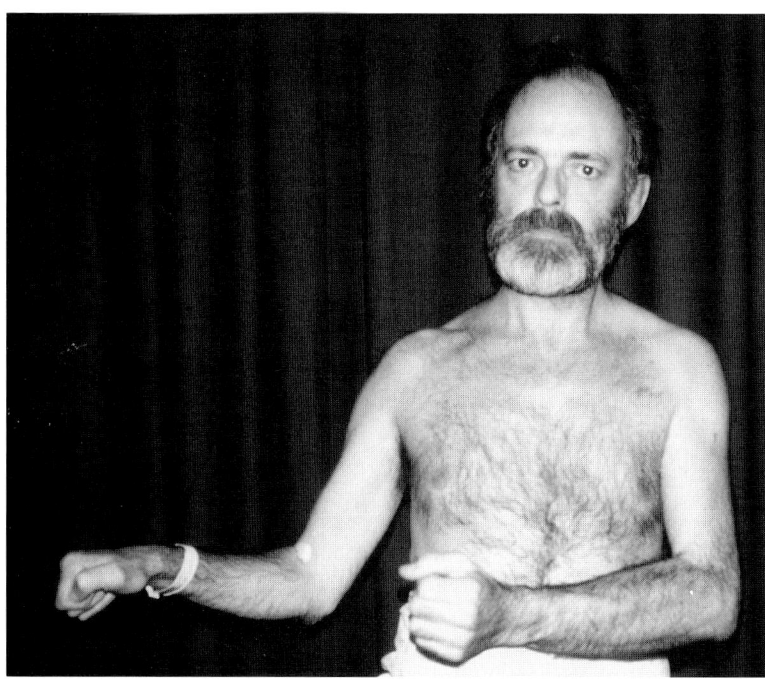

Figure 15-1. Internal rotation deformity in a patient with a locked posterior dislocation. This patient demonstrates an inability to externally rotate the arm.

combing their hair, washing their face, shaving, and even eating.[37] When physiotherapy does not improve their external rotation, these patients are often referred to the orthopaedic surgeon with the diagnosis of "frozen shoulder."

Physical Examination

On clinical inspection, the humeral head appears prominent posteriorly, while the coracoid process is prominent anteriorly. The acromion process may appear squared off anteriorly and laterally. The key physical sign in establishing the diagnosis is the internal rotation deformity (Fig. 15-1).[20,21] The size of the impression defect correlates directly with the magnitude of the internal rotation deformity. This loss of external rotation significantly limits function of the extremity at the level of the head and neck. Rowe and Zarins[37] also reported the inability of these patients to supinate the forearm when the arm is flexed forward.

Radiographic Examination

Routine radiographs obtained initially in the absence of an axillary view may be interpreted as normal.[21] Frequently, radiographs are not obtained at the time of injury, especially if associated with seizure or alcoholism. The trauma series, as previously described, is essential in establishing the diagnosis of a locked posterior dislocation. The axillary view remains the key investigation to clearly demonstrate the posterior subluxation and delineate the size of the impression defect (Fig. 15-2). The true anteroposterior and scapular lateral view are often difficult to interpret. The reason is that this is only a subluxation (some of the head in; some out). Several signs have been described on the anteroposterior view that suggest the diagnosis. These include internal rotation of the humerus, the vacant glenoid sign (reflecting a void in the anterior half of the glenoid fossa), and a "trough" line due to impaction of the humeral head. Nearly half these patients will exhibit an undisplaced fracture of the greater tuberosity or proximal humerus.[20] These fractures may divert attention from the glenohumeral joint. Computed tomography may be useful to elucidate the extent of the impression defect, as well as to delineate associated glenoid changes (Fig. 15-3).

Treatment

Appropriate management of a locked posterior dislocation depends on a variety of factors, including the duration of the dislocation, the size of the impression defect, the presence of changes in the glenoid, the functional disability of the patient, pain, and the general condition of the patient. Operative intervention is usually indicated in the active patient (Table 15-2).

When the duration of the dislocation is less than 6 weeks and the impression defect involves less than 20 percent of the articular surface, a gentle closed reduction as described in the previous section may be attempted. This reduction method may be successful in up to 50 percent of these delayed cases.[21] If stability is restored after reduction, the extremity might be immobilized in slight external rotation for 4 to 6 weeks. Perhaps immobilization is unnecessary. If instability with internal rotation persists after closed reduction, surgical reconstruction may be entertained.

When surgical reconstruction is necessary, the type of procedure depends on the amount of intact articular cartilage remaining to be reduced into the glenoid fossa. If more than 50 percent of the articular cartilage is viable and can be reduced, a subscapularis transfer (described by McLaughlin and modified by Neer to include a portion of the tuberosity) is indicated.[25] Using an anterior approach, the subscapularis insertion is identified and osteotomized from the lesser tuberosity. The humeral head is inspected and gently manipulated into the glenoid fossa. The subscapularis is then sutured into the defect via drill holes in bone. Postoperatively, immobilization in slight external rotation is maintained for 6 weeks.

With dislocation of greater than 6 months duration, progressive degeneration of the humeral head may ensue. When this occurs or when the impression defect involves more than 50 percent of the articular surface, hemiarthroplasty may be indicated. When concomitant glenoid erosion with secondary degenerative changes is present, total shoulder arthroplasty may be warranted. To ensure stability, when inserting the humeral component, retroversion should be decreased from the normal 35 to 40 degrees. In general, if the posterior dislocation has been present less than 6 months, the component might be positioned in approximately 20 degrees of retroversion. If the dislocation has been present for greater than 6 months, the humeral component might be placed in neutral version.[21] Using these guidelines, final version can be adjusted with trial components in place. Plication of the posterior capsule may be necessary to augment stability, preventing posterior subluxation or dislocation of the humeral component. If stability is achieved after arthroplasty, early motion may be initiated. If there is concern regarding stability of the implant, immobilization in external rotation is indicated.

Recurrent Posterior Subluxation

History

Recurrent posterior subluxation is the most common form of posterior instability and may be symptomatic, especially with athletic endeavors. Reports in the literature have referred to this entity as recurrent dislocation when, in fact, in most circumstances, it represents only a subluxation. Unlike recurrent anterior instability, most patients with recurrent posterior instability do not present with an initial

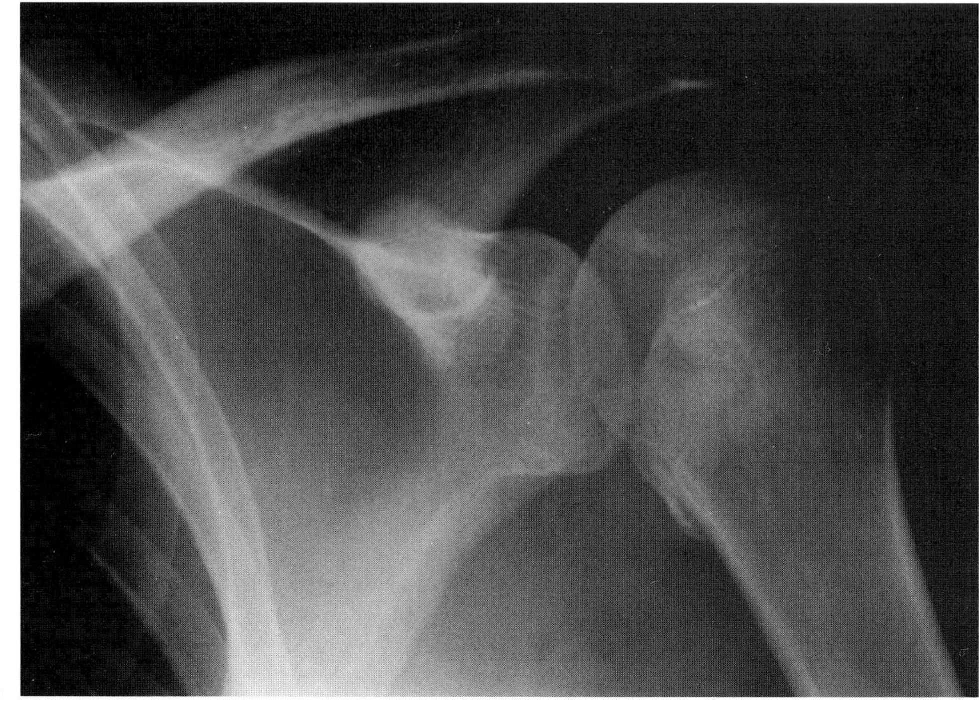

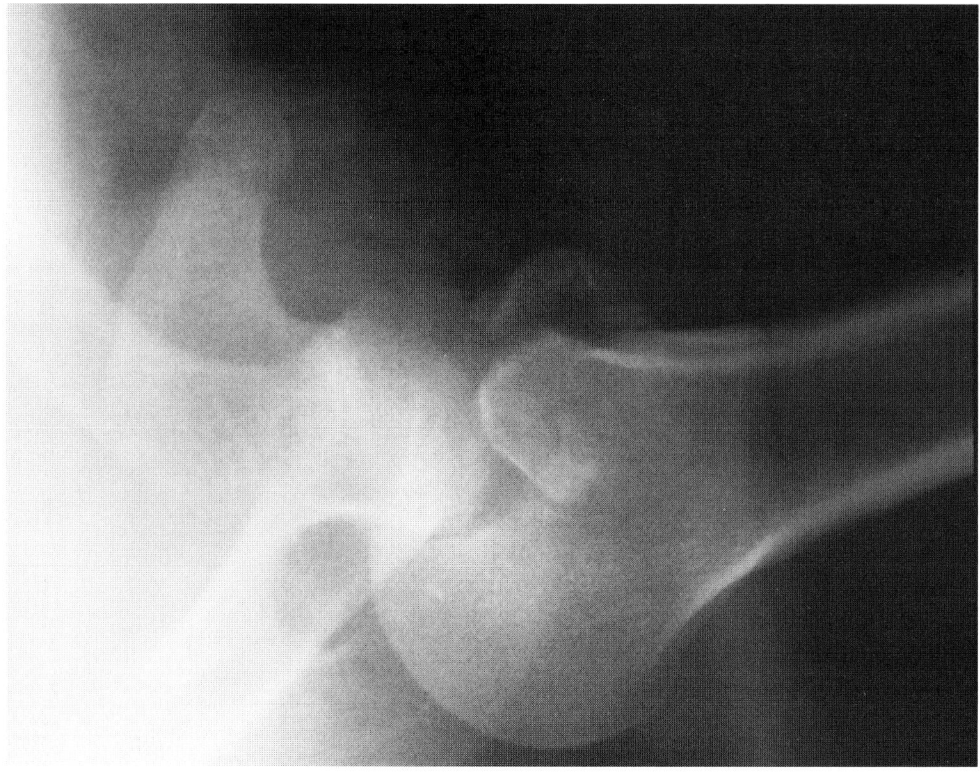

Figure 15-2. Locked posterior dislocation. (**A**) Anteroposterior radiograph. (**B**) Axillary radiograph demonstrates an impression defect of the humeral head.

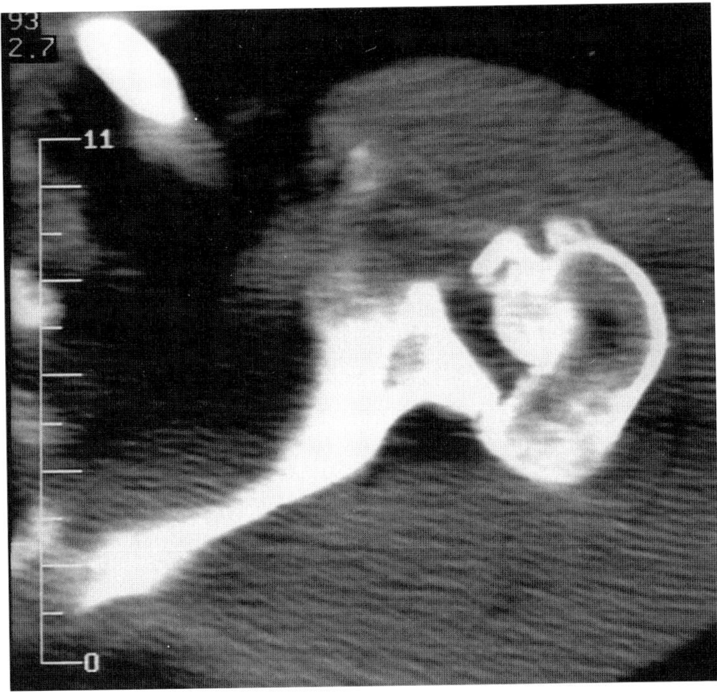

Figure 15-3. Computed tomography demonstrates posterior subluxation with an associated impression defect.

episode of significant trauma requiring reduction.[19,36] The most common scenario is that of an overuse endeavor with the shoulder, followed by an appreciation that it is slipping out of joint with arm positioning. With time, patients often learn to duplicate this maneuver and demonstrate the instability. Occasionally, it may progress so that the patient can sublux the shoulder with muscular contraction posteriorly. Most patients are only mildly symptomatic, and rehabilitation is the appropriate treatment regimen. Clinical laxity or excessive translation may be present in both shoulders, but it is usually the dominant shoulder that is symptomatic.[34] Patients often present to the physician because of painful tendinitis of the shoulder associated with instability. This is especially so in overhead athletes such as throwers, swimmers, and volleyball players.[39] In the rare patient refractory to rehabilitation, surgery may be warranted.

Physical Examination

In contrast to anterior instability, some patients with recurrent posterior subluxation can demonstrate the instability. This is either by a muscular contraction, termed *voluntary,* or by arm positioning, termed *involuntary.* In the usual situation, as the patient elevates the arm, the shoulder subluxes posteriorly, and as it approaches the coronal plane of the body, either in elevation or horizontal abduction, the shoulder visibly reduces (Fig. 15-4). Scapular winging is very common with posterior instability, especially as the joint subluxes. Sometimes patients cannot demonstrate the instability, and further testing is performed to determine direction. Also, in contrast to anterior instability, patients with recurrent posterior subluxation do not usually exhibit an apprehension sign. Frequently, when

Table 15-2. Treatment Recommendations for Chronic Posterior Dislocation

Size of Impression Defect (%)	Duration of Dislocation	Treatment
20	<6 Weeks	Closed reduction immobilization[a]
20–50	6 Weeks to 6 months	Subscapularis transfer
>50	<6 Months	Hemiarthroplasty[b] (20° retroversion)
>50	>6 Months	Hemiarthroplasty[b] (0° retroversion)

[a] If unstable postreduction, you should proceed to subscapularis transfer.
[b] If significant concomitant glenoid erosion, total shoulder arthroplasty may be required.

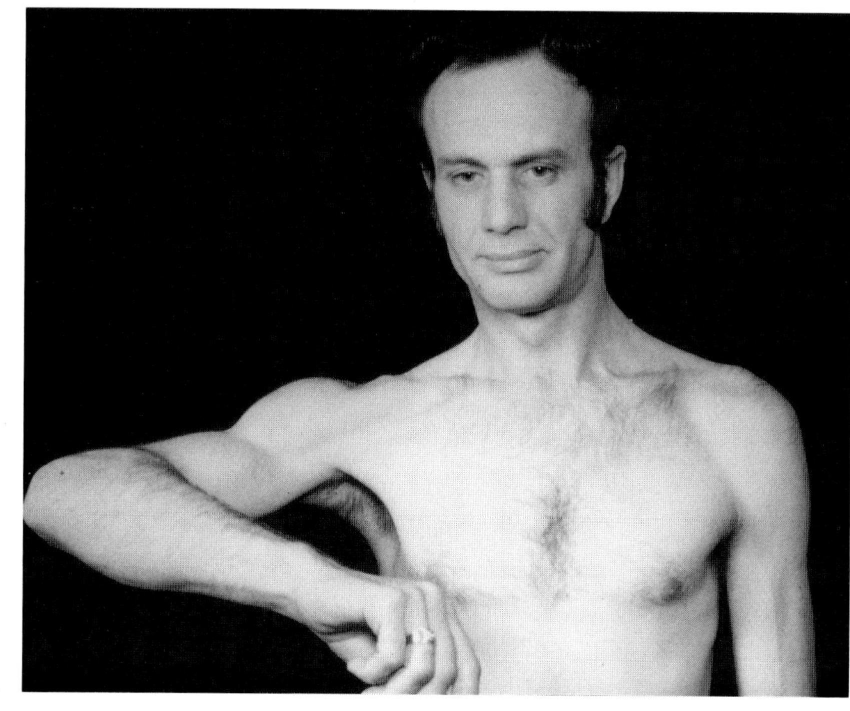

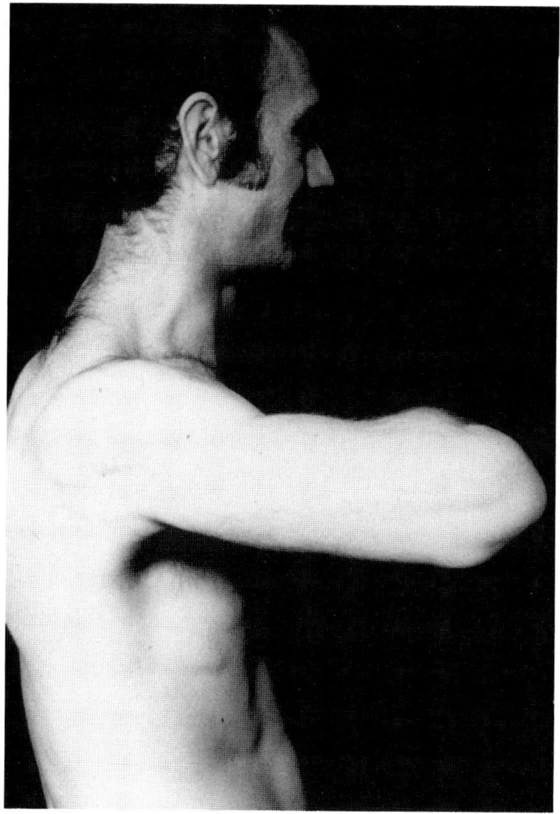

Figure 15-4. Recurrent posterior subluxation demonstrated by arm positioning. The provocative position is that of adduction, internal rotation, and forward flexion. (**A**) Frontal view; (**B**) lateral view.

stressed posteriorly, they are uncomfortable but usually not apprehensive as applied to anterior instability. Patients who have voluntary posterior instability and cannot demonstrate it by any means usually have a reproduction of their symptom complex when the humeral head is translated posteriorly in the glenoid fossa. When performing the "load-and-shift" maneuver, they often have a greater degree of posterior translation going at least to the rim when compared with the normal population but not as excessive as one might expect. There is no muscle wasting, usually a full range of motion, minimal tenderness, and very occasional crepitus, particularly with translation maneuvers. Occasionally, these patients have excessive flexibility in their joints, probably best assessed by abducting the thumb toward the forearm. Strength is often normal, but if there is a painful tendinitis, there may be pain-related weakness.

Assessment of posterior translation is carried out with the load-and-shift maneuver. With the patient sitting, the examiner grasps the humeral head between the thumb and index finger. While gently applying a compressive load to the glenoid with the humeral head, an attempt is made to translate the humeral head posterior and anteriorly. The extent of translation is then compared with the contralateral shoulder. Symptomatic posterior translation is helpful in confirming the diagnosis of posterior instability. When the humeral head is translated posteriorly, almost all patients with posterior instability appreciate that translation is their problem. Excessive translation in the absence of symptomatic reproduction must be interpreted cautiously. It is not uncommon for many normal patients to translate posteriorly almost to the glenoid rim.[27] The sulcus sign is determined by longitudinal traction on the upper arm, noting how far the humeral head moves away from the undersurface of the acromion. It is important to examine for this sign because it may be suggestive of an associated multidirectional instability pattern rather than unidirectional posterior instability.

Other parameters for hyperflexibility in such patients include extension of the middle finger parallel to upper arm, hypertension of the elbows, patellar hypermobility, and an ability to touch the palms to the floor without bending the knees.

Radiographic Examination

There are seldom any plain film radiographic changes, although posterior rim erosive defects may rarely be observed. Stress radiographs are often useful in that an axillary view with the shoulder subluxed helps determine excessive translation. This can also be documented fluoroscopically. Computed axial tomography and magnetic resonance imaging (MRI) have not proved to date very helpful, although there are recent publications of MRI changes with posterior instability located in the posterior capsular area. In difficult cases, diagnostic arthroscopy, associated with an examination under anesthesia, may be helpful.

Treatment

Fortunately, most patients with recurrent posterior subluxation of the shoulder have minimal pain and functional disability. Physiotherapy continues to form the cornerstone of treatment, consisting of a rotational and scapular strengthening program. Rotational strengthening may be achieved using a resistant rubber cord, emphasizing eccentric and concentric, external and internal rotation of the shoulder. Scapular strengthening may be achieved with seated rows for serratus and the rhomboids and shrugs for the trapezius, both in a concentric and eccentric mode. Rockwood,[34] along with Fronek et al[12] and Farek et al[10] have reported success of a structured rehabilitation program in the treatment of recurrent posterior instability.

Operative treatment may be considered in patients who remain symptomatic and functionally disabled despite an adequate trial of physiotherapy and activity modification. This may be particularly applicable in the athlete who has difficulty with overhead throwing, swimming, volleyball, and other sporting endeavors because of posterior instability. Pain may be an associated component, increasing the disability of the instability. These patients either present to the orthopaedic surgeon as a painful shoulder with a disability or a functional disability related to the instability, or a combination of the two. The usual indication for surgical treatment is pain. It is important for the surgeon to identify habitual or willful voluntary subluxors, because these patients will thwart any surgical intervention.

Arthroscopy may be useful diagnostically and sometimes therapeutically, especially in throwing athletes who have posterior instability.[39] Frequently, other findings in the joint exist in the overhead athlete, and sometimes minor labral debridement may prove beneficial, at least temporarily, in terms of relieving pain. However, it seldom affects the instability pattern.

As noted previously, several operative procedures are described in the literature, all with varying success.[2] Furthermore, it is essential that the surgeon rule out multidirectional instability in the preoperative evaluation. In the patient with multidirectional instability, a capsular shift is indicated to address the inferior capsular redundancy. In situations in which there is excessive glenoid version or glenoid deficiency, glenoid osteotomy and posterior bone block augmentation have been described. Unlike anterior instability, in which many surgeons correct the pathology, frequently with unidirectional posterior instability, most surgeons perform one operative procedure, with which they have achieved favorable results. However, in certain circumstances, associated pathology must be addressed. For example, if one performs a capsular tenodesis posteriorly and there is an associated reverse Bankart lesion, it also requires correction.

The operative procedures that we have applied for posterior unidirectional instability include posterior capsulorrhaphy (i.e., a modified ''reverse'' Putti-Platt) or a posterior glenoid osteomy. A posterior inferior capsular shift is reserved for patients who have multidirectional instability with an associated inferior component.

SURGICAL PROCEDURES

Posterior Capsular Infraspinatus Tenodesis

It is our preference in a patient who has recurrent unidirectional posterior subluxation to perform a soft tissue procedure using the capsule and infraspinatus tendon (Figs. 15-5 to 15-7). At the joint level, with the arm in neutral position, the posterior capsule is often thin and translucent and the infraspinatus muscular. It is essential when performing this procedure to move more laterally toward the greater tuberosity where the capsule is thicker and the infraspinatus more tendinous.

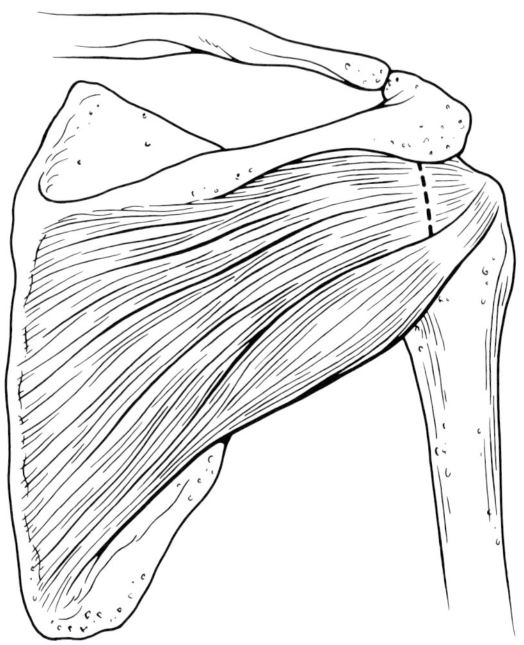

Figure 15-6. The deltoid fibers are bluntly split, and with the arm positioned in neutral rotation, a vertical incision is made directly through both the infraspinatus and the capsule approximately 4 mm lateral to the glenoid surface.

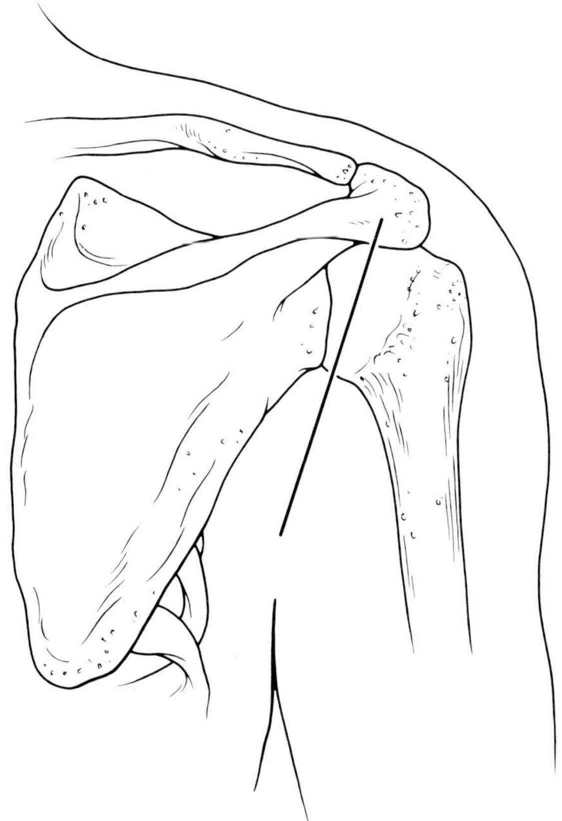

Figure 15-5. Posterior capsular infraspinatus tenodesis. A posterior longitudinal incision commences approximately 2 cm medial to the posterolateral corner of the acromion and extends to the posterior axillary crease.

Preoperatively, the patient may be placed into an outrigger shoulder spica cast with a long-arm component and a detachable spica bar. Immediately postoperatively while in the operating suite, the spica bar can be incorporated with the arm positioned in 5 degree extension, 10 to 20 degree abduction, and 20 degrees of external rotation. The difficulty in doing this is that the weight of the cast on the arm sometimes interferes with the surgery. It also poses some difficulties in draping, so frequently we put on only the waist band portion of the spica preoperatively.

The surgery is performed in the lateral decubitus position with the operative shoulder draped free. A longitudinal incision commences just at the posterolateral corner of the acromion and extends distally to the posterior axillary crease (Fig. 15-5). The underlying deltoid is identified and split in line with its fibers using blunt digital dissection. Appropriate retractors are placed under the deltoid, under the acromion, to retract superiorly, and a large right angle retractor to retract inferiorly. This reveals the underlying infraspinatus and teres minor fibers, which run at right angles to the deltoid. With the arm positioned in neutral rotation, a vertical incision approximately 3 to 4 mm parallel to the glenoid is made directly through the infraspinatus tendon and through the capsule to identify the joint surfaces (Fig. 15-6). It is critical that the incision not be made too far

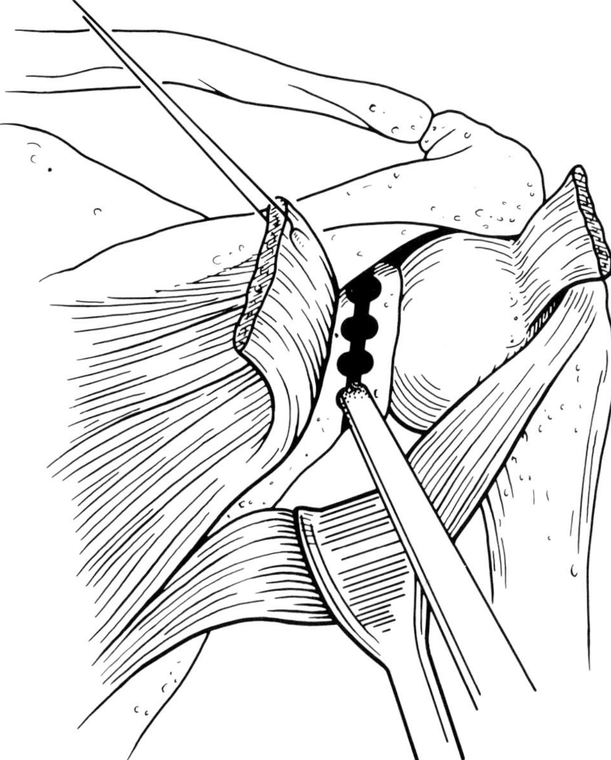

Figure 15-10. A 6-mm osteotome is used to gently hinge open the osteotomy site. The integrity of the anterior cortex and its periosteal attachments is maintained.

removal of the spica cast. Phase I consists of gentle passive motion emphasizing internal rotation, external rotation, and forward elevation and proceeds for approximately 4 weeks. Phase II follows and consists of active motion with terminal stretch, again emphasizing external rotation, internal rotation, and forward elevation. This phase continues for 2 to 4 weeks. Phase III consists of a strengthening program using an elastic resistance cord, usually beginning 10 to 12 weeks postoperatively. This strengthening program includes external rotators, internal rotators, shoulder shrugs, and narrow grip seated rows and emphasizes the eccentric as well as the concentric contraction phase. Overhead athletic activity is allowed at 4 months postoperatively, with return to contact sports permitted at 6 months.

SUMMARY

An acute traumatic posterior dislocation without an impression defect requiring reduction is rare.

Locked posterior dislocation with an impression defect requires special clinical examination, and an axillary view for diagnosis and its treatment depends on the size of the impression defect and the duration of the dislocation. It is very rare in the athletic population, but if diagnosed, appropriate treatment will, it is hoped, restore function.

Recurrent posterior subluxation is the most common form of posterior instability, perhaps not as uncommon as previously thought in the athlete. Fortunately, most patients

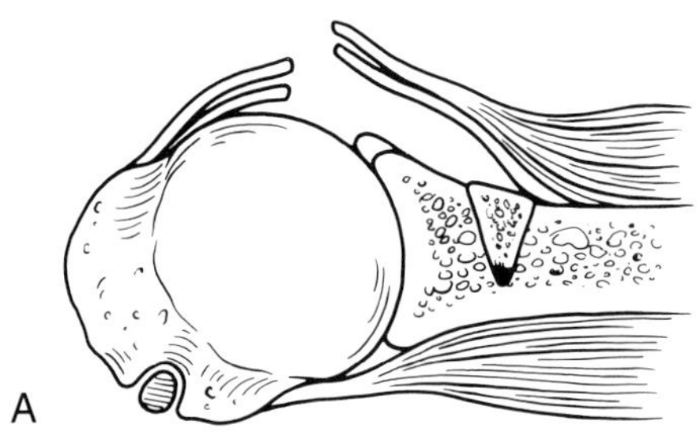

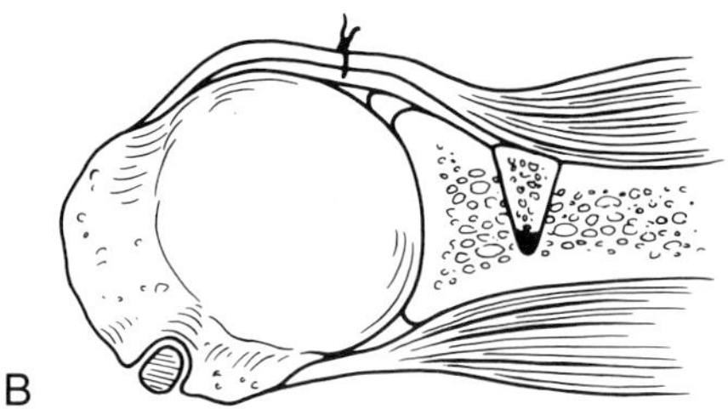

Figure 15-11. A tricortical graft is harvested from the posterior acromion and inserted into the osteotomy site. The capsule and infraspinatus are then overlapped to the posterior labrum.

with this pathology respond to a regimen of physiotherapy and activity modification. In those patients who remain functionally disabled despite an adequate trial of conservative treatment, operative intervention may prove helpful. Careful patient selection is essential in that the voluntary willful subluxor will not be helped by surgery. The best results are obtained by normal patients with normal tissues who have a traumatic onset to their instability pattern.

Our preference in patients with unidirectional posterior instability is to perform a capsular and infraspinatus tenodesis-type operation to the posterior glenoid labrum, using the tissue near the greater tuberosity, which is of better quality. Glenoid osteotomy is preferred by some but is of concern because of potential complications. Multidirectional instability must be ruled out, and if present, an alternative procedure is performed (i.e., capsular shift) to address the inferior capsular component.

Successful management for recurrent posterior subluxation requires accurate diagnosis, an adequate trial of physiotherapy, and judicious application of surgical reconstruction.

REFERENCES

1. Ahlgren SA, Hedlund T, Nistor L: Idiopathic posterior instability of the shoulder joint: results of operation with posterior bone graft. Acta Orthop Scand 49:600, 1978
2. Bell RH, Noble JS: An appreciation of posterior instability of the shoulder. Clin Sports Med 10:887, 1991
3. Bestasrd E: Glenoplasty: a simple reliable method of correcting recurrent posterior dislocation of the shoulder. Orthop Rev 5:29, 1976
4. Bigliani LU, Endrizzi DP, McIlveen SJ: Operative management of posterior shoulder instability. Orthop Trans 13:232, 1989
5. Boyd HB, Sisk TD: Recurrent posterior dislocation of the shoulder. J Bone Joint Surg [Am] 54:779–86, 1972
6. Brewer BJ, Wubbern RC, Carrera GF: Excessive retroversion of the glenoid cavity. J Bone Joint Surg [Am] 68:724, 1986
7. Chaudhuri GK, Sengupta A, Saha AK: Rotation osteotomy of the shaft of the humerus for recurrent dislocation of the shoulder. Acta Orthop Scand 45:193, 1974
8. Dugas RW, Scerpella TA, Clancy WG: Surgical treatment of symptomatic posterior shoulder instability. Orthop Trans 14:245, 1990
9. English E, Macnab I: Recurrent posterior dislocation of the shoulder. Can J Surg 17:147, 1974
10. Farek J, Pavlov BH, Warren RF: Posterior subluxation of the glenohumeral joint: nonsurgical and surgical treatment. Orthop Trans 10:220, 1986
11. Fried A: Habitual posterior dislocation of the shoulder joint: a report on five operated cases. Acta Orthop Scand 18:329, 1949
12. Fronek J, Warren RF, Bower M: Posterior subluxation of the glenohumeral joint. J Bone Joint Surg [Am] 71:205, 1989
13. Gerber C, Ganz R, Vinh TS: Glenoplasty for recurrent posterior shoulder instability. Clin Orthop 216:70, 1987
14. Gibb Td, Sidles JA, Harryman DT II et al: The effect of capsular venting on glenohumeral laxity. Clin Orthop 268:120–7, 1991
15. Goss TP, Costello G: Recurrent symptomatic posterior glenohumeral subluxation. Orthop Rev 17:1024, 1988
16. Greenhill BJ: Persistent posterior shoulder dislocation: its diagnosis and treatment by posterior Putti-Platt repair. J Bone Joint Surg [Br] 54:763, 1972
17. Harryman DT II, Sidles JA, Harris SL et al: Role of the rotator interval capsule in passive motion and stability of the shoulder. J Bone Joint Surg [Am] 74:53–66, 1992
18. Hawkins RJ: Unrecognized dislocations of the shoulder. Instr Course Lect 34:258, 1984
19. Hawkins RJ, Koppert G, Johnston G: Recurrent posterior instability of the shoulder. J Bone Joint Surg [Am] 66:169, 1984
20. Hawkins RJ, McCormack RG: Posterior shoulder instability. Orthopaedics 11:101, 1988
21. Hawkins RJ, Neer CS, Planta RM et al: Locked posterior dislocation of the shoulder. J Bone Joint Surg [Am] 69:9, 1987
22. Hindenach JCR: Recurrent posterior dislocation of the shoulder. J Bone Joint Surg [Am] 29:582–6, 1947
23. Johnston GH, Hawkins RJ, Haddad R et al: A complication of posterior glenoid osteotomy for recurrent posterior shoulder instability. Clin Orthop 187:147, 1984
24. Kretzler HH Jr: Scapular osteotomy for posterior shoulder dislocation. Proceedings of the Western Orthopaedic Association. J Bone Joint Surg [Am] 56:197, 1974
25. McLaughlin HL: Posterior dislocation of the shoulder. J Bone Joint Surg [Am] 34:584, 1952
26. McLaughlin HL: Locked posterior subluxation of the shoulder: diagnosis and treatment. Surg Clin North Am 43:1621, 1963
27. Morton KS: The unstable shoulder: recurring subluxation. Injury 10:304, 1978
28. Mowery CA, Garfin SR, Booth RE et al: Recurrent posterior dislocation of the shoulder: treatment using a bone block. J Bone Joint Surg [Am] 67:777, 1985
29. Neer CS, Foster CR: Inferior capsular shift for involuntary inferior and multidirectional instability of the shoulder. J Bone Joint Surg [Am] 62:897, 1980
30. Nobuhara K, Ikeda H: Rotator interval lesion. Clin Orthop 223:44–50, 1987
31. Norwood LA, Terry GL: Posterior shoulder subluxation. Am J Sports Med 12:25, 1984
32. Roberts A, Wickstrom J: Prognosis of posterior dislocation of the shoulder. Acta Orthop Scand 42:328, 1971
33. Rockwood CA Jr: The diagnosis of acute posterior dislocation of the shoulder. J Bone Joint Surg [Am] 48:1220, 1966
34. Rockwood CA Jr: Subluxation and dislocations about the shoulder. pp. 722–860. In Rockwood CA, Green DP (eds): Fracture in Adults. JB Lippincott, Philadelphia, 1984
35. Rowe CR: Prognosis in dislocations of the shoulder. J Bone Joint Surg [Am] 38:957–77, 1956
36. Rowe CR, Pierce DS, Clark JG et al: Voluntary dislocation

of the shoulder: a preliminary report on a clinical, electromyographic and psychiatric study of 26 patients. J Bone Joint Surg [Am] 55:445, 1973
37. Rowe CR, Zarins B: Chronic unreduced dislocations of the shoulder. J Bone Joint Surg [Am] 64:494, 1982
38. Schwartz E, O'Brien SJ, Warren FR et al: Capsular restraints to anterior-posterior motion of the shoulder. Orthop Trans 12:727, 1988
39. Schwartz E, Warren RF, O'Brien SJ et al: Posterior shoulder instability. Orthop Clin North Am 18:L409–19, 1987
40. Scott DJ Jr: Treatment of recurrent posterior dislocations of the shoulder by glenoplasty. J Bone Joint Surg [Am] 49:471, 1967
41. Severin E: Anterior and posterior recurrent dislocation of the shoulder: the Putti-Platt operation. Acta Orthop Scand 23:14, 1953
42. Surin V, Blader S, Boras, GM: Rotational osteotomy of the humerus for posterior instability of the shoulder. J Bone Joint Surg [Am] 72:181, 1990
43. Tibone JE, Prietto C, Jobe FW: Staple capsulorrhaphy for recurrent posterior shoulder dislocation. Am J Sports Med 9:135, 1981
44. Tibone JE, Ting A: Capsulorrhaphy with a staple for recurrent posterior subluxation of the shoulder. J Bone Joint Surg [Am] 72:999, 1990
45. Vegter J, Marti RK: Treatment of posterior dislocation of the shoulder by osteotomy of the neck of the scapula. J Bone Joint Surg [Br] 63:288, 1981
46. Warren RF, Kornblatt IB, Marchand R: Static factors affecting posterior shoulder stability. Orthop Trans 8:89, 1984
47. Weber SC, Caspari RB: A biomechanical evaluation of the restraints to posterior shoulder dislocation. Arthroscopy 5:115–21, 1989

CHAPTER SIXTEEN

Surgical Treatment of Multidirectional Instability of the Shoulder

Gary W. Misamore
Robert E. FitzGibbons

Surgical management of multidirectional instability of the shoulder represents the last exit on a long road of conservative treatment using an educational and rehabilitation program. Most patients with multidirectional instability can be treated successfully by patient education, shoulder girdle strengthening exercises, and occasionally modification of a patient's activity. Cooper and Brems[4] treated less than 16 percent of their patients with multidirectional instability by surgical intervention. Burkhead and Rockwood[3] achieved good or excellent results using a strengthening program in 29 of 33 shoulders classified as atraumatic multidirectional instability. Our clinical data support this finding in that less than 20 percent of our patients diagnosed with atraumatic multidirectional instability ultimately elect surgery for stabilization of the shoulder.

As we study the published literature on the subject of surgical treatment of multidirectional instability, it is difficult to reach solid conclusions. Only a few retrospective studies have been published to date that specifically review results of capsulorrhaphy for shoulders afflicted with multidirectional instability. The most confusing issue one encounters in studying these reports is trying to understand the specific type of instability being reviewed. This problem arises due to the lack of a uniformly accepted definition of multidirectional instability. This lack of a clear-cut definition results in heterogeneous patient populations in the published reports, thus making interstudy, and even intrastudy, comparisons and contrasts difficult.

Lippitt et al[6] and Thomas and Matsen[8] have introduced a classification of shoulder instability described by the acronyms of TUBS and AMBRI. As described in Chapter 11 of this book, TUBS represents instability resulting from a *t*raumatic etiology, which is *u*nidirectional, and in which a *b*ankart lesion is usually present, and most often requires *s*urgery for successful resolution of the patient's symptoms. By contrast, AMBRI represents instability that is *a*traumatic in etiology, whose associated laxity is *m*ultidirectional and often *b*ilateral, most frequently responds favorably to a *r*ehabilitation program, and when surgical intervention is required, is best addressed with an *i*nferior capsular shift.

Although this classification is useful in delineating the two opposite poles of shoulder instability, it does not describe all the variations of shoulder instability that lie somewhere between these two extremes. Not all patients with shoulder instability can be placed neatly into one or the other category in this classification system. There are many shades of gray between the two black-and-white extremes.

It is this problem that makes a review of the literature confusing. Without a clear and uniformly accepted definition of multidirectional instability in place, we must read prior reports with a critical eye. Are the authors of these reports discussing AMBRI patients, TUBS patients who develop secondary laxity in additional directions after an initial traumatic lesion in one direction, or some other variation or combination?

Neer and Foster[7] were the first to report on the inferior capsular shift for multidirectional instability in 1980. They reported on 40 shoulders in 36 patients who underwent surgery during a 5-year period. However, 29 of the 36 patients suffered moderate or severe trauma associated with their initial dislocation. Although all 36 patients had some degree of inferior laxity on examination, 5 were found to have a Bankart lesion at the time of surgery. Patient's ages ranged from 15 to 55 years. Seventeen of the patients had generalized ligamentous laxity. In some aspects, many of these patients fit the AMBRI classification; however, certainly not all the patients did.

In 1991, Altchek et al[1] reported on 40 patients treated surgically for multidirectional instability over 7 years. Thirty-nine of the 40 patients suffered a traumatic onset, with 36 of those suffering a frank dislocation. Twenty-eight of the 40 had no evidence of laxity in the opposite shoulder, and 20 of the 40 had no evidence of generalized laxity on examination. All but two shoulders had a Bankart lesion, and 24 had a Hill-Sachs lesion. Certainly, these do not fit in the AMBRI category and, in fact, seem much more like TUBS patients.

Cooper and Brems[4] reported surgical results of 38 patients treated over a 6-year period. Twenty-eight of these had laxity in the opposite shoulder, and 29 had generalized ligament laxity. No discussion of the role of trauma in the etiology of the instability in these patients was offered. However, seven of the shoulders were found to have a Bankart lesion. These patients likely represented a population close to the AMBRI grouping, although it may still not be a pure group.

Lebar and Alexander[5] reported on 10 patients treated surgically for multidirectional instability during a 4-year period. All these had inferior laxity on examination. Only three patients had generalized ligamentous laxity. Four suffered an initial significant traumatic onset. At surgery, three Bankart and two Hill-Sachs lesions were found. Six of the 10 patients had prior surgery on the shoulder for instability. From the information available, it is difficult to categorize these patients. However, it seems likely that these patients did not all fit the AMBRI or the TUBS classifications.

Considering the results in these prior reports, one must again view these critically. Neer and Foster[7] reported 97 percent "satisfactory" results in the 36 patients with follow-up of at least 1 year. Four patients returned to full sports. Three patients suffered axillary nerve injury during surgery. Altchek et al[1] reported that 90 percent of the 40 patients with at least 2-year follow-up had relief of instability with surgery, whereas 82 percent returned to sports. Cooper and Brems[4] reported that of 38 patients with 2-year follow-up, 90 percent were "subjectively better" although 20 percent had to limit some activities secondary to pain and 20 percent had some apprehension. Ten percent still had significant instability, and more than 25 percent had decreased their activity level postoperatively (five were disabled secondary to problems with the shoulder). Thirty-seven returned to some sports (not all at the same level as preoperatively), but this study included no high-level athletes. Lebar and Alexander[5] reported that of the 10 patients with 1-year follow-up, 8 were "happy with their surgery" and had an "overall improvement." One-half of the patients received a "medical discharge with disability." Of the five patients who returned to military duty, three continued to have "physical restrictions which made continued active duty difficult."

In summary, those reports suggest that "satisfactory" results were achieved in approximately 90 percent of cases (Neer and Foster, 97 percent[7]; Altchek et al, 90 percent[1]; Cooper and Brems, 90 percent[4]; Lebar and Alexander, 80 percent[5]). However, it would seem that even in those "satisfactory" results, the shoulder was often not normal for stressful activities. Regarding return to sports-level activities, Neer and Foster[7] reported 12 percent returned to full sports, whereas Altchek et al[1] reported 82 percent returned to sports. Cooper and Brems[4] reported 37 percent returned to "some sports" (although not all the same level as preoperatively). Lebar and Alexander[5] did not address sports return but did report that 50 percent returned to military duty postoperatively. However, only 20 percent returned to duty without some restriction of their activity.

Reports of surgical treatment of multidirectional instability seemingly suggest satisfactory results in approximately 90 percent of patients. However, as pointed out in this discussion, these reports are difficult to interpret and compare because it is not clear that all authors are describing the same type of instability patterns. The criteria for a satisfactory result are arbitrary, not clearly defined, and not consistent among the reports.

Because there are no clear criteria for diagnosis of multidirectional instability nor any standard measure for determining a successful outcome from surgery, we must view the limited reports available with a cautious and critical eye.

DIAGNOSIS

An individual diagnosed with multidirectional shoulder instability must have laxity in more than one direction, of which a component is inferior instability as demonstrated by the sulcus sign on physical examination. A patient with true multidirectional instability can present a diagnostic challenge. Repeat clinical examinations are sometimes needed to provide the clinician with a better opportunity to delineate the patients instability pattern. Patients often have vague shoulder complaints that are chronic in nature and not often associated with a single provocative position. They may complain of dysesthesias in the involved extremity. Their symptoms may be initiated by a traumatic event, repetitive activity, or simply activities of daily living. These may represent separate subsets under the general heading of multidirectional instability. Many patients will demonstrate evidence of generalized connective tissue laxity such as knee recurvatum, elbow hyperextension, and the ability to touch the thumb to the forearm with the wrist in flexion.

Patients with multidirectional instability are generally younger than 30 years of age. There is a higher percentage of women than men, in contrast to traumatic unidirectional instability in which there is a higher percentage of men than women. There usually is laxity of the opposite shoulder, although that laxity may not be symptomatic. Often, there is generalized ligamentous laxity as discussed in the previous paragraph. In addition to complaints of instability, these patients often complain of constant aching in the affected shoulder, likely because they suffer frequent minor subluxations. Often the instability is such a problem that the shoulder subluxes almost continuously throughout each day and often throughout each night. This results in a more continuous aching for many of these patients, in contrast to patients with traumatic unidirectional instability who typically experience infrequent but more intense bouts of pain during episodes of subluxation or dislocation. Also, patients with multidirectional instability frequently complain of paresthesias, dysesthesias, and heaviness through the entire extremity.

Because of the general irritability of the shoulder, examination can be difficult and confusing. The instability can often be difficult to demonstrate on examination due to voluntary guarding by the patient in an effort to protect the shoulder from pain. It is not uncommon for these patients to be initially treated for what is thought to be rotator cuff tendonitis. Often, it is not until the general tendonitis and capsulitis are resolved that the instability can be demonstrated on subsequent examinations. The details of examination for instability are covered in Chapter 2.

TREATMENT

When conservative treatment fails for true multidirectional instability, surgical intervention to decrease the redundant capsular tissue can be considered. The loose static restraints that are present in multidirectional instability place a greater demand on the dynamic restraints, resulting in the fatigue of the rotator cuff and scapular stabilizers. Bowen and Warren[2] postulated that the redundant capsule with its increased joint volume may result in the development of smaller intra-articular negative pressures and thus circumvent one of the shoulder's important passive restraints, allowing greater translation to occur.

With careful selection of patients for surgical intervention and careful attention to detail during surgery, reasonably good results from surgical reconstruction can result. The goal of the inferior capsular shift is to achieve global tightening of the entire shoulder capsule. In most cases, this can be accomplished through an anterior approach. Even in those cases with significant posterior laxity, that instability can be eliminated by an anterior approach through which the rotator cuff interval and anterior superior capsule are imbricated while the anterior, inferior, and posterior capsule is shifted to achieve global tightening. It is our practice to perform a posterior capsular shift only for patients with only posterior or posteroinferior instability or in those infrequent cases in which the instability is so severe that we think that posterior capsular tightening needs to be combined with an anteroinferior capsular shift.

Generally, the capsular tissue is more substantial anteriorly, and the anterior approach to the shoulder is more familiar to most surgeons. By extensive, but cautious, release of the capsule from its insertion onto the humeral neck, even most of the posterior capsule can be mobilized such that an adequate shift of the anterior, inferior, and posterior capsule can be performed from the anterior aspect of the shoulder.

SURGICAL OPTIONS

The surgical treatment for multidirectional instability attempts to correct the excessive laxity of the shoulder capsule. Neer and Foster[7] first described the inferior capsular shift. Altchek et al[1] modified this procedure by doing their "shift" on the glenoid side because most of their patients had a traumatic etiology with a Bankart lesion. Some clinicians are attempting arthroscopic capsular shifts in appropriately selected patients, but at this time this technique cannot be recommended as the standard of care for this complex problem. Laser treatment or capsular laxity has emerged as an additional surgical option. This procedure is in its infancy at this time and can only be viewed as an experimental procedure. With further time and study, we will be able to judge arthroscopic repair and laser treatment and their role in the management of multidirectional instability.

SURGICAL TECHNIQUE FOR OPEN INFERIOR CAPSULAR SHIFT

At the time of open reconstruction, a diagnostic shoulder arthroscopy may be carried out. This allows for the identification of a Bankart lesion that may require repair as well as treatment of associated pathology, including partial rotator cuff tears or labral tears opposite the side of the incision. Pathology of this type is usually easier to deal with arthroscopically than open.

For open anterior capsular reconstruction, the patient is placed in a supine position with the head of the bed elevated 20 degrees and a small pad placed posteriorly under the scapula to elevate the shoulder off the bed. The patient is positioned so that the shoulder is off the edge of the table. A short arm board is placed at the level of the elbow to support the shoulder and prevent extension, which may sublux the humeral head anteriorly and make repair difficult. The fore quarter is draped in an appropriate manner that allows free movement of the arm and provides anterior and posterior access to the shoulder. Before proceeding, the range of motion of the shoulder is measured for reference after the capsular shift.

We place our skin incision in the most prominent skin fold that extends vertically from the anterior portion of the axilla. The incision begins in the axilla (for cosmetic purposes) and extends approximately 7 cm. The skin is undermined to expose the deltopectoral interval. When using the axillary incision, generous subcutaneous tissue mobilization is needed for appropriate exposure (Fig. 16-1).

The cephalic vein, with most of its tributaries, is retracted laterally with the deltoid. The pectoralis is retracted medially. The clavipectoral fascia is then opened along the lateral edge of the short flexor tendons, and these tendons are retracted medially along with the pectoralis.

Occasionally, a small accessory band of the pectoralis major tendon may limit exposure inferiorly, and this may be partially released. Proximally, we release the clavipectoral fascia up to the coracoacromial ligament. We use a modified curved blunt deltoid retractor under the deltoid and over the humerus to aid with retraction of the deltoid laterally. A large right angle retractor is placed medially. Altchek et al[1] release the coracoacromial ligament to avoid impingement problems during the postoperative rehabilitation, but we have not found this to be necessary.

The margins of the subscapularis are identified by palpating the rotator cuff interval superiorly and identifying the circumflex vessels at the inferior border. The vessels are exposed, clamped, and coagulated to allow adequate exposure at the time of the inferior capsular shift.

The subscapularis is taken down using a combination of sharp dissection and blunt elevation to peel the tendon off the capsule. We take the subscapularis directly off the capsule whereas Neer and Foster[7] prefer to leave the deep half of the subscapularis tendon on the capsule to provide re-enforcement at the time of the capsular shift. The capsular foramen noted superiorly between the middle glenohumeral ligament and the superior glenohumeral ligament is closed with nonabsorbable sutures (Fig. 16-2). Occasionally, if the capsular rent is close to the equator of the glenoid (not usually the case), it can simply be incorporated into the horizontal component of the capsulotomy.

A transverse capsulotomy is carried to the center of the glenoid rim, with care taken not to damage the articular surface or the glenoid labrum (Fig. 16-2). If a significant

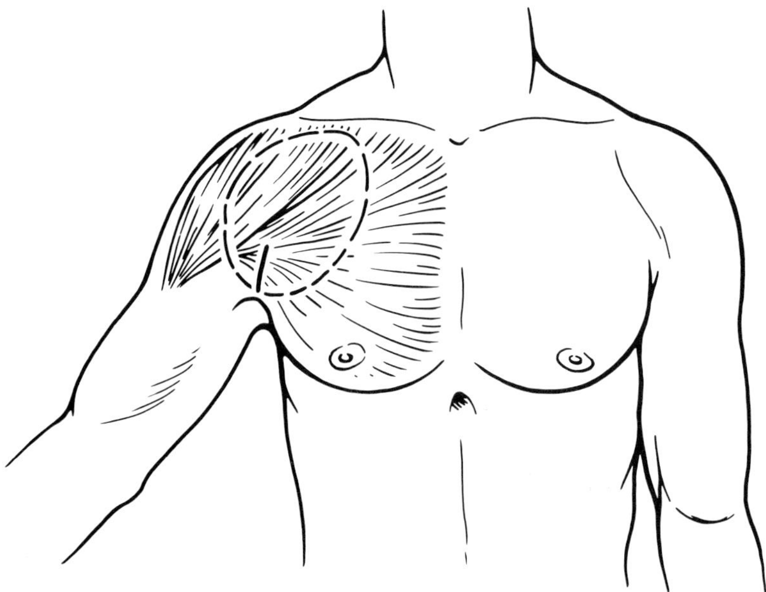

Figure 16-1. Anterior capsular shift. Placement of the anterior axillary incision is indicated. The tissues must be undermined superiorly to expose the deltopectoral interval.

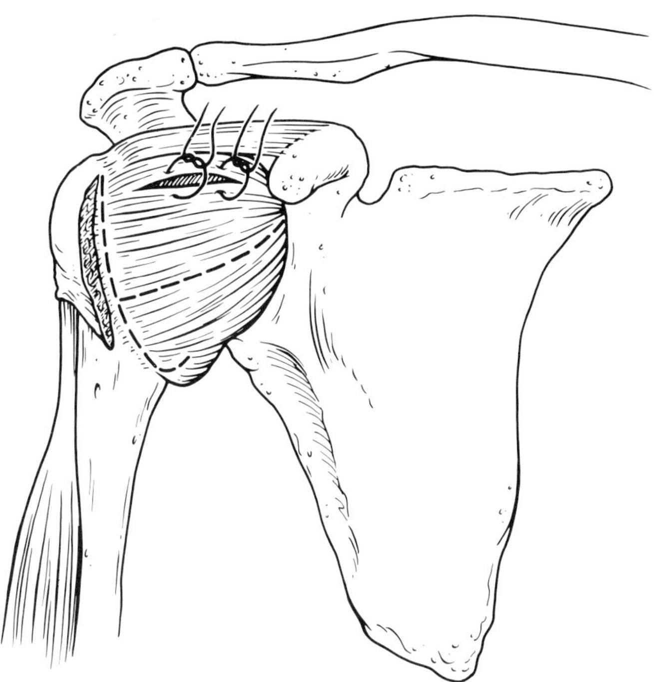

Figure 16-2. Anterior capsular shift. The capsular foramen superiorly is closed with sutures. Inferior and superior flaps are created by a T incision in the capsule with the vertical incision placed near the humeral insertion of the capsule.

Bankart lesion is identified, this may be addressed in one of two ways. The first option is that the Bankart lesion may be repaired along the glenoid margin, followed by a standard capsular shift made on the humeral side. The second option is to do the capsular shift on the glenoid side so that a simultaneous repair may be carried out. However, it has been our experience that it is much easier to aggressively mobilize the inferior capsule when the release is performed on the humeral side. Performance of the capsular release and repair along the glenoid has been useful in our experience only when the instability is primarily in an anteroinferior direction.

The vertical limb of the T capsulotomy is made laterally, taking care to leave a cuff (1 cm) of capsule attached to the humerus for later repair (Fig. 16-2). Neer and Foster[7] described the release of the capsule at its insertion and made a shallow trough along the inferior neck of the humerus to create a raw cancellous surface to aid the healing of the capsular tissue after the shift. It is our opinion that this trough is not necessary because the capsular tissue heals well and often the shifted flap of capsule does not appose the trough well anyway. A marking stitch can be placed at the superior lateral corner of the inferior capsular flap to aid with orientation at the time of the capsular shift. Also, the intersection of the horizontal and vertical limbs is marked on the humerus with electrocautery to aid in determining the amount of capsular advancement being achieved during closure of the capsule.

To accomplish an appropriate capsular shift for multidirectional instability, the capsule must be completely released inferiorly and as far posteriorly as deemed necessary to eliminate the posterior component of instability (Fig. 16-3). A blunt retractor or elevator can be placed under the inferior margin of the capsule to help protect the axillary nerve. Using moderate external rotation to expose the capsule, it is released inferiorly and posteriorly near the neck of the humerus. This will only be possible and safe if all soft tissue (i.e., subscapularis tendon/muscle) has been carefully dissected off the inferior capsule for adequate exposure. The capsular release is performed by carefully using a combination of elevators, scissors, and scalpel dissection under direct visualization. Obviously, great caution must be used in this area due to the close proximity of the axillary nerve.

The amount of capsular advancement must be individualized depending on the overall laxity of the tissue present and the degree of instability. The inferior flap is advanced proximally and to a lesser extent laterally to reduce the anterior, inferior, and posterior capsular redundancy (Fig. 16-4). This inferior flap is sutured into the lateral capsule stump remaining attached along the neck of the humerus. We perform this repair with numerous size 1 or 2 nonabsorbable sutures. The free ends of these sutures are not cut after the sutures have been tied but, rather, are preserved so that those sutures can be used for repair of the superior flap as it is advanced over the repaired inferior flap. The

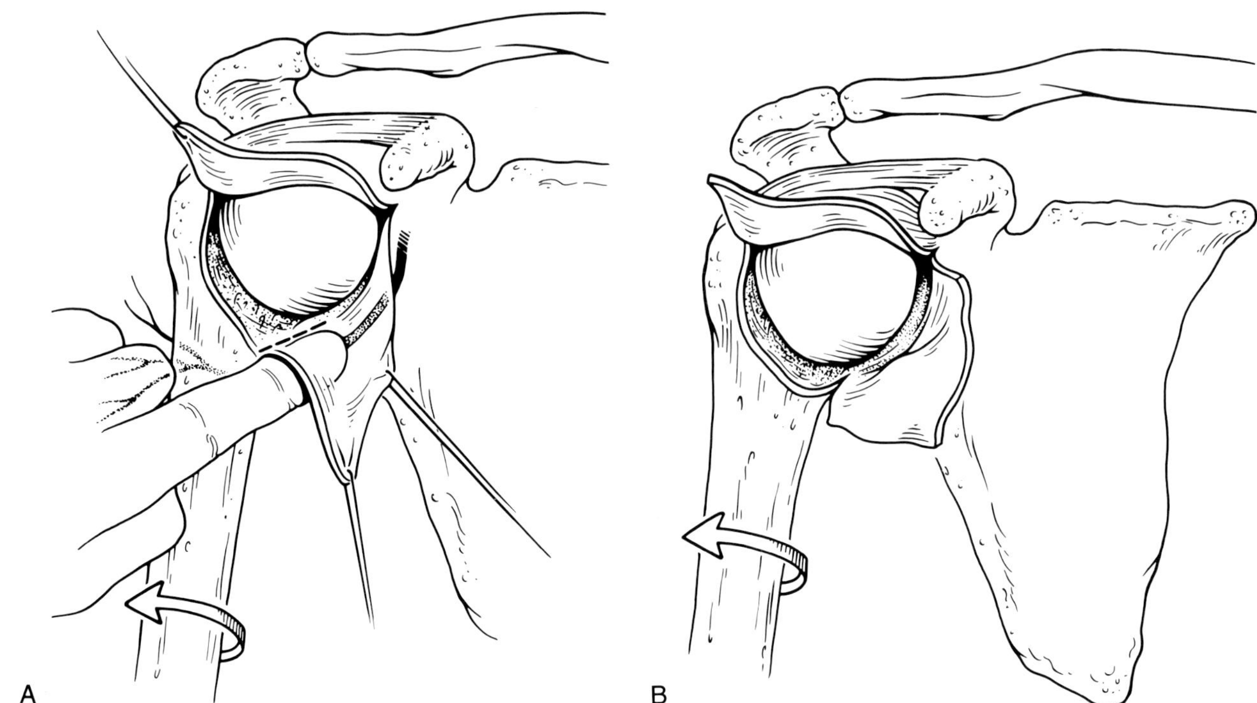

Figure 16-3. Anterior capsular shift. (**A**) The capsular incision extends inferior and posterior. (**B**) Posterior exposure is achieved by external rotation of the arm.

mark made on the anatomic neck with electrocautery before release of the capsule can be used to judge how much advancement has been accomplished. The superior flap is then advanced inferiorly and laterally in a similar fashion to re-enforce the inferior capsule flap. Great care is taken not to advance either flap too far laterally, as this may significantly decrease external rotation. The transverse incision in the anterior capsule is then sutured in an imbricated fashion. This is usually performed with moderate overlap because the flaps are typically advanced superiorly and inferiorly quite significantly. We place the arm in the position that provides optimal exposure at the time of the capsular shift. Altchek et al[1] recommended holding the arm 45 degrees of external rotation and 45 degrees of abduction at the time of the capsular shift. We have found that the tension of our shift is dependent on the placement of our sutures in the capsule as well as the amount of capsule released from the humeral neck and that arm position is not as significant a factor. Positioning of the arm is important if it allows the surgeon to better judge the placement of sutures.

At this point, the inferior capsular shift must be assessed. Unfortunately, a certain degree of ''artistic license'' must be exercised. Many factors must be considered including the age of the patient, the degree of generalized ligamentous laxity, and the ultimate goals of the patient (sport, occupation, or activities of daily living). The passive anterior, inferior, and posterior translation as well as the change in rotation can be compared with that present before performing the shift. There should be little or no residual passive translation present. Typically, the external rotation is reduced moderately but is quite variable and dependent on multiple factors including the postoperative desires of the patient as well as the generalized soft tissue make-up.

The subscapularis is anatomically repaired with nonabsorbable sutures. The deltoid and pectoralis are allowed to fall together to close the deep wound. Subcutaneous tissue and skin are closed in a standard fashion. In most cases, hemostasis is adequate, and we have found it unnecessary to use a drain.

POSTERIOR CAPSULAR SHIFT

In a few of our patients with atraumatic multidirectional instability (AMBRI) that fail conservative treatment, we have identified a pattern in which the posterior direction is most symptomatic. We briefly delineate our surgical technique for the posterior capsular shift.

The patient is placed in the lateral decubitus position with the affected shoulder up. A vertical incision is made from just medial to the posterolateral corner of the acromion toward the posterior axillary fold approximately

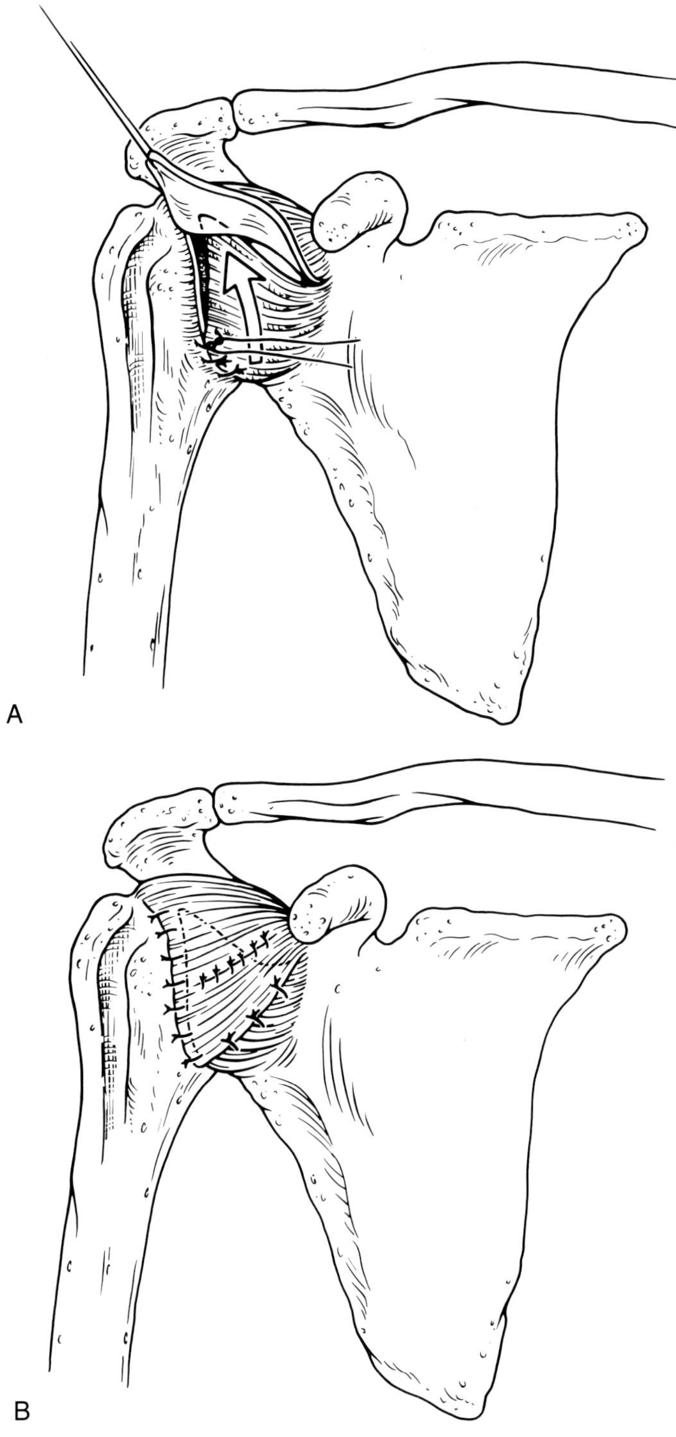

Figure 16-4. (**A & B**) Anterior capsular shift. Capsular repair is performed by superior and lateral advancement of the inferior flap and inferior and lateral advancement of the superior flap.

7 cm long and centered over the posterior glenohumeral joint. The fascia overlying the deltoid is more robust than anteriorly and requires sharp dissection. The deltoid is split in line with its fibers, and a deep self-retaining retractor is inserted (Fig. 16-5A). We have found it easier to split the fibers of the infraspinatus (not greater than 3 cm from the glenoid rim) for greater ease of exposure rather than developing the interval between the infraspinatus and teres minor (Fig. 16-5B). We have not noted any significant atrophy of the infraspinatus with this approach. In general,

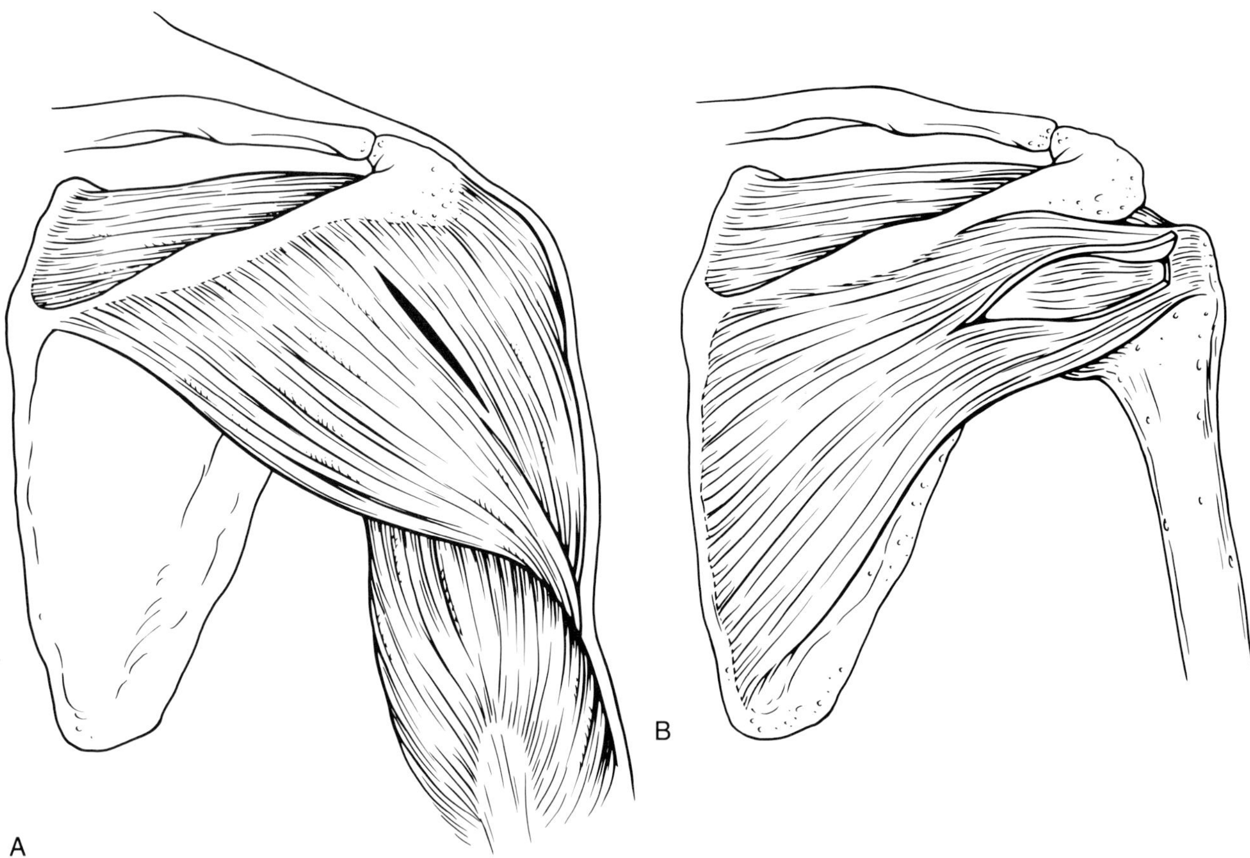

Figure 16-5. Posterior capsular shift. (**A**) The deltoid is split directly over the joint in the line of the muscle fibers. (**B**) The intraspinatus is split directly over the midlevel of the joint in the line of the muscle fibers. A short vertical incision in the tendon near its humeral insertion may be added to improve exposure of the capsule.

the tendons and muscle fibers peel off the posterior capsule with little difficulty. The capsular tissue is better on the glenoid side, and for that reason we prefer to do a modified capsular shift by release and repair of the capsule on the glenoid rather than on the humerus. Superior and inferior flaps are created in a fashion similar to that described for the anterior approach, except that the vertical incision is made along the glenoid margin (Fig. 16-6A). The capsule is incised lateral to the labrum so that the labrum is left attached securely to the glenoid rim. Only very rarely is a detachment of the labrum found posteriorly; thus, repair of the capsule posteriorly can be performed by suturing of the capsule to the labral tissue. After creation of the superior and inferior flaps, those flaps are advanced and prepared in the same menner as described for the anterior capsular shift (Fig. 16-6B). As noted, the difference in the posterior capsular shift is that we perform the procedure such that the flaps are repaired medially to the glenoid labrum. It is somewhat more difficult to tighten the capsule globally from the posterior approach. Rarely, after a posterior capsular shift, the anterior instability is still significant enough that we must do an anterior capsular shift in conjunction with the posterior procedure.

POSTOPERATIVE

Each patient is placed in a prefabricated orthosis (which has been fitted preoperatively) before leaving the operating room (Fig. 16-7). The splint places the shoulder in minimal abduction and neutral rotation in most cases. The arm position can be modified depending on the type of repair performed. A patient with predominantly posterior instability will be placed in slight external rotation to prevent stress on the posterior capsule. Patients are usually hospitalized overnight for observation, prophylactic antibiotics, and analgesics as necessary; however, most of these patients require very little pain medication.

We use the prefabricated orthosis for several reasons. The capsular shift requires a fair amount of dissection, and much of the tissue is quite fragile. The splint supports the arm in a cephalad direction, and thus the force of gravity

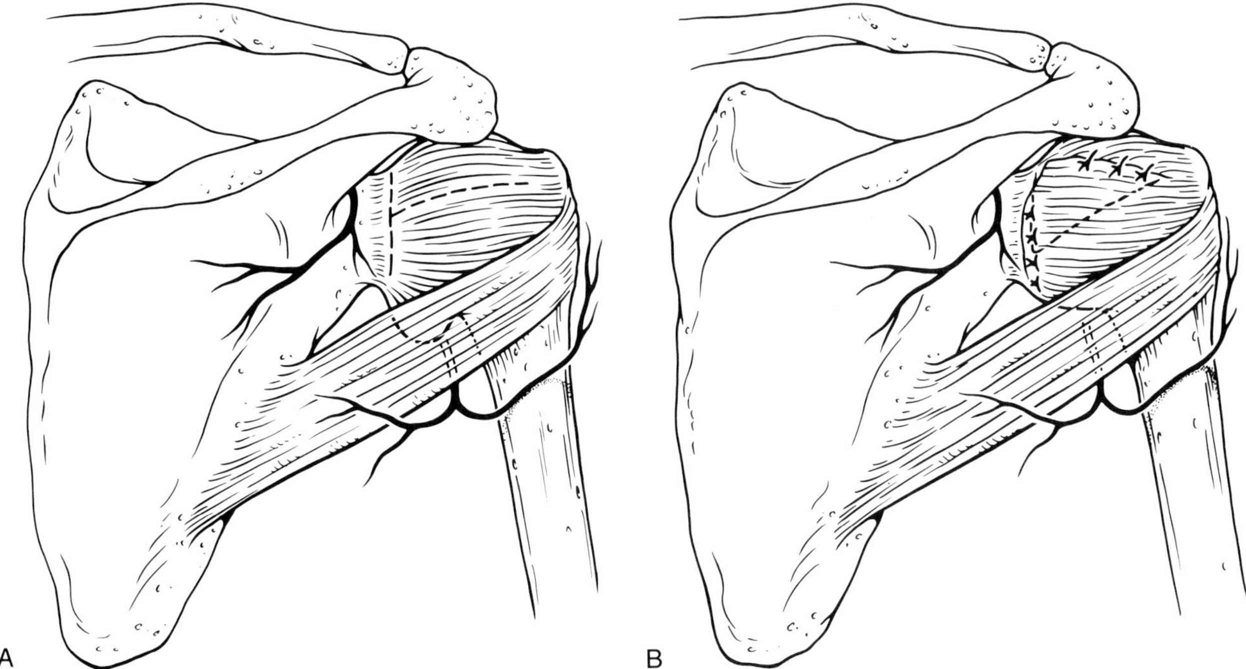

Figure 16-6. (**A**) Posterior capsular shift. A T capsulotomy is made in the posterior capsule with the vertical incision near the glenoid labrum. (**B**) Posterior capsular shift. Capsular repair is performed by superior and medial advancement of the inferior flap and inferior and medial advancement of the superior flap.

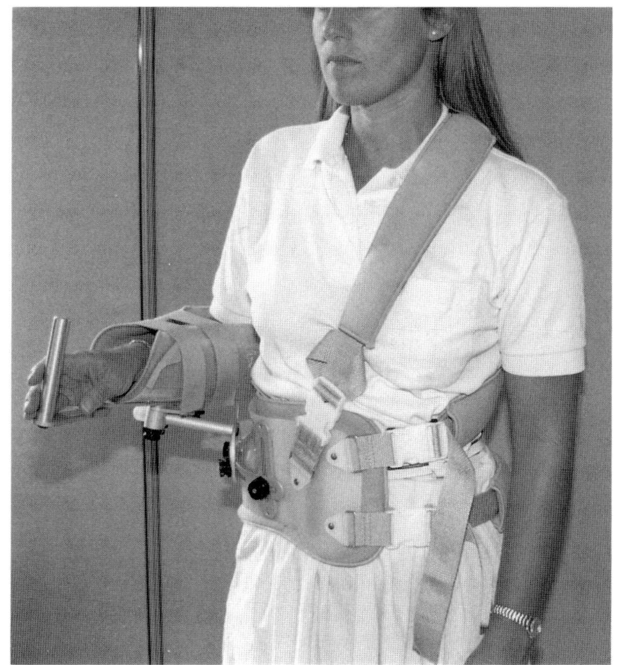

Figure 16-7. A prefabricated orthosis immobilizes the arm after surgery. Usually the arm is positioned in neutral rotation, but after a posterior capsular shift, more external rotation may be desired. Note that the orthosis lifts the affected extremity to prevent inferior stress on the capsular repair.

on the arm does not stress (or stretch) the inferior capsule during the healing phase. Commercially available orthosis are usually much easier to apply during surgery than are casts. These orthosis are tolerated well by patients and, in our experience, have been more comfortable for the patients and are more easily adjusted than casts. In occasional circumstances, we have used a simple arm immobilizer postoperatively rather than a cast or orthosis. However, this has been done only when the capsular tissues and the quality of the repair are both deemed to be quite good such that the concern for postoperative stretching of the repair is low.

We typically perform follow-up examination at monthly intervals. At each visit the stability of the repair is tested. During the first couple of months, stress testing is performed quite gently to avoid strain on the repair. A great deal of clinical judgment must be exercised to determine how fast/slow to progress the rehabilitation process after an inferior capsular shift for multidirectional instability. There is no "cookbook recipe" for how long to immobilize these patients. Variability in the technique used at the time of the capsular shift must be considered. We use immobilization as short as 4 weeks to as long as 4 months as required based on the individual and the tissue composition.

When the healing is thought to be satisfactory, the orthosis is discontinued, and the patient is placed in a shoulder immobilizer for comfort. The patient is allowed to use the affected arm for activities of daily living over the subsequent 4 weeks. Patients are allowed to wean themselves from the immobilizer as the discomfort subsides and they regain voluntary control of the shoulder. Most commonly, by 3 to 4 weeks after discontinuation of the orthosis, patients are ready to begin formal rehabilitation. If examination at that time reveals the shoulder irritation to be resolving and stability to be good, the patient is progressed to a program of gentle stretching and strengthening exercises. As the shoulder improves, gradual advances in the aggressiveness of the exercise regimen are made. Most patients can be given an appropriate home program and do not require regular visits to a physical therapist or athletic trainer. In general, we prefer elastic tubing and dumbbells and do not like to use any form of isokinetic therapy in the early rehabilitation process.

During the rehabilitation phase, the physician must constantly monitor the condition of the shoulder. The rehabilitation program must be adjusted for each individual patient. In the absence of significant generalized laxity and when a secure repair is accomplished at the time of surgery, the period of postoperative immobilization can be shortened and the aggressiveness of the rehabilitation exercises increased. By contrast, when the capsular tissues are poor and the repair is tenuous, the period of immobilization must be increased and the aggressiveness of the rehabilitation decreased. There is no "routine" postoperative management for this problem, and thus each case must be adjusted based on the ongoing assessment by the physician at the time of each examination.

Return to activities must be assessed individually also. Return to strenuous use of the arm, such as sports, varies from 6 to 12 months. For most patients, however, such recovery is typically in the range of 9 to 12 months.

PROGNOSIS

It has been our experience that greater than 90 percent of individuals with atraumatic multidirectional instability who undergo an inferior capsular shift attain good results with good stability and are able to function quite well with activities of daily living. Approximately two-thirds are able to return to sporting activities, but less than half are able to return to a high level of sports participation.

SURGICAL FAILURES

Any time revision surgery is contemplated, the reason for the initial failure must be determined to try to avoid repeating the same mistake. Determining the most symptomatic (i.e., anterior or posterior) direction of instability can often be made by careful history and repeat physical examinations on subsequent office visits. It is not uncommon for a patient to present with a failed anterior reconstruction for traumatic anterior instability when the underlying cause was multidirectional.

Possibly, the patient was not immobilized for a long enough period to allow the repair to heal adequately, or the early rehabilitation was too aggressive. Conversely, the patient may have been tightened excessively at the time of surgery, and then this was compounded by prolonged immobilization leading to a tight anterior capsule resulting in the humeral head going out the back.

Doing a revision of an inferior capsular shift is no different from any other type of revision orthopaedic case. The fascial planes are much more difficult to develop and, in most cases, must be performed by sharp dissection. The tissues can be distorted, and this is most important when attempting to release the inferior capsule due to the close proximity of the axillary nerve. Originally, Neer and Foster[7] reported three axillary nerve neuropraxias but did not delineate whether these patients had a previous shoulder procedure before the inferior capsular shift.

SUMMARY

Multidirectional instability can be a difficult shoulder ailment to diagnose correctly. Fortunately, most of these patients improve with rehabilitation and do not require surgical intervention. When rehabilitation fails, surgical reconstruction in the form of an inferior capsular shift can provide good to excellent results for activities of daily living but highly variable results for an athlete trying to get back to a high level of competition.

REFERENCES

1. Altchek DW, Warren RF, Skyhar MJ, Ortiz G: T-Plasty modification of the Bankart procedure for multidirectional instability of the anterior and inferior types. J Bone Joint Surg [Am] 73:105, 1991
2. Bowen MK, Warren RF: Ligamentous control of shoulder stability on selective cutting and static translation experiments. Clin Sports Med 10:757, 1991
3. Burkhead WZ Jr, Rockwood CA Jr: Treatment of instability of the shoulder with an exercise program. J Bone Joint Surg [Am] 74:890, 1992
4. Cooper RA, Brems JJ: The inferior capsular-shift procedure for multidirectional instability of the shoulder. J Bone Joint Surg [Am] 74:1516, 1992

5. Lebar RD, Alexander AH: Multidirectional instability. Am J Sports Med 20:193, 1992
6. Lippitt SB, Harryman DT, Sidles JA, Matsen FA: Diagnosis and management of AMBRI syndrome. Techniques Orthop 6:61, 1991
7. Neer CS, Foster CR: Inferior capsular shift for involuntary inferior and multidirectional instability of the shoulder. A preliminary report. J Bone Joint Surg [Am] 62:897, 1980
8. Thomas SC, Matsen FA: An approach to the repair of avulsion of the glenohumeral ligaments in the management of traumatic anterior glenohumeral instability. J Bone Joint Surg [Am] 71:506, 1989

CHAPTER SEVENTEEN

Acromioclavicular Joint Separations

Larry D. Field
Russell F. Warren

Subluxation or dislocation of the acromioclavicular joint is common after trauma to the shoulder. The extent of injury to the ligaments responsible for acromioclavicular joint stability along with trapezius and deltoid muscle attachments determines the direction and degree of instability. Treatment of certain types of acromioclavicular joint injuries remains controversial, and a clear understanding of the relevant anatomy and mechanisms of injury along with an effective classification system can assist the clinician in tailoring a treatment to a particular patient and injury.

ANATOMY

The acromioclavicular joint is classified as a diarthrodial joint averaging 9 mm by 19 mm in the adult.[12] Several investigators[16,40,53] have shown great variability in the angle of inclination of this joint (Fig. 17-1). No correlation between joint inclination and acromioclavicular joint injury[40] has been shown, but this variability should be kept in mind when performing a distal clavicle resection. Inman et al[26] noted that the acromioclavicular joint is capable of 20 degrees of total motion, with most of this motion occurring during the first 30 degrees of abduction. They also showed that the clavicle is capable of 40 degrees of upward rotation during shoulder flexion. Also, Kennedy and Cameron[30] noted that as the clavicle rotates upward the scapular rotates downward, resulting in synchronous motion that allows for placement of a lag screw between the clavicle and scapula without significantly affecting shoulder motion.

The acromioclavicular joint is stabilized by the strong superior and weaker inferior acromioclavicular ligaments. Additional but weak anterior and posterior ligaments are present as well. Fukuda et al[18] noted in a biomechanical study that the acromioclavicular ligament contributed approximately 90 percent of the ligamentous restraint to posterior displacement. This finding supports a classic study by Urist,[53] in which it was demonstrated that acromioclavicular joint stability was maintained even after cutting the trapezoid and conoid ligaments (Fig. 17-2A). In a second specimen, after both the superior acromioclavicular ligament and entire joint capsule were cut, subluxation of approximately 50 percent of the acromioclavicular joint developed (Fig. 17-2B and C). The incision was then extended to include the outer end of the clavicle, resulting in dissection of the muscles from the clavicle. This resulted in complete posterior dislocation but only in subluxation of the joint superiorly (Fig. 17-2D and E). Superior dislocation of the acromioclavicular joint occurred only after both the conoid and the more anterolaterally positioned trapezoid ligament were divided (Fig. 17-2F and G). Therefore, the conoid and trapezoid ligaments are the prime stabilizers, preventing superior dislocation, whereas the acromioclavicular ligament primarily resists horizontal translation.[42] Also, we have noted that the trapezoid and conoid ligaments tighten reciprocally with clavicle rotation, so that the trapezoid tightens on superior rotation and the conoid with inferior rotation.

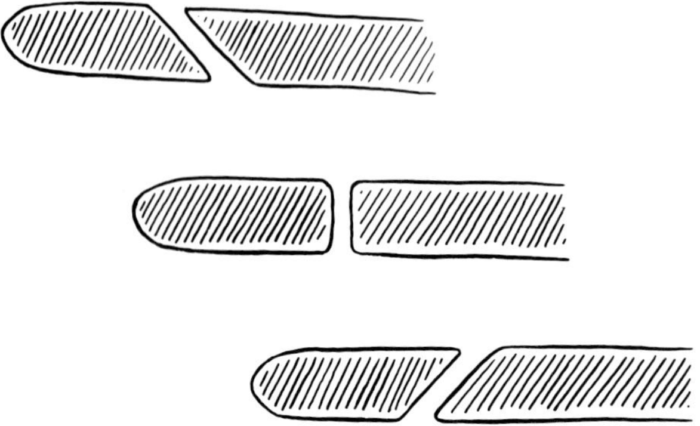

Figure 17-1. Angle of inclination of the acromioclavicular joint.

MECHANISM OF INJURY

Acromioclavicular joint injuries occur as a result of force applied directly to the shoulder or indirectly through the humerus. These injuries occur most commonly in the third and fourth decade and account for 12 percent of dislocations about the shoulder.[44] The direct mechanism of injury usually involves a fall onto the shoulder with the arm in an adducted position (Fig. 17-3A). Bearn[8] has shown through cadaveric studies that the sternoclavicular joint ligaments resist downward displacement of the distal clavicle. Also, Watkins[56] noted that the first rib limited downward displacement of the clavicle after application of a direct force (Fig. 17-3A). Continued depression of the acromion relative to the distal clavicle will result in either injury to the supporting ligaments about the acromioclavicular joint or a clavicle fracture. Also ipsilateral fracture of the clavicle[31,59] and the coracoid process[10,58] as well as sternoclavicular joint dislocations[45] can occur along with an acromioclavicular dislocation. When the acromioclavicular joint injury occurs without any associated fractures or other dislocations, then initial failure of the acromioclavicular ligaments is followed by disruption of the coracoclavicular ligaments. Failure of the coracoclavicular ligaments leads to loss of the primary suspension system of the arm, allowing the scapula to sag inferiorly relative to the clavicle. Continued force results in tearing of the deltoid and trapezius muscle attachments to the distal clavicle, increasing the deformity.[24,53]

The indirect mechanism of injury to the acromioclavicular joint occurs with transmission of a superiorly directed force through the humeral head to the undersurface of the acromion, as would occur with a fall onto the elbow or outstretched hand (Fig. 17-3B). Application of such a force would push the scapula superiorly relative to the clavicle, resulting in relaxation of the coracoclavicular ligaments as the distance between the coracoid and clavicle is reduced. The acromioclavicular ligaments, however, are eventually disrupted as acromial translation continues. Also, partial injuries to the acromioclavicular joint may occur in this setting, combined with rotator cuff contusions or tears.

CLASSIFICATION OF INJURIES

Classification systems as noted by Allman[2] and by Toss et al[52] have in the past subdivided acromioclavicular joint injuries into three grades based on anteroposterior (AP) radiographs and examination (Fig. 17-4). Grade I injuries constitute a sprain of the acromioclavicular ligaments and are characterized by no observable instability either radiographically or clinically. Grade II injuries represent incomplete stability of the acromioclavicular joint as illustrated by subluxation noted on AP radiographs. Grade III injuries represent complete acromioclavicular joint dislocations and often present both clinically and on AP radiographs with no contact at the joint surfaces. This occurs secondary to complete disruption of the coracoclavicular ligaments with subsequent loss of these ligaments' suspensory function that maintains approximation of the scapula with the clavicle.

These grading systems, however, have failed to include distinct variations of these injuries. In an effort to account for these variations, we have used an expanded classification system[55] based on a standard grading of ligament injuries from grades I to III (Table 17-1). To better classify patients with posterior subluxation of the clavicle on the acromion, grade II injuries have been subdivided. Grade IIA injuries represent the previously described inferior subluxations of the acromion at the acromioclavicular joint and are identified on radiographs. Grade IIB injuries represent posterior subluxations and are best visualized on axillary lateral radiographs. These grade IIB injuries result from complete disruption of the acromioclavicular ligaments, with stripping of the tissues of the outer clavicle.[53] Standard AP radiographs may fail to reveal the posterior subluxation present in grade IIB injuries and may only show slight widening of the acromioclavicular joint. Dislocations of the clavicle posteriorly on the acromion have been reported by Barber et al[5] and others.[48] Grade III injuries have also been subdivided to account for significant variations in displacement at the acromioclavicular joint. This subdivision of complete acromioclavicular joint dislocations into those with superior clavicular displacements of less than twice the width of the acromion (grade IIIA) and more than twice the width of the acromion (grade IIIB) represents degrees of soft tissue injury that may have significant implications with regard to treatment (Table 17-1). Finally, other subtypes such as inferior or subcoracoid dislocation of the clavicle[21] occur uncommonly.

AP radiographs alone may illustrate the extent of an acromioclavicular joint injury but commonly fail to define accurately the true degree of instability. Stress radiographs

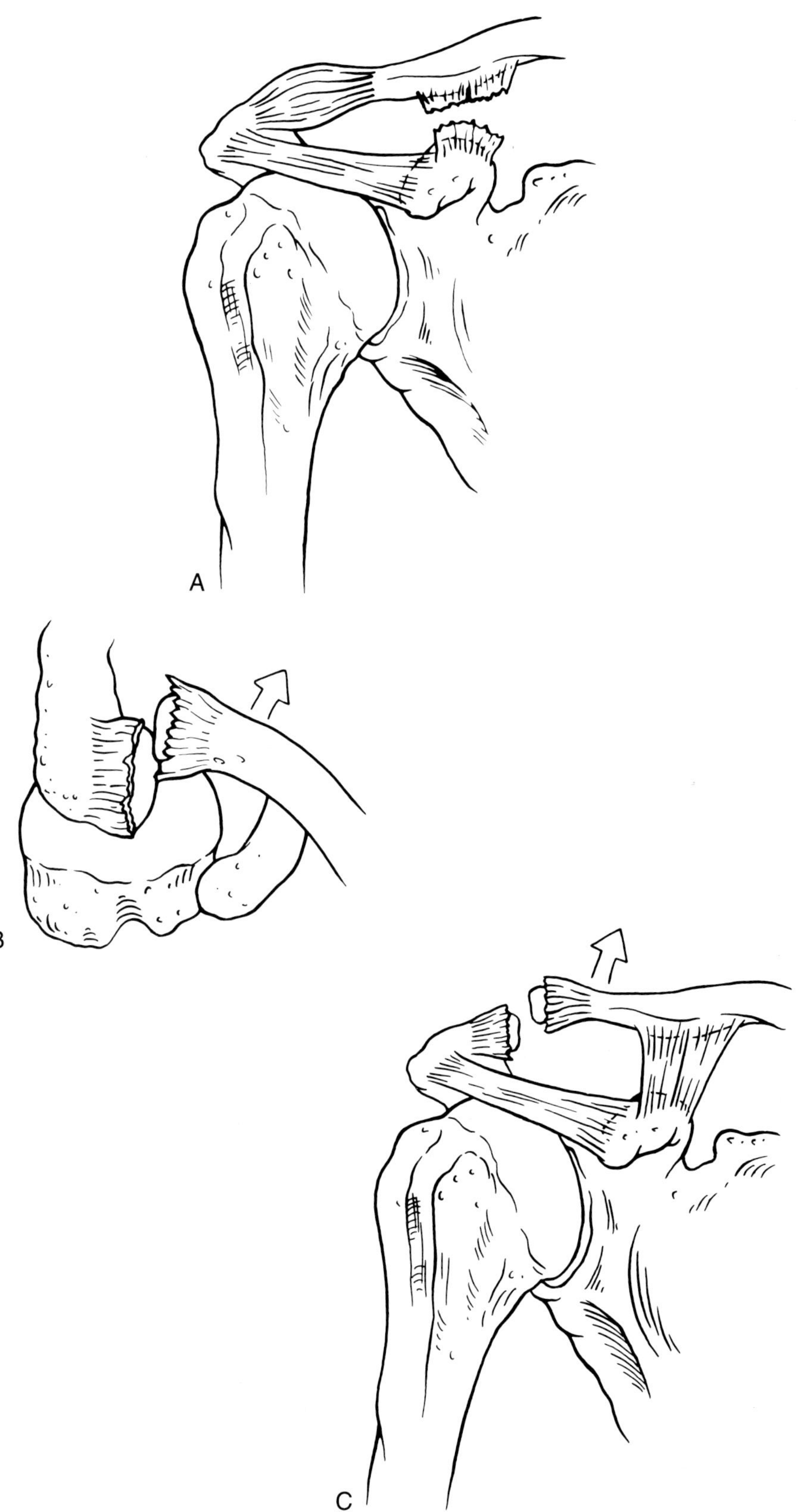

Figure 17-2. (**A**) Acromioclavicular instability after resection of the coracoclavicular ligaments. (**B & C**) Acromioclavicular ligaments and capsule. (*Figure continues.*)

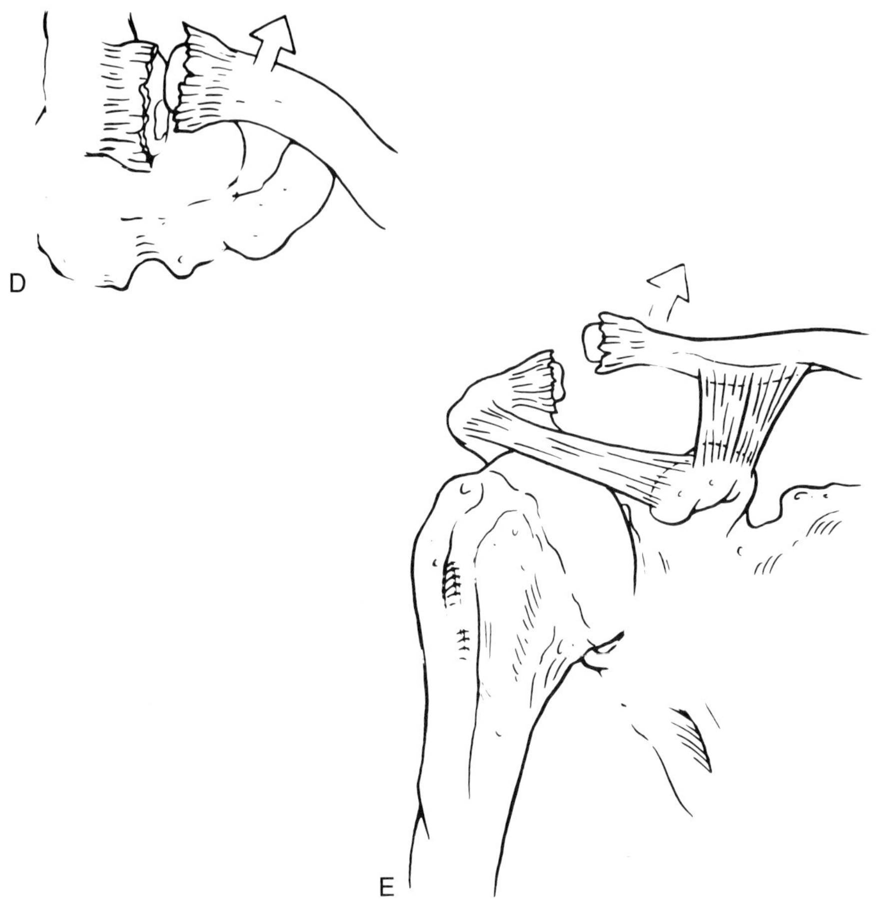

Figure 17-2. (*Continued*). (**D & E**) Resection of acromioclavicular ligaments and muscle attachment with resulting posterior dislocation of the acromioclavicular joint and mild scapular subluxation. (*Figure continues.*)

of both shoulders using 10 to 15 lb of weight attached to the wrists and performed with the patient sitting or standing are useful in helping to differentiate between a partial or complete disruption of the coracoclavicular ligaments and in defining the degree of displacement possible. These are no longer used routinely but only when a question as to treatment is raised. AP radiographs with a 15 degree cephalad tilt as recommended by Zanca[60] effectively avoid superimposition of the acromioclavicular joint onto the spine of the scapula and can help avoid overlooking intra-articular fractures at the acromioclavicular joint (Fig. 17-5). The average distance between the superior tip of the coracoid and the inferior margin of the clavicle should normally measure 1.1 to 1.3 cm[7,13] on an AP radiograph. However, comparison of radiographs from the injured and uninjured shoulder is important in helping to define the injury[42] Rockwood and Green[41] have suggested that widening of this coracoclavicular interval by 5 mm or 50 percent indicates a complete tear of the coracoclavicular ligament, but Rockwood and Matsen[42] have documented a complete disruption of the coracoclavicular ligaments, with a 25 percent difference in measurement. The axillary lateral radiograph is also an important view that can identify posterior displacement if present, as can the scapular lateral view.[1] Finally, radiographic technique specifically indicated for the acromioclavicular joint should be used to avoid the dark overpenetrated radiograph of the acromioclavicular joint obtained when radiographic technique designed for the glenohumeral joint is carried out.

SIGNS AND SYMPTOMS

Local tenderness and swelling over the acromioclavicular joint is present in acute injuries. The degree of tenderness may be mild as in grade I injuries or moderate-to-severe as in complete acromioclavicular joint dislocations. Also, tenderness at the coracoclavicular interspace is present when this ligament is significantly injured. Painful

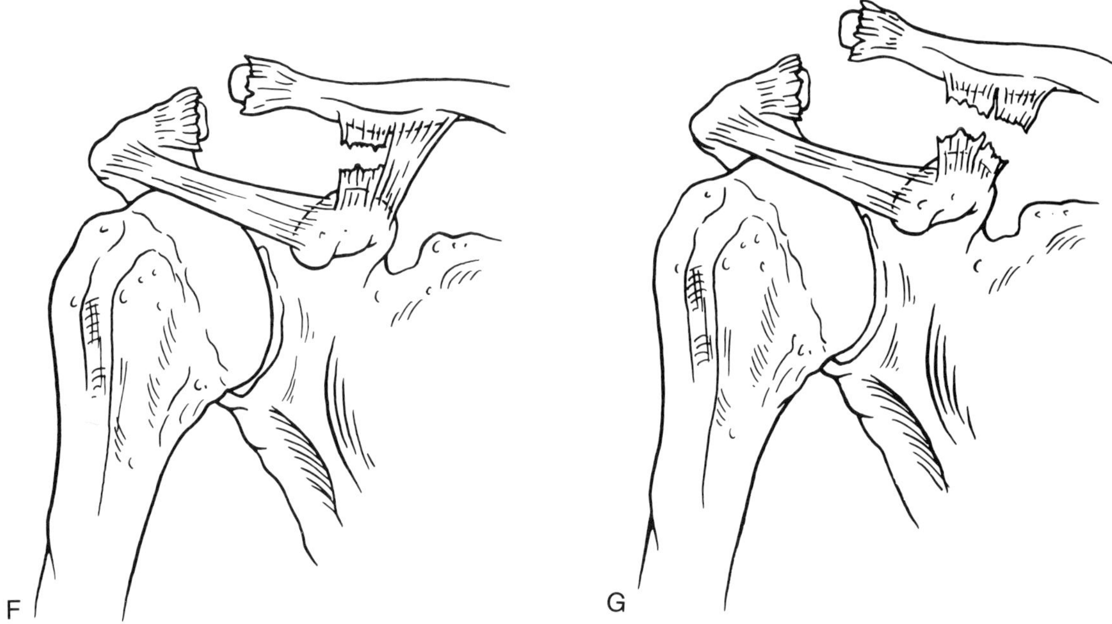

Figure 17-2. (*Continued*). (**F & G**) After completion of acromioclavicular ligament incision, only subluxation superiorly was present until the coracoclavicular ligaments were completely incised, allowing complete dislocation (Fig. G).

range of motion of the shoulder is present, especially after significant soft tissue disruption. Manipulation of the clavicle in the horizontal plane, especially if prominent, can help to assess the degree of posterior instability present. Also, pulling the arm inferiorly may assist in more accurately assessing the degree of displacement possible. The clavicle remains in its normal anatomic position while the acromion is displaced inferiorly in these injuries. Also, skin abrasions are common and should be carefully considered before any surgical intervention and monitored throughout treatment if a sling is used.

INDICATIONS FOR SURGERY

Grade I injuries of the acromioclavicular joint do not result in disruption of either the acromioclavicular or coracoclavicular ligaments, and little controversy exists regarding their appropriate treatment. There is no joint subluxation present, and simple arm sling immobilization for a short period until symptoms abate is often all that is necessary.

Subluxation exists at the acromioclavicular joint in grade IIA injuries, demonstrating some degree of ligament disruption. Most authors have recommended nonoperative treatment of these injuries. However, a study by Bergfeld et al[9] illustrated a 23 percent prevalance of persistent symptoms after nonoperative treatment. Also, Cox,[15] in a detailed study at Annapolis, reported on 164 acromioclavicular injuries, of which 60 percent were grade I, 32 percent were grade II, and 8 percent were grade III. Grade II injuries frequently resulted in symptoms at follow-up. Cox classified these symptoms as major in 13 percent and minor in 35 percent. Use of a Kenny-Howard type of immobilization significantly reduced this incidence when used for 4 to 6 weeks. Of 32 patients with grade II injuries that were not immobilized, 20 patients were symptomatic at follow-up; of 20 patients immobilized, only 5 were symptomatic.

Grade IIB injuries in which there is posterior subluxation are uncommon but will often require surgical intervention. Dislocation of the distal clavicle posterior to the acromion can occur,[5,48] and closed reduction may not be possible as the distal clavicle can become wedged between the posterior acromion and the scapular spine. Closed reduction can be attempted by displacing the scapula posteriorly to increase its distance from the sternum. If closed reduction fails, open reduction is indicated.

Treatment of grade III injuries of the acromioclavicular joint remains controverisal. Many articles promoting either nonoperative or operative treatment of these injuries have been published. Also, among those authors preferring nonoperative management, there have been many techniques for maintaining a reduction from adhesive bandages and

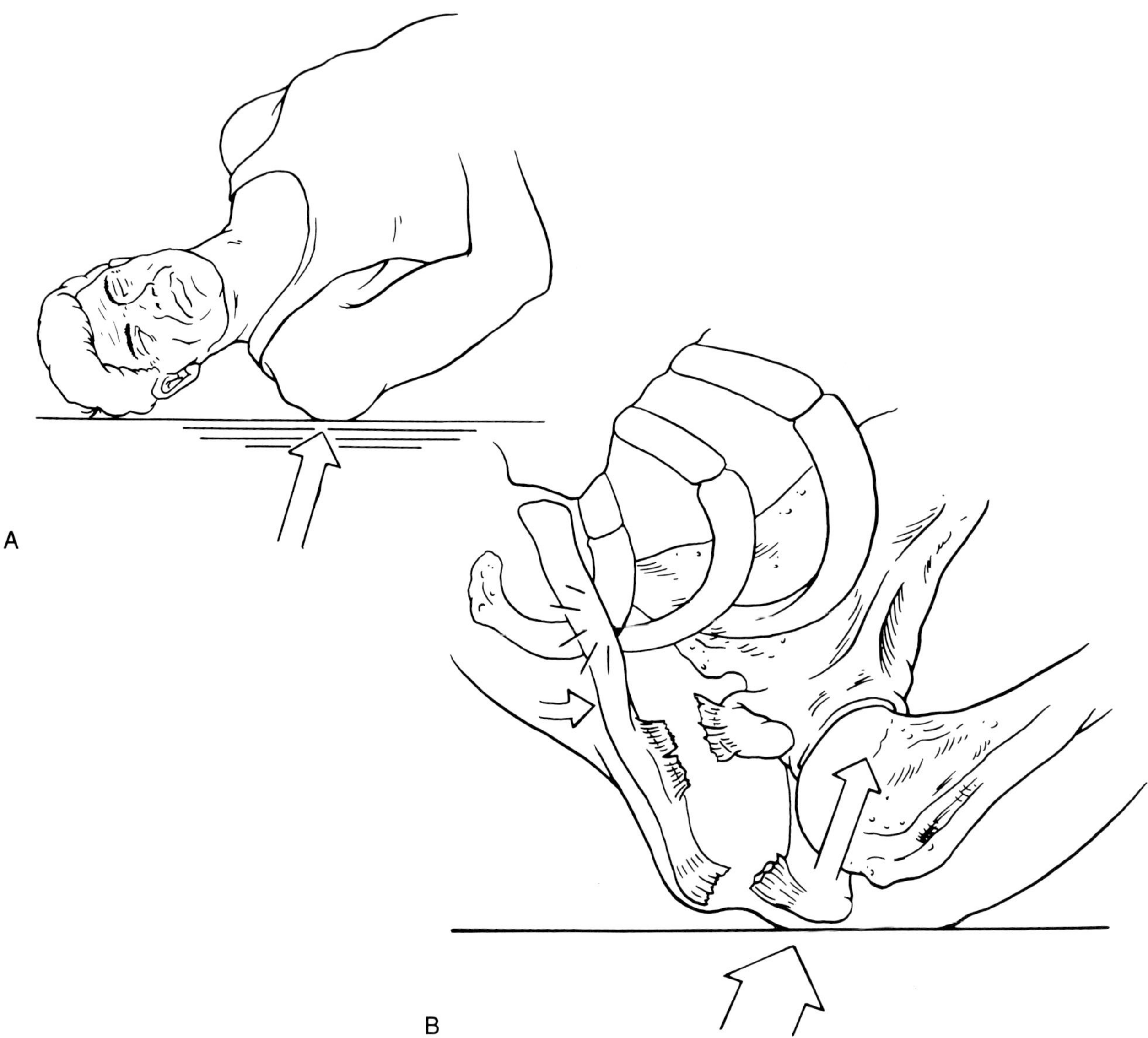

Figure 17-3. (**A & B**) Direct mechanism of acromioclavicular joint injury. (*Figure continues.*)

strapping to spica cast immobilization and the more modern Kenny-Howard sling.

Operative treatment for grade IIIA injuries to the acromioclavicular joint has been justified in the past at least partly on the contention that significant deficits in strength result from nonoperative treatment. However, several studies[23,34,51,54] have shown shoulder strength in nonoperative patients to be equal to either the uninjured arm or to patients undergoing operative treatment. Walsh and colleagues[54] evaluated 17 patients using the Cybex Isokinetic Dynamometer and reported that nine operatively treated patients who had greater deficits of abduction torque (19.8 percent) than the nonoperative patients, but external rotation was normal. Galpin et al[20] noted in a study comparing 21 nonoperatively treated patients with 16 patients treated using a Bosworth screw no significant strength differences as measured by a cable tensiometer. These studies do seem to contradict effectively the argument for surgical intervention on the grounds of strength maintenance alone. These studies, along with other investigations comparing functional outcomes of operatively and nonoperatively treated groups of patients,[4,25,27,32,49] found little difference between the groups. Based on the studies available, it is difficult to definitively support a specific form of treatment for all injuries. In our opinion, grade IIIA injuries, which by definition have displacements of less than twice the width of the acromion, usually may be treated nonoperatively by closed reduction. Treatment plans must be individualized,

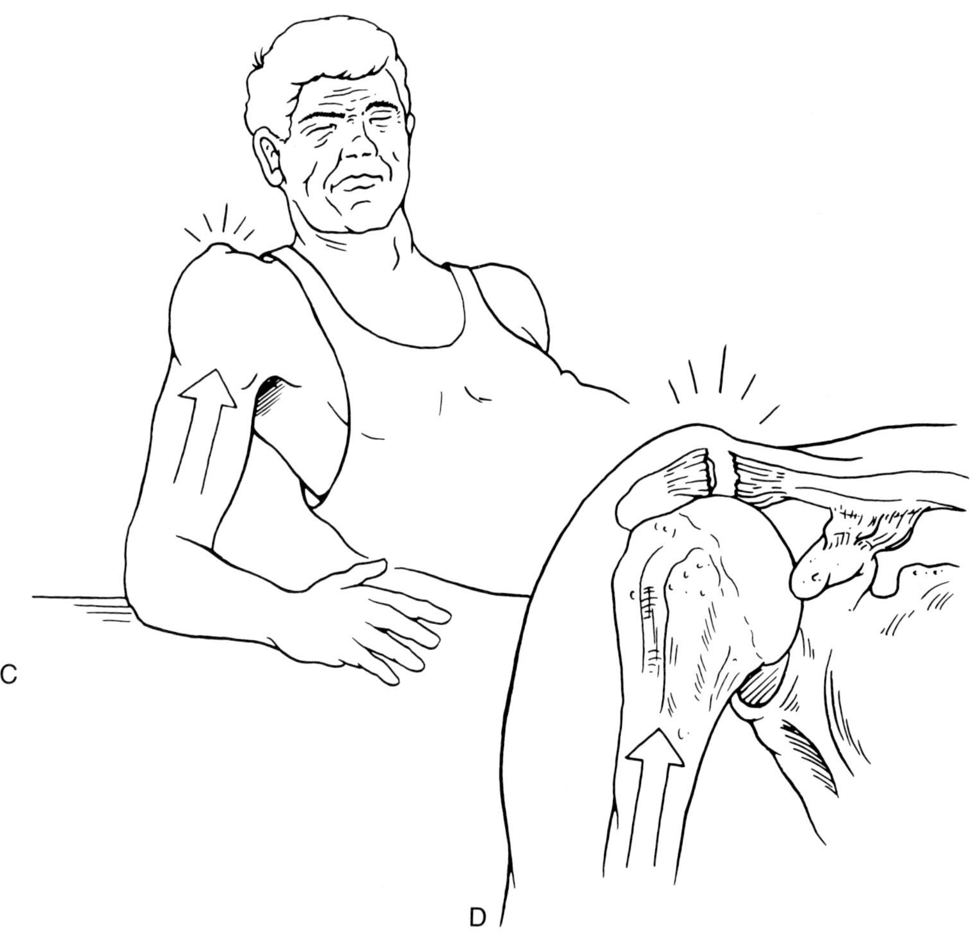

Figure 17-3. *(Continued).* (**C & D**) Indirect mechanism of acromioclavicular joint injury.

however, and in some cases, the possibility of surgery could be entertained if the patient is greatly concerned about the prominence and desires a more cosmetically pleasing appearance. Grade IIIB injuries, with gross displacement associated with muscle stripping and marked prominence of the distal clavicle, would be better served by an open procedure.

Patients with chronic acromioclavicular joint injuries may seek treatment for a painful acromioclavicular joint or due to a longstanding prominence. The acromioclavicular joint can become painful and degenerate after injury regardless of initial treatment or grade of injury. The original insult to the joint can result in intra-articular fragments of cartilage, an unstable meniscus, or persistent instability that can lead to chronic symptoms.

Arthritic changes after acromioclavicular joint injury and the need for subsequent joint resection occur in nearly equal frequency in operative and nonoperative patients. Taft et al,[49] in a study of 127 patients with acromioclavicular dislocations of whom 52 were treated operatively at a 10-year follow-up, noted that arthritis occurred in 42 percent of untreated patients and in 43 percent of those treated operatively. There was a suggestion in their study that arthritis after fixation with pins through the acromioclavicular joint was more ''severe'' than after coracoclavicular fixation techniques. Overall, 13 of 127 patients in their study required lateral clavicle resection. Treatment of these patients should consist initially of nonsteroidal antiinflammatory medications in conjunction with strengthening exercises and the avoidance of overhead activities. If there is no improvement, injection of an anti-inflammatory medication and Xylocaine into the acromioclavicular joint may be helpful. One should note the response to the injection as a confirmatory test. If symptoms continue to persist, excision of the outer end of the clavicle alone, as described by Gurd[22] and by Mumford[37] or by an arthroscopic technique,[36] can be performed when minor degrees of displacement at the acromioclavicular joint exist. When a grade III injury associated with a prominent distal clavicle is present, however, we recommend stabilization of the clavi-

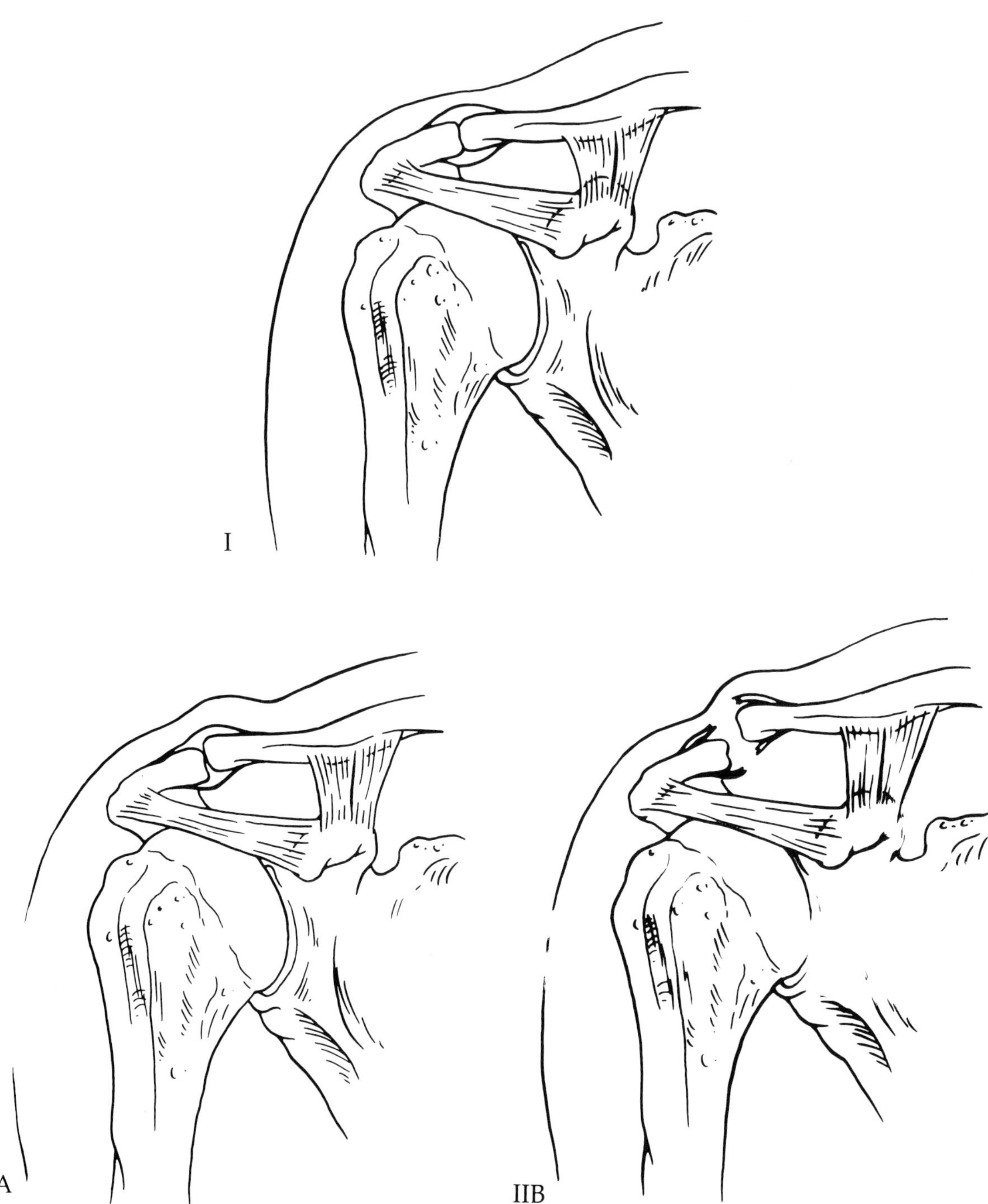

Figure 17-4. Classification of acromioclavicular joint injuries based on the degree of clavicular displacement resulting from ligament disruption. Grade I: mild sprain of acromioclavicular ligament with no instability. Grade II: subluxation of the acromioclavicular joint less than the width of the acromion. A subtype of grade II is posterior subluxation (IIB). This will have a similar appearance on an AP view except for widening of the joint space. Both IIA and IIB will have intact or slightly stretched coracoclavicular ligaments. (*Figure continues.*)

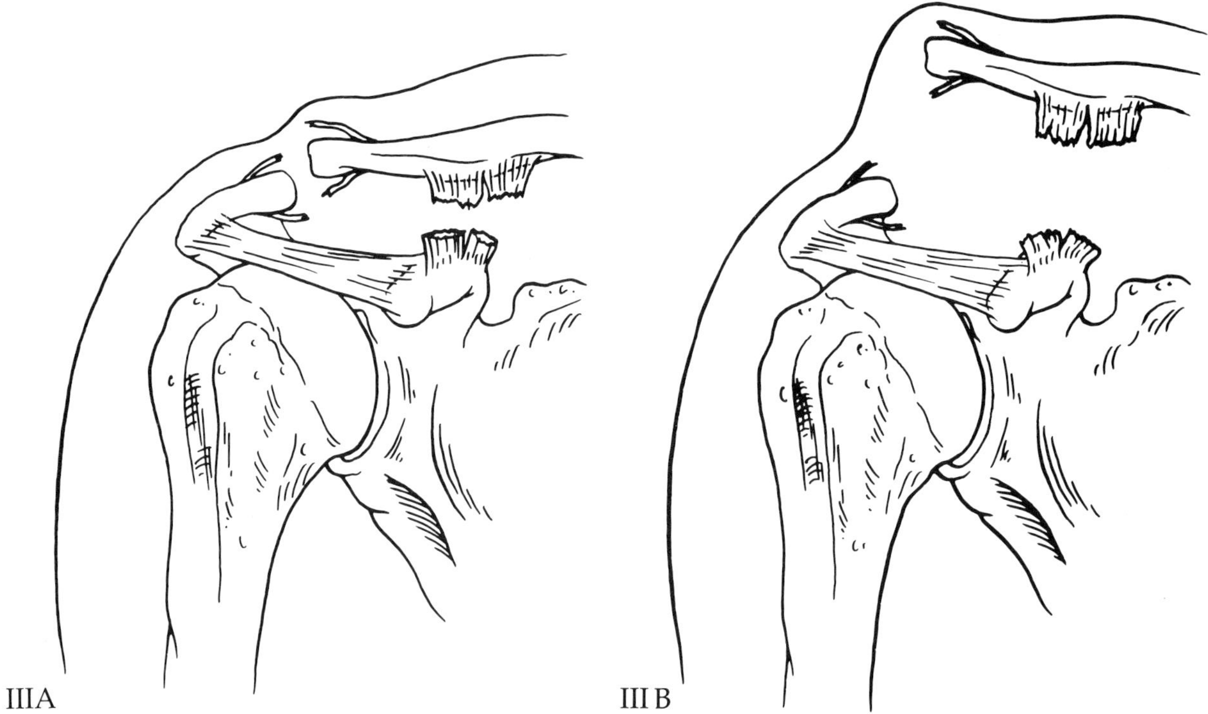

Figure 17-4. (*Continued*). Grade III: sprain with disruption of both the acromioclavicular ligaments and the coracoclavicular ligaments. This results in superior displacement of the clavicle, which in grade IIIA is greater than 1 but less than twice the width of the acromion and in IIIB is greater than twice the width of the acromion.

cle to the coracoid after distal clavicle excision, as symptoms from the inferior displacement of the scapula may persist.

NONOPERATIVE TREATMENT

After the decision to manage a patient with an acromioclavicular joint injury nonoperatively, a specific form of treatment must be selected. Various methods of immobilization have been reported and are often based on the degree of injury to the acromioclavicular joint. The primary goal in the treatment of these injuries regardless of grade is to return the patient to full activities as quickly as possible.

Grade I injuries are treated with a simple arm sling usually for 1 week or less followed by range of motion and strengthening exercises as symptoms abate. Grade IIA injuries are likewise treated with simple arm sling immobilization and an ice pack for the first 24 hours postinjury. The period of immobilization in the arm sling can be individualized but generally continues for 7 to 14 days. During this time and subsequently, an exercise program is instituted with athletic activities resumed after 3 to 6 weeks. Contact sports may be delayed until relatively pain-free motion and strength are present. We have not seen a grade IIA injury converted to a grade III injury by early return to athletics.

Nonoperative treatment of grade IIIA injuries has been accomplished through a variety of means. The Kenny-Howard sling[14] is designed to maintain reduction of the acromioclavicular joint dislocation by transferring the weight of the arm through the padded strap over the clavicle and is positioned medial to the acromioclavicular joint. Taft et al[49] recommended use of the Kenny-Howard sling continuously for 5 to 6 weeks. This sling, however, must be tight enough to maintain the reduction and must be used continuously to ensure stability and prevent late displacement at the acromioclavicular joint. We no longer use the Kenny-Howard sling as the primary method of closed treatment after noting the tendency of the acromioclavicular joint to sublux after treatment. The sling, however, can be helpful, especially early in the course of treatment by decreasing pain through a temporary reduction in acromioclavicular joint displacement. It is important to carefully monitor the skin for breakdown throughout treatment by removing the strap each day. We prefer use of a simple arm sling to be worn usually for 1 to 2 weeks as symptoms dictate. Gentle range of motion exercises are generally started after 1 week, followed by light strengthening exercises using elastic bands on the second week. A progressive exercise program that includes strengthening of the deltoid, trapezius, and rotator cuff muscles is then advanced

Table 17-1. Classification of Acromioclavicular Joint Injuries

Grade	AC Ligament	CC Ligament	Radiographic Findings
I	Injured, intact	Intact	No displacement of AC joint
IIA	Ruptured	Intact	Superior clavicle less than width of acromion
IIB	Torn with muscle dissection at end of clavicle	Intact	Joint widened. Axillary view shows posterior displacement
IIIA	Ruptured	Ruptured	Superior clavicular displacement more than width of acromion but less than twice the width of acromion
IIIB	Ruptured, with increased soft tissue detachment from the clavicle	Ruptured	Superior clavicular displacement more than twice the width of acromion

Abbreviations: AC, acromioclavicular, CC, coracoclavicular.

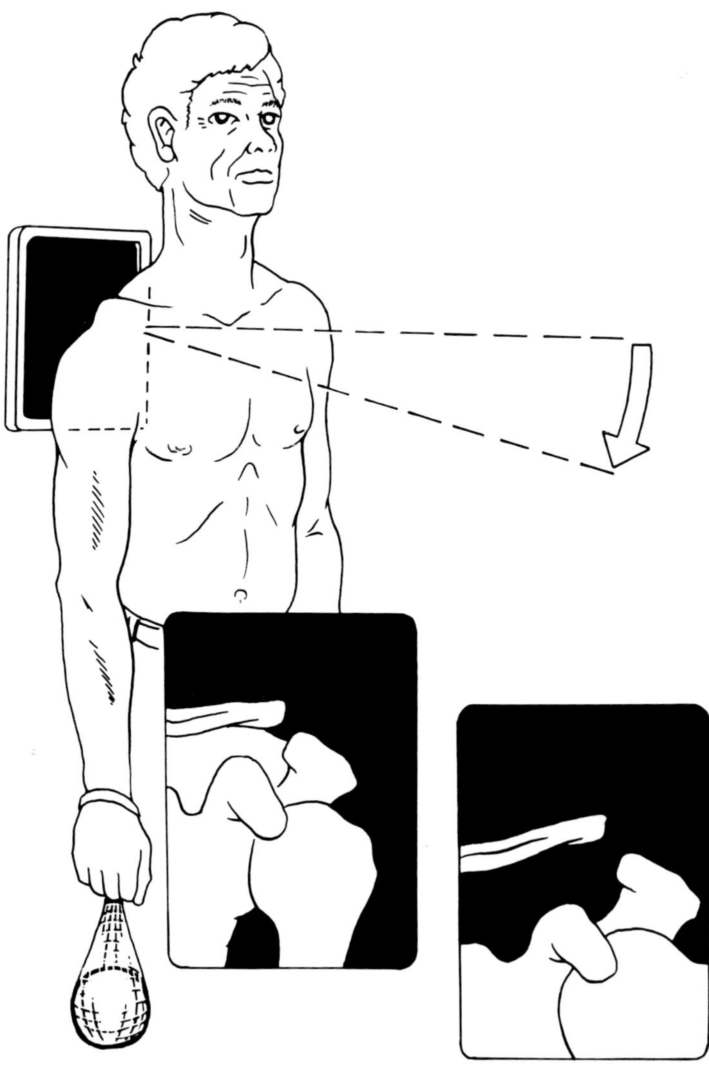

Figure 17-5. Radiographic technique for demonstrating acromioclavicular joint dislocation.

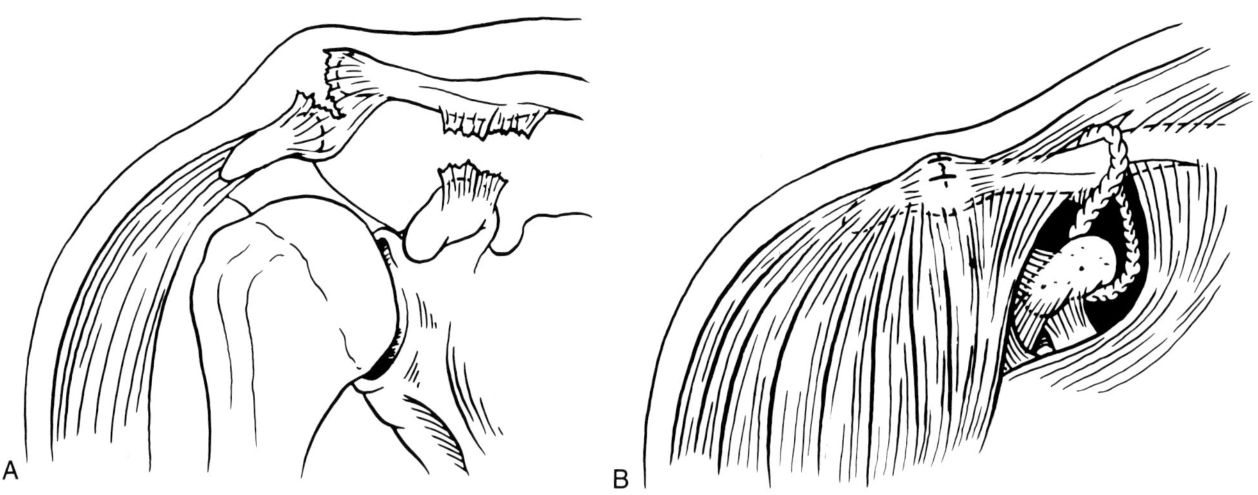

Figure 17-6. (**A & B**) In acute dislocations, reduction and stabilization are achieved by using PDS absorbable suture (Ethicon). Nine strands of suture are braided and passed under the base of the coracoid and over the clavicle and tied after reduction. Subsequent healing of the coracoclavicular ligaments will maintain the reduction.

through the sixth week. Sports activities can often be restarted on the third or fourth week in these patients. A prominence, if one persists after recovery, is generally not of concern to the patient. Also, after recovery, these patients can generally return within 6 to 8 weeks to their preinjury level of activity without limitation.

SURGICAL TREATMENT

Many operative procedures designed to repair or reconstruct acute grade IIB, grade IIIA, and grade IIIB acromioclavicular joint dislocations have been used. These various techniques can, however, be loosely grouped into the following categories: (1) direct acromioclavicular joint stabilization[43] with ligament repair; (2) reduction of the acromioclavicular joint by means of extra-articular stabilization from the clavicle to the coracoid by means of a Bosworth screw,[13] silk sutures,[56] wire loops,[7] Dacron tape,[6,28,39,50] or Ethicon PDS absorbable suture; (3) excision of the distal clavicle with transfer of the coracoacromial ligament to the remaining distal clavicle[67]; and (4) dynamic muscle transfers.[11,17,46] These procedures are all designed to reduce the acromioclavicular joint dislocation and allow for soft tissue healing in a more anatomic position, but mild deformity often remains.

Stabilization of the acromioclavicular joint with Kirschner wires or pins can often maintain reduction of acromioclavicular ligament dislocations. The risk of wire breakage and migration[33] has decreased the popularity of this technique. Placement of a lag screw from the clavicle to the base of the coracoid along with acromioclavicular joint debridement[29] has also been performed commonly. The screw is generally removed at about 8 weeks postoperatively. Dacron tape has been used for coracoclavicular stabilization. However, the tape has led to erosion and fractures, and failure of the tape has been reported as well.[19] Weaver and Dunn[57] reported on a technique involving excision of the distal clavicle followed by transfer of the coracoacromial ligament to the interamedullary canal of the resected distal clavicle. It is our preference to save the outer end of the clavicle in a acute injury unless there is an associated clavicle fracture very near or involving the acromioclavicular joint. Lastly, transfer of the tip of the coracoid with its attached short head of the biceps and coracobrachialis to the clavicle has also been performed.[11,17,46] This muscle transfer is designed to act as a dynamic stabilizer of the clavicle and maintain reduction at the acromioclavicular joint.

OUR PREFERRED TECHNIQUES

Acute Injuries

Surgical repair of an acute grade III injury is accomplished through an incision directed vertically and inferiorly from the posterior border of the clavicle toward the coracoid for approximately 4 cm. The acromioclavicular joint is then explored and debrided of any osteochondral fracture fragments. Excision of the meniscus is performed only if it is torn. Reduction of the acromioclavicular joint is then accomplished by passing an absorbable tape composed of nine strands of size 0 braided PDS (Ethicon) suture around the base of the coracoid and then over the clavicle (Fig. 17-6). The base of the coracoid is identified by spearation of the deltoid in line with its fibers for a distance of about 4 cm. Subperiosteal dissection around the base of the coracoid is then carried out, and a right angle clamp is then used to pull the braided PDS around the coracoid. Passage of this braided suture very near to the coracoid base is important to prevent anterior translation of the distal clavicle as the PDS braid is tightened. An alternative approach, which may decrease the tendency for anterior translation of the clavicle, is to drill a 1/4-in. hole in the clavicle and pass the braid through this hole before tightening. After reduction of the acromioclavicular joint is confirmed, the PDS braid is tied down with the knot anterior and inferior on the clavicle to avoid prominence of the knot. Coracoclavicular ligament repair is generally not performed unless direct and complete avulsion from the bone is noted, in which case reattachment is performed.

After stabilization of the acromioclavicular joint, the acromioclavicular ligaments are reapproximated when possible along with trapezius and deltoid muscle attachments. The wound is then irrigated and closed with a subcuticular pullout suture. Postoperatively, an arm sling is used for approximately 1 week, during which time pendulum exercises are performed. After 1 week, range of motion exercises to but not exceeding 90 degrees of elevation are encouraged. Internal and external rotation exercises using elastic bands are begun during the second week. Further elevation and aggressive rehabilitation and strengthening regimens are delayed until 6 weeks postoperatively. Also, heavy weight lifting is avoided for 3 months. In essence, the PDS braid acts as an internal splint allowing for ligamentous scarring until it is resorbed (56 days).

This procedure to date has resulted in excellent realignment with only occasional mild residual prominence. Neither clavicular erosion or fracture, as has been seen with the Dacron graft, has occurred.

Chronic Injuries

Symptomatic degenerative changes of the acromioclavicular joint occur after all grades of injury. Cox[15] found that 8 percent of patients with grade I injuries and 13 percent of patients with Grade II injuries continued to have major symptoms at follow-up. If conservative measures including nonsteroidal medications, strengthening exercises, and acromioclavicular joint injections fail to improve symptoms, then consideration should be given to distal clavicle excision. In the absence of significant displacement of the clavicle on the acromion, simple excision of approximately 1 to 1.5 cm is usually adequate toward alleviating symptoms. Both open and arthroscopic techniques have proved valuable.

Open excision of the distal aspect of the clavicle begins with a vertical incision over the lateral clavicle just medial to the acromioclavicular joint (Fig. 17-7A). A transverse

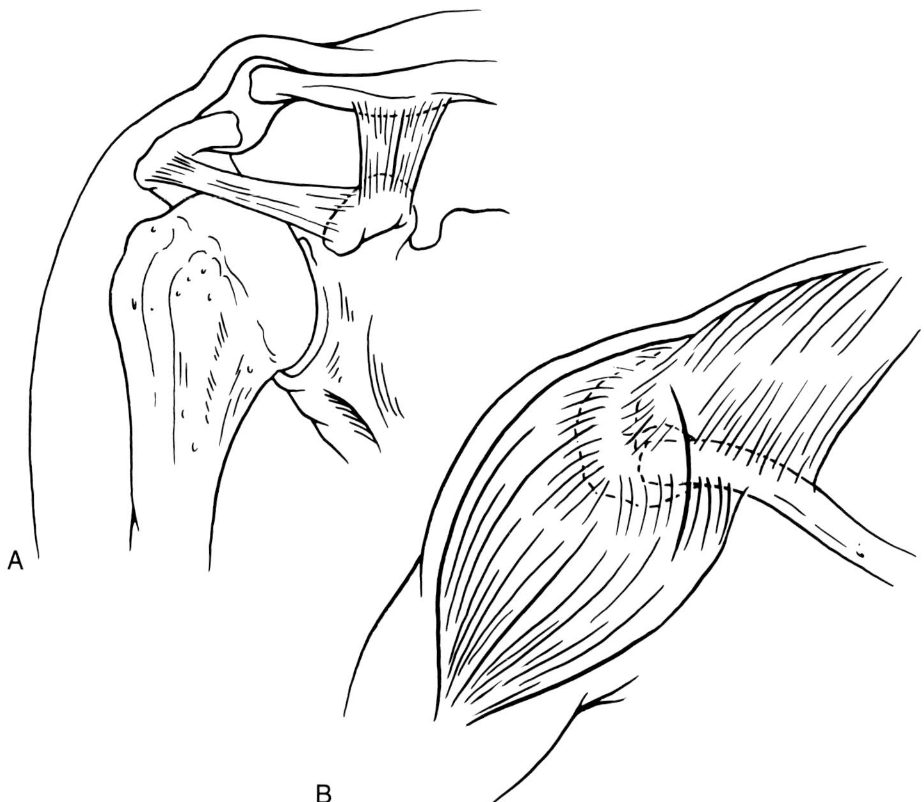

Figure 17-7. Technique for open distal clavicle resection. (**A & B**) Vertical incision allows for excellent exposure and cosmetic wound healing. (*Figure continues.*)

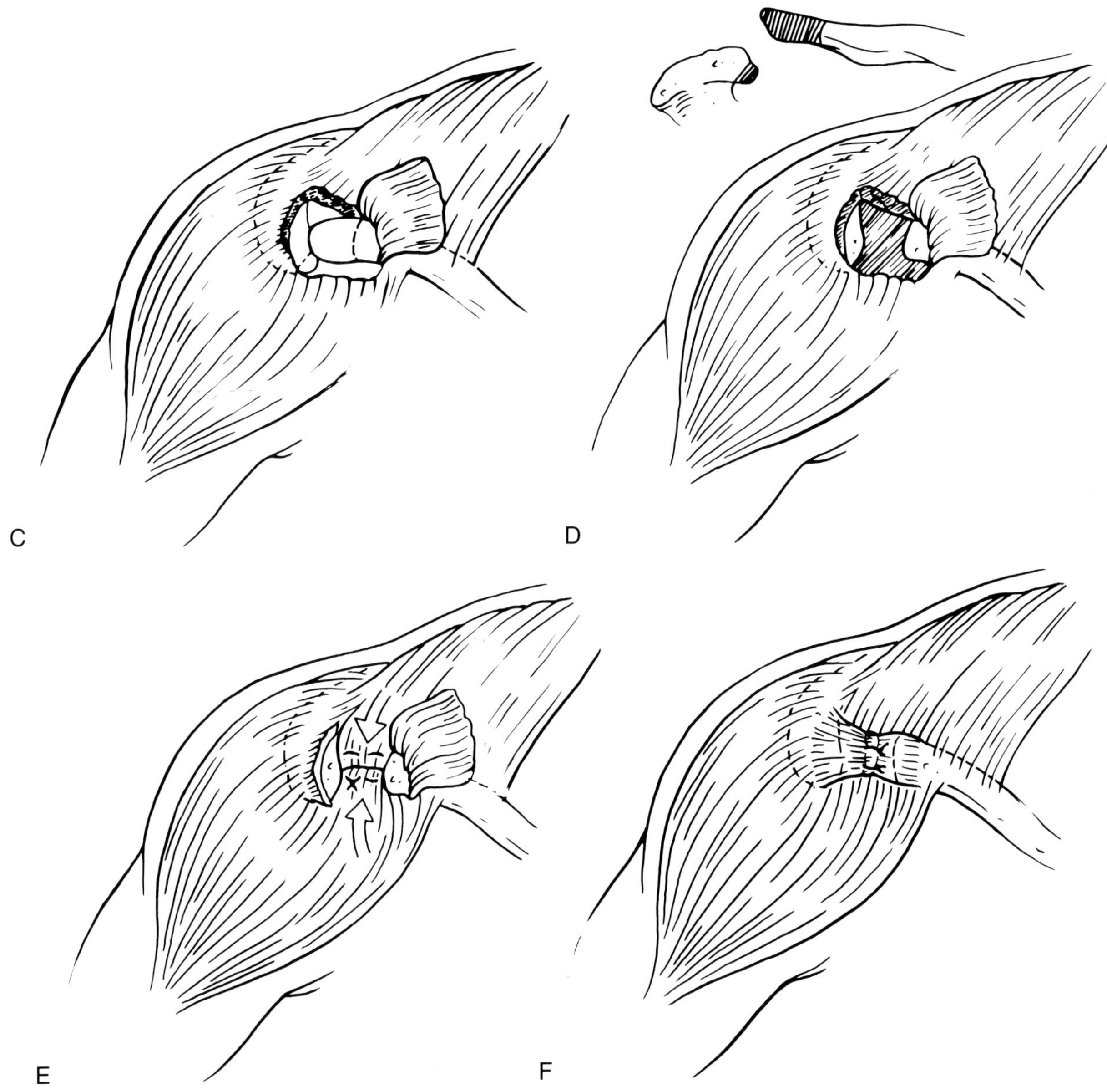

Figure 17-7. (*Continued*). (**C–F**) The distal clavicle is resected while preserving the acromioclavicular ligament muscular attachments to allow for muscle interposition within the defect.

incision directly over the joint is followed by subperiosteal dissection of the outer clavicle with preservation of the aponeurosis of the deltoid and trapezius as well as any remaining acromioclavicular joint to provide some stability to the outer clavicle. Small Bennett retractors are placed about the outer clavicle to protect the rotator cuff lying beneath the acromioclavicular joint. A power saw is used to remove the lateral clavicle. The osteotomy is performed in an oblique manner from anterior to posterior and lateral to medial (Fig. 17-7C). The amount of bone excised will vary with the angle of joint inclination (Fig. 17-1), but the resection should avoid injury to the coracoclavicular ligaments and allow clearance of the acromion during adduction and elevation of the arm. In checking the adequacy of the resection, a finger is placed in the defect while an adduction test is performed with the arm at 90 degrees. During this maneuver, the acromion should not be in contact with the clavicle. Possible causes of failure are inadequate resection of the posterolateral clavicle or failure to remove osteophytes on the deep surface of the acromial side of the joint. After resection of the distal clavicle, the defect is closed by pulling the deltoid and trapezius into the area of resection and overlapping them with the remaining joint capsule (Fig. 17-7D and E). Postoperatively, an arm sling is used as symptoms dictate. On the first postoperative day, pendulum exercises are initiated with range of motion exercises beginning on postoperative day 2 or 3. During the second or third postoperative week, resistance exercises using elastic bands are started and then advanced under supervision for 2 to 3 months.

Arthroscopic Technique

Excision of the distal clavicle using an arthroscopic technique can be accomplished with the patient either in the lateral decubitus position with the arm suspended at 60 degrees of abduction or with the patient positioned in the beach chair position.[47] The patient is placed supine using the beach chair position with the torso raised approximately 70 degrees and the patient shifted on the table toward the affected extremity. Once positioned, three primary portals—the posterior, anterior, and lateral—are used.[3] After arthroscopically directed examination of the glenohumeral joint, attention is turned to the subacromial space. If necessary, a partial bursectomy is performed to allow adequate visualization of the acromioclavicular joint. Next, with the inflow cannula in the posterior portal and the arthroscope in the lateral portal, excision of the distal end of the clavicle is accomplished using the arthroscopic burr through the anterior portal. Care should be taken to rcmove any osteophytes from the undersurface of the medial acromion at the acromioclavicular joint as well. After excision of approximately 1.5 cm of distal clavicle, the arthroscope is transferred to the anterior portal to confirm complete removal of the distal clavicle. If the excision is incomplete, the burr should again be placed through the anterior portal and removal of the distal clavicle completed. The protocol for postoperative management is the same as for the open technique of distal clavicle excision described previously.

Open Technique with Coracoclavicular Ligament Reconstruction

Significantly displaced chronic acromioclavicular joint injuries present a different challenge. We believe that in the presence of marked prominence of the clavicle, simple excision of the distal clavicle is usually inadequate. Stabilization of the clavicle to the coracoid helps re-establish the suspensory function of the coracoclavicular ligament. Occasionally, patients with marked prominence of the clavicle secondary to complete disruption of the coracoclavicular ligaments will present with symptoms suggestive of a throacic outlet syndrome. Vague complaints of weakness, fatigue, and parathesias aggravated by a dependent posture are not uncommon. Reconstruction of the coracoclavicular ligament at the time of surgical intervention may reduce this traction effect on the plexus that results from the lack of scapular suspension through the coracoclavicular ligaments.

Our preferred surgical technique for a chronically dislocated acromioclavicular joint begins with open distal clavicle excision as described for minimally displaced distal clavicles (see Fig. 17-7). However, before closure of the muscle defect, the remaining clavicle is reduced, and the coracoacromial ligament, if available, or a strip of conjoined tendon is used to maintain this reduction. Both of these tendons have the mild disadvantage of an anterior inclination, but resection of the distal clavicle minimizes the effect of clavicular translation.

If the coracacromial ligament is used, dissection of tissue from the undersurface of the acromion should be attempted to maximize length, and a fragment of bone from the coracoacromial ligament insertion should be removed to facilitate fixation to the resected end of the clavicle (Fig. 17-8A and B). When the conjoined tendon is used, the skin incision is extended inferiorly for 4 cm, being careful to avoid the musculcutaneous nerve (Fig. 17-8B). In taking part of the conjoined tendon, a strip of about 8 mm in width allows closure of the tendinous defect. Regardless of which tissue is used, it is then placed in the medullary canal of the distal end of the clavicle and secured to the clavicle with sutures through drill holes. To add support while this tissue is healing, the previously described PDS braid is added to the construct to help protect the tissue during the first 6 weeks and allow for early motion (Fig. 17-8B).

Postoperative management after clavicular stabilization is somewhat dependent on the strength of the reconstruction. An arm sling is used initially but is generally discontinued at 1 week, after which time pendulum exercises are started. Overhead activities are avoided for 6 weeks and weights avoided for 4 months. We have found this procedure to effectively re-establish the suspensory function of the clavicle and reduce clavicular prominence.

COMPLICATIONS

Complications of both operative and nonoperative treatment of acromioclavicular joint injuries can result in pain, prominence, or both. Pain unresponsive to conservative measures usually requires distal clavicle excision performed either arthroscopically or using an open technique. However, when there is marked prominence, excision of the distal clavicle should be followed by clavicular stabilization. Complications after operative treatment are most often due to persistent pain or prominence. Residual pain is often the result of inadequate distal clavicle excision, and care should be taken at the time of surgery to ensure that sufficient bone is removed. Mild prominence after surgical repair or reconstruction is common, but failure of the fixation itself can result in a markedly prominent distal clavicle. Reoperation may be necessary and should include

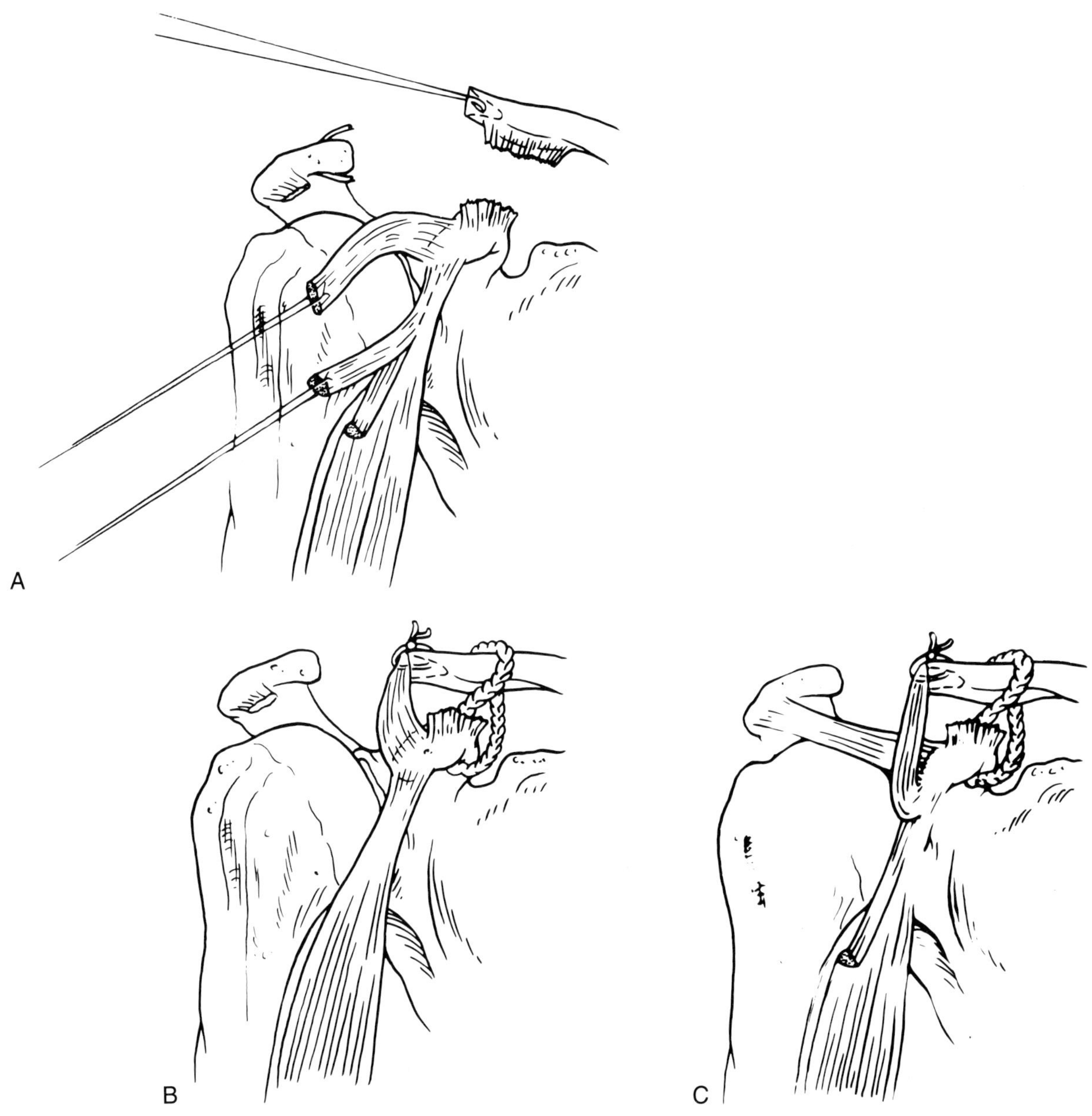

Figure 17-8. (**A**) Procedure for stabilization of the clavicle after lateral clavicular excision. The coracoacromial ligament is used, and if possible, a portion of the acromion is left attached to facilitate attachment to the outer clavicle. (**B**) The reduction is backed up with the absorbable PDS braid during the healing phase. (**C**) If the coracoacromial ligament is inadequate, a strip of conjoined tendon can be carefully dissected out to maintain reduction of the clavicle.

not only distal clavicle excision but also stabilization of the coracoid to the clavicle with reconstruction of the coracoclavicular ligament using either the coracoacromial ligazment or a strip of conjoined tendon as described (Fig. 17-8).

Osteolysis of the clavicle[35,38] is another complication that can occur at any time after an acute acromioclavicular joint injury or after repetitive use, as by a weight lifter. There is generally a well-localized tenderness, which may be aggravated by an adduction test. This test is performed by adducting the arm while at 90 degrees of elevation and palpating the joint for tenderness, crepitation, or displacement. Stephen J. O'Brien, MD (personal communication), has described a test to confirm this finding that is sensitive but not highly specific. It is performed by placing the internally rotated arm at 90 degrees of elevation and 10 degrees of adduction, with the elbow fully extended. Resisting a downward directed force in this position results in reproduction of the patient's acromioclavicular joint pain. AP radiographs of the joint should be carefully evaluated for small lucencies typical of the early stages of post-traumatic osteolysis. Visualization of the films with a lamp or use of a bone scan may assist in early inflammatory medications and with injections combined with exercises. Unfortunately, it appears that most patients ultimately require excision of the distal clavicle to maintain their activity levels.

REFERENCES

1. Alexander OM: Dislocation of the acromioclavicular joint. Radiography 15:260, 1949
2. Allman FL Jr: Fractures and ligamentous injuries of the clavicle and its articulations. J Bone Joint Surg [Am] 49a:774, 1967
3. Altchek DW, Warren RF, Wickiewicz TL, et al: Arthroscopic acromioplasty. J Bone Joint Surg [Am] 72a:1198, 1990
4. Bannister GC, Wallace AW, Stableforth PG, Hutson MA: The management of acute acromioclavicular dislocation. In Post M, Morrey BF, Hawkins RJ (eds): Surgery of the Shoulder. Mosby Year Book, St. Louis, 1990
5. Barber FA: Complete posterior acromioclavicular dislocation. Orthopedics 10:493, 1987
6. Bargren JH, Erlanger S, Dick HM: Biomechanics and comparison of two operative methods of treatment of complete acromioclavicular separation. Clin Orthop 130:267, 1978
7. Beardon JM, Hughston JC, Whattey GS: Acromioclavicular dislocation: method of treatment. Am J Sports Med 1:5, 1973
8. Bearn JG: Direct observations on the function of the capsule of the sternoclavicular joint in clavicle support. J Anat 101:159, 1967
9. Bergfeld JA, Andrish JT, Clancy WG: Evaluation of the acromioclavicular joint following first- and second-degree sprains. Am J Sports Med 6:153, 1978
10. Bernard TN, Brunet ME, Haddad RJ: Fractured coracoid process in acromioclavicular dislocation. Clin Orthop 175:227, 1983
11. Berson BL, Gilbert MS, Green S: Acromioclavicular dislocations: treatment by transfer of the conjoined tendon and distal end of the coracoid process to the clavicle. Clin Orthop 135:157, 1978
12. Bosworth BM: Acromioclavicular separation: new method of repair. Surg Gynecol Obstet 73:866, 1941
13. Bosworth BM: Complete acromioclavicular dislocation. N Engl J Med 241:221, 1949
14. Browner BD, Jupiter JB, Levine AM, Trafton PG (eds): Skeletal Trauma. WB Saunders, Philadelphia, 1992
15. Cox JS: The fate of the acromioclavicular joint in athletic injuries. Am J Sports Med 9:50, 1981
16. Depalma AF: Surgery of the Shoulder. 2nd Ed. JB Lippincott, Philadelphia, 1973
17. Ferris BD, Bhamra M, Paton DF: Coracoid process transfer for acromioclavicular dislocation. Clin Orthop 242:184, 1989
18. Fukuda K, Craig EV, An K et al: Biomechanical study of the ligamentous system of the acromioclavicular joint. J Bone Joint Surg [Am] 68a:434, 1986
19. Fullerton LR: Recurrent third degree acromioclavicular joint separation after failure of a Dacron ligament prosthesis. Am J Sports Med 18:106, 1990
20. Galpin RD, Hawkins RJ, Grainger RW: A comparative analysis of operative versus nonoperative treatment of grade III acromioclavicular separations. Clin Orthop 193:150, 1985
21. Gerber C, Rockwood CA: Subcoracoid dislocation of the lateral end of the clavicle. J Bone Joint Surg [Am] 69a:924, 1987
22. Gurd FB: The treatment of complete dislocation of the outer end of the clavicular joint: an hitherto undescribed operation. Ann Surg 113:1094, 1941
23. Hawkins RJ: The acromioclavicular joint. American Academy of Orthopaedic Surgeons Lecture, Summer Institute, Chicago, 1980
24. Horn JS: The traumatic anatomy and treatment of acute acromioclavicular dislocations. J Bone Joint Surg [Br] 36b:194, 1954
25. Imatani RJ, Hamlon J, Cody GW: Acute complete acromioclavicular separation. J Bone Joint Surg [Am] 57a:328, 1975
26. Inman VT, Saunders JB, Abbott LC: Observation on the function of the shoulder joint. J Bone Joint Surg 26:1, 1944
27. Jacobs B, Wade PA: Acromioclavicular joint injury. J Bone Joint Surg [Am] 48a:475, 1966
28. Kappakas GS, McMaster JH: Repair of acromioclavicular separation using a Dacron prosthesis graft. Clin Orthop 131:247, 1978
29. Kennedy JC: Complete dislocation of the acromioclavicular joint: 14 years later. J Trauma 8:311, 1968
30. Kennedy JC, Cameron H: Complete dislocation of the acromioclavicular joint. J Bone Joint Surg [Br] 36b:202, 1954
31. Lancourt JE: Acromioclavicular dislocation with adjacent clavicular fracture in a horseback rider. Am J Sports Med 18:321, 1990
32. Larsen E, Bjerg-Nielsen A, Christensen P: Conservative or surgical treatment of acromioclavicular dislocation. J Bone Joint Surg [Am] 68a:552, 1986
33. Lindsey RW, Gutowski WT: The migration of a broken pin following fixation of the acromioclavicular joint. Orthopedics 9:413, 1986
34. MacDonald PB, Alexander MJ, Frejuk J, Johnson GE: Comprehensive functional analysis of shoulders following complete acromioclavicular separation. Am J. Sports Med 16:475, 1988
35. Madsen B: Osteolysis of the acromial end of the clavicle following trauma. Br J Radiol 36:822, 1963
36. Meyers JF: Arthroscopic debridement of the acromioclavicu-

lar joint and distal clavicle resection. In McGinty JB (ed): Operative Arthroscopy. Raven Press, New York, 1991
37. Mumford EB: Acromioclavicular dislocation. J Bone Joint Surg 23:799, 1941
38. Murphy OB, Bellamy R, Wheeler et al: Posttraumatic osteolysis of the distal clavicle. Clin Orthop 109:108, 1975
39. Park JP, Arnold JA, Coker TP et al: Treatment of acromioclavicular separations. Am J Sports Med 8:251, 1980
40. Pettrone FA, Nirschl RP: Acromioclavicular dislocation. Am J Sports Med 6:160, 1978
41. Rockwood CA, Green DP: Fractures. Vols. 1 and 2. JB Lippincott, Philadelphia, 1975
42. Rockwood CA, Matsen FA (eds): The Shoulder. Vol. 1. WB Saunders, Philadelphia, 1990
43. Roper BA, Levack B: The surgical treatment of acromioclavicular dislocation. J Bone Joint Surg [Br] 64b:597, 1982
44. Rowe CR: Symposium on surgical lesions of the shoulder. Acute and recurrent dislocation of the shoulder. J Bone Joint Surg [Am] 44a:997, 1962
45. Sanders JO, Lyons FA, Rockwood CA: Management of dislocations of both ends of the clavicle. J Bone Joint Surg [Am] 72a:399, 1990
46. Skjeldal S, Lundblad R, Dullerud R: Coracoid process transfer for acromioclavicular dislocation. Acta Orthop Scand 59:180, 1988
47. Skyhar MJ, Altchek DW, Warren RF et al: Shoulder arthroscopy with the patient in the beach-chair position. Arthroscopy 4:256, 1988
48. Sondergard-Petersen P, Mikkelsen P: Posterior acromioclavicular dislocation. J Bone Joint Surg [Br] 64b:52, 1982
49. Taft TN, Wilson FC, Oglesby JW: Dislocation of the acromioclavicular joint. J Bone Joint Surg [Am] 69a:1045, 1987
50. Takagishi K, Yonemoto K, Tsukamoto Y, Yamamoto M: Treatment of complete acromioclavicular dislocation using synthetic materials. In Post M, Morrey BF, Hawkins RJ (eds): Surgery of the Shoulder. Mosby Year Book, St. Louis, 1990
51. Tibone J, Sellers R, Tonino P: Strength testing after third-degree acromioclavicular dislocations. Am J Sports Med 20:328, 1992
52. Tossy JD, Mead NC, Sigmond AM: Acromioclavicular separation: useful and practical classification for treatment. Clin Orthop 28:111, 1963
53. Urist MR: Complete dislocations of the acromioclavicular joint. J Bone Joint Surg 28:813, 1946
54. Walsh WM, Peterson DA, Shelton G, Neumann RD: Shoulder strength following acromioclavicular injury. Am J Sports Med 13:153, 1985
55. Warren RF: The acromioclavicular and sternoclavicular joints. p. 1502–23. In Evarts CM (ed): Surgery of the Musculoskeletal System. 2nd Ed. Churchill Livingstone, New York, 1990
56. Watkins JT: An operation for the relief of acromioclavicular subluxations. J Bone Joint Surg 7:790, 1925
57. Weaver JK, Dunn HL: Treatment of acromioclavicular injuries, especially complete acromioclavicular separation. J Bone Joint Surg [Am] 54a:1187, 1972
58. Wilson KM, Colwill JC: Combined acromioclavicular dislocation with coracoclavicular ligament disruption and coracoid process fracture. Am J Sports Med 17:697, 1989
59. Wurtz LD, Lyons FA, Rockwood CA: Fracture of the middle third of the clavicle and dislocation of the acromioclavicular joint. J Bone Joint Surg [Am] 74a:133, 1992
60. Zanca P: Shoulder pain: involvement of the acromioclavicular joint: analysis of 1,000 cases. AJR 112:493, 1971

CHAPTER EIGHTEEN

Fractures of the Shoulder Girdle

Theodore F. Schlegel
Richard J. Hawkins

PROXIMAL HUMERUS FRACTURES

Anatomy

Bony Architecture

The proximal humerus consists of four well-defined parts that include the humeral head, the lesser and greater tuberosities, and the proximal humeral shaft. A well-defined relationship exists between these parts, with the neck shaft inclination angle measuring an average of 145 degrees in relationship to the shaft and retroverted an average of 30 degrees. The proximal humerus arises from three distinct ossification centers, including one for the humeral head and one each for the lesser and greater tuberosities. The fusion of the ossification centers creates a weakened area in the construct, known as the epiphyseal scar, making these regions of the proximal humerus susceptible to fracture.

Rotator Cuff and Girdle Muscles

The rotator cuff and shoulder girdle muscles create forces on the proximal humerus as a result of their inherent pull (Fig. 18-1). These forces are in equilibrium when the proximal humerus is intact. This balance is disrupted when one or several parts of the proximal humerus are fractured.

The pectoralis major and deltoid will be most influential on the distal shaft fracture segment, although the proximal fragments, consisting of the articular head segment as well as the lesser and greater tuberosities, will be most influenced by the rotator cuff musculature. Understanding these deforming forces will facilitate treatment.[17,35]

Arterial Contributions

Disruption of the arterial blood supply to the proximal humerus from trauma or surgical intervention can result in avascular necrosis of the humeral head. There are three main arterial contributions to the proximal humerus[18,36] (Fig. 18-2). The major arterial contribution to the humeral head segment is the anterior humeral circumflex artery. The terminal portion of this vessel, the arcuate artery, is interosseous in nature and perfuses the entire epiphysis.[18,36] If this vessel is injured, only an anastomosis distal to the lesion can compensate for the resulting loss of blood supply.

Less significant blood supply to the proximal humeral head is delivered by a branch of the posterior humeral circumflex artery, as well as the small vessels entering through the rotator cuff insertions. The posterior humeral circumflex artery, which penetrates the posteromedial cortex of the humeral head, is thought to supply only a small portion of the posteroinferior part of the articular surface of the humerus compared with the arcuate artery. The vessels that enter the epiphysis via the rotator cuff insertions are also thought to be inconsequential as well as inconsistent in their vascular supply to the humeral head.

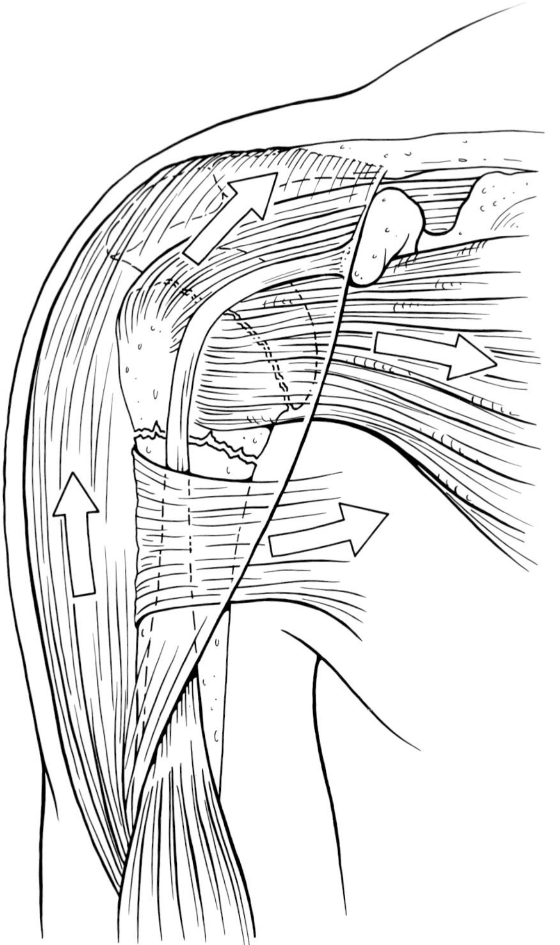

Figure 18-1. Displacement of a fracture fragment is due to the pull of muscles attached to various bony components: (*1*) the head, (*2*) the lesser tuberosity, (*3*) the greater tuberosity, and (*4*) the shaft. The subscapularis inserts on the lesser tuberosity: it's unopposed pull causes medial displacement. The supraspinatus and infraspinatus insert on the greater tuberosity: unopposed pole can cause superior and posterior displacement. The superior and posterior displacement. The pectoralis major inserts on the humeral shaft: it's unopposed pull can cause medial displacement.

Radiographic Evaluation

Accurate diagnosis is essential for the proper treatment of proximal humeral fractures. Three radiographic views are required in most shoulder injuries to ensure consistent identification of fracture types (Fig. 18-3). Radiographs of the injured shoulder are taken both perpendicular and parallel to the scapular plane.[46] Although fracture fragments may be shifted with any movement of the patient's arm, we would nevertheless consider the axillary view best taken in 20 to 40 degrees of abduction essential as a third view for the following reasons. First, it contributes valuable additional information regarding the fracture configuration, because it is oriented at right angles to the two previous views. Second, it is the most reliable means of detecting a locked posterior dislocation with an impression fracture. Third, it provides an assessment of the glenoid margin. Each of these views may be obtained with the patient in a standing, sitting, or supine position. If a sling has been previously applied, it does not need to be removed. When the patient is too uncomfortable to have the arm abducted, a Velpeau axillary[7] can be obtained. In this situation, the patient is seated and tilted obliquely backward 45 degrees while the plate is placed below and the radiograph taken comes from above. These three plain radiographs are sufficient to make an accurate diagnosis. On occasion, computed tomography (CT) will be helpful in further defining the magnitude of humeral head defects in head-splitting fractures, impression fractures, or chronic fracture dislocations. CT scans can also be helpful in determining the amount of displacement of greater tuberosity fractures[44] as well as assessing glenoid pathologies.

Classification

For a classification system to be functional, it must be designed to provide a means for an accurate reproducible diagnosis, allow for ease of communication, and direct treatment. The system must be comprehensive enough to encompass all factors, yet specific enough to allow for an accurate diagnosis and treatment.[6] Over the years, a wide array of classification systems has been proposed. In the

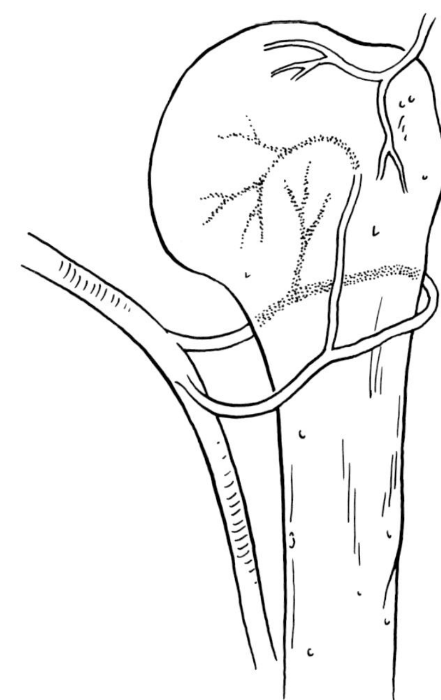

Figure 18-2. Blood supply of the proximal humerus.

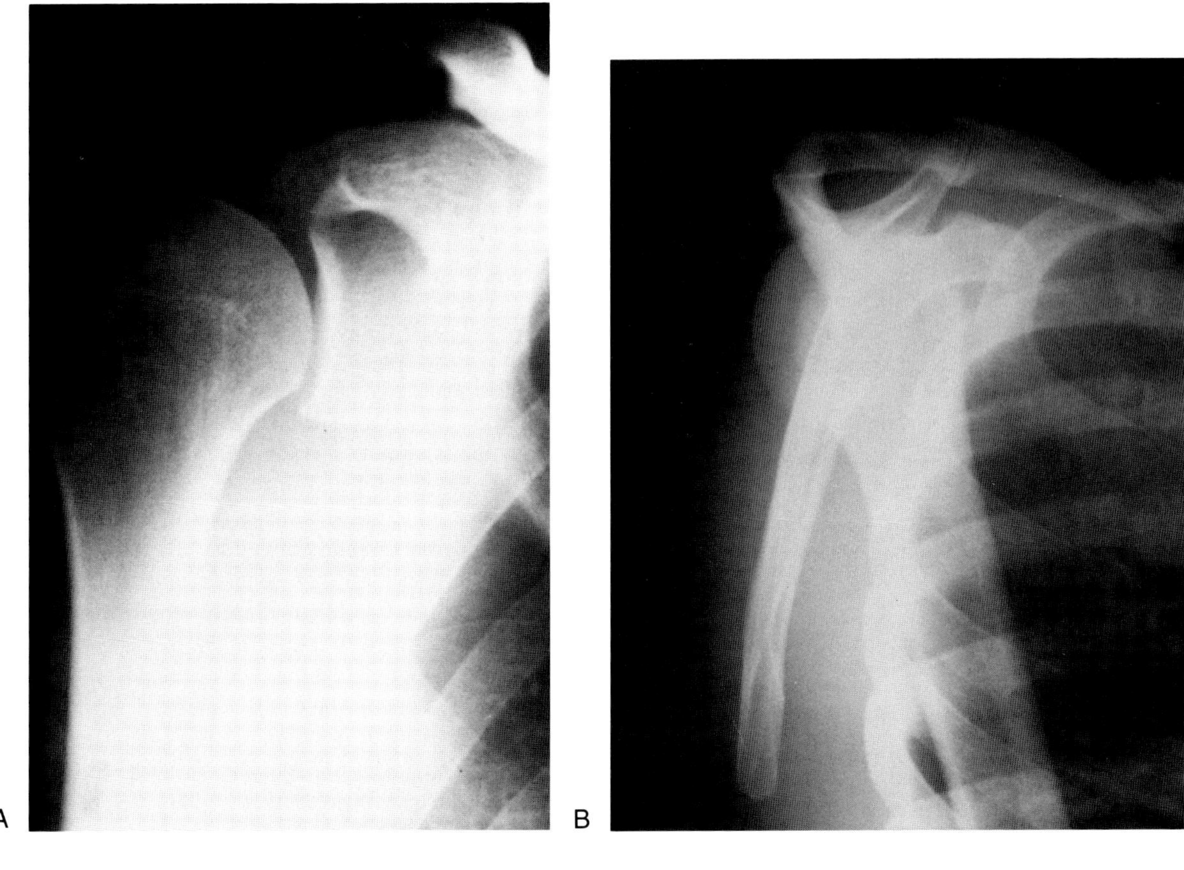

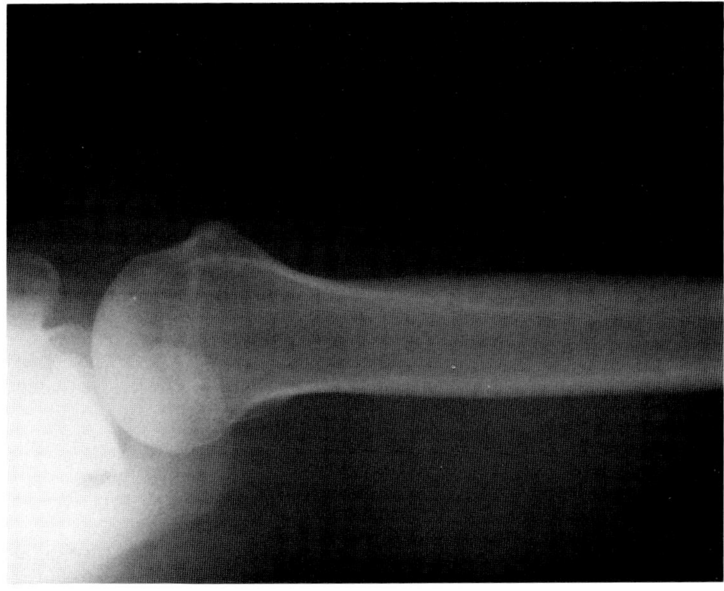

Figure 18-3. Standard radiographic examination of the shoulder. (**A**) anteroposterior view; (**B**) lateral scapular view; (**C**) lateral axillary view.

past, they have been based on the anatomic level of location of the fracture, mechanism of injury, amount of contact by fracture fragments, degree of displacement, and vascular status of the articular segment.[31,62] These systems have failed in their ability to provide a functional classification system with an inability to reproduce diagnosis and treat these complex injuries.

In 1970, Neer[22] described a classification based on the displacement of these four segments. Later, he eliminated numbered groups and detailed the application of the simplified version referring only to the segments involved. A segment is considered to be displaced if it is separated from its neighboring segment by more than 1 cm or angulated more than 45 degrees from its original position. The fracture pattern refers to the number of displaced parts (segments, e.g., two-part, three-part, or four-part). Comminution or the number of fracture fragments or lines is irrelevant unless they fit into the previously described classification. Unfortunately, Neer's system does not consider all the various subpatterns that affect treatment, but it is the accepted standardized classification, at least in North America.

The terminology used to identify proximal humeral fractures denotes first the ''pattern of displacement'' and, second, the ''key segment'' displaced. For example, in a three-part pattern, a displaced tuberosity is always considered the key segment even though a displaced shaft segment is also present (e.g., three-part greater tuberosity displacement). With fracture-dislocations, the fracture pattern is first identified, but the direction of the dislocation replaces the key segment in the description. A fractured tuberosity segment is always displaced in the direction opposite the dislocation. Therefore, a three-part anterior fracture-dislocation would refer to anterior dislocation of the head and attached lesser tuberosity and posterior displacement of the greater tuberosity. The position of the associated displaced shaft segment is variable.

Jakob[23] and the AO group have proposed an alternative classification scheme that emphasizes the vascular supply to the articular segment. This system was developed in an attempt to predict the risk of avascular necrosis after these fractures. This classification scheme is divided into three categories according to the severity of the injury. Type A represents the least severe fracture with no vascular interruption to the articular segment. It is unlikely in these fractures that avascular necrosis will occur. Type B represents a more severe injury with an increased risk of avascular necrosis, and type C is the most severe fracture, representing an injury in which total vascular isolation of the articular segment occurs with a high risk of avascular necrosis. Each group is then subdivided into a numerical scheme to further delineate severity. Because the AO classification system is more complicated and no long-term results regarding treatment of various fractures have been published, most surgeons continue to use Neer's system.

Methods of Treatments

Minimally Displaced Fractures

Many methods of treatment of proximal humeral fractures have been proposed. Fortunately, most (85 percent) proximal humeral fractures are minimally displaced and therefore can be treated nonoperatively with a sling for comfort and early range of motion. The periosteum, capsule, and rotator cuff limit fracture displacement so that reduction is unnecessary. The unconstrained design of the glenohumeral joint and the global range of the shoulder motion provide the advantage that it can compensate for even moderate amounts of residual fracture displacement. Successful treatment has been documented when a sling is provided for comfort and early mobilization once pain subsides and there is some fracture security.[7,44,47]

Assisted motion exercises may begin when the fragments move in unison. This can be determined by the examiner grasping the humeral head between the thumb and index finger of one hand and rotating the elbow with the opposite hand. The absence of pain, crepitus, and movement between the shaft and the proximal humerus suggests clinical continuity. Once this is documented, passive range of motion may begin as early as 2 but more often 3 weeks after the fracture. Overly aggressive activity before this stage may distract the minimally displaced fracture, resulting in either a malunion/nonunion of the humerus. Intermittent radiographs are necessary to confirm that there is no displacement of the fracture during healing and physical therapy exercises.

As the fracture becomes more stable, it is then possible to progress therapy to include active exercises with terminal stretch and eventually resisted strengthening exercises. This program should be well designed and carefully monitored and continued until union. Satisfactory functional outcome often takes between 6 and 12 months.

Two-Part Fractures

Two-Part Anatomic Neck Fractures

One two-part fracture occurs through the anatomic (not surgical) neck. The anatomic neck represents the old epiphyseal plate, whereas the surgical neck represents the weakened area below the tuberosity and head, which is approximately 2 cm distal to the anatomic neck.

This pattern is extremely rare, and there are little published data to suggest the ideal method of management.[12,25] Some authors have recommended an attempt at preserving the fragment, especially in the young active patient. Closed reduction is difficult because the articular head segment is usually angulated or rotated. Open reduction and internal fixation with interfragmentary screws is an option but due to the small head fragment, it may prove difficult to obtain adequate screw purchase in the head fragment without violating the articular surface. Most authors agree that in these cases, prosthetic hemiarthroplasty provides the most predictable result. Unfortunately, this method of treatment almost certainly precludes an athlete's chance to return to high-demand activities.

A deltopectoral approach with release of the subscapularis tendon from the lesser tuberosity affords excellent exposure to these fractures. Once the fracture is visualized, the appropriate form of treatment can be instituted. The rehabilitation program after surgery is based on the method of treatment used.

Two-Part Greater Tuberosity Fractures

Two-part displaced fractures of the greater tuberosity are relatively uncommon. When they occur, they are often associated with an anterior glenohumeral dislocation. After closed reduction, there is commonly residual displacement of the greater tuberosity (Fig. 18-4). Neer reported that when the fragment was displaced greater than 1 cm, it was pathognomonic for a longitudinal tear of the rotator cuff. In most cases, the greater tuberosity is displaced superiorly and posteriorly by the unopposed pull of the rotator cuff. If the fracture heals in a displaced position, it will cause impingement on the acromion or posterior glenoid, limiting forward elevation and external rotation, respectively, interfering with overhead activities.

Radiographic findings can be subtle because of the small size of the fragment. Plain film radiographs frequently underestimate the residual posterior displacement and may be the reason for the low reported incidence of two-part greater tuberosity fractures. Therefore, CT scans or magnetic resonance imaging (MRI) are often warranted to assess the residual displacement of the fragment.

McLaughlin[43] found that outcomes correlated closely with the amount of residual fragment displacement. Those fractures that healed with more than 1 cm of displacement resulted in permanent disability, although those with less than 0.5 cm of residual displacement did well. If there was 0.5 to 1 cm of displacement, there was often a prolonged convalescence, and many patients had persistent pain, with 20 percent requiring revision surgery.

An explanation for these results may be partially answered by reviewing the results of a prospective study of 14 consecutive patients with radiographic evidence of acute isolated greater tuberosity fractures (TF Schlegel et al,

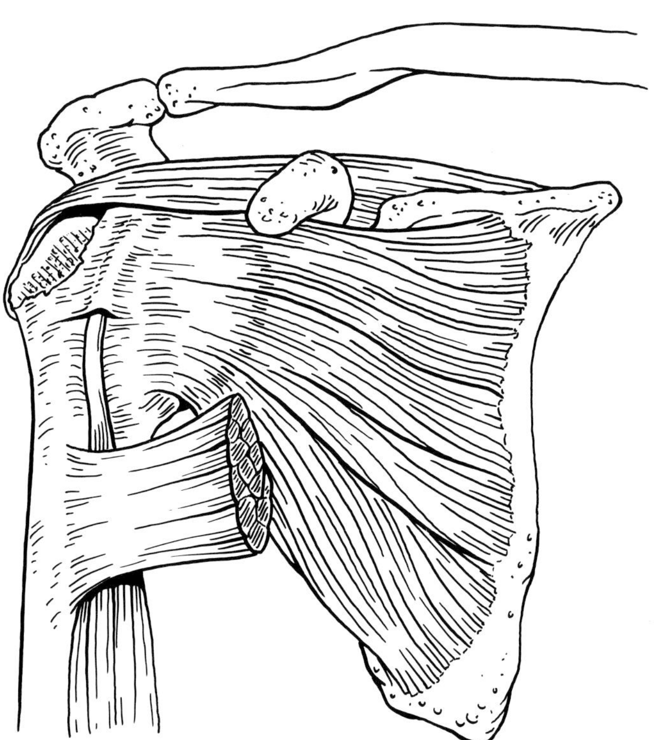

Figure 18-4. Displaced two-part greater tuberosity fracture.

unpublished data). MRIs were obtained to document intra-articular structures, integrity of the rotator cuff, and size and amount of greater tuberosity displacement. Rotator cuff tears were documented in 6 of the 14 patients. Of these six patients, two had greater than 1 cm of residual fracture displacement, one had 5 mm of displacement, and the remaining three individuals had nondisplaced fractures. The incidence of rotator cuff tears was 100 percent if there was more than 5 mm of fracture displacement. The incidence of rotator cuff tears was dramatically less (22 percent) in nondisplaced fractures. Although this is a relatively small percentage, it is higher than would be expected for nondisplaced fractures. These results would suggest that isolated nondisplaced or minimally displaced greater tuberosity fractures may not be as innocuous as previously considered.

If closed reduction of the fracture fragment is attempted, longitudinal traction should be applied to the extremity while the arm is flexed and adducted to the neutral position. If a reduction is obtained, there may still be problems with maintaining the reduction. If this method of treatment is used, serial radiographs are needed to check for subsequent displacement, and sequential examinations are required to document rotator cuff muscle strength.

If there is residual displacement greater than 5 mm in an athlete, open reduction and internal fixation should be considered. Because there is a chance that the fracture will heal in a displaced position, there is concern that late impingement will occur. This may preclude the athlete's return to sports. Open reduction and internal fixation of the fragment allows for an anatomic reduction and an accelerated rehabilitation and, it is hoped, an early return to sports.

Repair of the greater tuberosity with multiple heavy nonabsorbable sutures incorporated into the rotator cuff tendon has produced favorable results[16] (Fig. 18-5A). If the fragment is large enough, the fracture can be stabilized with a screw and washer[51] (Fig. 18-5B). Despite the method of treatments, a meticulous repair of the rotator cuff tendon should be performed if a tear is present. Rehabilitation can be started when the fragments move in unison.

Two-Part Surgical Neck Fractures

Another type of two-part fracture occurs through the surgical neck, and the shaft is displaced more than 1 cm or angulated more than 45 degrees from its original position. The tuberosities are both attached to the head so that it often remains in a neutral position. A posterior hinge is frequently present and contributes to the apex anterior angulation of the proximal shaft. If the head fragment is left significantly angulated, limitation of forward elevation may occur and compromise eventual function.

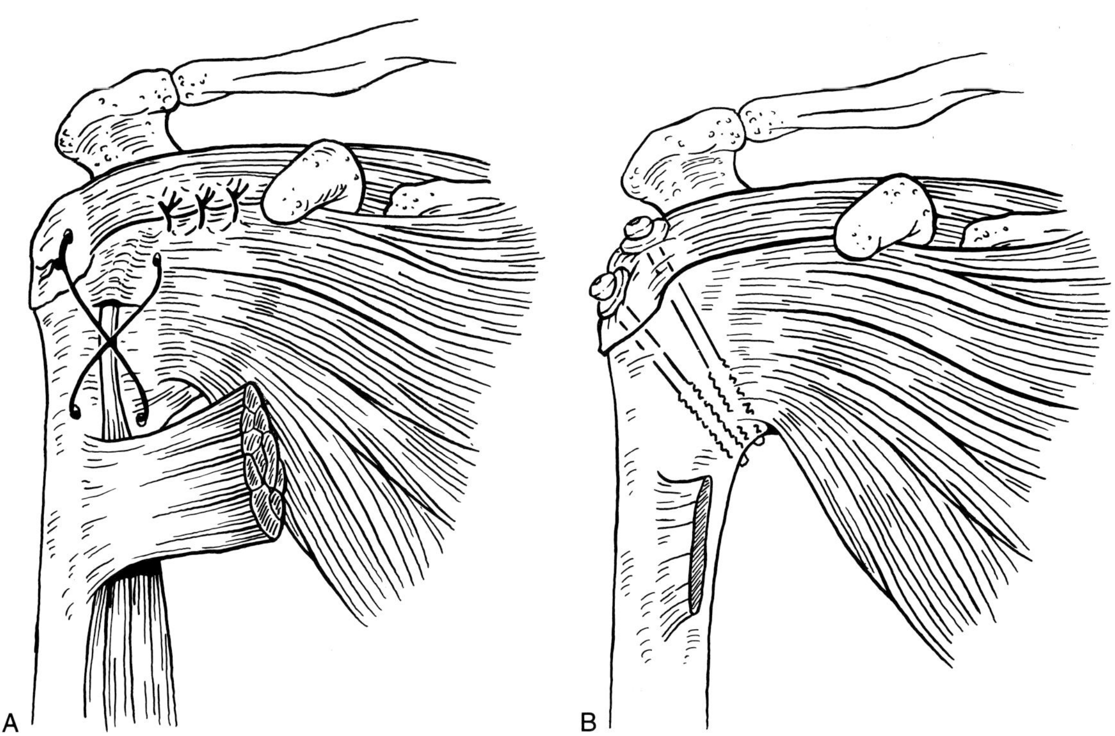

Figure 18-5. Methods of open reduction and internal fixation and a two-part surgical-neck fracture. (**A**) Figure-of-8 with heavy nonabsorbable sutures; (**B**) screw-and-washer fixation.

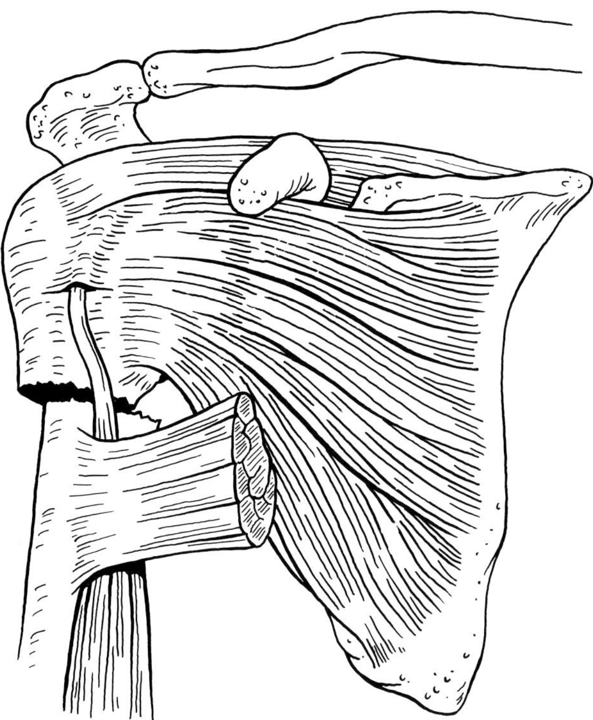

Figure 18-6. Displaced two-part surgical-neck fracture.

Most displaced two-part surgical neck fractures are unimpacted, and the shaft is displaced anteromedially by the pull of the pectoralis major (Fig. 18-6). Although closed reduction may be attempted, repeated and forcible attempts at closed reduction may be prevented by interposition between the bone fragment of periosteum, biceps tendon, or deltoid muscle between the bone fragments or by buttonholing of the shaft through the deltoid, pectoralis major, or fascia. If the first attempt is unsuccessful, it is usually best to attempt the next reduction under general anesthesia with assistance of an image intensifier. Fluoroscopy will allow for visualization of the fracture fragments. The technique of closed reduction involves distal traction and lateral displacement with simultaneous flexion of the shaft. Traction is then released to lock the fragments together. If an acceptable reduction is achieved, sling immobilization for 3 to 4 weeks is adequate. However, without fixation, angulation often reoccurs. With closed means it is not obtaining but rather maintaining the reduction, which presents the challenge.

In many cases, the fracture is reducible but unstable, and percutaneous pin fixation may be used. Under fluoroscopic control, Steinmann pins (2.5-mm terminally threaded) can be advanced across the reduced fracture from the anterior and lateral cortex of the shaft into the proximal segment (Fig. 18-7). It is often easier to skewer the head from above through the greater tuberosity adjacent to the acromion, passing the pins into the distal segment. Fixation may not be rigid, and therefore sling immobilization for 3 to 4 weeks is required while the fracture segments become secure. The pins may be removed at that time and rehabilitation commenced. This form of fixation is less optional than others in allowing for early rehabilitation.

In certain cases, obtaining a closed reduction may be too difficult or the reduction of the fracture may be too unstable to effectively maintain it with percutaneous pinning. In these patients, it may be necessary to proceed with open reduction and internal fixation. Our preferred method of fixation involves the use of some form of intramedullary fixation in conjunction with the tension-band technique (Fig. 18-8). The tension-band technique for this type of two-part fracture is inadequate alone, in that it does not provide a decent construct.[32] However, when the tension-band technique incorporates the rotator cuff tendon and is used in conjunction with intramedullary fixation, adequate stability is achieved. This allows for early passive range of motion exercises after surgery.

Many other methods of open reduction and internal fixation have been proposed. In young patients with good bone stalk, the use of an AO buttress plate and screws has been associated with good results. Reported complications include impingement of the plate if it is positioned too

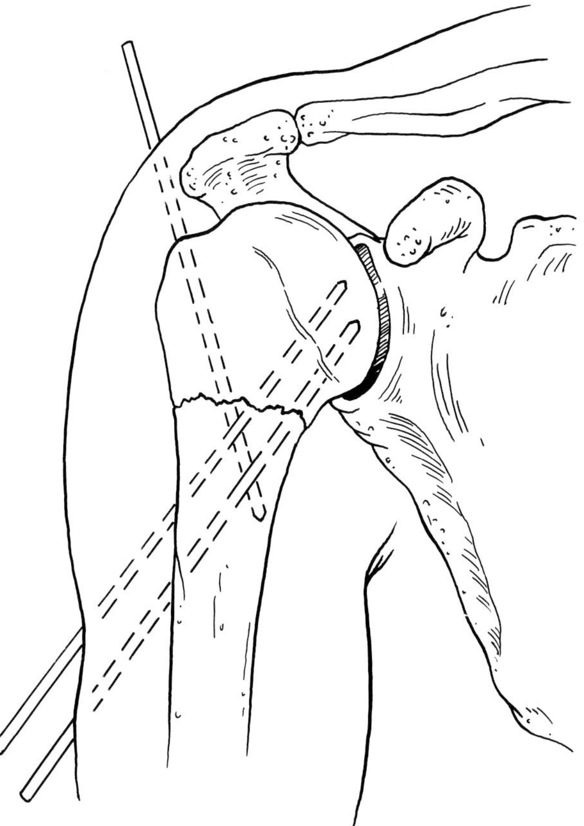

Figure 18-7. Percutaneous pinning of a two-part surgical-neck fracture.

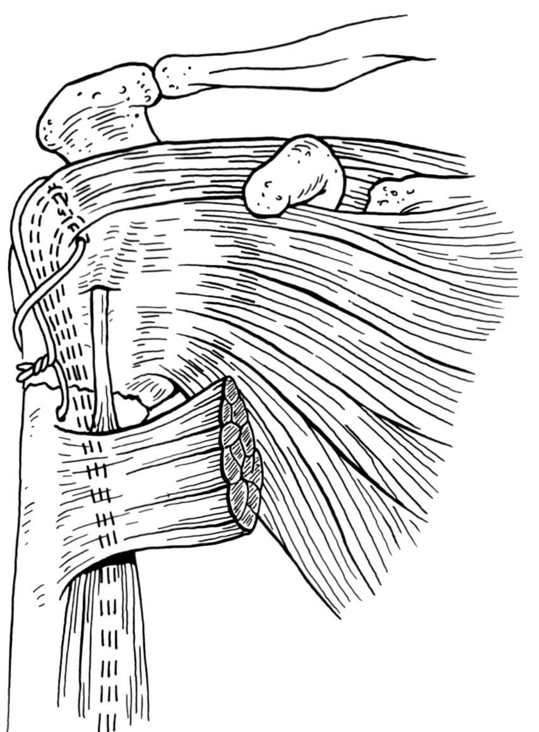

Figure 18-8. Combination of intermedullary rod fixation and tension-band technique of a two-part surgical-neck fracture.

proximal and persistent varus deformity.[51] Screws may also violate the articular surface or limit motion if left protruding laterally. If this method of fixation is used, great attention to detail needs to be implemented to avoid the above-noted complication.

The use of an intramedullary rod alone is another alternative means of internal fixation. Ender nails or Rush rods have been used in the past. This technique can be performed through a very limited incision. A small split is made through the deltoid and rotator cuff to insert the hardware. The disadvantage with this technique is that it may not provide rigid fixation and control rotational displacement. Also, a second surgical procedure is often required to remove the hardware because it can produce impingement on the undersurface of the acromion. Other intramedullary devices have been developed to provide greater rigidity as well as provide rotational control with the use of an interlocking proximal screw (Fig. 18-9). These devices have solved many of the previous difficulties with Rush rod fixation. A Mouradian nail or some form of fixation from below into the head has also been described.

Three-Part Fractures

Three-part fractures are difficult to manage closed from both the perspectives of obtaining and maintaining a reduction (Fig. 18-10). In the active patient, they are usually best treated with open reduction and internal fixation. Because of problems in obtaining and maintaining reduction by closed means, conservative treatment, by simply accepting the deformity, may result in malunion and stiffness of the shoulder.[37,47,64]

Closed reduction and percutaneous pinning has been proposed as a means of achieving acceptable results with minimal disruption of the surrounding blood supply and soft tissues. Jarberg et al[23] reported on results of this method of treatment for unstable fractures (mostly two-part but a few three-part) of the proximal humerus. This treatment is based on the premise that an acceptable closed reduction of the fracture fragments can be obtained. Although the head shaft segment can be reduced, the difficulty and obvious challenge are to reduce the tuberosity segment as well.

Open reduction and internal fixation with a buttress T plate was once popular, but several recent studies have reported inferior results with high rates of failure.[34,51,59] There are several disadvantages of this method of treatment. This technique involves extensive soft tissue dissection, which may potentially disrupt the remaining blood supply to the humeral head, leading to necrosis. There is also a tendency to place the hardware too proximal, which

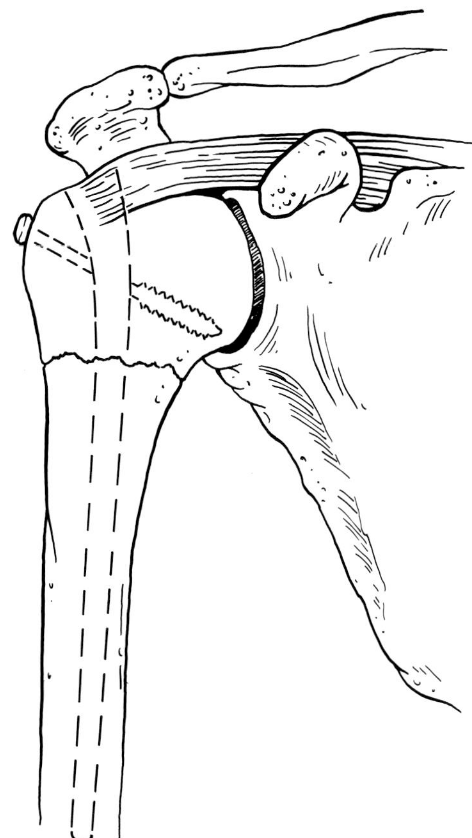

Figure 18-9. Use of intermedullary rod with a proximal interlocking screw for a two-part surgical-neck fracture.

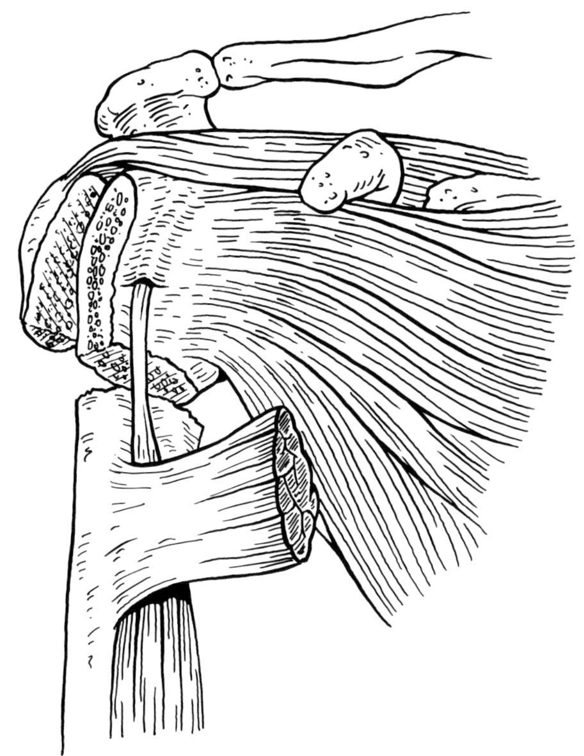

Figure 18-10. Three-part displaced greater tuberosity fracture.

may result in secondary impingement, necessitating a second surgical procedure to remove the hardware. It is for these reasons that this technique has fallen out of favor for the treatment of most displaced three-part proximal humeral fractures.

Figure-of-eight tension-band wiring was popularized by Hawkins et al,[20] who reported satisfactory results in a series of 14 patients with three-part proximal humeral fractures. The advantages of this method of management include adequate visualization of the fracture fragments ensuring anatomic reduction with minimal soft tissue stripping, preservation of the vascular supply to the humeral head, and secure fixation of the fracture fragments, relying on soft tissue and not bone. Complications with this treatment have been reported to be minimal. Avascular necrosis of the humeral head did develop in two patients, only one of whom was symptomatic enough to require revision to hemiarthroplasty. Tension-band wiring is an excellent method of treatment for three-part proximal humerus fractures because it provides reduction and secure enough fixation of the fracture fragments to allow early passive range of motion. An 18-gauge wire or size 5 nonabsorbable suture provides stability. The suture or wire is passed through or under the rotator cuff as well as through the tuberosity. A colpotomy needle is helpful in the passage of the wire or suture. A drill hole is made in the shaft of the humerus, approximately 1 cm below the fracture site, and the wire or suture can be passed through the hole and looped back in a figure-of-eight fashion (Fig. 18-11). Early rehabilitation can be implemented if adequate fixation of the fracture fragments is achieved.

Four-Part Fractures

Displaced four-part proximal humeral fractures can occur in any age group. A bimodel distribution exists, with peaks occurring in the adolescent or young male and in the upper middle-aged or elderly group.[22,54] Regardless of the age group, displaced four-part fractures, with or without associated dislocation, have been reported to have up to a 90 percent incidence of avascular necrosis[25] (Fig. 18-12). It is for this reason that unless the patient is young and active, immediate arthroplasty has been recommended as the treatment of choice.[60]

In the athlete, it is critical to review the radiographs carefully to ensure that the fracture has not been mistaken for a four-part valgus impacted pattern. Jakob et al[24] have stressed that the management of these fractures deserves special consideration because the rate of avascular necrosis has been found to be significantly lower (20 percent) than the classically described four-part fracture. In these special cases, closed reduction or limited open reduction and minimal internal fixation has produced satisfactory results.[24] The difficulty is to establish this diagnosis.

Even if the diagnosis of a displaced four-part fracture is confirmed in the young athlete, an attempt at open reduction and internal fixation is warranted. These fractures can be treated with the same methods of fixation used for the three-part fracture. The success of treatment is related to obtaining an anatomic reduction and repair of the rotator cuff. Even when there has been strict attention to surgical detail, review of published series demonstrates high failure rates, most often secondary to avascular necrosis.[37,47,51,59] The number of patients who develop symptomatic osseous necrosis is unknown. If the patient develops a painful shoulder secondary to avascular necrosis, a delayed hemiarthroplasty can alway be performed.

Fracture Dislocations

These injuries are probably more common in the athletic population than in the general population. Fracture dislocations require reduction of the humeral head and are often managed according to the remaining fracture pattern as previously described. A dislocation, if left untreated, almost condemns the patient to a poor functional result. Management of these injuries can often be complicated by associated neurologic compromise such as axillary or brachial nerve injury. Vascular disruption in the case of the axillary artery, if unrecognized, can prove catastrophic. Angiography should be performed without delay because early diagnosis and repair are crucial to outcome.

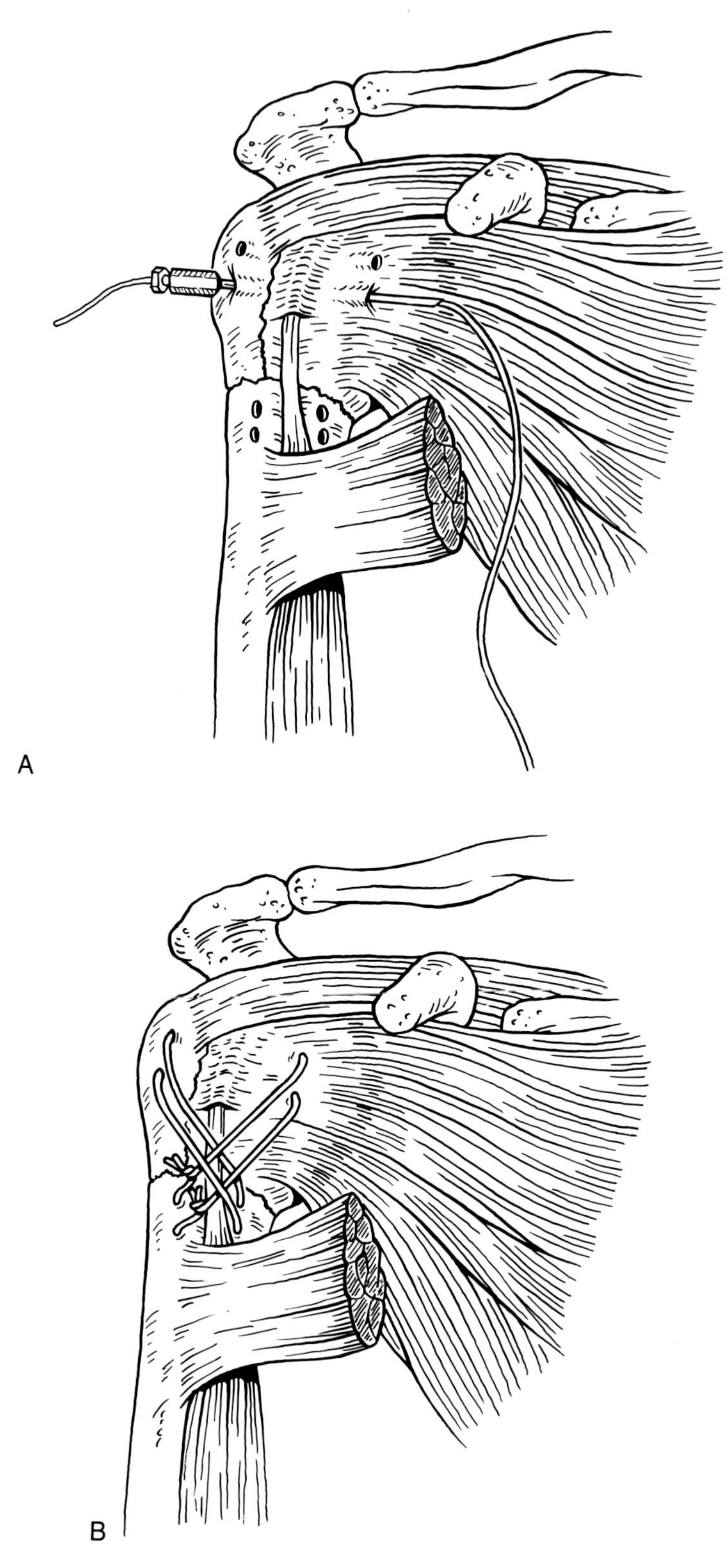

Figure 18-11. Repair of a three-part displaced greater tuberosity fracture. (**A**) Reduction of a three-part fracture with preparation for tension-band technique. Colopotomy needle is helpful in passage of wire or suture. (**B**) Figure-of-eight tension-band wiring technique.

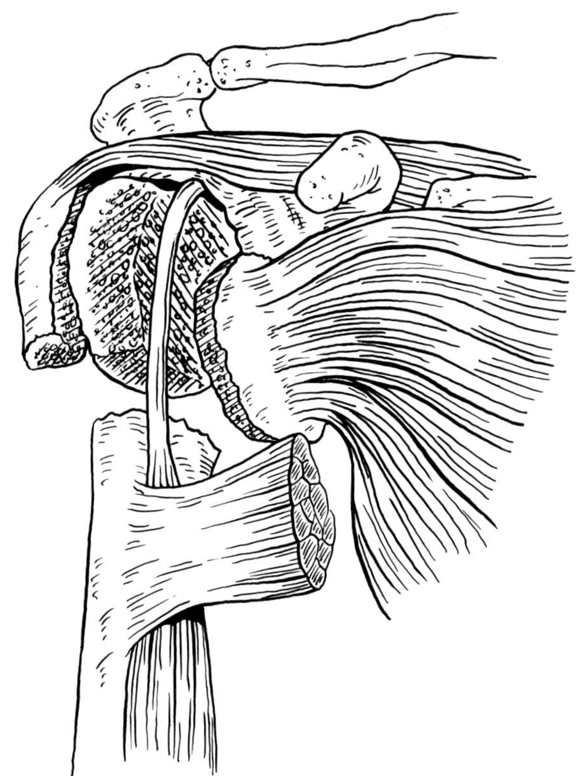

Figure 18-12. Displaced four-part proximal humeral fracture.

Articular-Surface Fractures

Impression defects or head-splitting fractures may result when the humeral head has been severely impacted against the glenoid rim. This most often occurs with posterior dislocations, some of which still go unrecognized, as originally described by McLaughlin.[43] This is described as a locked posterior dislocation with an impression fracture in the area of the lesser tuberosity. Management of this injury is determined by the size of the impression defect and the time the locked posterior dislocation has been present. After an acute injury with less than a 20 percent impression fracture, the joint will usually be stable after closed reduction.[21] Postoperative immobilization for 6 weeks in external rotation will restore long-term stability. In the presence of a 20 to 45 percent defect present for less than 6 months, the McLaughlin procedure or Neer's modification of the McLaughlin transfer fixes the lesser tuberosity and its attached subscapularis tendon with a screw into the head defect. Spica immobilization or gunslinger splint in external rotation is used postoperatively. With a greater than 45 percent impression defect or a greater than 6 months' dislocation, there may be no alternative but to perform a hemiarthroplasty.

The rare head-splitting fracture may occasionally be reduced closed if it consists of two large fragments. It usually requires open reduction and screw fixation if there are two or three large segments. Comminution with multiple segments may require hemiarthroplasty.

Proximal Humeral Physeal Fractures

In the pediatric athlete, fractures of the upper extremity are the most common injury encountered. Fractures of the glenohumeral joint, however, are relatively uncommon. Most of the fractures that occur in this group involve the distal, not the proximal, humerus. Even though this represents a relatively small number of injuries, it is important to be able to recognize and appropriately treat the fracture of the proximal humeral physis. This knowledge will ensure optimal results in the competitive athlete.

The incidence of physeal fractures involving the proximal humerus has been reported to be approximately 3 percent of all physeal fractures.[45,52,] Landin[36] reported that most of these resulted from a traumatic injury. Horseback riding was determined to be the greatest culprit. This study revealed that less than one-quarter of these fractures occurred in organized sports. However, as the participation in team sports increases in the younger patient population, one would expect a greater number of these fractures to be seen in the future.

The physeal plate is usually the weakest link in the proximal humeral construct. The strength of the physeal plate varies with age. Before maturity, the physis and perichondral ring weaken, allowing for injury to occur. Peterson and Peterson[52] confirmed this hypothesis when they reported that most of the injuries occurred between 11 and 12 years in girls and between 13 and 14 years in boys.

Physeal plate injuries can occur from either micro- or macrotrauma. Microtrauma is responsible for the stress fracture or failure of the proximal humeral physeal plate, which occurs in the throwing athlete. Repetitive high loads often lead to physeal weakening. Dotter[13] first described this injury in 1953 as "Little League shoulder." Since that time, there have been many reports in the literature on this injury. All cases have occurred in high-performance male pitchers who are between 11 and 13 years of age. Tullos and King[61] found that the pitching patterns in adolescence are similar to those in adults. Internal rotational torque forces are generated as high as 1,400 in./lb before ball release and as high as 2,700 in./lb at ball release.[1] These forces are four times that generated by the lower extremity while kicking a ball. A common radiographic finding in stress physeal fractures involves widening of the proximal humeral physeal plate. The treatment for this disorder would initially involve cessation of throwing. After an adequate period of rest, it may be possible to gradually work back into a well-designed shoulder strengthening program. This treatment protocol was successful in all but one of the cases reported. Lipscomb[38] described an individual who required operative treatment for a loose body after developing avascular necrosis of the epiphysis from a stress fracture of the physis. Prevention of this injury can occur by teaching proper pitching mechanics.[1] For the immature pitcher, emphasis should be placed on the development of skill and control.[58] With maturity, speed can then be considered a goal.

The second cause of a physeal fracture is macrotrauma. Higher-energy injuries from football and wrestling produce the greatest number of physeal fractures in high school sports. Almost all physeal fractures are either Salter-Harris I, through the growth plate, or Salter-Harris II, a fracture that travels traversely through the growth plate before exiting through the metaphysis on the side opposite the fracture's initiation. Salter-Harris type I are less common and usually occur in younger children, younger than the age of 10 years.[4,10,30] Salter-Harris II fractures are more common and usually involve children older than the age of 10 years. Salter-Harris III and IV fractures of the proximal humerus are extremely rare.[10,30] This relates to the fact that forces applied directly against the articular surface or perpendicular to the physis rarely occur. The exact mechanism of the Salter-Harris I and II proximal physeal injuries is not fully understood. The periosteum of the anterolateral aspect of the proximal humerus is thought to be architecturally weak. In this fracture pattern, the distal fragment is usually forced anteriorly and lateral, causing a fracture through the physis. The classification of these injuries relates to location, degree of displacement, and stability. The stability usually depends on the degree of initial displacement and the magnitude of injury. Near and Horowitz[45] described the most commonly accepted system for grading fracture displacement, and it is as follows: grade I, involves less than 5 mm of shaft displacement as related to the epiphysis; grade II, up to one-third of the width of the shaft is displaced; grade III, up to two-thirds of the width of the shaft is displaced; and grade IV, greater than two-thirds of the width of the shaft is displaced. The treatment relates to the amount of displacement. With displacement there is often a rotational deformity of the proximal segment, which can affect functional outcome. Fortunately, the proximal humeral physis is responsible for 80 percent of the longitudinal growth in the entire upper arm, allowing for tremendous remodeling potential. This, coupled with the great mobility of the glenohumeral joint, explains the favorable outcome in most of these injuries. Excessive residual varus angulation can occasionally cause functional limitations. Closed treatment is the standard of care. In Neer type I and II fractures, a shoulder immobilizer can be used for the first several days until the patient is comfortable. At that point, the patient is placed in a sling for comfort only. Circumduction exercises can be started. At 3 weeks, when callous formation occurs, active abduction can be included. At 6 weeks, when there is healing, a formal rehabilitation exercise program is started. In noncollision athletes, return to sports can occur when muscle strength and range of motion are equal to the unaffected extremity. In collision athletes, sufficient bone healing must occur. With Neer type III and IV, which involve marked displacement of the fracture, one must ensure that a sufficient reduction exists to prevent limitation of motion after fracture healing. This is especially true in the high-performance athlete who requires full range of motion for throwing, gymnastics, and swimming. High-performance throwing athletes may require more aggressive treatment. In displaced fractures, operative treatment is occasionally required. This usually involves a closed reduction and percutaneous pinning under an image intensifier. Once the fracture is properly reduced, reduction can be maintained using percutaneous threaded pins. The patient is placed in a shoulder immobilizer while the wounds heal. Early gentle circumduction exercises can be started. Pins are removed at 3 to 4 weeks. Primary open reduction to improve fracture position has no role in the treatment of this injury. The outcome of this treatment, when compared with closed reduction and percutaneous pinning, has led to inferior results.[4,41,49] The only case for open reduction of fracture would be an open fracture, a fracture with a severe vascular injury, or when there is soft tissue such as periosteum or biceps tendon interposed between the fragments.

Rehabilitation

Progression of the rehabilitation program must be individualized to optimize the recovery of the shoulder function. The surgeon and the physical therapist must convey to the patient a clear understanding of what is expected for short- and long-term goals. The postoperative management program has three well-defined phases. Phase I consists of passive or assisted range of motion; phase II is active range of motion with terminal stretching; phase III is a resisted program with ongoing active motion and terminal stretching.

Phase I begins on day 1, especially with the aid of an interscalene block for early pain control, and continues for 6 weeks. It is essential to confirm that the fracture fragments move in unison, signifying fracture stability. This phase may rarely need to be delayed for up to 4 weeks in some cases if the fixation is not rigid. This phase consists of passive forward elevation and external rotation of the involved shoulder with the assistance of the contralateral extremity. Assisted exercises begin in the supine position, with early emphasis on elevation and external rotation. Internal rotation exercises are included if the rotator cuff is intact (i.e., surgical neck fractures) or when secure fixation has been achieved by internal fixation in cases of tuberosity fractures. This exercise is frequently avoided in the early period after hemiarthroplasty with tuberosity repair for four-part fractures to avoid tension on the greater tuberosity segment. Pendulum exercises are used as a warm-up after a few days. Several days later, those exercises are performed sitting or standing. Toward the end of this initial 6-week phase, isometric strengthening may be added. These are performed by applying gentle resistance to inward and outward rotation when the arm is at the side and the elbow is flexed to 90 degrees. Similar exercises are performed for flexion and extension. These activities need to be monitored carefully by the physician and the physical therapist. These are taught to the patient and the patient's spouse so that they can be carried out at home.

Phase II, commencing at 6 weeks, consists of active range of motion exercises with terminal stretching, beginning once early union has been achieved and confirmed clinically and radiographically. When commencing phase II, resumption of the supine position permits concentration on forward elevation and outward rotation and is often advisable when starting the second phase of the program, at least for a few days. Full active range of motion in all planes is sought during this phase.

Phase III, resisted strengthening, begins 10 weeks after surgery when union is ensured and adequate range of motion has been obtained. The challenge to achieve normal shoulder function is met with greater resistance during the strengthening exercises and the ongoing terminal stretching program. Maximal recovery is rarely achieved before the first postoperative year.

Complications

Many complications have been reported after closed and open treatment of displaced proximal humerus fractures. These can be thought of as nonspecific or specific to proximal humeral fractures. Infection, neurovascular injury, malunion/nonunion, hardware failure, joint stiffness, and heterotopic ossification can result after the treatment of any fracture. Avascular necrosis, however, is specific to significantly displaced proximal humeral fractures.[47]

Infection does occur infrequently with open reduction and internal fixation of displaced proximal humerus fractures. Fortunately, the proximal humerus has adequate soft tissue coverage, with good vascular supply to the tissues decreasing the risk of infection. However, infections still do occur, and it is for this reason that care should be taken to maintain sterility, administer prophylactic antibiotics, and prevent excessive soft tissue dissection when these fractures require surgery. Obtaining hemostasis at the time of closure and appropriately draining the wound are also important to prevent hematoma formation, which increases the potential risk for infection.

Neurovascular injuries have been well documented after displaced proximal humeral fractures. Stableforth[58] reported a 5 percent incidence of axillary artery compromise and a 6.2 percent incidence of brachial plexus injuries. Vascular injuries most often are associated with penetrating or violent blunt trauma caused by the initial injury but can also occur after open reduction and internal fixation.[65] If a vascular injury occurs, the lesion is usually found at the junction of the anterior humeral circumflex and axillary artery. The diagnosis is often difficult to make, because peripheral pulses are often normal as a result of collateral circulation. Expanding hematoma pallor and paresthesias are all suspicious for a vascular injury. Paresthesias in the corresponding neurologic distribution are often the most reliable clinical sign. Because early diagnosis and repair are crucial to the outcome, angiography should be performed without delay when a vascular injury is suspected.

The axillary nerve is the most susceptible neurologic structure to injury after fractures with and without dislocation of the proximal humerus. The axillary nerve provides motor supply to the deltoid and teres major, with sensory distribution over the lateral aspect of the upper arm. A normal sensory examination of the skin overlying the lateral deltoid is not always indicative of an intact axillary nerve. A more reliable means of testing the integrity of the axillary nerve is by palpating for active contraction of all three slips of the deltoid muscle. However, this too is sometimes difficult to assess accurately in an acute fracture when there is associated pain. An electromyogram should be obtained if a nerve injury is suspected. This study should be obtained no earlier than 4 weeks after the injury when the results are most accurate and can be used as a baseline for further comparisons of recovery of function. Most of these injuries are secondary to a neuropraxia and will improve with time. If a complete axillary nerve injury does not improve within a 3- to 6-month period, surgical exploration is warranted.

Malunion of the proximal humerus can cause significant functional limitations. In the case in which the greater tuberosity heals in a superior or medial position, the space beneath the subacromial arch will be limited, and impingement will occur when the arm is abducted or externally rotated. This problem can be corrected with a salvage surgical procedure that requires an osteotomy of the greater tuberosity and mobilization of the rotator cuff. This is often difficult because the anatomy is quite distorted and there is often extensive searing. Secondary arthritis can occur in certain cases if the malunion is not properly treated.

Nonunion at the surgical neck is not an infrequent complication, particularly of two-part displaced shaft fractures and three-part fractures. Interposition of soft tissue, excessive soft tissue dissection, inadequate immobilization, poor patient compliance, or overaggressive physical therapy all contribute to nonunion. Treatment in these cases includes open reduction and internal fixation, autogenous bone grafting, and spica cast immobilization. Rush nails with tension-band wiring is a preferred method of internal fixation for these difficult cases.

Joint stiffness can occur as a result of either closed or open treatment. Prolonged immobilization with other means of management can result in bursal or capsular adhesions. Prominent hardware (i.e., rods/plates) can contribute to limited mobility. Persistence with daily terminal stretching programs is the best management but may require up to 18 months for full benefit. Forced manipulation risks refracture and is rarely required.

Heterotopic ossification appears to be related to both repetitive forceful attempts at closed reduction and delay in open reduction beyond 1 week for fracture-dislocations. Inadequate irrigation to wash out bony fragments after open reduction and internal fixation may also increase the risk. Exercises to maintain range of motion should be the mainstay of treatment. After 1 year, if a negative bone scan indicates quiescence, excision of the heterotopic bone with soft tissue releases may be considered.

Osseous necrosis is one of the most severe complications after displaced three-part proximal humerus fractures. It results from disruption of the vascular supply to the humeral head. This is generally considered to be a complication of four-part fractures but is also common after three-part fractures and can occur in some two-part fractures.[47] Rates of osseous necrosis range from 3 to 25 percent in three-part fractures and as high as 90 percent in four-part fractures.[18,47] The incidence of avascular necrosis has been noted to be slightly higher in those patients undergoing open reduction and internal fixation compared with closed treatment. Factors responsible for disruption of blood supply may be from the inital trauma of the injury or as a result of extensive soft tissue dissection for open reduction and internal fixation. It is uncertain how many individuals who develop avascular necrosis will become symptomatic enough to warrant further surgery. If resorption or collapse of the articular segment occurs, pain and loss of motion may result. In these cases, hemiarthroplasty can provide significant functional improvement. Total shoulder arthroplasty may be necessary if joint incongruity involves the glenoid surface.[46]

CLAVICLE FRACTURES

Anatomy

Bony Architecture

The embryologic development of the clavicle occurs through a combination of intramembranous and endochondral ossification. The central portion is the first area of ossification and is responsible for the growth of the clavicle up until the age of 5 years.[11,15] Medial and lateral epiphyseal growth plates eventually develop, with only the sternal ossification center being visible radiographically.[11] The medial clavicular epiphysis is the most important to longitudinal growth and contributes as much as 80 percent of the entire length.[50] The physis fuses between the ages of 22 and 25 years.

The clavicle is the only bone that connects the trunk to the shoulder girdle. It is attached medially to the sternum and laterally to the scapula by a combination of extra-articular and capsular ligaments. The bony architecture is not only important to its function but also provides an explanation for the pattern of fractures encountered. The clavicle has a double S-shaped curve that varies in cross-sectional area along its length. The medial portion is tubular and resists axial loading. This portion of the clavicle protects the costoclavicular space, where the medial cord and origin of the ulnar nerve are at risk for injury with medial clavicle fractures, clavicular nonunions, and healed fractures with exuberant callus.[5,8,28,39,56] The flat lateral portion functions to resist the muscular and ligament forces. The weakened junction of the medial tubular and flattened lateral clavicle places the middle clavicle at risk for fracture.[39]

Muscle Attachments

It is important to understand the relationship of the soft tissue structures to the clavicle. This knowledge will lessen the risk of damage to vital structures during treatment. The clavicle is a bony framework for muscle origins and insertions. The soft tissue structures that surround the bony clavicle can be divided into the areas above, below, and behind this structure. Above the clavicle, the cervical fascia, sternocleidomastoid muscle, omohyoid, and upper third of the trapezius insert from medial to lateral onto the superior aspect of the clavicle. Below the clavicle, the clavicular head of the pectoralis major and minor attaches medially while the anterior deltoid is attached laterally. Finally, behind the clavicle, although no muscles directly insert, there is a continuous myofascial layer that lies in front of the large vessels and nerves as they pass from the root of the neck to the axilla. Behind the medial clavicle, the internal jugular and subclavian veins join to form the innominate vein. Behind the midportion are both the subclavian and axillary veins.

Radiographic Evaluation

The anteroposterior view is the most beneficial screening examination for shaft fractures. Rowe[10] has suggested that when an anteroposterior radiograph is obtained, the films should include the upper third of the humerus, the shoulder

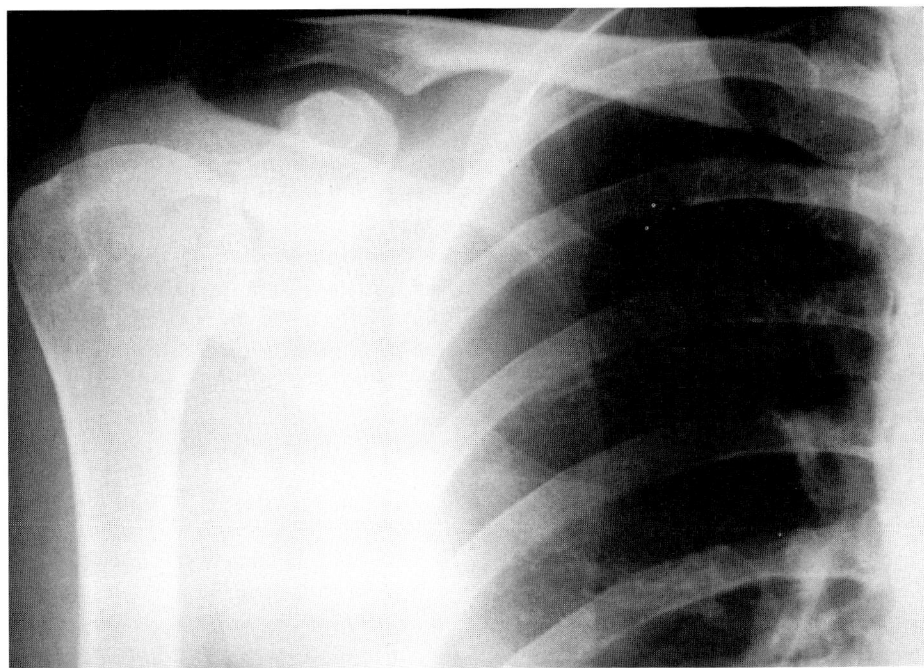

Figure 18-13. Anteroposterior view of the clavicle.

girdle, and the upper lung fields so that other girdle fractures or a pneumothorax can be quickly identified (Fig. 18-13). When a high-energy injury occurs, a chest x-ray should be obtained to evaluate for a potential pneumothorax or rib fractures. The configuration of the fracture may suggest other associated injuries. Additional views at right angles to each other, such as 45 degree superior and inferior anteroposterior tilt radiographs, can be useful adjuncts in delineating fracture position. Fracture of the medial clavicle may be particularly difficult to detect on plain film radiographs. In certain situations in which there is a high suspicion for a medical clavicle injury or there is an articular component, CT scan may be useful. For lateral clavicle fractures, a 15 degree cephalic tilt radiograph can assist in evaluating the lateral articular segment and acromioclavicular joint (Fig. 18-14).

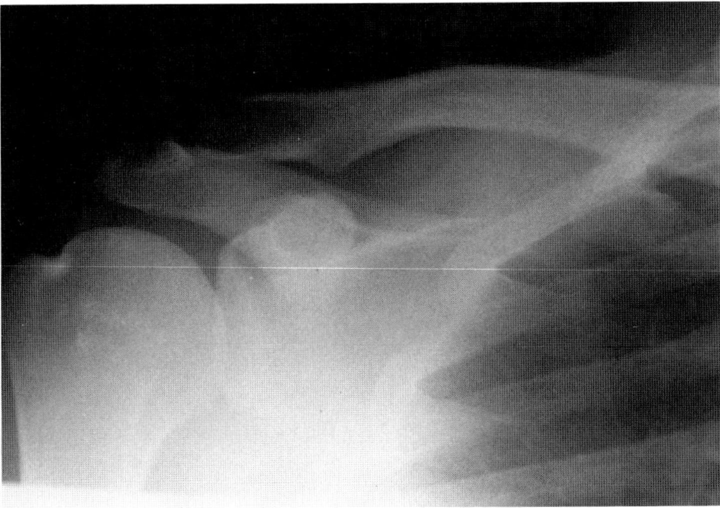

Figure 18-14. Fifteen-degree cephalic tilt view for evaluation of lateral clavicle fractures.

Classification

Clavicle fractures are most commonly classified according to location. Although there is not one generally accepted classification scheme, Craig's system[9] appears to be the most useful in assisting our understanding of fracture anatomy, mechanism of injury, clinical presentation, and alternative methods of treatment. In this system, three groups exist, depending on fracture location. Group I involves fractures of the diaphyseal midshaft portion and carries a high union rate. Group II fractures involve the distal third of the clavicle. Neer recognized the difficulties in treating this group and proposed a further subdivision into three types (Fig. 18-15). Type I is a distal third clavicle fracture with minimal displacement. Type II involves a displaced fracture that occurs at the attachment of the coracoclavicular ligaments to the clavicle. This type is then further subdivided into type IIA and IIB, depending on whether the ligaments remain intact. Type IIA fractures are those in which the coronoid and trapezoid ligaments remain attached to the distal segment. In this case, because the medial fragment has no attached ligaments, it becomes unstable and displaces superiorly as a result of the pull of the sternocleidomastoid muscle. This fracture pattern results in a greater rate of nonunions. A type IIB fracture occurs within the area of the coracoclavicular ligament attachment. In these fractures, the coracoid ligament is disrupted while the trapezoid ligament remains attached to the distal segment. This pattern is more stable than the type IIA fracture. Type IIIC are fractures that are intraarticular at the acromioclavicular joint. Finally, group III fractures involve the medial end of the clavicle near the sternoclavicular articulation and are seldom seen.

Methods of Treatment

Treatment is based on fracture location, displacement, and associated injuries. Fortunately, the vast majority of clavicle fractures may be treated conservatively with anticipation of union and good functional return. As with other fractures, the basic principles are to (1) achieve a satisfactory reduction, (2) maintain the reduction, and (3) minimize immobilization of the adjacent joints.

Midshaft Diaphyseal Fractures (Group I)

Most midshaft diaphyseal fractures are treated nonoperatively. Fracture reduction is rarely indicated. Options for nonoperative fracture immobilization include a figure-of-eight bandage or an arm sling. Anderson et al[2] found no differences in healing or functional or cosmetic results when comparing immobilization using a simple sling and figure-of-eight bandage. Regardless of the type of immobilization, shortening and residual deformity result. In most cases, this does not represent a functional problem. If a figure-of-eight bandage is used, care should be taken not to increase fracture displacement with improper placement of the straps.

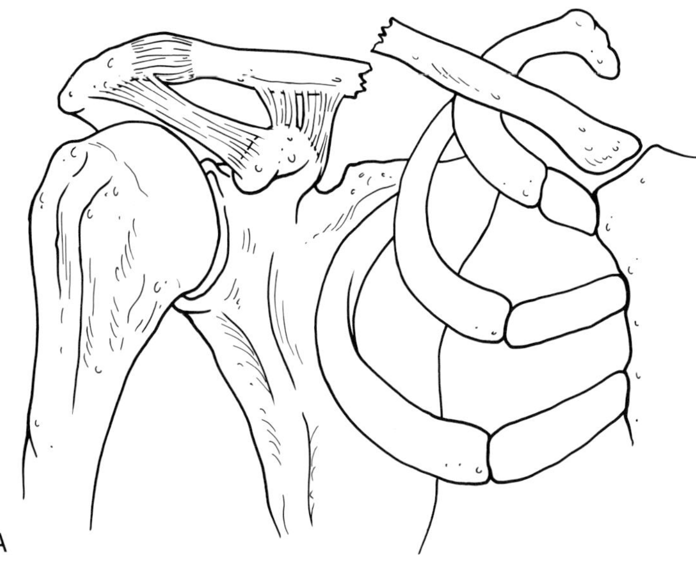

Figure 18-15. Craig's classification system for clavicle fractures. (**A**) Group 1: midshaft diaphyseal fracture. (**B**) Group 2: distal third clavicle fractures. In subclassification type I fractures the ligaments are intact and there is minimal displacement of the distal clavicle fracture. In type IIA, the fracture is medial to the acromioclavicular (AC) ligaments with both ligaments intact. In type IIB, the fracture is between the AC ligaments with the coronoid ligament disrupted. Type III is an interarticular fracture of the distal clavicle. (**C**) Group 3: medial end fracture.

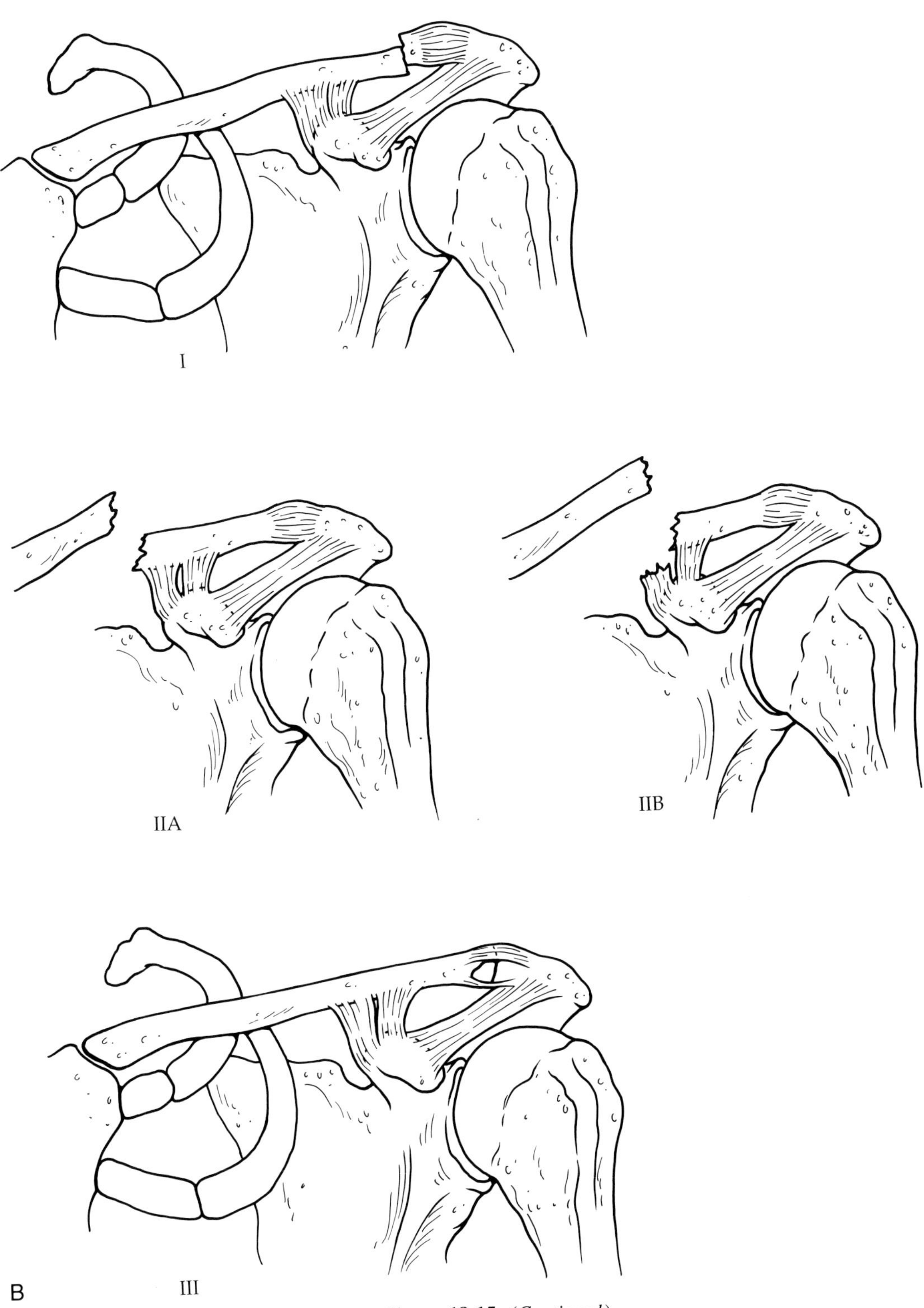

Figure 18-15. (*Continued*)

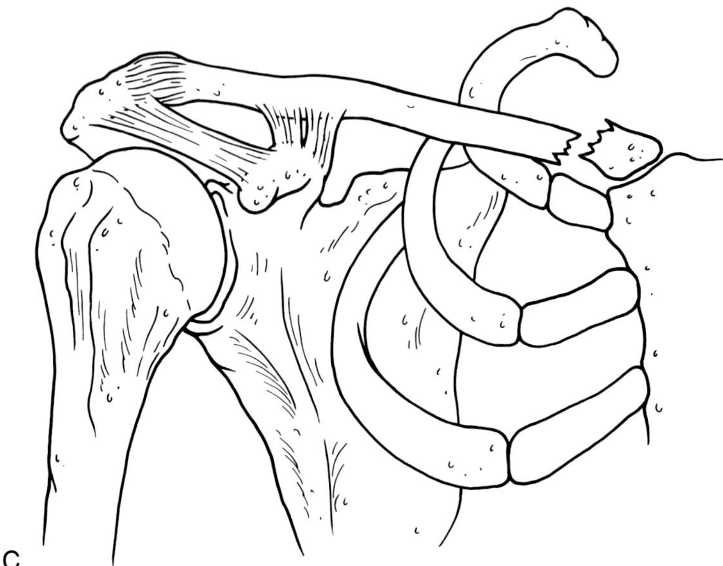

Figure 18-15. *(Continued)*

The indications for surgery in this group include open fractures, displaced fractures with potential compromise of the overlying skin, and fractures with associated neurovascular injury. In cases of severe fracture displacement, without an open wound or neurovascular compromise, an attempt at closed reduction may be warranted. When there is greater than 100 percent overlap of the fracture fragments, a higher incidence of nonunion exists. In the athlete, this may represent an indication for surgery in an attempt to prevent a prolonged convalescence. Typically, a 3.5 AO reconstruction compression plate or some form of intramedullary fixation is the most appropriate form of immobilization.

AO plates are malleable, allowing them to be contoured to the curved shape of the clavicle. By contrast, intramedullary devices, by their nature, avoid the irregular exterior of the clavicle, achieving their stability internally by three-point fixation. Smooth pins should be avoided because of the risk of migration. In general, if surgery is required, we prefer the use of a plate. Exceptions include thin individuals in whom the plate may lead to skin erosion or when there is extensive fracture comminution that precludes good screw purchase. The hardware should be removed in athletes returning to collision sports.

Distal Clavicle Fractures (Group II)

Nondisplaced (type I) and intra-articular (type III) fractures are generally treated nonoperatively with a sling for comfort and early rehabilitation. Good results should be anticipated. In displaced fractures (types IIA and IIB), a controversy still remains regarding the ideal method of treatment. This fracture type has an increased incidence of nonunion with closed treatment. The weight of the arm pulls the distal fragment inferiorly, while the trapezius pulls the proximal fragment superiorly, creating a gross displacement of the fracture.

It may be possible to achieve a closed reduction; however, the difficulty comes in maintaining the reduction. The standard figure-of-eight bandage is almost always inadequate. A Kenny Howard sling may be used to hold the distal clavicle reduced in a manner similar to its use with high-degree acromioclavicular separations. This device, however, requires continual wear for optimal results. For this reason, compliance is often poor. If a nonunion occurs, the patient is often asymptomatic, and no further treatment is required. If the nonunion is painful, a salvage procedure such as a Mumford or a Weaver-Dunn reconstruction can be performed.

Some authors advocate primary open reduction for these injuries. Multiple methods exist for treatment. In cases in which the outer clavicle segment is small and comminuted, the distal fragment can be excised and the clavicle can be fixed to the coracoid in a similar fashion to the Weaver-Dunn procedure. When the distal segment is larger, a plate may be a consideration. With this method, caution must be taken to ensure that at least four secure cortices can be achieved in the lateral fragment. If this is not possible, failure of the fixation will almost surely occur. Proper surgical intervention does not always ensure a satisfactory outcome. A recent study documented a 17 percent failure rate with operative management.[31] For this reason, the distal fractures remain the most challenging clavicle fracture to treat.

Over the years, our surgical approach to these fractures has evolved. Our first choice would be rigid fixation of the fracture with a plate-and-screw technique supplemented by clavicle fixation to the coracoid. Bone grafting can increase the rate of healing in these difficult fractures. If the distal fragment is too small for plate-and-screw fixation, then we have elected to excise the distal fragment and perform a Weaver-Dunn procedure, securing the distal medial end of the fragment to the coracoid using the transfered coracoid-acromial ligament as an autogenous graft. The postoperative rehabilitation for both procedures involves 3 to 4 weeks of immobilization in a sling, followed by a passive program that is eventually advanced to active motion. Strengthening begins after 6 weeks, when healing of the repair is adequate. With this approach, good results should be expected.

Medial Clavicle Fractures (Group III)

Group III represents approximately 5 percent of all clavicle fractures. In most of these cases, symptomatic support is the treatment of choice. Indications for surgery would include severe neurovascular compromise or injury. If an operation is warranted, open reduction and internal fixation with either an intramedullary device or plate are the two options. When using intramedullary devices, threaded pins are imperative to prevent the potentially catastrophic results associated with migration.

When these fractures occur in children, they usually represent an epiphyseal fracture.[11] Symptomatic treatment using a sling for support is the method of choice. These fractures are very rare and are not often significantly displaced. Good results should be expected.

Rehabilitation

It is critical after fixation of such fractures to have some temporary immobilization in a sling for between 2 and 4 weeks. This is especially so with intramedullary fixation and especially applicable to fractures of the outer fracture, such as type II fractures. Occasionally, passive motion may be commenced below the horizontal plane immediately. Active motion is usually delayed until callus is present at approximately 5 to 6 weeks. Resisted exercises are not commenced for approximately 8 to 10 weeks.

Complications

Several known complications have been reported after closed and open treatment of clavicle fractures. As previously discussed in the section on proximal humeral fractures, all these can occur after the treatment of any fracture regardless of location. Complications include infection, neurovascular injury, malunion/nonunion, hardware failure, joint stiffness, arthritis, and heterotopic ossification. The most common complication with clavicle fractures is nonunion. Despite the frequency of these fractures, the incidence is very low and reported to be less than 5 percent.[3,14,26,27,48,55] In adults, most fractures should be expected to heal in 6 weeks. Nonunion is generally determined when the fracture has failed to show clinical or radiographic progression of healing at 4 to 6 months.[27] Factors predisposing to this problem include inadequate immobilization, fracture location, severity of trauma, soft tissue interposition, refracture, and primary open reduction and internal fixation. Proper immobilization is difficult to achieve in any clavicle fracture. Distal clavicle fractures have a higher incidence of nonunion and account for more than one-half of the ununited fractures after closed treatment.[48] Increased severity of trauma has been reported to be responsible for up to 50 percent of the nonunions.[27] Healed clavicle fractures are thought to have an altered blood supply, making them susceptible to a nonunion. If a fracture occurs through this previously healed area, it is thought that further alteration of the vascularity occurs.[63] With increasing degrees of displacement, there is a higher likelihood of soft tissue interposition, which alters healing.[27] Finally, several authors have reported an increased incidence of nonunions in those who undergo primary open reduction and fixation.[48,55] Poor internal fixation, rather than surgery itself, may play the primary role of increased incidence of nonunion. Fortunately, nonunions are often asymptomatic. When they are symptomatic, they can cause pain, dysfunction, or neurovascular compromise. In these cases, open reduction and internal fixation and bone grafting are needed.[27] When a nonunion occurs in a contact athlete, even if he or she is asymptomatic, union should be achieved before the athlete returns to sports to prevent further and more serious injuries.

Malunion is common but rarely symptomatic. These usually represent a cosmetic problem. Occasionally, when it becomes symptomatic, it is secondary to significant shortening, leading to muscular dystrophy. When they are a problem, treatment includes contouring the bone or performing an osteotomy, internal fixation, and bone grafting to achieve a more acceptable position.

Neurovascular compromise often is the result of abundant callus, malunion, or fracture displacement. The vascular structures that have been reported to be involved in compression syndromes include the carotid artery, subclavian vein, and subclavian artery. The brachial plexus can be injured as a result of a neuropraxia or progressive compression affecting the medial cord, which often produces primarily ulnar nerve symptoms.

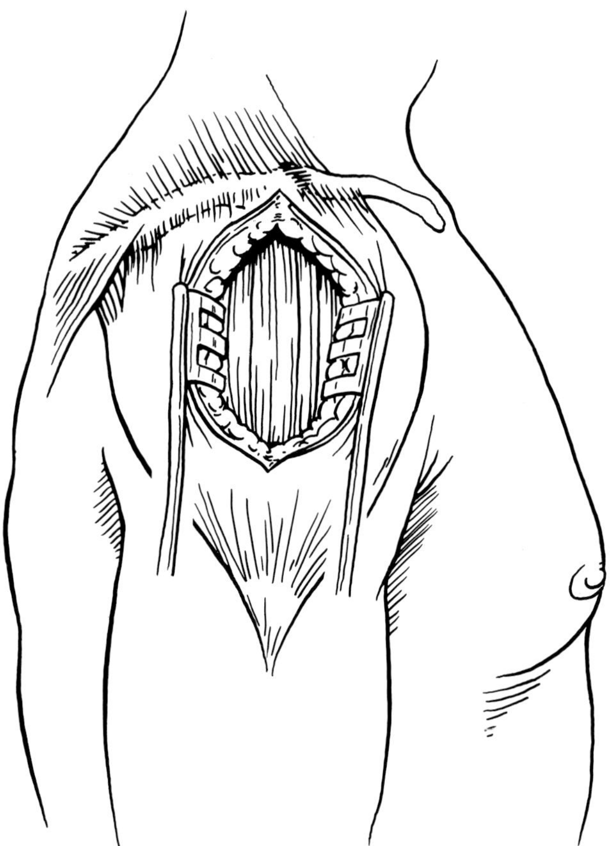

Figure 18-16. Limited deltoid splitting approach.

Finally, post-traumatic symptoms of the joint may follow intra-articular injuries of both the sternoclavicular and acromioclavicular joints. Degenerative disease of the distal clavicle is much more common. This is often the result of an unrecognized type III distal clavicle fracture.

SHOULDER GIRDLE SURGERY

Positioning for Surgery

Most patients are positioned on the operating room table in a semisitting "beach chair" position, with the head rotated to the contralateral side. Either regional or general anesthesia can be used, depending on the surgeon's preference. To prevent the patient from sliding down the operating room table, a pillow is placed behind the knees, with a seat belt across the patient's thighs. The bladder of a blood pressure cuff may be positioned underneath the ipsilateral scapula and inflated to bring the shoulder into the most advantageous position for surgical approach. Rarely in complex fracture patterns, especially in the presence of a posterior dislocation when there may be a need for an additional posterior approach, the patient should be positioned lateral decubitus. A sterile drape is placed across the neck to prevent hair and saliva from contaminating the wound. Intravenous antibiotics are administered to the patient 30 minutes before surgical incision and two doses postoperatively. Preoperatively, the patient is instructed to scrub the shoulder and axillary region for a total of 5 minutes with an antiseptic solution. This allows for the use of a single-step preparation, consisting of a Betadine solution in an alcohol base, to provide antimicrobial properties as well as enhancing the ability for the drapes to stick to the patient, maintaining a sterile field. A sterile stockinette allows for free manipulation of the arm. A large sterile drape is applied anteriorly and then wrapped completely and circumferentially to seal off the axilla and to hold the drapes in the appropriate position.

Surgical Approach for Proximal Humeral Fractures

Two utilitarian approaches are available for the surgical treatment of most proximal humeral fractures. The first is a limited deltoid split, useful for isolated greater tuberosity fractures and two-part surgical neck fractures treated with intramedullary nailing. A supralateral incision is made, beginning at the anterolateral aspect of the acromion and

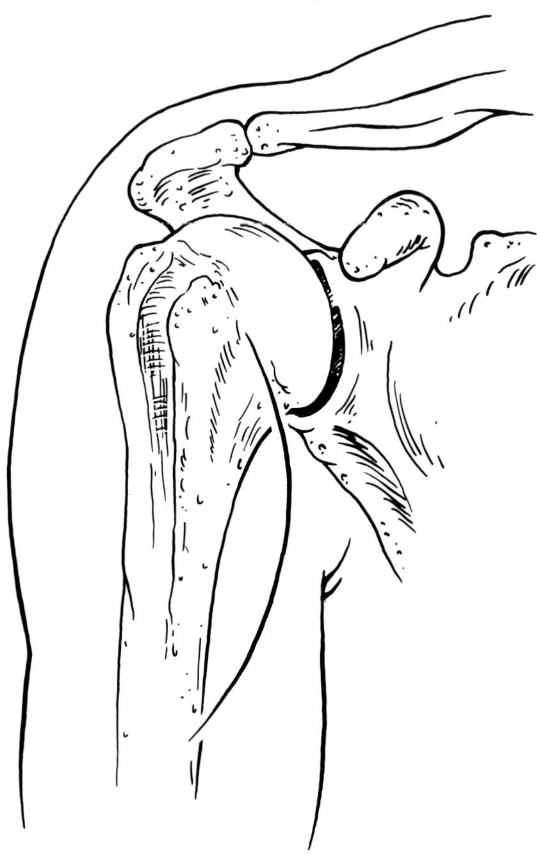

Figure 18-17. Extended deltoid pectoral approach.

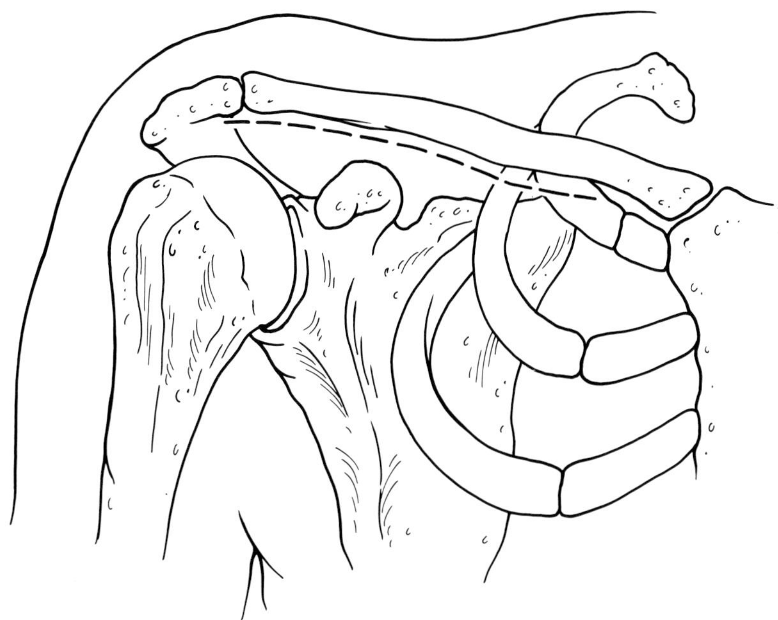

Figure 18-18. Surgical approach to the clavicle.

coursing distally for 4 to 5 cm (Fig. 18-16). The deltoid fibers are split bluntly and the fracture identified. One must remember during the deltoid split that the axillary nerve courses laterally, lying approximately 3 to 5 cm distal to the lateral margin of the acromion.

The second approach uses an extended deltopectoral incision measuring 12 to 15 cm in length, originating at the anterolateral corner of the acromion, curving toward the coracoid, and ending at the deltoid insertion (Fig. 18-17). The cephalic vein can be taken center medially or laterally during the dissection. If the vein is taken laterally, often excessive tension is placed on the vein, leading to rupture. The insertion of the pectoralis major is partially released for exposure. Adducting the humerus during the procedure aids in relaxing the deltoid. If excessive deltoid tension is present, a transverse division of the anterior 1 cm of the deltoid insertion lessens damage to the deltoid. Blunt dissection is then carried out in the subacromial space to free up any adhesions. A deltoid retractor is placed deep to the deltoid and acromion and superficial to the rotator cuff and humeral head. The coracoacromial ligament may be released superiorly for improved exposure.

Surgical Approach for Clavicle Fractures

Displaced midshaft fractures are exposed using a curvilinear incision 1 cm anterior, and therefore inferior, to the clavicle (Fig. 18-18). This is taken down through subcutaneous tissue to the platysma and trapezial fascia.

The fracture is subperiosteally exposed and reduced. Standard AO technique is used to achieve fixation. A 3.5-mm reconstruction plate is used, allowing contouring to clavicular shape. Extreme care is necessary to avoid the neurovascular structures inferior and posterior to the clavicle, especially during the drilling and determination of screw length. The plate is ideally placed superior on the clavicle, which represents the tension side of this fracture. Unfortunately, this often leads to skin problems postoperatively due to the limited subcutaneous tissue. We prefer the plate on the anteroinferior aspect of the clavicle. This has the advantages of less skin compromise and potentially decreasing the risk of injury to the neurovascular structures. If fracture orientation allows, the plate in this position will allow the direction of the drill, tap, and screw to be from anteroinferior to posterosuperior, providing the least opportunity for neurovascular compromise.

If one wishes to use intramedullary fixation, a similar but shorter incision is made and the fracture exposed. The lateral or distal fragment is elevated, exposing its medullary canal. A guide wire is then placed from the fracture toward the acromioclavicular joint retrograde, exiting at the posterior wall of the lateral fragment. The fracture is reduced and held in position while the guide wire is passed antegrade, back across the fracture, to an appropriate depth. Alternative forms of intramedullary fixation consist of Knowles, Steinmann, or Rockwood pins. In both these situations, the pin itself is brought back from the fracture site and then, with the fracture reduced, is drilled into the medial clavicular fragment. All these fixation devices have a threaded shaft and, as such, resist migration. The cannulated screw, as well as the Knowles and Rockwood pins, will further resist medial migration with their nuts.

Once the fracture has been stabilized with the fixation device, the screw is left just within the subcutaneous tissue so that it may be later removed once union has been achieved. If not needed, the nut or screw should not be used because it may cause significant irritation just under the skin.

REFERENCES

1. Albright JA et al: Clinical study of baseball pitchers. Correlation of injury to the throwing arm with method of delivery. Am J Sports Med 6:15–21, 1978
2. Anderson K, Jensen P, Lauritzen J: Treatment of clavicular fractures. Figure-of-eight bandage vs. a simple sling. Acta Orthop Scand 57:71–74, 1987
3. Apeli L, Burch HB: Study on the pseudoarthrosis of the clavicle. p. 188. In Chapchal G (ed): Pseudarthroses and Their Treatment. Eighth International Symposium on Topical Problems in Orthopaedic Surgery. Thieme, Stuttgart, 1979
4. Baxter MP, Wiley J: Fractures of the proximal humeral epiphysis: their influence on humeral growth. J Bone Joint Surg [Br] 68:570–3, 1986
5. Berkheise EJ: Old ununited clavicular fractures in the adult. Surg Gynecol Obstet 64:1064–72, 1937
6. Bigliani LU: Fractures of the proximal humerus. In Rockwood CA, Matsen FA (eds): The Shoulder. W.B. Saunders, Philadelphia, 1990
7. Bloom MH, Carter W: Diagnosis of posterior dislocation of the shoulder with the use of Velpeau axillary and angle-up roentgenographic views. J Bone Joint Surg [Am] 49: 943–9, 1967
8. Cook T: Reduction and external fixation of fractures of the clavicle in recumbency. J Bone Joint Surg [Am] 36: 878–80, 1954
9. Craig EV: Fractures of the clavicle. In Rockwood CA Jr, Matsen FA (eds): The Shoulder. W.B. Saunders, Philadelphia, 1990
10. Dameron TB Jr, Reibel DB: Fractures involving the proximal humeral epiphyseal plate. J Bone Joint Surg [Am] 51:289–98, 1969
11. Dameron TB Jr, Rockwood CA Jr: Fractures of the shaft of the clavicle. p. 608. In Rockwood CA, Wilkins KE, King RE (eds): Fractures in Children. JB Lippincott, Philadelphia, 1984
12. DePalma AF, Cautilli RA: Fractures of the upper end of the humerus. Clin Orthop 20:73, 1961
13. Dotter WE: Little Leaguer's shoulder—a fracture of the proximal epiphyseal cartilage of the humerus due to baseball pitching. Guthrie Clin Bull 223:68–72, 1953
14. Eskola A, Vainionpaa S, Myllynen P: Surgery for ununited clavicular fracture. Acta Orthop Scand 57:366–7, 1986
15. Fawcett J: The development and ossification of the human clavicle. J Anat 47:225–34, 1913
16. Flatow EL, Cuomo F, Madaz MG et al: Open reduction and internal fixation of two-part displaced fractures of the greater tuberosity of the proximal part of the humerus. J Bone Joint Surg [Am] 73:1213, 1991
17. Gerber C, Schneeberger AG, Vinh T: The arterial vascularization of the humeral head. J Bone Joint Surg 1486, 1990
18. Hagg O, Lundberg G: Aspects of prognostic factors of comminuted and dislocated proximal humeral fractures. In Bateman JE, Welsh RP (eds): Surgery of the Shoulder. BC Decker, Philadelphia, 1984
19. Hall MC, Rosser M: The structure of the upper end of the humerus with reference to osteoporotic changes with senescence leading to fractures. Can Med Assoc J 88:290, 1963
20. Hawkins RJ, Bell RH, Gurr K: The three-part fracture of the proximal part of the humerus: operative treatment. J Bone Joint Surg [Am] 68:1410, 1986
21. Hawkins RJ, Neer CS, Pianta RM, Mendoza FX: Locked posterior dislocation of the shoulder. J Bone Joint Surg [Am] 69:9, 1987
22. Horak J, Nilsson BE: Epidemiology of fracture of the upper end of the humerus. Clin Orthop 112:250, 1975
23. Jaberg H, Warner JP, Jakob R: Percutaneous stabilization of unstable fractures of the humerus. J Bone Joint Surg [Am] 74:508, 1992
24. Jakob R, Miniaci A, Auson P: Four part valgus impacted fractures of the proximal humerus. J Bone Joint Surg [Br] 73:295, 1991
25. Jakob RP, Kristiansen T, Mayo K et al: Classification and aspects of treatment of fractures of the proximal humerus. p. 330. In Bateman JE, Welsh RP (eds): Surgery of the Shoulder. Dechin, Philadelphia, 1984
26. Johnson EW Jr, Collins HR: Nonunion of the clavicle. Arch Surg 87:963–6, 1963
27. Jupiter JB, Leffert RD: Nonunion of the clavicle. J Bone Joint Surg [Am] 69:753–60, 1987
28. Kay SP, Eckardt JJ: Bracial plexus palsy secondary to clavicular nonunion. A case report and literature survey. Clin Orthop 206:219–22, 1986
29. Knight RA, Mayne JA: Comminuted fractures and fracture/dislocations involving the articular surface of the humeral head. J Bone Joint Surg [Am] 39:1343, 1957
30. Kohler R, Trillaud JM: Fracture and fracture separation of the proximal humerus in children: report of 136 cases. J Pediatr Orthop 3:326–32, 1983
31. Kona J, Bosse MJ, Staeheli JW et al: Type II distal clavicle fractures: a retrospective review of surgical treatment. J Orthop Trauma 4:115–20, 1990
32. Koval KJ, Sanders R, Zuckerman JD et al: Modified tension band wiring of displaced surgical neck fractures of the humerus. J Shoulder Elbow Surg March/April 1993
33. Kristiansen B, Barfod G, Bredesen J et al: Epidemiology of proximal humeral fractures. Acta Orthop Scand 50:75, 1987
34. Kristiansen B, Christensen SW: Plate fixation of proximal humeral fractures. Acta Orthop Scand 57:320, 1982
35. Laing PG: The arterial supply of the adult humerus. J Bone Joint Surg [Am] 38:1105, 1956
36. Landin LA: Fracture patterns in children. Acta Orthop Scand, suppl. 202:1–109, 1983

37. Leyshon RL: Closed treatment of fractures of the proximal humerus. Acta Orthop Scand 55:48, 1984
38. Lipscom AB: Baseball pitching injuries in growing athletes. J Sports Med 3:25–34, 1975
39. Ljunggren AE: Clavicular function. Acta Orthop Scand 50:261–8, 1979
40. Lusskin R, Weiss CA, Winer J: The role of the subclavius muscle in the subclavian vein syndrome (costoclavicular syndrome) following fracture of the clavicle. Clin Orthop 54:75–84, 1967
41. McBride EO, Sisler J: Fractures of the proximal humeral epiphysis and juxta-epiphyseal humeral shaft. Clin Orthop 38:143–53, 1965
42. McLaughlin H: Trauma. WB Saunders, Philadelphia, 1956
43. McLaughlin HL: Dislocation of the shoulder with tuberosity fractures. Surg Clin North Am 43:1615, 1963
44. Morris MF, Kilcoyne RF, Shuinan W: Humeral tuberosity fractures evaluation by CT scan and management of nonunion. Orthop Trans 11:242, 1987
45. Neer CS, Horowitz BS: Fractures of the proximal humeral epiphyseal plate. Clin Orthop 41:24–31, 1965
46. Neer CS II: Displaced proximal humeral fractures, part I: classification and evaluation of three-part and four-part displacement. J Bone Joint Surg [Am] 52:1077, 1970
47. Neer CS II: Displaced proximal humeral fractures, part II: treatment of three-part and four-part displacement. J Bone Joint Surg [Am] 52:1080, 1970
48. Neer CS II: Nonunion of the clavicle. JAMA 172: 10006–1011, 1960
49. Nilsson S, Svartholm F: Fracture of the upper end of the humerus in children. Acta Chir Scand 130:433–9, 1965
50. Ogden JA, Conologue GJ, Bronson NL: Radiology of postnatal skeletal development. Vol. 3. The clavicle. Skeletal Radiol 4:196–203, 1979
51. Paavolainen P, Bjorkenheim JM, Slatis P et al: Operative treatment of severe proximal humeral fractures. Acta Orthop Scand 54:374, 1983
52. Peterson CA, Peterson HA: Analysis of the incidence of injuries to the epiphyseal growth plate. J Trauma 12: 275–81, 1972
53. Quesana F: Technique for the roentgen. Diagnosis of fractures of the clavicle. Surg Gynecol Obstet 42:4261–81, 1926
54. Rose SH, Melton J III, Morrey BF: Epidemiologic features of humeral fractures. Clin Orthop 168:24–30, 1982
55. Rowe CR: An atlas of anatomy and treatment of mid-clavicular fractures. Clin Orthop 58:29–42, 1968
56. Sakellarides H: Pseudoarthrosis of the clavicle. J Bone Joint Surg [Am] 43:130–8, 1961
57. Slager RF: From Little League to big league, the weak spot is the arm. Am J Sports Med 5:37–48, 1977
58. Stableforth PG: Four-part fractures of the neck of the humerus. J Bone Joint Surg [Br] 66:104, 1954
59. Sturzenegger M, Fornaro E, Jakob RP: Results of surgical treatment of multi-fragmented fractures of the humeral head. Arch Orthop Trauma Surg 100:249, 1982
60. Tanner MW, Cofield RH: Prosthetic arthroplasty for fracture and fracture-dislocations of the proximal humerus. Clin Orthop 179:116, 1983
61. Tullos HS, King JW: Lesions of the pitching arm in adolescents. JAMA 220:264–71, 1972
62. Watson-Jones R: Fractures and Joint Injuries. 5th Ed. Williams & Wilkins, Baltimore, 1955
63. Wilkins RM, Johnston RM: Ununited fractures of the clavicle. J Bone Joint Surg [Am] 65:773–8, 1983
64. Young TB, Wallace WA: Conservative treatment of fractures and fracture dislocations of the upper end of the humerus. J Bone Joint Surg [Br] 67:373, 1925
65. Zuckerman JD, Flugstad DL, Teitz CC, King HA: Axillary artery injury as a complication of proximal humeral fractures. Clin Orthop 189:234, 1984

CHAPTER NINETEEN

Neurologic Disorders

Xavier A. Duralde
Louis U. Bigliani

GENERAL CONSIDERATIONS

The shoulder is vulnerable to a wide variety of injuries through athletic participation, including injuries to the acromioclavicular joint and rotator cuff, as well as those that result in glenohumeral instability and subacromial impingement. Injuries to the peripheral nerves are less common, and some may be subtle and difficult to detect by the clinician.

As interest in recreational athletics has increased in recent years, so has the incidence of sports-related injuries, including those to the peripheral nerves about the shoulder.[62] Upper extremity nerve injuries far outnumber those seen in the lower extremities in sports.[61,62,153] Poor training techniques and early specialization in one sport by young athletes have contributed to this increase in sports-related nerve injuries.[46,55,110] Although contact sports such as football and wrestling continue to cause many peripheral nerve injuries about the shoulder, almost every sport has been implicated, including bowling, golf, backpacking, and rope skipping.[50,58,115,149]

Injuries to the axillary, suprascapular, musculocutaneous, long thoracic, and spinal accessory nerves produce distinct clinical syndromes.[75,133,138,140,143] Prompt recognition of these conditions can facilitate treatment and rehabilitation, leading to a safe return to athletics.

Nerves about the shoulder are susceptible to injury from compression, stretch, and friction,[140] all of which can result from either a one-time excessive uncontrolled stress or persistent, repetitive, submaximal stresses.[110,134] Bateman[8] has identified certain common mechanisms of one-time excessive uncontrolled stress, including projectile falls, shoulder-angle blows, frontal-force injuries, axillary injuries, and twisting injuries. Nerve injuries secondary to entrapment syndromes from chronic repetitive stress about the shoulder present more insidiously but with characteristic patterns. Although debate continues as to the exact pathophysiology of these syndromes,[15,134,141] the most common presentation is pain, followed by atrophy and weakness in the affected muscle groups.

The degrees of nerve injuries have been well described by Seddon[133] in ascending order of severity as neuropraxia, axonotmesis, and neurotmesis. Most peripheral nerve injuries about the shoulder in sports are neuropraxias, consisting of a conduction block with intact neural elements, including axons and their connective tissue sheaths. The prognosis for complete recovery in these cases is excellent. The second degree of nerve injury, axonotmesis, follows more severe trauma and results in axonal injury and distal axon degeneration without disruption of the connective tissue sheaths. The ultimate prognosis in these cases is good, but recovery time may be extended depending on the length of the nerve that must regenerate. Injuries to the short nerves about the shoulder (e.g., the axillary and suprascapular nerves) fare better after axonotmesis-type injuries than do the longer nerves to the forearm (e.g., the radial and ulner nerves) because of the generally shorter distance from the lesion to the site of muscle innervation. Neurotmesis, or complete nerve disruption, carries a poor prognosis for regeneration but, fortunately, is rare in the athlete. It is more often associated with high-energy trauma, fractures, and penetrating injuries.[61]

Electromyelograph Evaluation

The electromyelogram (EMG) is a valuable tool in the diagnosis and treatment of peripheral nerve injuries about the shoulder in athletes.[19,73,134,153] The evaluation consists of two complementary parts: the needle electrode examination (NEE) and the nerve conduction velocity (NCV) study. The NEE records electrical potentials produced by muscle fibers. Characteristic patterns can be observed in normal muscle, acutely denervated, and reinnervated fibers. Because a single nerve fiber innervates many muscle fibers, injury to one nerve fiber can be detected from abnormal depolarization in multiple muscle fibers. This examination can be very sensitive in detecting partial denervation within a muscle.

The NCV study records the conduction velocity of nerve fiber action potentials by myelinated fibers. Action potentials are evoked in a nerve by electrical stimulation, and the response is measured at a distance from the stimulation site with either surface electrodes or needles inserted into the affected muscles. The NCV study is useful in localizing the site of nerve compression. Normal latencies for all the nerves about the shoulder have been described,[71,76,86,115] although some authors recommend the use of the contralateral side as a control.[109]

Despite its unquestioned usefulness, however, the EMG has certain limitations in the athletic setting. Wallerian degeneration and muscle surface membrane changes that result in the abnormal impulses recorded by NEE do not occur for approximately 2 to 3 weeks after nerve injury. Therefore, both the athlete and the physician must wait several weeks after injury before the degree of nerve damage can be determined. Another problem is that the EMG cannot adequately differentiate between axonotmesis and neurotmesis, two lesions whose prognosis differ markedly.

An experienced electromyographer who can interpret the EMG in the light of the athlete's history and clinical presentation is essential. This is especially important in cases of partial injury or chronic compression, in which the electromyographer must evaluate muscle activity in relation to motor-unit potentials on NEE, as well as the size of compound muscle action potentials in relation to stimulation on NCV. The overlap of multiple muscle groups in the shoulder further complicates these EMG studies, demanding expert technique and interpretation.

Despite these limitations, however, the EMG is an invaluable tool in diagnosing nerve injuries about the shoulder. It helps the physician to distinguish between atrophy secondary to pain and that secondary to nerve injury, and it reveals associated nerve injuries that occur commonly about the shoulder.[3,82,133] The EMG can also reveal subclinical healing, thus assisting prognotication.

Differential Diagnosis

The differential diagnosis in the evaluation of peripheral nerve injuries about the shoulder always includes injuries to the cervical roots and the brachial plexus. In the acute setting on the playing field, one must maintain a high degree of suspicion for cervical spine injuries, especially when associated nerve injuries are suspected, and provide adequate protection of the cervical spine until this diagnosis can be ruled out. Fortunately, cervical spine injuries are much less common in sports than peripheral nerve injuries about the shoulder.[8]

Injuries to the brachial plexus in athletes can take on many forms, including "burners," true supraclavicular nerve injuries, thoracic outlet syndromes, and acute brachial neuritis. Burners are brief episodes of burning dysesthesia that frequently involve the entire upper extremity and are sometimes accompanied by momentary weakness. Burners are caused by a forceful increase of the acromiomastoid distance when the head is forced in the direction of the contralateral shoulder, occurring typically in young athletes participating in contact sports.[8,117,153,156] The muscles most often involved are the deltoid, biceps, spinati, and brachioradialis. Although the exact location of this nerve injury remains uncertain, burners are characterized by a rapid return of sensation and strength. Return to play can be allowed as soon as the athlete's neurologic examination normalizes, which usually occurs before the sporting event is over.[8,153]

True supraclavicular brachial plexus injury is suspected when multiple muscle groups innervated by different peripheral nerves are affected. This type of injury has a much poorer prognosis than peripheral nerve injury, and the athlete must be thoroughly evaluated for associated vascular injuries.[3,59,74,82,92,117]

Less dramatic in presentation is thoracic outlet syndrome, which can have an insidious onset in the athlete. This occurs most often in racquet sports, in which players commonly have unilateral hypertrophy and a resultant abnormally low carriage of the shoulder.[59,69,77,82,120,123] Although these athletes typically complain of pain with overhead activities, their neurologic findings usually involve the lower brachial plexus and affect the forearm and hand. However, an increasing incidence of high radial palsy has been noted in tennis players with triceps weakness secondary to thoracic outlet syndrome.[100,120] Thoracic outlet syndrome has also been associated with exuberant callus from a comminuted clavicular fracture in a college football player,[92] was well as cervical ribs in adolescent athletes.[123] Postural training and specific exercises to strength the periscapular muscles usually lead to resolution of symptoms.[120,123]

Acute brachial neuritis, a syndrome of unknown origin, can present in the athlete, although it is not a true athletic injury. This condition, first described by Parsonage and Turner,[113,147] is characterized by the onset of shoulder pain (which may be severe) followed by weakness. Acute brachial neuritis is best differentiated from other causes of brachial plexus and peripheral nerve injuries by EMG evaluation, which may show the involvement of muscles not innervated by the brachial plexus, or severe denervation restricted to a single muscle, but excluding other muscles innervated by the same peripheral nerve.[59,153]

Finally, the differential diagnosis in injuries in peripheral nerve injuries about the shoulder should include muscle injuries, which often mimic denervation.[39,57]

Preventive Measures

It is important to emphasize the value of proper conditioning and preventive measures in the avoidance of peripheral nerve injuries about the shoulder. Most peripheral nerve injuries about the shoulder occur in inexperienced athletes.[46,50,51,55,61,62,97,110,134] Prevention of these types of injuries includes the following: adequate preseason physical examinations; matching of competitors for age, weight, and skill levels; proper conditioning; the avoidance of excessive training at too early an age; the thorough rehabilitation of injuries before players return to sport; appropriate and properly maintained equipment and playing fields; adequate supervision; and rule changes as necessary. Although in the United States football, basketball, gymnastics, baseball, and roller skating have the highest injury rates[46] among adolescent populations, in Japan mountain climbing was the single most common sport resulting in nerve injury, secondary to excessive weight in the backpacks of novice mountain climbers. The common thread in all these studies is that inexperience and lack of conditioning result in nerve injuries about the shoulder. Rather than pinpoint a specific sport as unsafe because of a high incidence of injuries, emphasis should be on proper training techniques in all sports to reduce the incidence of all injuries.[106]

Prognosis

Most injuries to the peripheral nerves about the shoulder in sports have a good overall prognosis.[8,61,62] Treatment consisting of observation, physical therapy, and cross-conditioning of the athlete will generally result in resolution of the nerve injury. Bracing is sometimes required during this period for symptomatic relief and to decrease stress on the regenerating nerve.[42,50,70,146,158] Electrical stimulation has also been advocated,[8] although its efficacy has not been confirmed. In cases that do not resolve spontaneously, surgical exploration with neurolysis and possible muscle transfers may be indicated. Specific indications for operative intervention are discussed in relation to each specific nerve. The following sections discuss the anatomy of each of the peripheral nerves about the shoulder, the clinical presentation on injury, treatment, and prognosis.

AXILLARY NERVE INJURY

Pertinent Anatomy

The axillary nerve is the most commonly injury nerve about the shoulder in both athletic and nonathletic injuries.[82,133] The axillary (or circumflex) nerve is composed of fibers from the 5th and 6th cervical nerve roots and originates from the posterior cord of the brachial plexus near the level of the coracoid process[140] (Fig. 19-1). It passes laterally onto the inferolateral border of the subscapularis tendon and rests approximately 3 to 5 mm medial to the musculotendinous junction, where (accompanied by the posterior circumflex humeral artery) it enters the quadrilateral space.[87] The axillary nerve maintains a close anatomic relationship to the inferior capsule by sending two articular twigs to it while passing through the quadrilateral space into the posterior aspect of the shoulder (Fig. 19-2). The axillary nerve then divides into anterior and posterior branches, which supply the anterior and posterior portions of the deltoid muscle. A small branch that arises posteriorly innervates the teres minor and posterior deltoid muscles and supplies the skin overlying the deltoid muscle. The posterior branch terminates as the lateral brachial cutaneous nerve of the arm. The anterior branch continues to wind around the surgical neck of the humerus under the deltoid muscle and extends to the anterior border of the deltoid. The axillary nerve has points of relative fixation at the posterior cord of the brachial plexus, the quadrilateral space, and the nerve's insertion into the deltoid muscle.[3]

The short length of the axillary nerve renders it vulnerable to stretch injuries, especially in the presence of a dislocation, and the nerve's close relationship to the capsule makes it susceptible to injury during surgical capsular procedures for shoulder instability.[20,103] The quadrilateral space, which is bounded by the teres minor superiorly, long head of triceps medially, teres major inferiorly, and humeral neck laterally, forms a potential site of compression of the axillary nerve as it passes from the anterior to the posterior aspect of the shoulder.[23,28,96,124]

Mechanism of Injury

Axillary nerve injuries occur most commonly as a result of anterior shoulder dislocation, a common athletic injury.[8,14,18,62,66,82,84,88,93,94,99,104,114] The exact incidence of nerve palsy with acute dislocation ranges from 9 to 18 percent,[14,114] although Bateman[8] stated that approximately one-

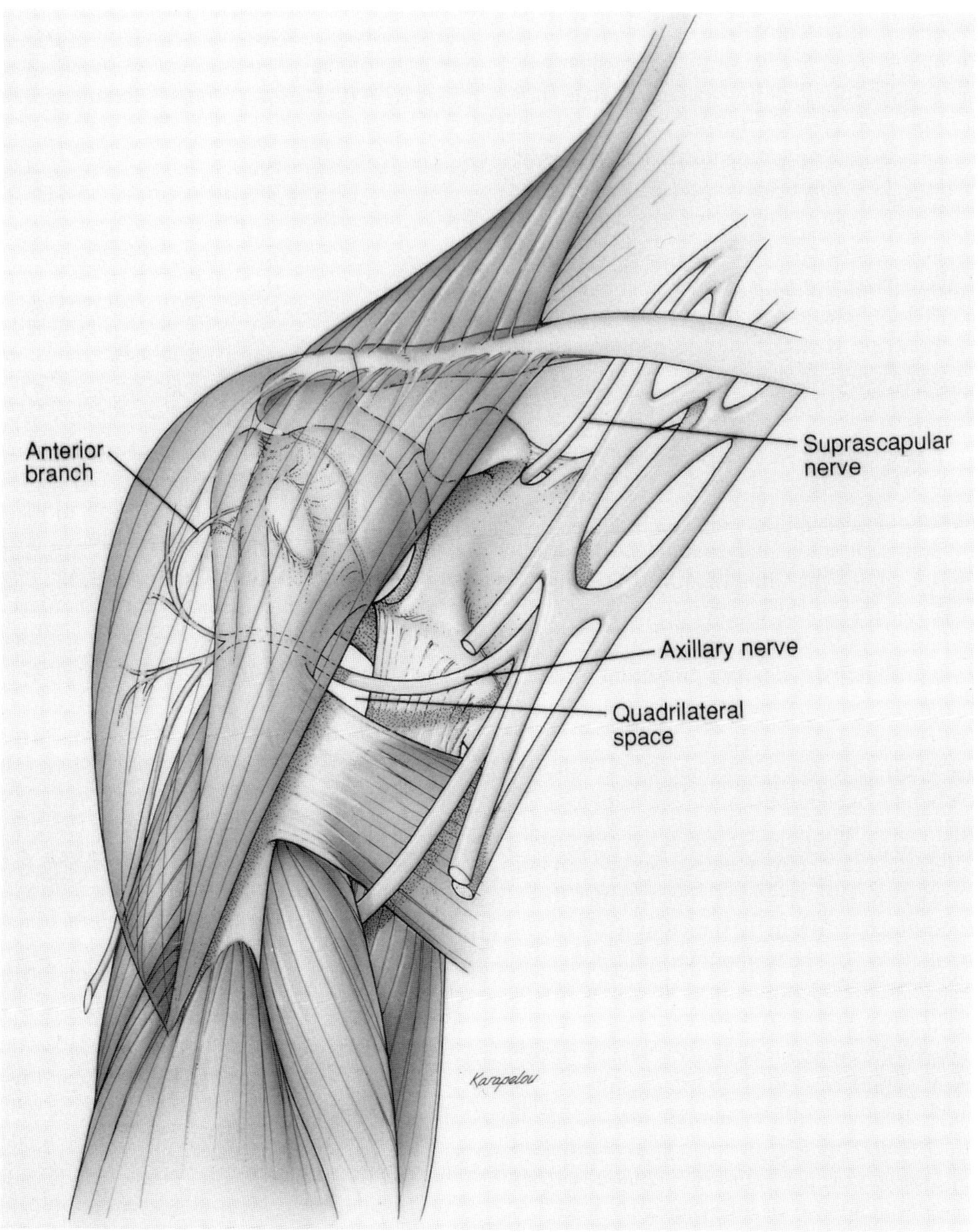

Figure 19-1. Anterior view of axillary nerve. The axillary nerve takes its origin from the posterior cord of the brachial plexus near the level of the coracoid process, passes along the anterior border of the subscapularis muscle, and then courses posteriorly and inferiorly to the border of the subscapularis and enters the quadrilateral space.

third of dislocations result in some form of axillary nerve palsy. Pure inferior dislocations, luxatio erectae, have an even higher incidence of axillary nerve palsy, which has been reported to be as high as 60 percent.[88]

Blunt trauma to the anterior aspect of the shoulder in the absence of dislocation occurs often in certain athletic activities such as football, wrestling, and gymnastics and may result in axillary nerve injury.[8,10,62,93,94] The prognosis following blunt trauma is worse than with axillary nerve palsy following shoulder dislocation or humeral fractures.[10,14,140] Axillary trauma from a direct blow has similarly been implicated in axillary nerve injury.[8,62] This type of trauma may result in hematoma formation and subsequent fibrosis, leading to nerve compression. Acute axillary neuropathy has also been associated with backpacking (''rucksack palsy''), usually in inexperienced hikers carrying packs that are too heavy.[62] The etiology is thought to be secondary to a traction injury on the axillary nerve caused by depression of the shoulder.

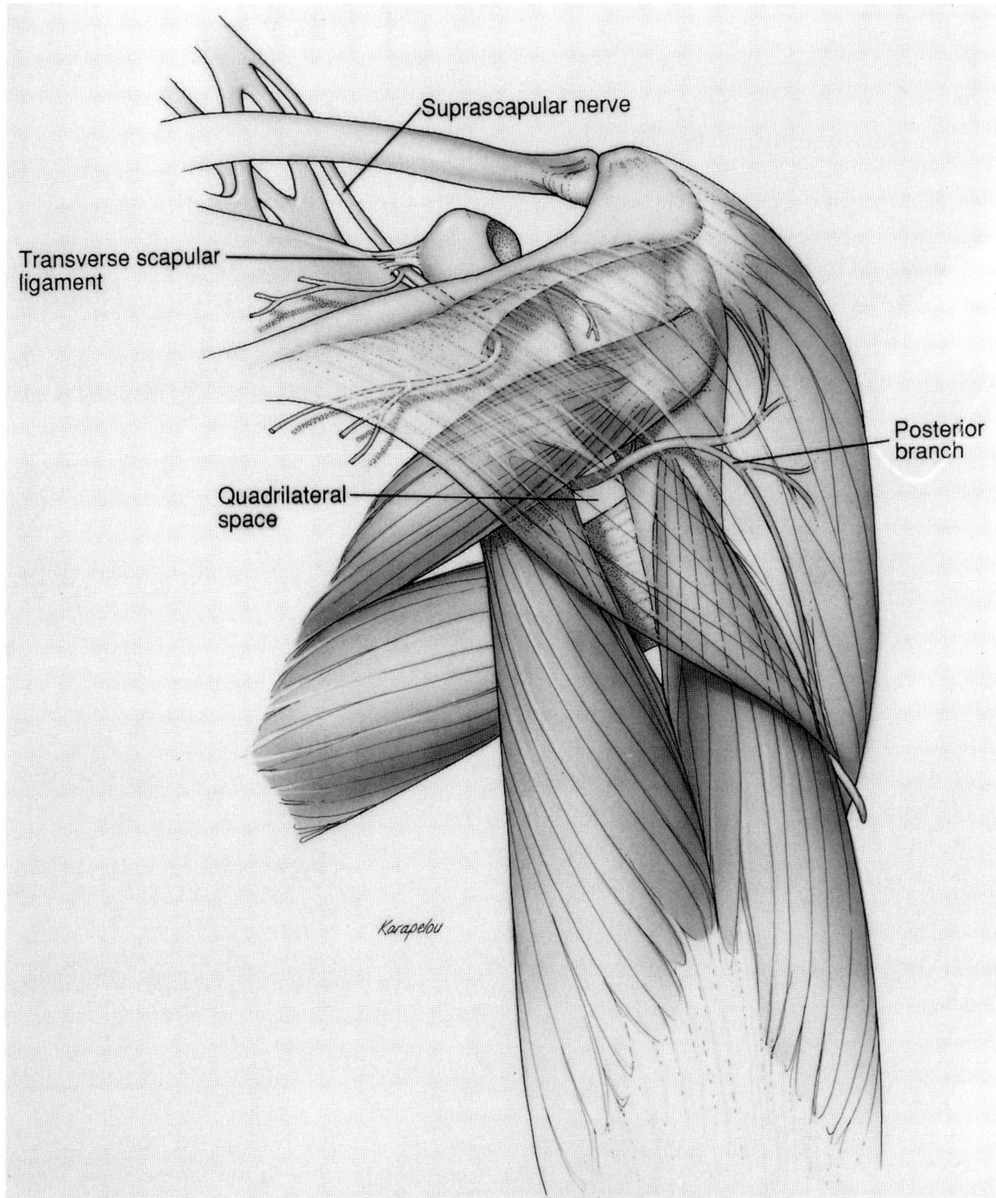

Figure 19-2. Posterior view of axillary nerve. After the axillary nerve passes through the quadrilateral space, it divides into anterior and posterior branches, which supply the anterior and posterior portions of the deltoid muscle. A branch to the teres minor also arises from the posterior axillary branch and also supplies the skin overlying the deltoid.

Quadrilateral space syndrome, a chronic compression involving the axillary nerve, has been described in throwing athletes. This form of axillary nerve entrapment arises insidiously, without a history of trauma. Fibrous bands at the inferior edge of the teres minor muscle have been implicated, as well as randomly oriented fibrous bands found in the quadrilateral space. In this syndrome, the abducted, externally rotated position causes compression at the quadrilateral space, compromising both the axillary nerve and posterior humeral circumflex artery.[23,28,96,124] A chronic compression syndrome has been described in this area in a baseball player secondary to inferior osteophytes on the humeral head.[9] An acute entrapment of the axillary nerve has also been described in an arm wrestler's quadrilateral space, secondary to violent contraction of the muscles surrounding the quadrilateral space.[47]

Finally, the axillary nerve is susceptible to injury during surgery for instability, which is commonly performed in overhead athletes.[20,87,103] The surgeon must be careful to protect the nerve during the inferior portion of the capsular dissection. The main trunk of the nerve is also at risk during arthroscopy because of its usual location 2 cm from the posterior portal.[20] Inferior placement of the posterior portal should be avoided.

Clinical Presentation

Axillary nerve palsy in the acute setting in the athlete can be subtle, and careful physical examination and EMG evaluation are necessary to make an accurate diagnosis.[43] Evaluation of strength is often hampered by pain,[84] and partial axillary nerve injury may present as weakness without complete paralysis.

In the acute setting, the athlete classically presents with weakness in abduction, decreased sensation along the deltoid muscle insertion, atrophy of the deltoid muscle, and subluxation of the glenohumeral joint. Pain is not a prominent complaint. Surrounding muscle groups, however, can compensate for lost deltoid muscle function.[3,43,89,136] The pectoralis and supraspinatus muscles can permit abduction,[82] which is seen in up to 60 percent of patients with axillary neuropathy, and the supraspinatus and long head of the biceps muscles can prevent subluxation. Blom and Dahlback[14] reported normal sensation in 13 of 17 patients with total denervation of the axillary nerve.

In cases of chronic compression syndrome such as quadrilateral space syndrome, the patient typically presents with tenderness in the posterior shoulder in the area of the quadrilateral space. Symptoms are vague, consisting of a dull ache and weakness with progressive use, and are exacerbated by placing the arm in the hyperabducted and externally rotated position and resisting internal rotation.[124]

During physical examination, the deltoid muscle must be palpated carefully by the examiner while resisted abduction is attempted. The examiner should also be aware that a normal sensory examination does not preclude the diagnosis of axillary nerve injury.

Electromyelogram Evaluation

As with other peripheral nerve injuries, the EMG is critical in making the definitive diagnosis. The technique of EMG evaluation of the axillary nerve has been outlined by Kraft[76] and consists of stimulation at Erb's point with a recording by surface electrodes over the deltoid muscle. The recorded values are compared with standard latencies. Berry and Brill[10] found that in 15 percent of cases in which complete axillary nerve lesion was suspected based on clinical examination, an incomplete lesion was noted on EMG. EMG is also helpful in monitoring the recovery of nerve function that can precede clinical recovery and in excluding lesions that involve associated nerves or the brachial plexus, which occur more commonly than an isolated axillary nerve lesion.[116,140]

In cases of quadrilateral space syndrome, however, the EMG evaluation is often normal. The examination of choice in this case is an arteriogram performed with the arm held in the abducted, externally rotated position. A positive arteriogram shows occlusion of the posterior humeral circumflex artery.[28,96,124]

Differential Diagnosis

The differential diagnosis for axillary nerve lesions includes injury to the posterior cord that affects the radial nerve and the thoracodorsal nerve. Careful examination of the latissimus dorsi muscle, as well as the radially innervated nerves, will differentiate this condition from an isolated axillary nerve lesion.

Acute brachial neuritis involves the deltoid muscle alone in approximately 10 percent of cases, although usually the spinati are involved.[113] A diagnostic indicator of acute brachial neuritis is severe pain in the shoulder, which is usually not found with isolated axillary nerve injury.

Deltoid weakness also can be seen in more diffuse brachial plexus lesions and cervical root lesions involving C5 and C6. These two diagnoses can be differentiated from isolated axillary nerve lesions through careful physical examination and EMG evaluation.

Treatment

Axillary nerve lesion in athletes after either dislocation or blunt trauma[8,10] generally responds to a course of observation and physical therapy and does not require more aggressive management. An EMG evaluation confirms the diagnosis and indicates whether the injury to the axillary nerve is complete or incomplete. When the axillary nerve lesion has been demostrated to be incomplete by both clinical examination and EMG testing, the prognosis is favorable and gradual improvement is expected. Bateman[8] recommends splinting the shoulder in a position of partial abduction and pursuing a daily regimen of electrical stimulation and passive range of motion exercises to prevent stiffness. When the EMG reveals a complete axillary nerve lesion, the athlete should be re-evaluated at monthly intervals. Because the axillary nerve is relatively short, recovery should be seen between the third and fourth month after injury.[10]

Surgical exploration and grafting is generally recommended 2 to 4 months after injury if no return of function is noted.[3,10,61,116] The site of injury is generally in the area of the quadrilateral space and requires both anterior and posterior approaches. If a nerve injury in continuity is noted, simple neurolysis is advocated.[116] If the nerve is torn, the anterior portion of the axillary nerve is dissected through the anterior approach to the level of the quadrilateral space. Through a posterior approach, the posterior limb of the axillary nerve is similarly dissected and the neuroma excised. Sural nerve grafts are generally used because primary repair of the axillary nerve is generally not technically possible. The sural nerve is first grafted to the posterior limb of the axillary nerve and then passed through the quadrilateral space. The anterior anastomosis is then performed through the anterior incision. The results of this surgery are generally good,[116] but fortunately, surgery in the athletic population is seldom needed. Chronic axillary nerve compression in the quadrilateral space syndrome generally improves with change in pitching mechanics[124] and rest. Cahill and Palmer[23] showed excellent or satisfactory results in 16 of 18 cases treated this way. Cormier et al[28] similarly found improvement in 75 percent of cases with conservative management. The need for operative intervention is dictated by the failure of symptoms to resolve with conservative management. If surgery is deemed necessary, posterior approach to the shoulder is advocated for exposure of the quadrilateral space. The nerve to the teres minor muscle is located and traced back to the axillary nerve in the quadrilateral space. Release of fibrous bands on the teres minor muscle and aberrant bands crossing the quadrilateral space generally results in relief of symptoms.[28,96,124]

Prognosis and Return to Sport

The short length of the axillary nerve, which renders it susceptible to injury with shoulder dislocation, also gives the nerve a good prognosis for improvement because the distance from the site of injury to muscle end plates is relatively short. The recovery rate for the axillary nerve after dislocation of the shoulder has generally been in the range of 80 percent.[3,4] The result with blunt injury to the shoulder was worse in the series by Berry and Brill.[10] Other factors affecting prognosis are the degree of initial denervation on initial EMG,[93] as well as the level of injury in the brachial plexus,[82] with a worse prognosis noted in injuries involving a greater number of nerves. The prognosis in quadrilateral space syndrome is generally good, even in resistant cases in which surgery is required. No consensus exists in the literature as to the exact point at which return to sports should be allowed. In general, normalization of the EMG, as well as recovery of at least 80 percent of deltoid muscle strength, is recommended.

SUPRASCAPULAR NERVE

Pertinent Anatomy

Because of its anatomic location, the suprascapular nerve is susceptible to injury in athletes, and lesions of this nerve are more common than was previously thought.[71,81,151] The suprascapular nerve originates from the upper trunk of the brachial plexus and is formed from the spinal roots of C5 and C6, with a variable contribution from the C4 nerve root. It branches from the upper trunk of the brachial plexus at Erb's point and runs laterally, crossing the posterior triangle of the neck parallel and deep to the omohyoid muscle and deep to the trapezius muscle. The nerve then passes through the suprascapular notch of the scapula, which is bridged by a thick transverse scapular ligament (Fig. 19-3). The shape and size of the suprascapular notch varies significantly and has been classified into six varieties by Rengachary et al.[12] After entering the supraspinatus fossa, the nerve gives off two motor branches to the supraspinatus muscle and then passes laterally within the fossa, providing sensory branches to the posterior capsule of the glenohumeral joint and acromioclavicular joint. It then passes around the lateral border of the base of the spinous process to the infraspinatus fossa, where the nerve terminates, supplying motor branches to the infraspinatus muscle. Approximately 50 percent of individuals have a spinoglenoid ligament,[2,13] which is an aponeurotic band that separates the supraspinatus and infraspinatus muscles.[38,98] The suprascapular nerve has no cutaneous distribution or innervation.

The suprascapular nerve has a short course and several sites of relative fixation along the nerve, making it vulnerable to both traction and compressive forces.[133] The nerve is fixed at both its origin at Erb's point on the brachial plexus and at its terminal insertion on the infraspinatus.[98,125] Also, two critical points between these endpoints are implicated in injuries to the nerve: its passage through the suprascapular notch and around the base of the spine of the scapula in the spinoglenoid area.[98,125] The nerve is relatively fixed to the suprascapular notch, and anatomic studies have shown that motion does not occur at this point, even with extremes of motion.[32,81,126,133,140] Anomalous bifid transverse scapular ligaments have also been described.[5]

Mechanism of Injury

The mechanism of injury to the suprascapular nerve in sports (Table 19-1) is generally a traction injury, which can occur with an increase in acromiomastoid distance and stretching of the nerve between Erb's point and the suprascapular notch.[8,75,98,125] For this reason, suprascapular nerve injuries can be associated with acromioclavicular separations that occur by the same mechanism. Rengachary et al[125] have observed through anatomic dissection that depression, hyperabduction, and retraction of the scapula causes the suprascapular nerve to become opposed against the sharp inferior border of the transverse scapular ligament, creating an acute change of direction in the nerve at this point and resulting in nerve injury. This injury, therefore, does not occur secondary to friction of the nerve passing through the suprascapular foramen but from the so-called sling effect.

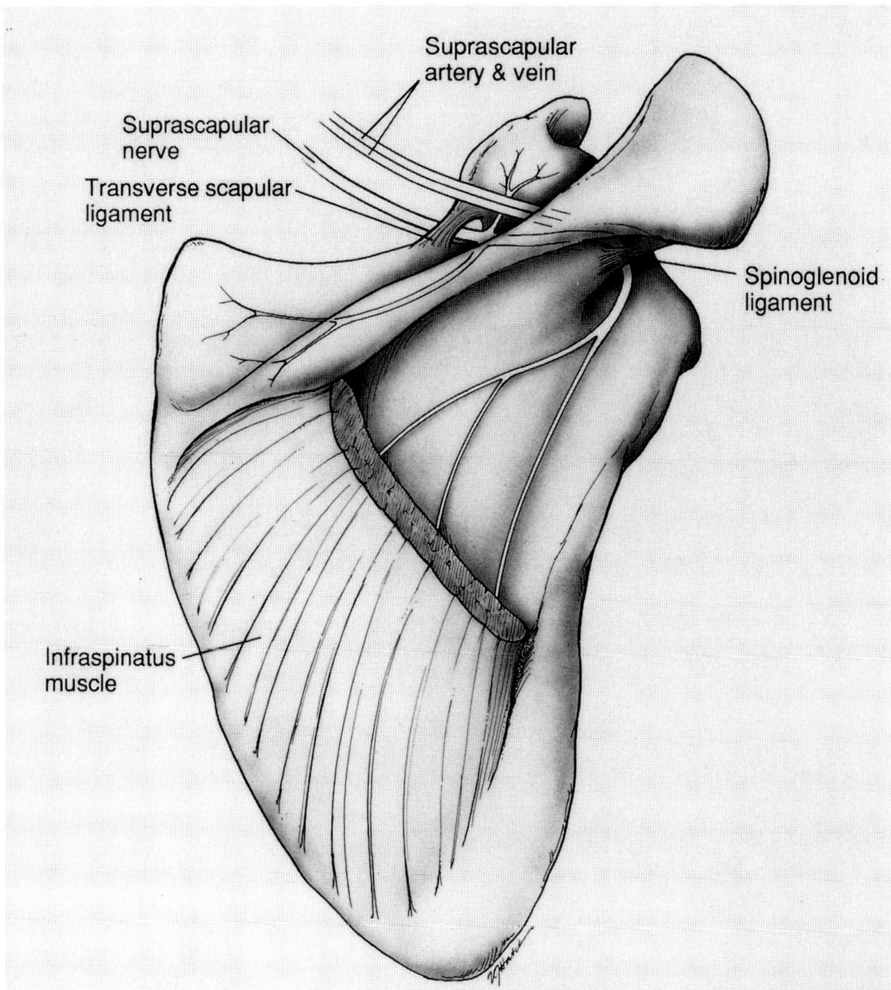

Figure 19-3. Posterior view of scapula with suprascapular nerve. The suprascapular nerve passes through the suprascapular notch of the scapula, which is bridged by the thick transverse scapular ligament. On entering the supraspinatus fossa, the nerve supplies the motor branches to the supraspinatus muscle. It then passes around the lateral border of the base of the spinous process to the infraspinatus fossa where the nerve terminates, supplying motor branches to the infraspinatus muscle. Approximately 50 percent of individuals have a spinoglenoid ligament, which is an aponeurotic band that separates the supraspinatus and infraspinatus muscles.

Cross-body adduction or protraction with forward flexion and rotation has also been found to maximally stretch the nerve.[98,122,131] This type of maneuver is commonly seen in fencing,[2] thowing sports,[8,21] racquet sports,[13,143,157] and weight lifting. Suprascapular nerve entrapment syndromes can follow either repetitive and prolonged motions or single acute events.[81] Entrapment can also occur more distally at the spinoglenoid area, and this is more commonly seen in sports requiring rapid, forceful, external rotation movements, such as volleyball.[38] The cocking motion for the serve results in rapid external rotation of the shoulder, and this rapid motion of the infraspinatus muscle pulls the suprascapular nerve against the base of the spine of the scapula or spinoglenoid ligament, resulting in injury to the nerve at this point. Injury to the nerve in this spinoglenoid area has also been noted secondary to ganglion cysts[44,52,63,143,159] (Fig. 19-4). The origin of these

Table 19-1. Sports Associated With Suprascapular Nerve Injury

Baseball[21]	Basketball[17,32]
Cycling[159]	Weight lifting[1,13,44,131]
Fencing[2]	Physical education[5]
Surfing[139]	Tennis[13,157]
Throwing[8]	Backpacking[52]
Volleyball[38,62]	Gymnastics[81]
Racquetball[144]	

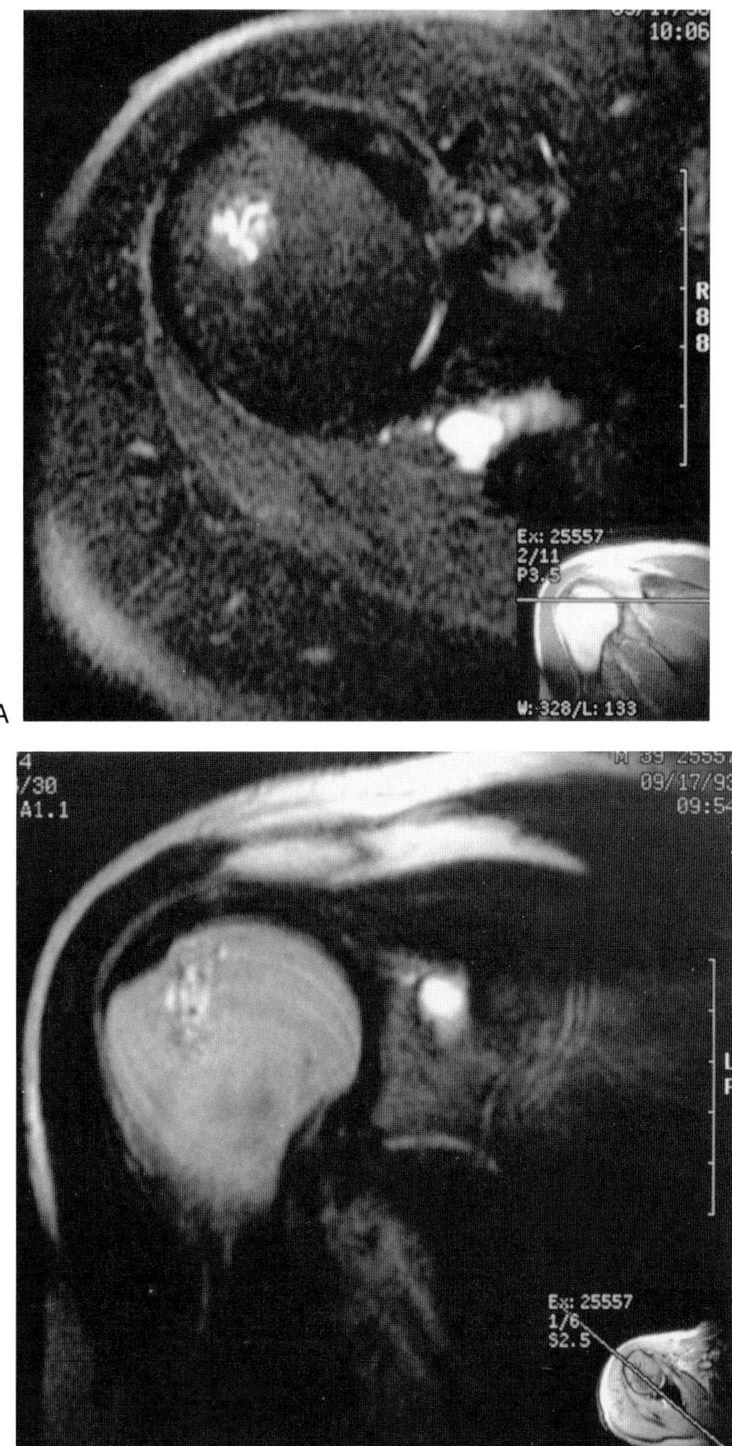

Figure 19-4. (**A & B**) Ganglion cyst impinging on suprascapular nerve and spinoglenoid area. Suprascapular nerve compression in the spinoglenoid area is characterized by isolated involvement of the infraspinatus muscle with sparing of the supraspinatus. Ganglion cysts can occur in this area, leading to compression of the nerve at this site. Magnetic resonance imaging can clearly define ganglion cysts in this area and direct surgery toward their removal.

ganglion cysts in athletes has not been adequately explained, but their presence should be suspected in cases of suprascapular nerve entrapment, and especially those affecting just the infraspinatus muscle. The suprascapular nerve is at risk for injury along the glenoid neck during arthroscopic stabilization procedures using transglenoid sutures.[11]

Clinical Presentation

The cardinal symptoms of suprascapular neuropathy are vague posterior shoulder pain, weakness of abduction, external rotation, and atrophy of the supraspinatus and infraspinatus muscles. Symptoms generally have an insidious onset[1] and are poorly localized.[2,5,52,75,81,101,119] Pain can also radiate down the radial axis of the arm.[75,132,151] Pain is an inconsistent finding with entrapment at the spinoglenoid area.[13,38,143] The source of the pain is thought to be the sensory fibers to the acromioclavicular and glenohumeral joints,[98] and because there is no dermal distribution to this nerve, the symptoms are poorly localized, leading commonly to a delay in diagnosis on the average of 12 months.[52]

Physical examination of the athlete with suprascapular neuropathy can be difficult because symptoms are vague and signs are often poorly localized. Atrophy of the supraspinatus and infraspinatus muscles is the hallmark of this neuropathy, but the supraspinatus muscle can be difficult to see because of the overlaying trapezius muscle. Wasting of the infraspinatus is the most likely diagnostic sign on physical examination.[81,131] Depending on the level of involvement, the athlete may have weakness in forward elevation and external rotation. A drop arm sign, in which the patient cannot maintain the arm in neutral rotation, may be seen with severe cases, although the teres minor muscle (which is innervated by the axillary nerve) usually allows some external rotation.[140] Full abduction is usually possible,[148] although loss of strength in abduction is usually noted. In laboratory studies, Strohm and Colachis[139] noted a 40 percent loss in abducation between 30 and 60 degrees with anesthetic block of the suprascapular nerve, although full abduction was still possible. Variable tenderness at the suprascapular notch has been reported,[75] and if a large ganglion is present, this can sometimes be palpated as well.[44] Frozen shoulder has presented in conjunction with suprascapular neuropathy,[75, 101] and glenohumeral subluxation has been reported as a complication after this neuropathy.[159] Skin sensation, however, is characteristically normal.

Laboratory Evaluation

The EMG remains the most reliable test for making the diagnosis of suprascapular nerve entrapment.[1,2,25,27,36,52,71,75,76,81,101,132] The technique of nerve conduction includes stimulation at Erb's point and recording over the supraspinatus and infraspinatus muscles using single coaxial needle electrodes, rather than surface electrodes.[119] This technique can also reveal the site of nerve conduction delay and differentiate between Erb's point, the transverse scapular ligament, and the spinoglenoid ligament.[1] The EMG also helps to exclude other neuropathies in cases in which diffuse shoulder atrophy is present and other muscle groups are involved.[52]

Rangachary has described an x-ray view to reveal the shape of the suprascapular notch using a 15 to 30 degree caudal tilt. This view is also helpful in cases of scapular fracture to detect deformation of the suprascapular notch.[36,97] In the cases of suspected ganglion cyst, a computed tomographic or magnetic resonance imaging scan is helpful in visualizing the site and extent of the cyst.[44] Bryan and Wild[21] recommend the computer-assisted tomographic scan to evaluate the degree of infraspinatus muscle atrophy and the appropriateness of surgical intervention. They have found poor postoperative results in athletes who have severe preoperative atrophy. Because shoulder pain and weakness in external rotation and forward elevation are also characteristic of rotator cuff tears,[31,32,94,95,104,105] an arthrogram of the shoulder is helpful in excluding this diagnosis. Several authors have advocated the infiltration of local anesthetics under fluoroscopic guidance into the area of the suprascapular notch.[27,31,36,45,75,95,105,119,129,132,139,151] Pain relief with this injection confirms the diagnosis of suprascapular nerve entrapment at this point. Murray[101] discourages the use of this test because it is difficult to perform and unreliable.

Differential Diagnosis

The differential diagnosis for suprascapular nerve entrapment is extensive, and a variety of diagnoses should be excluded before an EMG is ordered. Rotator cuff tears are much more common than suprascapular nerve entrapment and present similarly.[31,32,94,95,105] Moreover, these two diagnoses can present simultaneously.[95,104] Cervical root lesions of C5 must be excluded,[8] as must injuries to the upper trunk of the brachial plexus.[1] If the supraspinatus and infraspinatus are the only muscles affected, however, these two diagnoses can generally be excluded.

Glenohumeral arthritis can present with posterior shoulder pain, weakness in external rotation secondary to pain, and diffuse atrophy. Vague pain about the shoulder with suprascapular nerve entrapment can also be confused with impingement syndrome,[131] as well as calcific bursitis.[157]

The concomitant presentation of frozen shoulder and suprascapular neuropathy has been well described by Koppel and Thompson.[75] The supraspinatus and infraspinatus muscles are affected in one-third to one-half of patients with acute brachial neuritis,[113,147] and occasionally these muscles are the only ones involved.

Treatment

A conservative regimen including observation, rest, and analgesics is generally recommended for suprascapular nerve entrapment.[1,13,17,32,38,75,81,97,119,131,159] Analgesics,[75] cortisone injections into the suprascapular notch,[45,75,157] and electrical stimulation[8,75,157] have also been advocated, although variable success has been obtained with these techniques.[38,81]

In cases of suprascapular nerve entrapment resistant to 3 to 6 months of conservative management, surgical decompression is indicated.[8,13,32,119,157] The area of compression can be determined by EMG, and then surgery can be directed to that site. Involvement of both the supraspinatus and infraspinatus muscles, with a conduction delay at the suprascapular notch, would be an indication for transverse scapular ligament release, whereas conduction delay at the spinoglenoid ligament with isolated involvement of the infraspinatus muscle would be an indication for surgical release at this more distal site.[2] If a ganglion cyst is present, it should be excised.[44,52,63,144,159]

The transverse scapular ligament is generally released via a posterior approach,[5,25,125,126] although an anterior approach has been advocated.[101] Notchplasty has been advocated by Rask[122] but is generally thought to put the patient at risk for postoperative heterotopic bone formation.[75,101,143] In most series, release of the transverse scapular ligament alone has achieved good results.[75,101,119,143]

Our surgical technique includes placement of the patient in the lateral decubitus position and a posterior approach over the superior border of the spine of the scapula. The trapezius is elevated from the spine of the scapula subperiosteally, and dissection is carried out between the trapezius and supraspinatus muscles. In cases of entrapment at the suprascapular notch, the supraspinatus muscle is retracted caudally to expose the transverse scapular ligament. The suprascapular artery and vein, which travel superiorly to the transverse scapular ligament, are retracted, and a blunt retractor is placed in the notch to protect the nerve. The transverse scapular ligament is excised, but the notch is not widened by excision of bone. In cases of entrapment by a ganglion cyst or a fibro-osseous tunnel in the spinoglenoid area, detachment of the origin of the deltoid muscle allows access to the base of the spine of the scapula, both superiorly and inferiorly, for wide exposure of the nerve. Through this approach, decompression of the nerve at the transverse scapular ligament, removal of a ganglion cyst, and decompression of the spinoglenoid area can all be performed. The trapezius and deltoid insertion are then attached to the spine of the scapula through drill holes, using nonabsorbable sutures. The athlete's arm is placed in a sling postoperatively, and early passive range of motion is started the day after surgery.

Prognosis

Prognosis for recovery in suprascapular neuropathy is good, both with conservative treatment and surgical intervention.[1,2,5,13,38,44,81,119,145,159] Postoperatively, most athletes note decreased pain and increased strength and endurance. However, continued atrophy despite normalization of the EMG has been the rule in most series.

Return to sports should be allowed on a symptomatic basis as strength of the shoulder improves and pain resolves. Good strength of external rotation is most important in throwing athletes, in whom it serves an important function of arm deceleration in the follow-through phase. Athletes who are allowed to return to throwing before good strength has returned to their external rotators are at risk for developing rotator cuff pathology secondary to inadequate deceleration, although Ferretti et al[38] found no significant problems in volleyball players who continued to play despite marked infraspinatus atrophy.

MUSCULOCUTANEOUS NERVE

Pertinent Anatomy

The musculocutaneous nerve is derived primarily from fibers of the C5 and C6 spinal roots, with occasional fibers from C7. It originates from the lateral cord of the brachial plexus near the inferior border of the pectoralis minor and continues distally between the axillary artery and the median nerve. It then enters the upper arm by passing obliquely and distally through the coracobrachialis muscle, between the biceps and brachialis muscles that it innervates (Fig. 19-5).

The musculocutaneous nerve penetrates the deep brachial fascia lateral to the biceps tendon approximately 2 to 5 cm above the elbow crease, and it terminates as the lateral antebrachial cutaneous nerve of the forearm, which then divides into anterior and posterior terminal cutaneous branches. These branches innervate the skin of the radial aspect of the forearm.

The musculocutaneous nerve is vulnerable to traction injury proximal in its course, where it lies on the subscapularis muscle.[65] Although the usual penetration point for the musculocutaneous nerve in the coracobrachialis muscle has been described as 5 cm distal to the coracoid, Bach et al[7] and Flatow et al[40] have shown through anatomic dissections that in a high percentage of patients penetration by either the main nerve trunk or small nerve twigs occurs

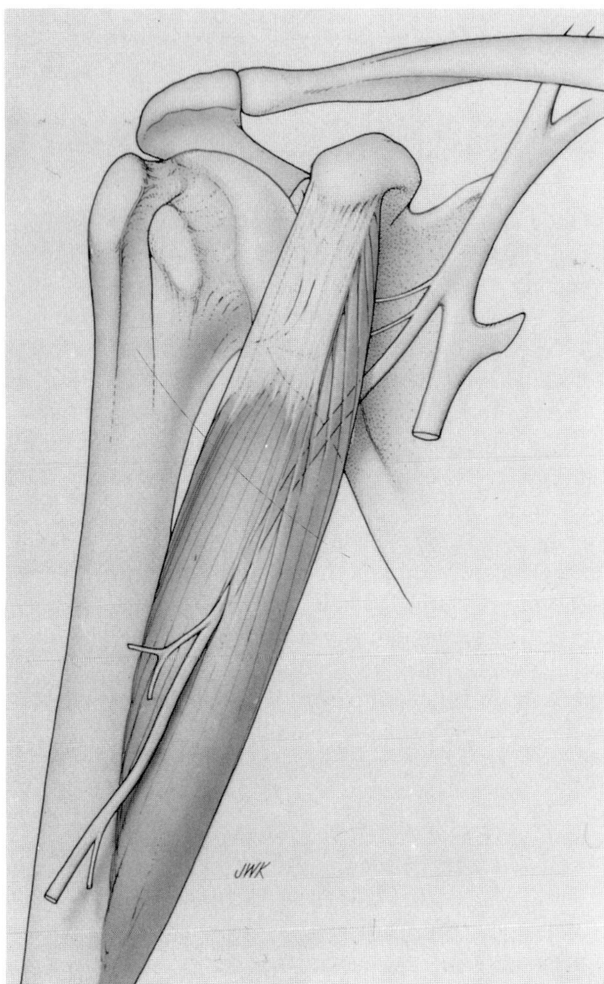

Figure 19-5. Anterior view of the musculocutaneous nerve. The musculocutaneous nerve originates from the lateral cord of the brachial plexus near the inferior border of the pectoralis minor. It enters the upper arm by passing obliquely and distally through the coracobrachialis and between the biceps and brachialis muscles, which it innervates.

much higher to the coracoid, with penetrations as close as 17 mm from the coracoid. Significant variation is common in the path of this nerve.[140]

Mechanism of Injury

Isolated musculocutaneous nerve injuries are not common but have been reported in a variety of clinical situations secondary to both direct and indirect trauma. Bateman[8] described a direct force to the anterior shoulder producing a musculocutaneous nerve injury. Indirect trauma to the musculocutaneous nerve has occurred with humeral and clavicular fractures[140] and anterior shoulder dislocations.[65,84,93,94,114] The musculocutaneous nerve is at risk for traction across the humeral head or coracoid with the arm in abduction and external rotation, and traction injuries have been described in competitive airplane flying,[47] as well as throwing a football. Compression of the nerve by a hypertrophied or engorged coracobrachialis muscle has been implicated in musculocutaneous nerve palsy in rowers and weight lifters.[16,72,91] Direct traction to the nerve by forceful extension of the forearm has also resulted in musculocutaneous nerve palsy.[8,145]

Surgical procedures on the anterior aspect of the shoulder for instability in athletes have been associated with musculocutaneous nerve palsy.[93,94] This has been especially true in the Bristow and Putti-Platt procedures.[7,127,128] Pittman et al[118] have pointed out the vulnerability of the musculocutaneous nerve to injury during shoulder arthroscopy due to traction on the nerve. Responsible factors included joint distension, excessive traction, and extravasation of fluid. Positioning for other operative procedures involving abduction, extension, and external rotation of the arm has also produced musculocutaneous nerve injury.[33]

Clinical Presentation

An athlete with a musculocutaneous nerve palsy presents with wasting of the biceps and brachialis muscles, as well as weakness in elbow flexion (Fig. 19-6). There is a variable loss of sensation on the lateral aspect of the forearm,[91] but generally there is no pain involved with musculocutaneous nerve palsy.

Examination of these athletes reveals atrophy of the biceps and brachialis muscles or, in the case of incomplete injuries, a decrease in tone of these muscles. There is a loss of the biceps tendon reflex, and hypoesthesias of the lateral forearm are usually present. Elbow flexion is weak or absent, although some flexion is possible using the brachioradialis muscle.

Differential Diagnosis

The differential diagnosis for musculocutaneous nerve injury includes rupture of the biceps tendon at the elbow, as well as more diffuse nerve injuries. With distal biceps tendon ruptures, a superiorly retracted biceps muscle can be seen and felt to contract in the upper arm, and a loss of contour is noted. In the acute phase, swelling and ecchymosis, as well as tenderness, are evident. Brachial plexus injury or lateral cord injuries must also be differentiated from isolated musculocutaneous nerve injuries. With lateral cord injuries, the wrist and finger flexors are also affected. C5 and C6 root injuries also affect the musculocutaneous nerve, but in these cases, the deltoid muscle and spinati muscles will also be involved. Brachial neuritis

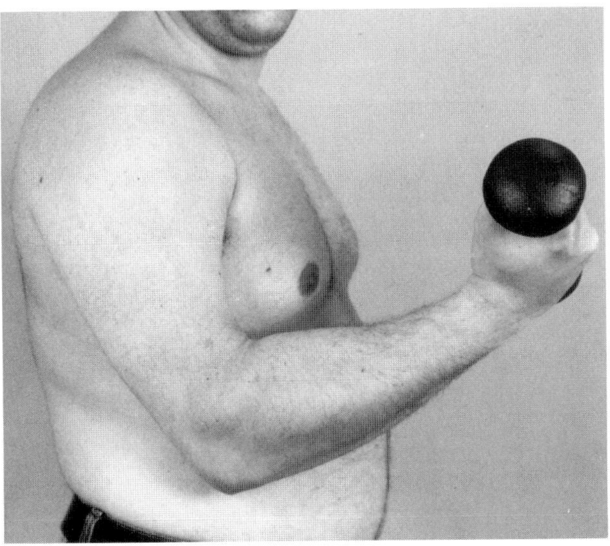

Figure 19-6. Severe biceps and brachialis atrophy secondary to musculocutaneous nerve injury. This patient demonstrates atrophy of the biceps and brachialis muscles due to complete musculocutaneous nerve palsy that occurred during a procedure for recurrent shoulder instability.

can involve the musculocutaneous nerve, but this usually occurs in association with other muscle groups. Another distinguishing feature is that brachial neuritis is painful, in contrast to isolated musculocutaneous nerve injury. Careful physical and EMG evaluation help to differentiate these entities.

Electromyelogram Evaluation

EMG evaluation is the easiest way to differentiate musculocutaneous nerve injuries from those associated with more diffuse nerve involvement. The musculocutaneous nerve is stimulated at Erb's point and impulses are recorded using surface electrodes over the biceps and brachialis muscle bellies. Kraft has defined normal latencies of nerve conduction, although the contralateral side can also be used as a control.[76]

Treatment

Closed injuries of the musculocutaneous nerve generally recover spontaneously without requiring surgical intervention.[91] For injuries of the musculocutaneous nerve associated with repetitive use or a frontal blow, observation, rest, and electrical stimulation generally yield good results.[8,16,72,91] Incomplete lesions of the musculocutaneous nerve can simply be monitored if they demonstrate progressive recovery; lesions that do not demonstrate recovery or that fail to recover completely within 3 months should be surgically explored.[74] Complete lesions are rare in the athletic population but may occur after repair for anterior shoulder instability. If there is no sign of early improvement, these lesions should be explored earlier than 3 months for appropriate repair.[16,22]

Prognosis and Return to Sport

The prognosis for musculocutaneous nerve injury in athletes is generally good; most players improve once the offending activity is eliminated.[16,72,91] Jerosch et al[65] found complete spontaneous recovery after shoulder dislocation, although dislocations associated with higher energy trauma and those associated with a greater number of nerve injuries have a worse prognosis. Return to sport may be allowed once the athlete is asymptomatic, with appropriate alteration in technique if the nerve lesion was secondary to repetitive use or positioning.

LONG THORACIC NERVE

Pertinent Anatomy

The long thoracic nerve (external respiratory nerve of Bell, or posterior thoracic nerve) is a pure motor nerve to one muscle originating directly from the spinal roots of C5, C6, and C7. The 5th and 6th cranial nerve roots join after they pierce the scalenus medius muscle and are then united with the C7 contribution to the muscle at the level of the first rib. The long thoracic nerve then passes laterally beneath the brachial plexus and clavicle dorsal to the axillary vessels and then continues down along the anterolateral aspect of the chest wall, supplying branches to all the digitations of the serratus anterior muscle[50,51,67,140,155] (Fig. 19-7). The long thoracic nerve is well protected to the level of the inferior portion of the pectoralis major. Gregg et al[50] think that the long thoracic nerve has two points of fixation, one at the scalenus medius muscle and the second at the superior muscle mass of the serratus anterior, and is susceptible to traction injury between these points.

Kauppila,[70] in recent anatomic studies, noted no significant motion in the nerve at the first through fourth digitations with either head or shoulder motion. The lower digitations of the serratus anterior muscle, however, were very mobile, and she thinks that the nerve is susceptible to tension and compression injuries with scapular motion at this level.[70] There is marked variation in the anatomy of this nerve, which may account for the variable susceptibility to injury noted in athletes.

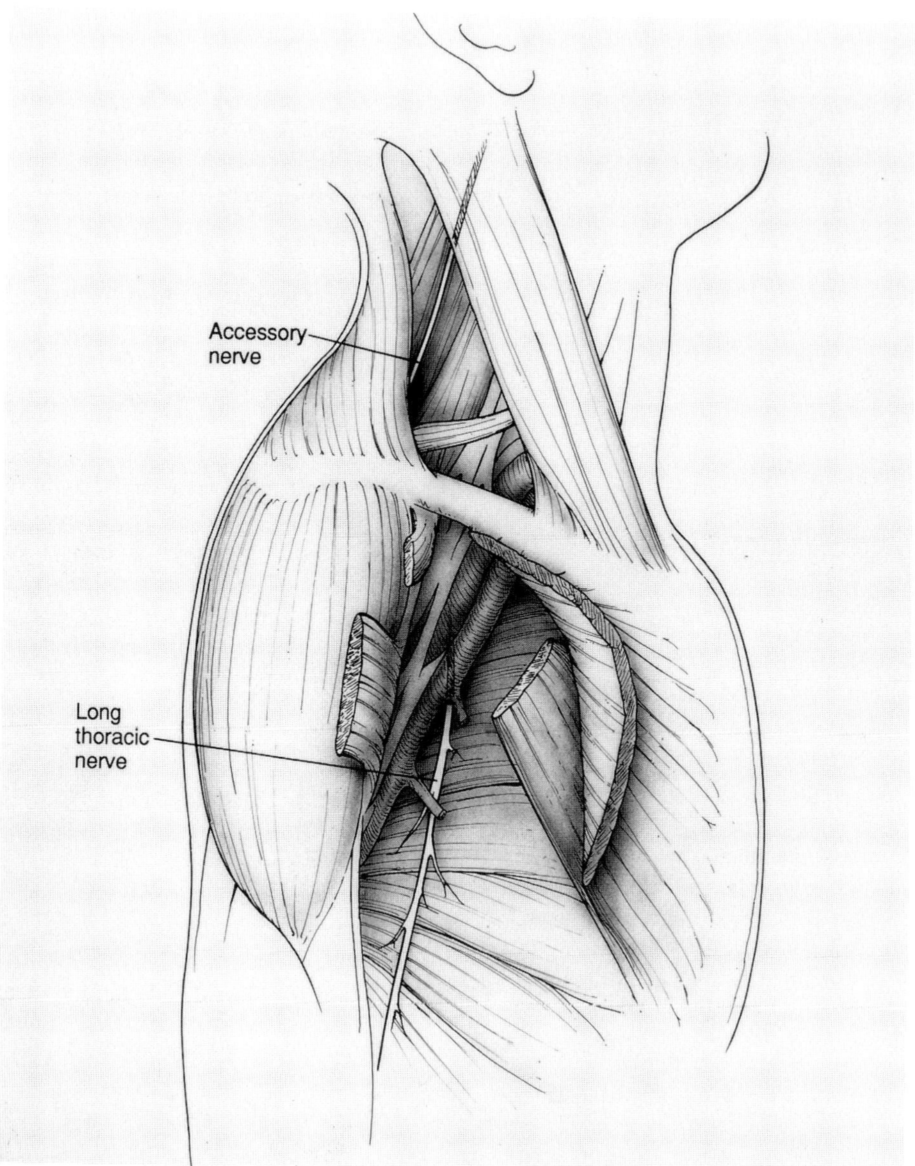

Figure 19-7. Lateral view of long thoracic nerve. The long thoracic nerve passes laterally beneath the brachial plexus and the clavicle and continues down along the anterior lateral aspect of the chest wall supplying branches to all the digitations of the serratus anterior muscle. This root level nerve is purely motor and supplies only one muscle, the serratus anterior.

Mechanism of Injury

First described by Velpeau in 1837,[150] isolated serratus anterior muscle paralysis due to a long thoracic nerve lesion can occur as a result of an acute injury, or more insidiously, as a result of repetitive motion, positioning, or repetitive strain. A wide variety of sports has been implicated (Table 19-2). In general, the lesion occurs secondary to asynchronous motion of the arm and scapula, which can occur with a missed shot in golf, handball, or tennis,[65] or in contact sports in which the arm is jerked into an abnormal position.[111] Gregg et al[50] have noted that tension is placed on the nerve when the head is rotated, flexed, and laterally tilted away from the shoulder with the arm overhead. In this position, the scapula moves posteriorly, laterally, and inferiorly, and it places tension on the nerve, which is fixed at the scalenus medius muscle. A blow to the shoulder is unlikely to cause an isolated injury to the long thoracic

Table 19-2. Sports Implicated in Long Thoracic Nerve Injury

Archery[41]	Hockey[50]
Backpacking[50,64,149]	Rope skipping[115]
Ballet[50]	Shooting[155]
Basketball[68,149]	Skiing[149]
Bowling[50]	Soccer[50]
Discus[8]	Squash[50]
Football[50,67]	Swimming[149]
Golf[50,149]	Tennis[50,51]
Gymnastics[50]	Weight lifting[50,56,135,149]
Handball[149]	Wrestling[48]

nerve without more diffuse involvement of the brachial plexus.[70,140]

Chronic repetitive motions in sports such as swimming and tennis, which result in movement of the scapula as described by Gregg et al,[51] can also cause long thoracic nerve traction injuries. The same position is maintained for extended periods in marksmen while shooting a rifle and may account for reported long thoracic nerve injuries in these athletes.[155] Fatigue of the periscapular muscles, such as is seen in backpacking, rope skipping, and weight lifting, can allow abnormal scapular motion on the chest wall and result in long thoracic nerve injury.[68,111] The weight lifting exercises most commonly associated with this lesion include behind-the-neck French curls[50] and bench press.[135,149]

Clinical Presentation

The serratus anterior muscle stabilizes the scapula on the chest wall to create a stable platform for glenohumeral motion.[138] It also functions to rotate the scapula forward as the arm is elevated above shoulder level. Symptoms of long thoracic nerve palsy can be attributed to loss of these two functions of the serratus anterior muscle. Athletes complain of an uncosmetic winging of the scapula and a decrease in forward elevation.[48,50,67] Weakness with overhead activity[50] and a vague posterior aching or burning shoulder pain are commonly reported. Patients may initially complain of severe pain, whereas winging does not become obvious until several weeks after the initial injury, when pain is resolving.[41,50]

Physical examination of the patient with long thoracic nerve palsy is characterized by winging and a decrease in active elevation, usually to less than 110 degrees. Scapular winging is best observed by having the patient flex the shoulders to 90 degrees, extend the elbows, and internally rotate the shoulders and then push against a wall with both hands.[50] Palpation of the serratus anterior muscle is sometimes possible just anterior to the latissimus dorsi muscle, although this test is not reliable.[48] Observation of the scapula during attempted active forward elevation reveals uncoordinated scapular motion. Despite scapular winging, careful observation of the scapula reveals it to be closer to the midline posteriorly and slightly elevated in relation to the contralateral normal scapula,[107] in distinction to spinal accessory nerve palsy.

Electromyelogram Evaluation

EMG evaluation confirms the diagnosis of long thoracic nerve palsy. The nerve is stimulated with a bipolar surface electrode in the supraclavicular fossa, and recordings are made using concentric needle electrodes along the 5th or 6th ribs anterior to the midaxillary line.[86,115] Normal conduction velocities have been described by Petrera and Trojaborg.[115]

Differential Diagnosis

The differential diagnosis of long thoracic nerve palsy is extensive. Winging of the scapula can occur secondary to trapezius muscle paralysis,[12] posterior shoulder instability, brachial plexus lesions,[74,138] and traumatic serratus anterior muscle avulsions[39,57] as well as scoliosis, malunions of the scapula, and chronic glenohumeral conditions.[97] Acute brachial neuropathy involving the long thoracic nerve,[41,113,147] diabetic amyotrophy, polio, multiple sclerosis, toxic agents, cold exposure, and infection have all been associated with long thoracic nerve palsy.[149]

Treatment

Although no other muscle can adequately substitute for the function of the serratus anterior muscle,[158] recovery of serratus anterior muscle function can occur over extended periods of up to 2 years, and therefore, observation is recommended.[41,50,67,158] If the lesion is thought to be secondary to a repetitive use injury, this activity should be stopped. Physical therapy is performed, including passive range of motion exercises to stretch the rhomboid and pectoralis minor muscles. Electrical stimulation of the nerve is also used to maintain muscle tone. Strengthening of the remaining periscapular muscles is encouraged. A brace to the scapula has been suggested by many authors,[50,70,146,158] although this may be cumbersome[41] and poorly accepted by the athlete. A brace, however, limits further winging of the scapula, thereby decreasing the stretch on the long thoracic nerve during recovery. Athletes are discouraged from reading in bed with the head propped on the hand, because this position results in traction on the long thoracic nerve.[50] If the athlete's symptoms and paralysis persist and become chronic, resulting in significant disability beyond the 1- to 2-year mark, operative intervention should be considered. Muscle transfer procedures to substitute for the serratus anterior muscle have been used with variable results. We favor transfer of the sternal head of the pectoralis major muscle, using a fascia lata graft into a hole made through the inferior angle of the scapula, as described by Marmor and Bechtol.[90] Transfers of the rhomboids, teres major, and pectoralis minor muscles have been described in the literature.[35,53,60,83,108,121,137]

The surgical technique for transfer of the sternal head of the pectoralis major muscle begins with placement of the athlete in the beach chair position, with a sandbag beneath the right medial border of the scapula to thrust it forward. A skin incision is begun along the inferior border of the deltopectoral groove and extended along the lateral border of the pectoralis major. Dissection is carried down to the pectoralis major muscle insertion and the biceps muscle and the division between the clavicular and sternal heads of the pectoralis major muscle is identified and developed (Fig. 19-8). The insertion of the sternal head is then detached from the humerus just anterior to the biceps tendon and dissected medially to its neurovascular bundle. Blunt dissection is then carried along the lateral chest wall and the serratus anterior and latissimus dorsi muscles to the level of the inferior border and tip of the scapula. At times, the inferior tip of the scapula can be well visualized through this one incision, although a second skin incision over the tip of the scapula is sometimes necessary. A large vascular anastomosis in this area is retracted posteriorly along with the teres major and minor muscles. A fascia lata graft measuring 15 by 5 cm is then harvested from the lateral thigh. This is fashioned into a tube and sutured to the end of the pectoralis tendon. This tendinous extension is then passed through a foramen made in the inferior tip of the scapula and then sutured back on itself at moderate tension. The incision is closed and a Velpeau dressing applied. A scapular brace is worn for the first 6 weeks postoperatively to stabilize the scapula during healing.

Prognosis

In general, the prognosis for recovery after long thoracic nerve palsy is excellent; the average recovery occurs by 8 months, with a range of 1 to 24 months.[50] In the series of Gregg et al,[50] all athletes with long thoracic nerve injuries demonstrated full symptomatic recovery, although residual weakness was noted on repeat physical examination. Goodman et al[48] noted that three of four patients with complete

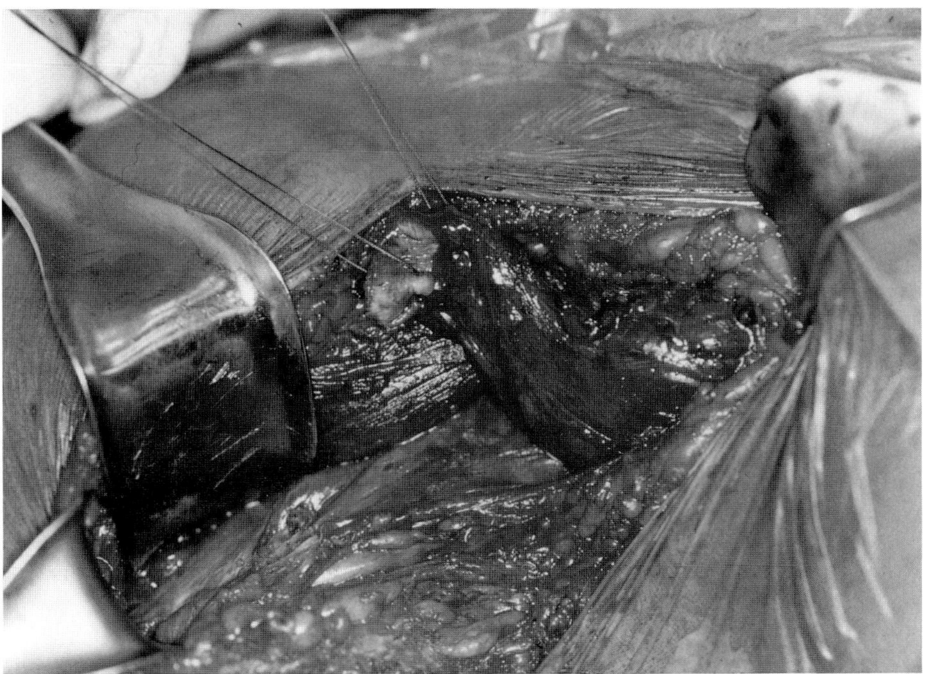

Figure 19-8. Operative view of pectoralis transfer. The sternal head of the pectoralis major is detached from the humerus and bluntly separated from its clavicular head. A fascial tube fashioned from fascia lata is then sutured to the pectoralis tendon and passed through a foramen made in the inferior border of the scapula. This is sutured back to itself at moderate tension to duplicate the function of the serratus anterior muscle.

palsy compensated for their disability and could abduct greater than 130 degrees. Foo and Swann[41] also noted a slight residual palsy at 2 years postinjury, although most of their patients thought that they had recovered completely. Overpeck and Ghormley[111] noted 11 of 15 patients with complete or good recovery after long thoracic nerve palsy. Critical evaluation in the series of Gregg et al,[50] however, revealed that 9 of 10 patients who had full symptomatic recovery showed signs of early fatiguing on testing.

A return to sporting activity is not recommended until the athlete's symptoms have resolved. Once symptomatic recovery has occurred, athletes can generally return to sport, even if early fatiguing is noted on physical examination.

SPINAL ACCESSORY NERVE

Pertinent Anatomy

The spinal accessory nerve (cranial nerve XI) is a motor nerve that innervates the trapezius muscle. It enters the neck by passing through the jugular foramen and then pierces the sternocleidomastoid muscle, which it supplies. It then courses obliquely and superficially across the floor of the posterior triangle of the neck to the ventral border of the trapezius muscle (Fig. 19-9). As it courses deep to the trapezius muscle, the accessory nerve communicates with C2, C3, and C4, and it forms a plexus that continues to the deep surface of the trapezius muscle. The nerve continues distally and crosses the medial border of the scapula to innervate the trapezius muscle on its deep surface.[140] Variations in the innervation of the trapezius muscle are frequent, and several authors have suggested that the inferior trapezius muscle receives innervation from C3 and C4.[85,107,109] Anderson and Flowers[6] have shown through EMG studies, however, that all motor innervation to the trapezius comes from the spinal accessory nerve. The trapezius muscle has three separate heads that function together to rotate the scapula on the chest wall and allow full abduction.[29,34,54,107] The superior portion of the trapezius elevates the scapula, whereas the middle portion draws the scapula toward the midline, and the inferior portion draws the angle of the scapula downward (Fig. 19-10).

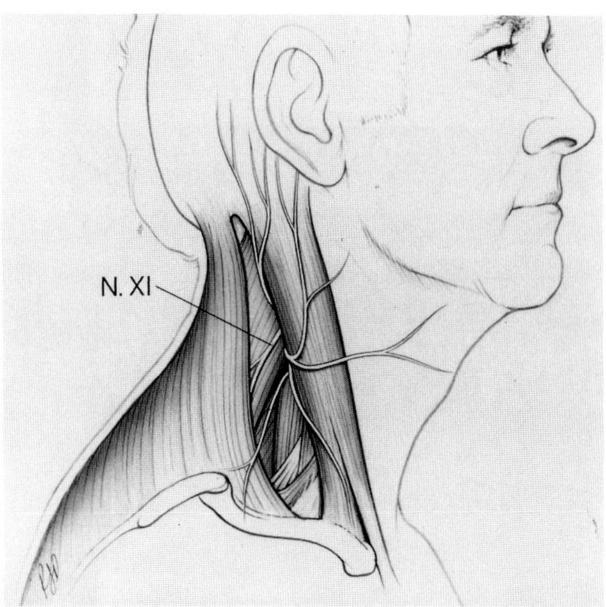

Figure 19-9. Lateral view of neck showing spinal accessory nerve (cranial nerve XI). The spinal accessory nerve passes out of the skull through the jugular foramen, piercing the sternocleidomastoid muscle, which it innervates. It then courses obliquely and superficially across the floor of the posterior triangle of the neck to the ventral border of the trapezius muscle. Its superficial location and close proximity to the deep lateral chain of nodes renders it susceptible to injury both by direct blow and by surgical biopsy of lymph nodes in this area.

Mechanism of Injury

The most common cause of injury to the spinal accessory nerve is not in athletic competition but rather from biopsy of a posterior cervical node, radical neck dissection, or penetrating injury to the base of the neck.[6,12,29,34,54,107,109,130,154] Isolated injuries to this nerve in sports, however, have been reported secondary to crush injuries and stretching injuries. Bateman[8] described a blow to the neck from a hockey stick resulting in an isolated spinal accessory nerve injury, and similar crush injuries to the neck have also resulted in isolated palsy of this nerve.[107,112] Bateman[8] described an isolated spinal accessory nerve injury with a fall on the point of the shoulder, which increases the acromiomastoid distance, and Cohn et al[26] and Mendoza and Main[97] have reported this injury during wrestling with the "cross-face maneuver," which results in the head being forcefully rotated in the opposite direction. Logigian et al[85] have reported stretch palsy of the spinal accessory nerve from lifting a heavy weight and simultaneously turning the head quickly.

Clinical Presentation

The athlete with trapezius muscle paralysis presents with a persistent ache in the posterior shoulder and medial scapula, often radiating down the arm.[12,80,107,109] This persistent ache is gradual in onset after injury and may represent stretching of the brachial plexus,[12,80,107] straining of the remaining periscapular muscles,[12,102] impingement secondary to forward rotation of the scapula,[12] or frozen shoulder.[12] Athletes typically complain of drooping of the affected

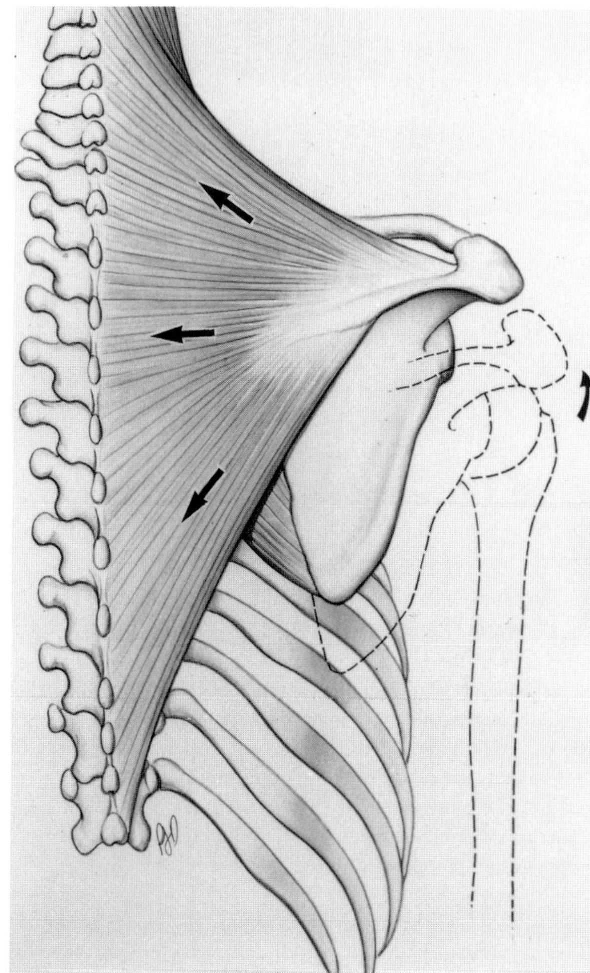

Figure 19-10. Posterior view showing functions of the trapezial heads. The three heads of the trapezius muscle serve to hold the scapula on the chest wall. The superior portion of the trapezius elevates the scapula, while the middle portion draws the scapula toward the midline, and the inferior portion draws the angle of the scapula downward. Trapezial paralysis allows drooping of the scapula with migration away from the midline and rotation and winging of the inferior pole of the scapula.

shoulder[12] and weakness with overhead use that begins several weeks after their shoulder injury.[12,107] They may also complain of weakness of other shoulder muscles, which is the result of the loss of scapular stabilization. Finally, variable complaints of paresthesias, including numbness that can radiate from the face to the hand and involving the radial and ulnar nerves, have been reported.[107]

Physical examination in the athlete with trapezial paralysis reveals drooping of the shoulder[12,107,109] and an asymmetric neck line[12] (Fig. 19-11). The scapula lowers and moves further from the midline, and its inferior angle is drawn upward by the rhomboid muscles. Winging is exacerbated by abduction more than flexion.[107] A loss of contour of the shoulder is noted, and the distal clavicle and acromion appear more prominent secondary to trapezial atrophy.[12,85] Anderson and Flowers[6] recommend a test of abduction strength to isolate the trapezius in which the patient internally rotates the upper arm and pronates the hand. In this position, without anterior flexion of the shoulder, the arm is carried through a complete arc of 180 degrees. This maneuver is impossible without an intact trapezius. However, if supination or flexion are allowed, the athlete can often forward elevate the arm fully. A shoulder shrug is not a reliable test of trapezial function because the levator scapulae can often perform this function.[6] Several authors have noted complete motion but weakness overhead on physical examination.[6,54,85]

Frozen shoulder is commonly associated with trapezial paralysis, and restricted motion of the glenohumeral joint may be found.[12] Other shoulder muscles may appear weak; so for accurate evaluation, the scapula should be manually

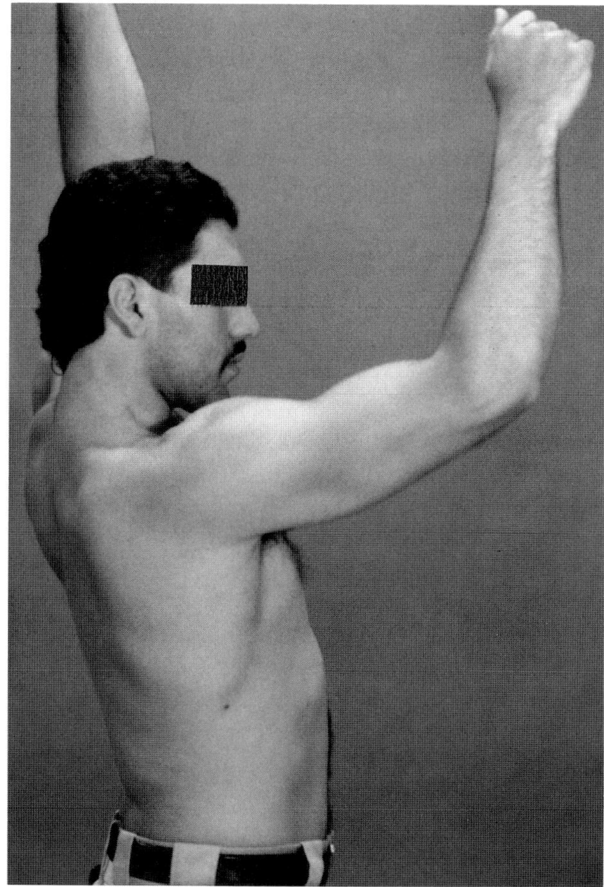

Figure 19-11. Anteroposterior view showing loss of contour of the neck. This patient with complete paralysis of the spinal accessory nerve reveals an asymmetric neck line with loss of the trapezial contour and drooping of the shoulder secondary to rotation of the scapula.

stabilized by the examiner on the chest wall while these muscles are being tested.[85]

Electromyelogram Evaluation

As with other nerve injuries, the EMG provides a definitive diagnosis of spinal accessory nerve palsy. The EMG is performed by stimulation at the midpoint of the posterior margin of the sternocleidomastoid muscle and the 3rd and 4th cervical roots. Measurements are taken at the superior, medial, and inferior trapezius muscle using concentric needle electrodes.[24,37,49] Normal latencies have been described for nerve conduction, although the contralateral side may be used for control. Olarte and Adams[109] prefer the NEE to make the diagnosis.

Differential Diagnosis

The differential diagnosis for spinal accessory nerve palsy includes root avulsion[74,85] and serratus anterior palsy.[6,12,29,80,107,109] In root avulsion, there is a lack of function of surrounding muscle groups. In serratus anterior palsy, the scapula moves closer to the midline and higher,[107] and winging of the scapula is accentuated more by forward flexion than by abduction.[85,109]

Treatment

For penetrating injuries or injuries resulting from neck surgery, immediate exploration and nerve grafting are indicated and usually provide good results.[54] Most athletic injuries, however, are closed injuries, which are treated initially with observation, application of a sling, nonsteroidal anti-inflammatory medications,[97] and electrical stimulation. This conservative treatment, unfortunately, is often unsuccessful, especially in active individuals.[12,109,140] If no improvement occurs clinically or on EMG in 6 weeks, surgical exploration and neurolysis are recommended.[8,34] Neurolysis delayed beyond 6 weeks has little chance of success in these cases.[109] Resistive exercises aimed at strengthening the adjacent scapular muscles are not sufficient to compensate or substitute for absent trapezius muscle function. Scapular stabilizing procedures have been used to substitute for the paralyzed trapezius muscle. Fixation of the medial border of the scapula to the spinous process by fascia lata as a static type of stabilization has been described,[30,58,142,152] but this procedure does not compensate for the complex dynamic function of the trapezius muscle.[85] Procedures involving transfer of the levator scapulae with fascia lata sling fixation have also been reported to be useful procedures,[29] but results deteriorate with fascial stretching.[12] Several series have reported successful results with a dynamic muscle transfer using the levator scapulae and rhomboid muscles.[78-80] Bigliani et al[12] have reported very favorable results using the transfer of the levator scapulae and rhomboid muscles, achieving a dynamic transfer to substitute for the paralyzed trapezius muscle.

Our surgical technique begins with the patient in the lateral decubitus position and a longitudinal incision parallel to the medial border of the scapula. The degenerated trapezius muscle is incised to expose the levator scapulae and rhomboid muscles. The levator scapulae, rhomboid minor, and rhomboid major are all detached from the scapula with a thin sliver of bone (Fig. 19-12). A separate skin incision is made along the lateral border of the posterior spine of the scapula, and the soft tissues are elevated from this incision to the medial incision. The levator scapulae is sutured through bony drill holes to the lateral spine of the scapula. The rhomboid minor and major are transferred

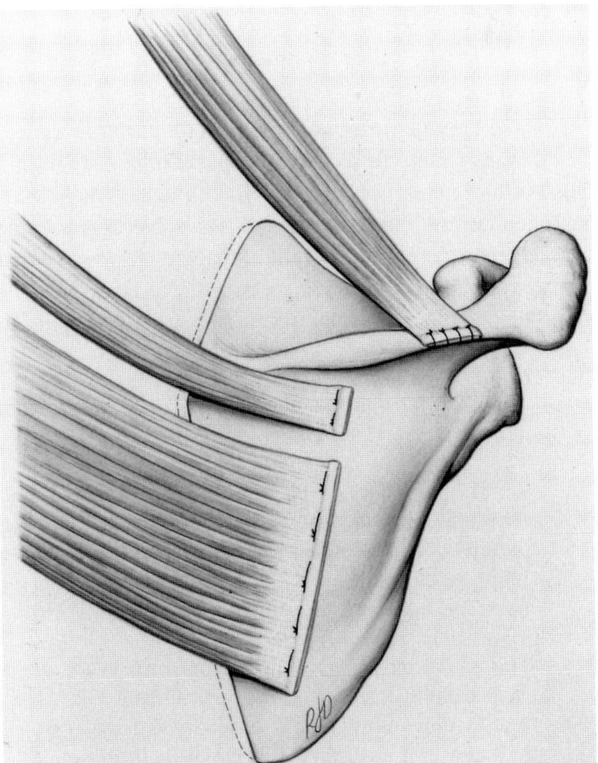

Figure 19-12. Levator scapulae and rhomboid major and minor transfer. The levator scapulae, rhomboid minor, and rhomboid major insertions on the medial border of the scapula are detached with a thin wafer of bone. The levator scapulae is transferred to the lateral border of the spine of the scapula through drill holes while the rhomboid minor and major are transferred onto the body of the scapula after subperiosteal elevation of the infraspinatus muscle. In this position, they serve to closely duplicate the function of the paralyzed trapezial muscle.

onto the body of the scapula lateral to their original insertion and are sutured under moderate tension, again through bony drill holes. The wounds are closed, and the athlete is placed in a brace or abduction pillow for 6 weeks postoperatively. This operation has resulted in diminished pain and improved function, yet it should not be performed as a primary procedure for spinal accessory nerve palsy but should follow unsuccessful neurolysis or nerve grafting.[12]

Prognosis

The rarity of spinal accessory nerve injury from closed injuries in athletes makes generalizations on prognosis difficult. In general, the prognosis with complete spinal accessory nerve palsy after open or closed injury is poor, with worsening of symptoms over time.[12,80] No other muscle groups around the scapula can adequately compensate for loss of trapezial muscle function, and the likelihood of a successful return to sports is small, no matter how the injury is treated. However, a relatively asymptomatic athlete may attempt to return to sports.

SUMMARY

Isolated nerve injuries about the shoulder in the athlete are rare, but symptoms secondary to nerve injury can mimic those of more common injuries. The clinician who evaluates shoulder injuries in athletes must be able to recognize and diagnose these injuries. In this chapter, clinical presentation, evaluation, and treatment of isolated nerve injuries about the shoulder are reviewed to assist the physician in the management of these often puzzling injuries.

REFERENCES

1. Agre JL, Ash N, Cameron MC, House J: Suprascapular neuropathy after intensive progressive resistive exercise: case report. Arch Phys Med Rehabil 68:236, 1987
2. Aiello I, Serra G, Traina CG, Tugnoli V: Entrapment of the suprascapular nerve at the spinoglenoid notch. Ann Neurol 23:314, 1982
3. Alnot JY: Traumatic brachial plexus palsy in the adult. Retro- and infraclavicular lesions. Clin Orthop 237:9, 1988
4. Alnot JY, Jolly A: Les lesions du nerf circonflexe. A propos de 19 cas. Re Chir Orthop 69:539, 1983
5. Alon M, Weiss S, Fishel B et al: Bilateral suprascapular nerve entrapment syndrome due to an anomalous transverse scapular ligament. Clin Orthop 234:31, 1988
6. Anderson R, Flowers RS: Free grafts of the spinal accessory nerve during radical neck dissection. Am J Surg 118:769, 1969
7. Bach BR, O'Brien SJ, Warren RF et al: An unusual neurologic complication of the Bristow procedure. J Bone Joint Surg [Am] 70:458, 1988
8. Bateman JE: Nerve injuries about the shoulder in sports. J Bone Joint Surg [Am] 49:785, 1967
9. Bennett GE: Shoulder and elbow lesions of the professional baseball pitcher. JAMA 117:510, 1941
10. Berry H, Brill V: Axillary nerve palsy following blunt trauma to the shoulder region. A clinical and electromyographic review. J Neurol Neurosurg Psychiatry 45:1027, 1982
11. Bigliani LU, Dalsey RM, McCann PD, April EW: An anatomic study of the suprascapular nerve. Arthroscopy 6:301, 1990
12. Bigliani LU, Perez-Snaz JR, Wolfe IN: Treatment of trapezius paralysis. J Bone Joint Surg [Am] 67:871, 1985
13. Black KP, Lombardo JA: Suprascapular nerve injuries with isolated paralysis of the infraspinatus. Am J Sports Med 18:225, 1990
14. Blom S, Dahlback LD: Nerve injuries in dislocations of the shoulder joint and fractures of the neck of the humerus. Acta Chir Scand 136:461, 1970
15. Bora FW, Pleausre DE, Didizian NA: A study of nerve regeneration and neuroma formation after nerve suture by various techniques. J Hand Surg 1:138, 1976
16. Braddom RL, Wolfe C: Musculocutaneous nerve injury after heavy exercise. Arch Phys Med Rehabil 59:290, 1978
17. Brogi M, Laterza A, Neri C: Entrapment neuropathy of the suprascapular nerve. Riv Neurobiol 25:318, 1979
18. Brown JT: Nerve injuries complicating dislocation of the shoulder. J Bone Joint Surg [Br] 34:526, 1952
19. Brumback RA, Bobele GB, Rayan GM: Electrodiagnosis of compressive nerve lesions. Hand Clin 8:241, 1992
20. Bryan WJ, Schander K, Tullos HS: The axillary nerve and its relationship to common sports medicine shoulder procedures. Am J Sports Med 14:113, 1986
21. Bryan WJ, Wild JJ: Isolated infraspinatus atrophy: a common cause of posterior shoulder pain and weakness in the throwing athlete. Am J Sports Med 17:130, 1989
22. Burge PD, Rushworth G, Watson NA: Patterns of injury to the terminal branches of the brachial plexus. J Bone Joint Surg [Br] 67:630, 1985
23. Cahill BR, Palmer RE: Quadrilateral space syndrome. J Hand Surg 8:65, 1983
24. Cherington M: Accessory nerve: conduction studies. Arch Neurol 18:708, 1968
25. Clein LJ: Suprascapular entrapment neuropathy. J Neurosurg 43:337, 1975
26. Cohn BT, Brahms MD, Cohn M: Injury to the eleventh cranial nerve in a high school wrestler. Orthop Rev 15:59, 1986
27. Colachis SC, Strohm BR: Effect of suprascapular and axillary nerve blocks on muscle force in upper extremity. Arch Phys Med Rehabil 52:22, 1971
28. Cormier PJ, Matalon TA, Wolin PM: Quadrilateral space syndrome: a rare cause of shoulder pain. Radiology 167:797, 1988
29. Dewar FP, Harris RI: Restoration of function of the shoulder following paralysis of the trapezius by fascial sling fixation and transplantation of the levator scapulae. Ann Surg 132:1111, 1950

30. Dickson FD: Fascial transplants in paralytic and other conditions. J Bone Joint Surg 19:405, 1937
31. Donovan WH, Kraft GH: Rotator cuff tears versus suprascapular nerve injury: a problem in differential diagnosis. Arch Phys Med Rehabil 55:424, 1974
32. Drez, D: Suprascapular neuropathy in the differential diagnosis of rotator cuff injuries. Am J Sports Med 4:43, 1976
33. Dundore DE, DeLisa JA: Musculocutaneous nerve palsy: an isolated complication of surgery. Arch Phys Med Rehabil 60:130, 1979
34. Dunn AW: Trapezius paralysis after minor surgical procedures in the posterior clavicle triangle. South Med J 67:312, 1974
35. Durman DC: An operation for paralysis of the serratus anterior. J Bone Joint Surg 27:380, 1945
36. Edeland HG, Zachrisson BE: Fracture of the scapular notch associated with lesion of the suprascapular nerve. Acta Orthop Scand 46:758, 1975
37. Fahrer H, Ludin HP, Mumenthaler M, Neiger M: The innervation of the trapezius muscle: an electrophysiological study. J Neurol 207:183, 1974
38. Ferretti A, Cerullo G, Russo G: Suprascapular neuropathy in volleyball players. J Bone Joint Surg [Am] 69:260, 1987
39. Fitchet SM: Injury of the serratus magnus (anterior) muscle. N Engl J Med 203:818, 1930
40. Flatow EL, Bigliani LU, April EW: An anatomic study of the musculocutaneous nerve and its relationship to the coracoid process. Clin Orthop 244:166, 1989
41. Foo CL, Swann M: Isolated paralysis of the serratus anterior. J Bone Joint Surg [Br] 65:552, 1983
42. Foucar HO: The "clover leaf" sling in paralysis of the serratus magnus. BMJ 2:865, 1933
43. Friedman AH, Nunley II JA, Urbaniak JR, Goldner RD: Repair of isolated axillary nerve lesions after infraclavicular brachial plexus injuries: case reports. Neurosurgery 27:403, 1990
44. Ganzhorn RW, Hocker JT, Horowitz M, Switzer H: Suprascapular nerve entrapment. J Bone Joint Surg [Am] 63:492, 1981
45. Garcia G, McQueen D: Bilateral suprascapular nerve entrapment. J Bone Joint Surg [Am] 63:491, 1981
46. Goldberg B: Injury patterns in youth sports. Phys Sports Med 7:175, 1989
47. Goodman CE: Unusual nerve injuries in recreational activities. Am J Sports Med 2:224, 1983
48. Goodman CE, Kenrick MM, Blum MV: Long thoracic nerve palsy: a follow-up study. Arch Phys Med Rehabil 56:352, 1975
49. Green RF, Brien M: Accessory nerve latency to the middle and lower trapezius. Arch Phys Med Rehabil 66:23, 1985
50. Gregg JR, Labosky D, Harty M et al: Serratus anterior paralysis in the young athlete. J Bone Joint Surg [Am] 61:825, 1979
51. Gregg JR, Torg E: Upper extremity injuries in adolescent tennis players. Clin Sports Med 7:37, 1988
52. Hadley MN, Jonntay UK, Pittman HW: Suprascapular nerve entrapment. J Neurosurg 64:843, 1986
53. Harmon PH: Surgical reconstruction of the paralytic shoulder by multiple muscle transplantations. J Bone Joint Surg [Am] 32:583, 1950
54. Harris HH, Dickey JR: Nerve grafting to restore function of trapezius muscle after radical neck dissection (a preliminary report). Ann Otol Rhinol Laryngol 74:880, 1965
55. Harvey JS: Overuse syndromes in young athletes. Clin Sports Med 2:595, 1983
56. Hauser CU, Martin WF: Two additional cases of traumatic winged scapula occurring in the armed forces. JAMA 121:667, 1943
57. Hayes JM, Zehr DJ: Traumatic muscle avulsion causing winging of the scapula. A case report. J Bone Joint Surg [Am] 63:495, 1981
58. Henry AK: An operation for slinging a dropped shoulder. Br J Surg 15:95, 1927
59. Hershman EB: Brachial plexus injuries. Clin Sports Med 9:311, 1990
60. Herzmark MH: Traumatic paralysis of the serratus anterior relieved by transplantation of rhomboidei. J Bone Joint Surg [Am] 33:235, 1951
61. Hirasawa Y: Injuries to peripheral nerve in sport. Semin Orthop 3:240, 1988
62. Hirasawa Y, Sakakida K: Sports and peripheral nerve injury. Am J Sports Med 11:420, 1983
63. Hirayama T, Takemitsu Y: Compression of the suprascapular nerve by a ganglion at the suprascapular notch. Clin Orthop 155:95, 1980
64. Ilfeld FW, Holder HG: Winged scapular: case occurring in soldier from knapsack. JAMA 120:448, 1942
65. Jerosch J, Castro WHM, Colemont J: A lesion of the musculocutaneous nerve. A rare complication of anterior shoulder dislocation. Acta Orthop Belg 55:230, 1989
66. Johnson JR, Bayley JIL: Early complications of acute anterior dislocation of the shoulder in middle-aged and elderly patients. Injury 13:431, 1965
67. Johnson JTH, Kendall HO: Isolated paralysis of the serratus anterior muscle. J Bone Joint Surg [Am] 37:567, 1955
68. Kaplan PE: Electrodiagnostic confirmation of long thoracic nerve palsy. J Neurol Neurosurg Psych 43:50, 1980
69. Karas SE: Thoracic outlet syndrome. Clin Sports Med 9:2, 1990
70. Kauppila LI: The long thoracic nerve: possible mechanisms of injury based on autopsy study. J Shoulder Elbow Surg 2:5, 1993
71. Khalili AA: Neuromuscular electrodiagnostic studies in entrapment neuropathy of the suprascapular nerve. Orthop Rev 3:12, 1974
72. Kim SM, Goodrich JA: Isolated proximal musculocutaneous nerve palsy. Arch Phys Med Rehabil 65:735, 1984
73. Kimura J: Electrodiagnosis in Diseases of Nerve and Muscle: Principles and Practice. 2nd Ed. FA Davis, Philadelphia, 1989
74. Kline DG, Hudson AR: Complications of nerve injury and nerve repair. p. 695. In Lazar S, Greenfield J (eds): Complications in Surgery and Trauma. JB Lippincott, Philadelphia, 1983
75. Koppel HP, Thompson WAL: Peripheral Entrapment Neuropathies. Williams & Wilkins, Baltimore, 1963

76. Kraft GN: Axillary musculocutaneous and suprascapular nerve latency studies. Arch Phys Med Rehabil 53:383, 1972
77. Kuland DN, McCue FC, Rockwell DA et al: Tennis injuries: prevention and treatment. Am J Sports Med 7:249, 1979
78. Lange M: Die behandlung der irreparablem trapeziuslahmung. Langenbecks Arch Klin Chir 270:437, 1951
79. Lange M: Die operative behandlung der irreparablem trapeziuslahmung. Tio Fakult Mecmuasim 22:137, 1959
80. Langenskiold A, Ryoppy S: Treatment of paralysis of the trapesius muscle by the Eden-Lange operation. Acta Orthop Scand 44:383, 1973
81. Lauland T, Fedders O, Sgaard I, Kornum M: Suprascapular nerve compression syndrome. Surg Neurol 22:308, 1984
82. Leffert RD, Seddon H: Infraclavicular brachial plexus injuries. J Bone Joint Surg [Br] 47:9, 1965
83. Lindstrom N, Danielsson L: Muscle transposition in serratus anterior paralysis. Acta Orthop Scand 32:369, 1962
84. Liveson JA: Nerve lesions associated with shoulder dislocation; an electrodiagnostic study of 11 cases. J Neurol Neurosurg Psych 47:742, 1984
85. Logigian EL, McInnes JM, Berger AR et al: Stretch-induced spinal accessory nerve palsy. Muscle Nerve 2:146, 1988
86. LoMonaco MD, Pasqua PG, Tonali P: Conduction studies along the accessory, long thoracic, dorsal scapular and thoracodorsal nerves. Acta Neurol Scand 68:171, 1983
87. Loomer R, Graham B: Anatomy of the axillary nerve and its relation to inferior capsular shift. Clin Orthop 243:100, 1989
88. Mallon WJ, Bassett FH III, Goldner RD: Lutatio erecta: the inferior glenohumeral dislocation. J Orthop Trauma 4:19, 1990
89. Markhede G, Monastyrski J, Stener B: Shoulder function after deltoid muscle removal. Acta Orthop Scand 56:242, 1985
90. Marmor L, Bechtol CO: Paralysis of the serratus anterior due to electric shock released by transplantation of the pectoralis major muscle. A case report. J Bone Joint Surg [Am] 45:156, 1963
91. Mastiglia FL: Musculocutaneous neuropathy after strenuous physical activity. Med J Aust 145:153, 1986
92. Matz SW, Welliver PS, Welliver DI: Brachial plexus neuropraxia complicating a comminuted clavicle fracture in a college football player. Am J Sports Med 17:581, 1989
93. McIlveen SJ, Bigliani LU, Duralde XA, D'Alessandro DF: Isolated nerve injuries about the shoulder. Orthop Trans 2:247, 1987
94. McIlveen SJ, Duralde XA: Isolated nerve injuries about the shoulder. p. 214. In Bigliani LU (ed): Complications of Shoulder Surgery. Williams & Wilkins, New York, 1993
95. McIlveen SJ, Steinmann SJ, Bigliani LU: Rotator cuff tears and associated nerve injury. Presented at the 58th Annual Meeting of the AAOS, Anaheim, CA, 1991
96. McKowen HC, Voorhies RM: Axillary nerve entrapment in the quadrilateral space. J Neurosurg 66:932, 1987
97. Mendoza FX, Main K: Peripheral nerve injuries of the shoulder in the athlete. Clin Sports Med 9:331, 1990
98. Mestdagh M, Drizenko A, Ghestem P: Anatomical basis of suprascapular nerve syndrome. Anat Clin 3:67, 1981
99. Milton GV: The mechanism of circumflex and other nerve injuries in dislocation of the shoulder and the possible mechanism of nerve injuries during reduction of dislocation. Aust NZ J Surg 23:24, 1976
100. Mitsunga MM, Nakano K: High radial nerve palsy following strenuous muscular activity. Clin Orthop 98:39, 1982
101. Murray JWG: A surgical approach for entrapment neuropathy of the suprascapular nerve. Orthop Rev 3:33–5, 1974
102. Nahum AM, Mullally W, Marmor L: A syndrome resulting from radical neck dissection. Arth Otolaryngol 74:424, 1961
103. Neer CS, Foster CR: Inferior capsular shift for involuntary and multidirectional instability of the shoulder. J Bone Joint Surg [Am] 62:897, 1980
104. Neviaser RJ, Neviaser TJ, Neviaser JS: Concurrent ruptures of the rotator cuff and anterior dislocation of the shoulder in the older patient. J Bone Joint Surg [Am] 70:1308, 1988
105. Neviaser TJ, Ain BR, Neviaser RJ: Suprascapular nerve degeneration secondary to an attenuation by a ganglionic cyst. J Bone Joint Surg [Am] 68:622, 1986
106. Nirschl RP: Prevention and treatment of elbow and shoulder injuries in the tennis player. Clin Sports Med 7:289, 1988
107. Norden A: Peripheral injuries to the spinal accessory nerve. Acta Chir Scand 94:515, 1946
108. Ober FR: Transplantation to improve the function of the shoulder joint and extensor function of the elbow joint. pp. 274–6. In Edwards JW (ed): Lectures on Reconstruction Surgery. The American Academy of Orthopaedic Surgeons, Ann Arbor, MI, 1944
109. Olarte M, Adams D: Accessory nerve palsy. J Neurol Neurosurg Psych 40:1113, 1977
110. O'Neill DB, Micheli LJ: Overuse injuries in the young athlete. Clin Sports Med 7:591, 1988
111. Overpeck DD, Ghormley RK: Paralysis of the serratus magnus muscle. JAMA 114:1995, 1940
112. Paljarvi L, Partanen J: Biting palsy of the accessory nerve. J Neurol Neurosurg Psych 43:744, 1980
113. Parsonage MJ, Turner JWA: Neurologic amyotrophy: shoulder girdle syndrome. Lancet 1:973, 1948
114. Pasila M, Jaroma H, Kaviluoto O, Sundholm, A: Early complications of primary shoulder dislocations. Acta Orthop Scand 49:260, 1978
115. Petrera JE, Trojaborg W: Conduction studies of the long thoracic nerve in serratus anterior palsy of different etiology. Neurology 34:1033, 1984
116. Petrucci FS, Morelli A, Raimondi PL: Axillary nerve injuries. Twenty-one cases treated by nerve graft and neurolysis. J Hand Surg 7:271, 1982
117. Pianka G, Hershman EB: Neurovascular injuries. In Nicholas JA, Hershman EB (eds): The Upper Extremity and Spine in Sports Medicine. Mosby, St. Louis, 1990
118. Pittman MI, Nainzadeh N, Ergas E, Springer S: The use of somatosensory evoked potentials for detection of neuropratia during shoulder arthroscopy. Arthroscopy 4:250, 1988
119. Post M, Mager J: Suprascapular nerve entrapment. Clin Orthop 223:126, 1987
120. Priest JD: The shoulder of the tennis player. Clin Sports Med 7:387, 1988
121. Rapp IH: Serratus anterior paralysis treated by transplantation of the pectoralis minor. J Bone Joint Surg [Am] 36:852, 1954

122. Rask MR: Suprascapular nerve entrapment: a report of two cases treated with suprascapular notch resection. Clin Orthop 123:73, 1977
123. Rayan GM: Lower trunk brachial plexus compression neuropathy due to cervical ribs in young athletes. Am J Sports Med 16:77, 1988
124. Redler MR, Ruland LJ III, McCue FC III: Quadrilateral space syndrome in a throwing athlete. Am J Sports Med 14:511, 1986
125. Rengachary SS, Burr D, Luca S et al: Suprascapular entrapment neuropathy; a clinical, anatomical and comparative study. II. Anatomical study. Neurosurgery 5:447, 1979
126. Rengachary SS, Neff JP, Singer PA et al: Suprascapular entrapment neuropathy: a clinical, anatomic and comparative study. I. Clinical study. Neurosurgery 5:441, 1979
127. Richards RR, Hudson AR, Bertoid JT et al: Injury to the brachial plexus during Putti-Platt and Bristow procedures. Am J Sports Med 15:374, 1987
128. Richards RR, Hudson AR, Waddell JP, Urbaniak JK: Injury to the brachial plexus during anterior shoulder repair. AAOS, 53rd Annual Meeting, New Orleans, 1986
129. Rose DL, Kelly CR: Shoulder pain. Suprascapular nerve block in shoulder pain. J Kans Med Soc 70:135, 1969
130. Roy PH, Bearhs OH: Spinal accessory nerve in radical neck dissections. Am J Surg 118:800, 1969
131. Saeed MA, Kraft GH: Bilateral suprascapular neuropathy. Orthop Rev 11:135, 1982
132. Sarno JB: Suprascapular nerve entrapment. Surg Neurol 20:493, 1983
133. Seedon H: Surgical Disorders of the Peripheral Nerves. Churchill Livingstone, Edingburgh, 1972
134. Sicuranza MJ, McCue FC III: Compressive neuropathies in the upper extremity of athletes. Hand Clin 8:263–73, 1992
135. Stanish WD, Lamb H: Isolated paralysis of the serratus anterior muscle: a weight training injury. Am J Sports Med 6:385, 1978
136. Staples OS, Watkins AL: Full active abduction in traumatic paralysis of the deltoid. J Bone Joint Surg 25:85, 1943
137. Steindler A: The Traumatic Deformities and Disabilities of the Upper Extremity. Charles C. Thomas, Springfield, Illinois, 1946
138. Stewart JD: Focal Peripheral Neuropathies. Elsevier, New York, 1987
139. Strohm BR, Colachis SC: Shoulder joint dysfunction following injury to the suprascapular nerve. J Am Phys Ther Assoc 45:106, 1965
140. Sunderland S: Nerves and Nerve Injuries. 2nd Ed. Churchill Livingstone, New York, 1978
141. Szabo RM, Gilberman RH: The pathophysiology of nerve entrapment syndromes. J Hand Surg 12A:880, 1987
142. Szubinski A: Ersatz des gelahmten trapezius durch fascienzugel. Zentralbl Chir 47:1172, 1920
143. Thompson RC, Schneider W, Kennedy T: Entrapment neuropathy of the inferior branch of the suprascapular nerve by ganglia. Clin Orthop 166:185, 1982
144. Thompson WAL, Koppell HP: Peripheral entrapment neuropathies of the upper extremity. N Engl J Med 260: 1261, 1959
145. Trojaborg W: Motor and sensory conduction in musculocutaneous nerve. J Neurol Neurosurg Psych 39:890, 1976
146. Truong XT, Rippel DV: Orthotic devices for serratus anterior palsy: some biomechanical considerations. Arch Phys Med Rehabil 60:66, 1979
147. Turner JWA, Parsonage MJ: Neurologic amyotrophy (paralytic brachial neuritis): with special reference to prognosis. Lancet 2:209, 1957
148. VanLinge B, Mulder J: Function of supraspinatus muscle and its relation to supraspinatus syndrome. J Bone Joint Surg [Br] 45:750, 1963
149. Vastamaki M, Kauppila LI: Etiologic factors in isolated paralysis of the serratus anterior muscle: a report of 197 cases. J Shoulder Elbow Surg 2:5, 1993
150. Velpeau AALM: Luxations de l'epaule. Arch Gen Med 14:269, 1837
151. Weaver HL: Isolated suprascapular nerve lesions. Br J Acc Surg 15:117, 1983
152. Whitman A: Congential elevation of scapula and paralysis of serratus magnus muscle. JAMA 99:1332, 1932
153. Wilbourn AJ: Electrodiagnostic testing of neurologic injuries in athletes. Clin Sports Med 9:229, 1990
154. Woodhall B: Trapesius paralysis following minor surgical procedure in the posterior cervical triangle. Results following cranial nerve suture. Am Surg 136:375, 1952
155. Woodhead AB: Paralysis of the serratus anterior in a world class marksman. Am J Sports Med 13:359, 1985
156. Wroble RR, Albright JP: Neck and low back injuries in wrestling. Clin Sports Med 5:295, 1986
157. Yoon TN, Grabois M: Scapular nerve injury following trauma to the shoulder. J Trauma 21:652, 1981
158. Zeier FG: The treatment of winged-scapula. Clin Orthop 91:128, 1973
159. Zoltan JD: Injury to the suprascapular nerve association with anterior dislocation of the shoulder. Case report and review of the literature. J Trauma 19:203, 1979

CHAPTER TWENTY

Biceps Disorders

Robert H. Bell
Jeffrey S. Noble

THE BICEPS TENDON

Long the neglected structure of the shoulder, the biceps tendon has over the past few years begun to receive greater attention. Although seldom a significant problem in the athletic population, the biceps is frequently a component of common shoulder problems in the older patient. This is due in great part to its location and tendency toward degenerative changes. However, this is not to say that there are not specific problems of this tendon that affect the athlete. In fact, as our population ages and yet remains ever active later in life, the number of older athletes increases and with it comes a greater number of problems with a degenerative component. With this in mind, it is the intent of this chapter to provide an overview of the biceps tendon, not just in the young athlete but also his or her older counterpart.

Anatomy

The biceps construct consists of two heads, the short and long. The long head of the biceps originates proximal at the apex of the glenoid, the supraglenoid tubercle. It is confluent with the superior aspect of the glenoid labrum and has its attachment at varying positions along the upper rim of the glenoid. Anatomic studies by Habermeyer et al[12] found the tendon originated from the supraglenoid tubercle 20 percent of the time and the posterior labrum 48 percent of the time. Twenty-eight percent had an origin from both sites. This would imply that most biceps attachments have an integral relationship with the glenoid labrum and, thus, may be involved in instability problems, as is discussed later.

Many individuals have addressed the issue of the biceps being intra-articular. As point of fact, it is an intra-articular tendon; however, it has a synovial sheath along its entire intra-articular course. This sheath represents a continuation of the synovial lining of the subacromial bursa, which winds its way down to the end of the bicipital groove, doubling back on itself, and heading retrograde into the joint along the tendon. It is this sheath that prevents the extravasation of contrast in normal arthrography.

Once exiting the joint, the tendon passes beneath several structures, the first of which is the coracohumeral ligament. The importance of this structure has been debated; however, most believe it provides strength to the rotator interval by reinforcing thc confluence of the supraspinatus and subscapularis tendons. Passing beneath this, the biceps enters the bicipital groove coursing beneath the transverse ligament. Several studies have been performed, looking at the various parameters of the groove.[5,13] They found the average depth of the groove to be 4.3 mm and the angle of the medial wall to be 56 degrees. The importance of this angle is the suspected greater tendency for medial tendon dislocation if the wall were shallow. This theory was not, however, proven statistically. Why then would there ever be a case of biceps subluxation? The belief is that the soft tissues provide the critical support and restraint to medialization.

Studies by both Meyer[23,24] and Paavolainen et al[26] indicate the area of the thickened rotator cuff, immediately beneath the coracohumeral ligament, provides the principal resistance to medial translation of the tendon. In Paavolainen's study, sectioning the transverse ligament at the groove did not allow any further translation medially. However, when the cuff overlying the biceps was also released, the biceps readily subluxed. In a cadaveric study, Peterson[27] examined 77 specimens and found only five cases of medial biceps subluxation. In all cases, there was a concomitant defect of the supraspinatus tendon. Hence, in cases of suspected biceps subluxation, one must be suspicious of a defect in and about the rotator cuff interval and or a subscapularis pull off.

Function

The actual biomechanics of the biceps originally included the concept of motion of the tendon within the groove with elbow flexion. However, Lippmann[18,19] and Hitchcock and Bechtol[14] have shown that the biceps does not slide within the groove but that the humerus moves relative to the fixed tendon. Lippmann[19] studied cadaveric specimens, noting that motion of the tendon in the groove could not be produced with elbow motion alone but required shoulder motion as well. This study helped initiate the concept of the biceps as a dynamic head depressor.

In another study of patients with large full-thickness tears of the rotator cuff, Rowe[29] found, in many cases, the biceps tendon had hypertrophied. He thought this was in response to the unrestricted superior humeral migration, thereby implicating the biceps as a head depressor. Kumar et al,[17] in a study of 15 cadaveric specimens, looked at the stabilizing effect of the biceps by comparing the amount of proximal migration of the humeral head while applying traction to both the short and long heads. With the long head released intra-articularly, the humeral head demonstrated significant upward migration.

Other authors have also looked at the function of the biceps in a dynamic fashion, using the technique of electromyelogram (EMG) analysis. From Ting[31] and Furlani[8] to Basmajian and Latif,[2] most of the studies demonstrated that the biceps acts as a contributing force in the motions of forward flexion and abduction. Furthermore, they have shown that in cuff-deficient shoulders, the biceps actually tends to provide a greater force than in an asymptomatic functioning shoulder with an intact cuff.[29] As one would anticipate, those shoulders found to be cuff-deficient also demonstrated significant hypertrophy of their intact biceps tendon, reinforcing the concept of the biceps as an active dynamic stabilizer of the shoulder.

Taking this one step farther, what role is played by the biceps in terms of stability in the throwing athlete's shoulder? Kumar et al,[17] in their cadaveric study, demonstrated the stabilizing effect of the biceps on the humeral head, preventing anterior translation during elbow flexion and forearm supination.

Similarly, Itoi et al[16] showed that both the long and short head of the biceps contribute to anterior stability of the shoulder and that this role increases as the degree of instability increases. The study of Glousman et al[11], using dynamic EMGs further demonstrated that the biceps is active during the throwing, especially in cases of associated instability. Hence, there would appear to be a role played by the biceps, especially in unstable shoulders, to help prevent further anterior translation.

Physical Examination

Most patients with findings of biceps pathology will have concomitant rotator cuff, impingement, instability, or acromioclavicular joint problems. Seldom is the biceps the principal source of discomfort but instead a manifestation of the underlying primary problem. Hence, the history and physical examination must be thorough, with attention directed at one, establishing the primary disorder, and two, the extent of associated biceps disease. Frequently, the patient's initial and chief complaint will be anterior shoulder pain in the region of the biceps. One must be sure to investigate further to rule out other problems so as not to miss the true etiology of the biceps problem. The history should be directed at determining the date of onset of symptoms, if there was a traumatic event, any prior treatment, and, if so, how effective, type of athletic participation, if throwing, what motion and when it hurts, any sounds associated with the pain, and lastly, how much it limits the patient. Remember, the biceps, owing to its relationship and involvement with many other shoulder functions, will often be part of other disease processes.

As in all musculoskeletal examinations, inspection of the involved extremity precedes all other maneuvers. The examiner should note asymmetry, discoloration, ecchymosis, and abnormal posturing. In the case of the biceps, simple inspection will demonstrate tears of the long head and the conjoined distal biceps tendon. Differentiation of these respective lesions is best accomplished by manual motor testing. Asking the patient to flex the elbow against resistance will cause a sharp demarcation at the site of the musculotendinous junction of the torn muscle (Fig. 20-1). Palpation is ineffective for proximal tears of the long head; however, distal tears of the conjoined tendon will result not only in proximal migration of the muscle body (Fig. 20-2) but also an absence of the normally palpable tendon in the antecubital fossa. Profound weakness on resisted supination (Yeargason's test) is pathognomonic of distal tears owing to the biceps' strong contribution to forearm supination with a flexed elbow.

The classic complaint in biceps tendinitis is that of anterior shoulder pain. Its location is over the distal portion of the bicipital groove in contrast to cuff impingement pain,

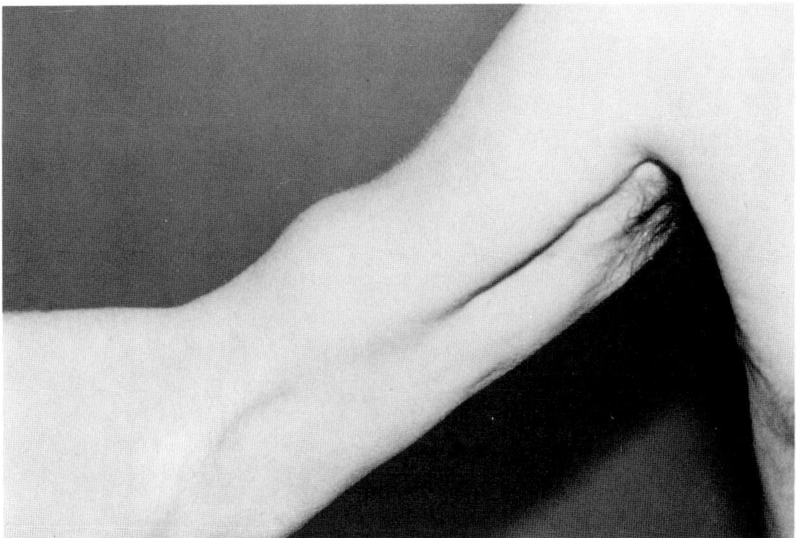

Figure 20-1. Patient with a tear of the long head of the biceps. Note the proximal change in the contour of the muscle body and the distal migration.

which tends to be more proximal, nearer the greater tuberosity. Cuff pain will also be referred to the middeltoid or its humeral insertion. In a test first described by Metsen and Kirby,[21] placing the arm in 10 degrees of internal rotation, the biceps is brought directly anterior for ease of palpation. The examiner flexes the elbow 90 degrees and holds the arm in 10 degrees of internal rotation, placing the index finger 2 cm distal to the anterior edge of the acromium in the midline of the humerus (Fig. 20-3). The patient with bicipital pathology will be tender in this position. However, due to anatomic variation, the groove may be medial or lateral to this location. Gentle internal and external rotation combined with palpation should help to localize the diseased tendon.

Several additional dynamic tests may be used to further evaluate the biceps. Speed's test[9] combines elbow exten-

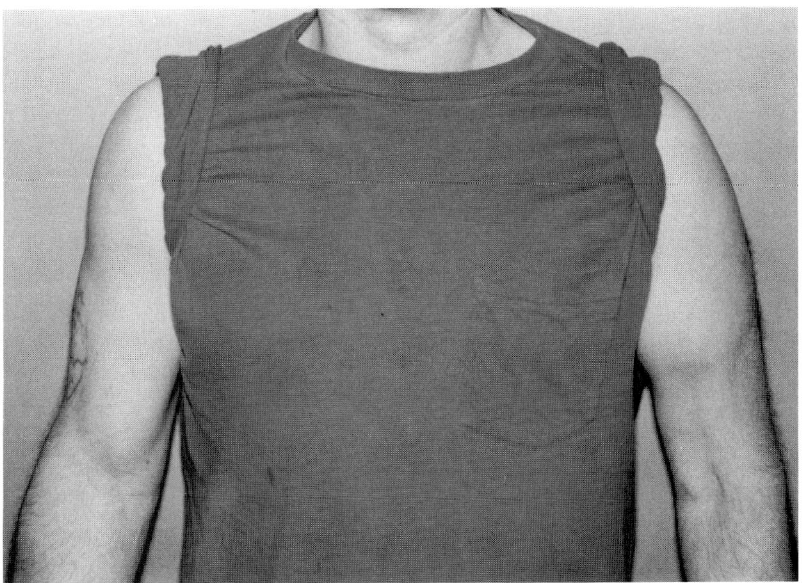

Figure 20-2. Patient with a prior distal biceps tear on the right and successful reconstruction presents with a distal tear of his left arm. Note the proximal migration and altered contour of the muscle body. The patient demonstrated a significant loss of strength on supination, a typical finding in such tears.

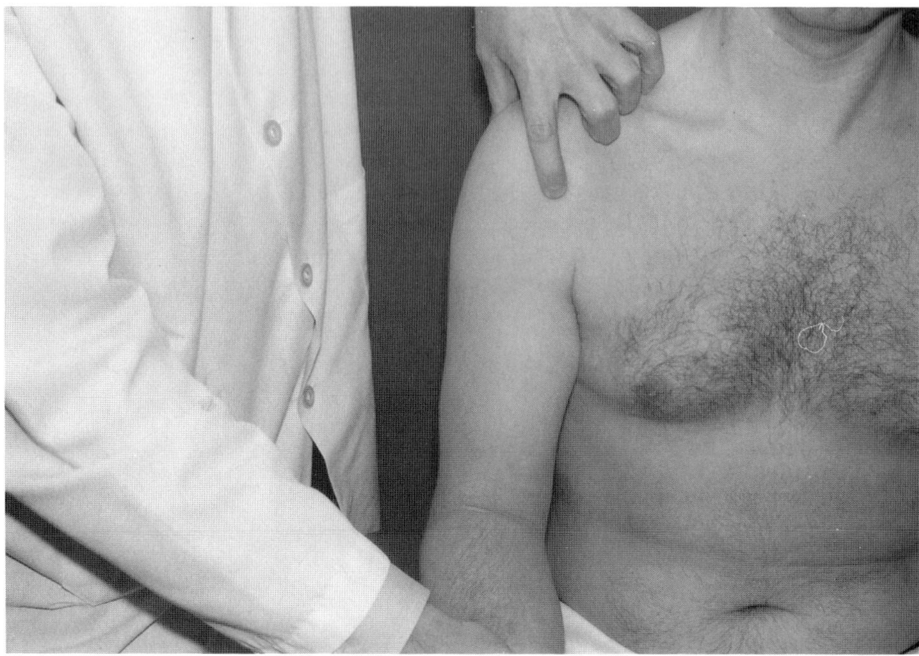

Figure 20-3. With the arm in 10 degrees of internal rotation, the biceps is best palpated at a point slightly inferior to the acromium and directly anterior.

sion with shoulder flexion to elicit anterior pain in the region of the groove (Fig. 20-4). A positive test should have pain well localized anteriorly and proximal with no evidence of asymmetry.

Yeargason's sign[32] begins by having the patient flex the elbow 90 degrees and then grasp the examiner's hand. The patient then supinates against resistance. Pain in the biceps region is indicative of pathology (Fig. 20-5).

Ludington's test[20] places the patient's arms behind the head in a position of abduction and external rotation. In

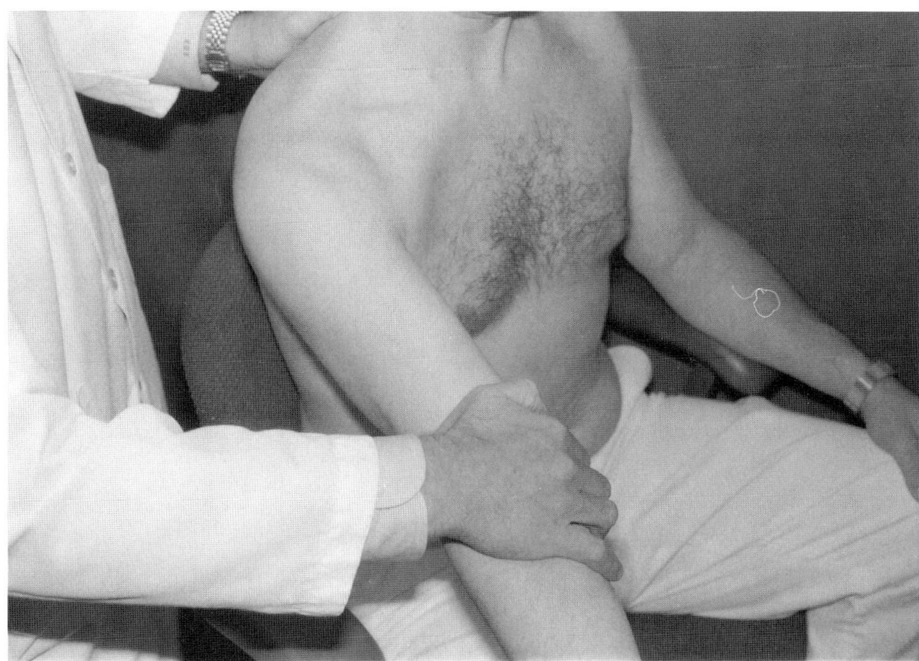

Figure 20-4. Speed's test. The patient extends the elbow, supinates the forearm, and attempts to forward elevate the arm against resistance. A positive test will cause anterior shoulder pain.

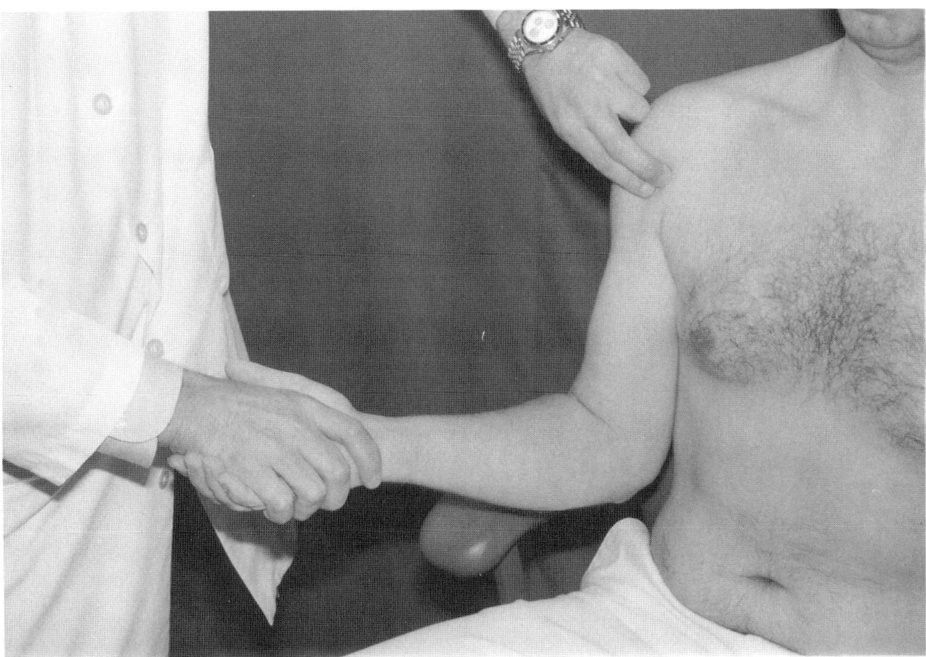

Figure 20-5. Yeargason's sign. With the elbow flexed, the patient grasps the examiner's hand and attempts to supinate against resistance. Pain anteriorly in the region of the biceps is a positive sign.

cases of long-head tears, the asymmetry will be readily apparent. If the tendon is intact but inflamed, contraction in this position will cause pain over the bicipital groove (Fig. 20-6).

Heuter's sign[15] tests the relative strength of the biceps as a forearm flexor and supinator. The patient is asked to flex the elbow against resistance with the forearm in supination and then in pronation (Fig. 20-7). In cases of biceps tears or inflammation, the normally stronger position of supination will be diminished.

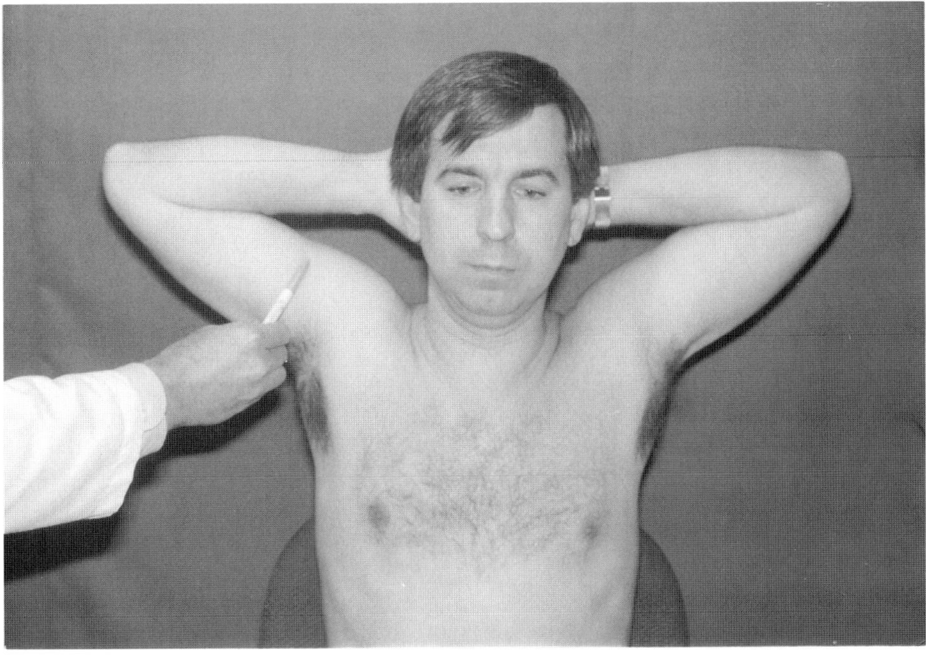

Figure 20-6. Ludington's test. The patient is asked to place both arms behind their head and gently flex their elbows to highlight the contour of the biceps bilaterally. Any proximal defects will stand out while viewed in profile.

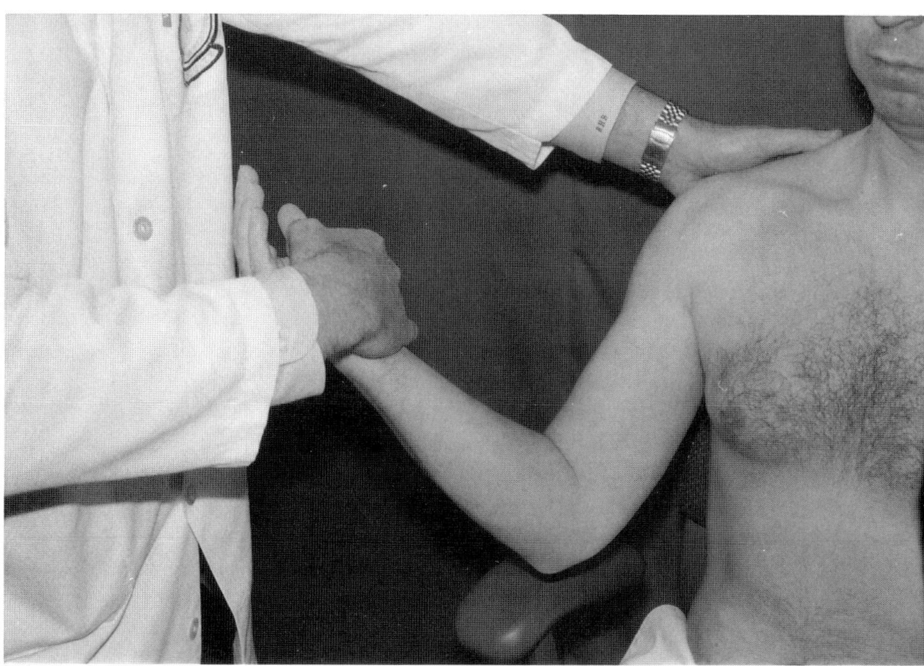

Figure 20-7. Heuter's sign. The patient supinates their forearm and then flexes the elbow against resistance. Much like Yeargason's test, this maneuver will elicit anterior pain in patients with biceps disease.

A test we call the abduction-extension test places the patient's arm in a position of marked extension, supination, and 30 degrees of abduction. This places the biceps on stretch, within the sheath, causing anterior pain (Fig. 20-8).

Owing to its rarity, few tests exist for biceps instability. The one most often used uses the position of the apprehension test for glenohumeral instability. The arm is placed in 90 degrees of abduction and comparable external rotation. As the arm is rotated, the examiner palpates the bicipital groove and notes any subluxation (Fig. 20-9).

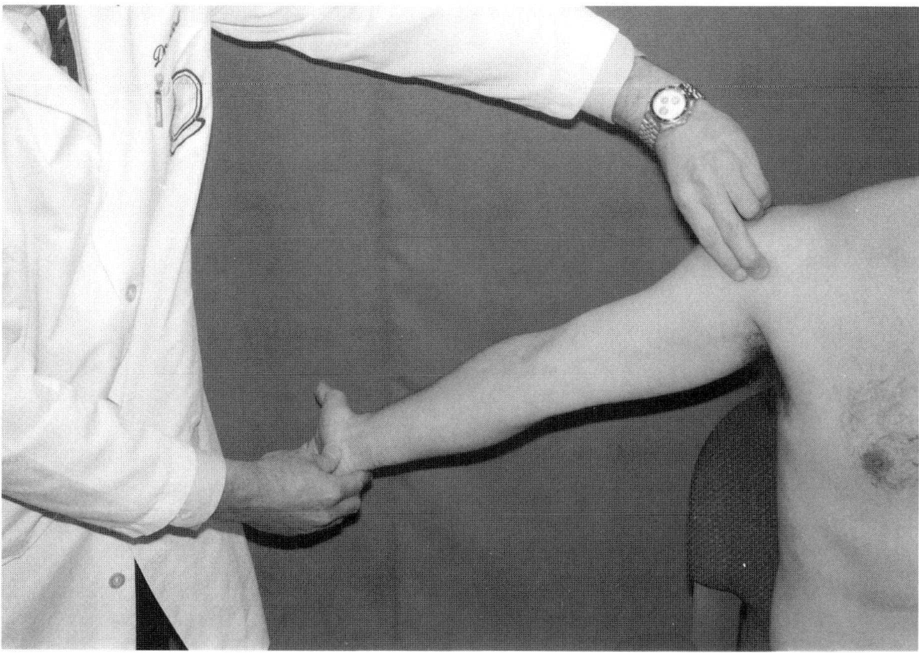

Figure 20-8. Abduction-extension test. The patient is asked to supinate the forearm, extend the elbow, and abduct and extend the shoulder. This maneuver places stress on the inflamed tendon and will cause anterior shoulder pain about the proximal biceps tendon.

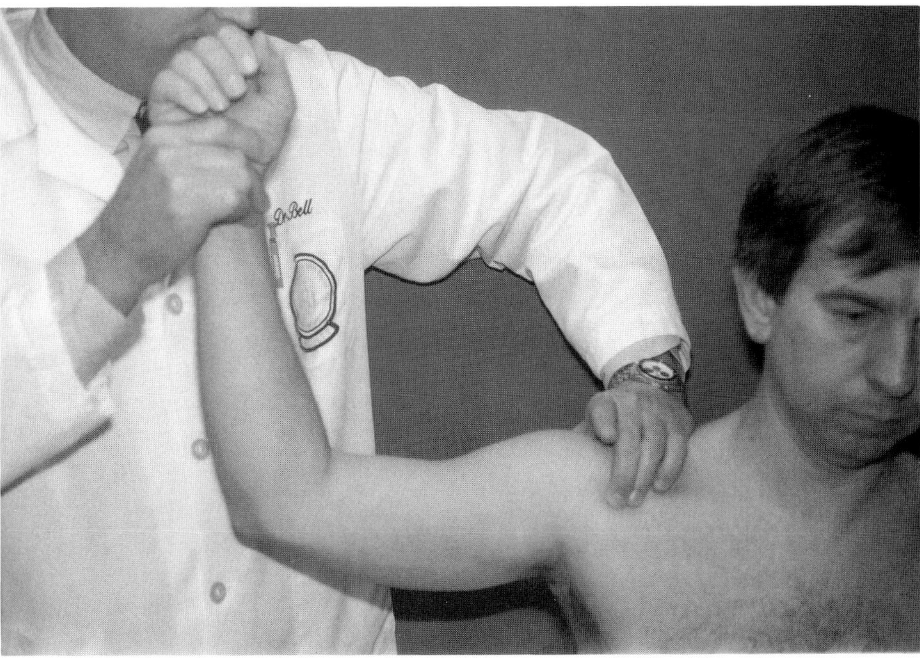

Figure 20-9. Instability test for the biceps. Much like the apprehension sign, the test requires the examiner to bring the patient's arm into 90 degrees of abduction and external rotation while simultaneously palpating the area of the bicipital groove. In patients with instability of the biceps, a palpable and occasionally audible clunk will be appreciated along the anterior edge of the acromium.

IMAGING STUDIES

Radiographs

Routine radiographic studies often fail to reveal changes of the bicipital groove. Several views specifically obtained will provide that information; however, all patients must first undergo routine radiographic studies to rule out other related problems such as impingement, rotator cuff tears, and degenerative arthritis. Our standard series includes a scapular anteroposterior, scapular lateral, and an outlet view. In suspected cases of biceps pathology, there are two additional views ordered. The first is the bicipital groove view of Cone. With the cassette held at the apex of the shoulder and the arm externally rotated, the beam is oriented along the coronal axis of the humerus and angled slightly medially. This view provides an excellent means of determining the presence of groove changes such as spurs or narrowing.

The Fisk view places the patient on the x-ray table, leaning on the elbows, holding the cassette in his or her hands. The beam is directed from above along the anterior aspect of the shoulder. This provides a tangential view of the groove and its pathology.

Ultrasound

The use of ultrasound for diagnostic purposes in the shoulder was popular during the late 1980s owing both to its low cost and noninvasive nature. However, its applicability was limited due to the problem of reader dependence. Only a few centers dealing in large quantities of studies became proficient in their interpreting. The principal application was for determining cuff pathology; however, the biceps was also studied. With the introduction of the magnetic resonance image (MRI) and improved specificity, the interest in ultrasonography for the shoulder wanted. This is not to say that it is no longer used. In fact, it remains a reliable, noninvasive, inexpensive technique for determining biceps integrity—its limit being the interpretation of other problems.

Arthrography

Unfortunately, routine arthrograms are often underused by today's orthopaedists. This study may provide not only information about the presence or absence of a rotator cuff tear but also the size and thickness of the residual tear. Furthermore, the status of the biceps, its presence, changes within the groove, and synovitis may be determined. Subluxations may be confined with arthrography, noting the intra-articular presence of the tendon proximally and its absence distally within the groove. Further information can be obtained with the addition of computed tomography (CT) cuts after the arthrogram.

Magnetic Resonance Imaging

In recent years, the use of MRI has grown enormously due in part to better machines, coils, and improved interpretation skills. As our ability to read this study increases, must more is being learned preoperatively about the biceps. Fissures of the intratendinous portion, partial tears within the groove, and laminations at its origin from the glenoid all may be detected on MRIs. Of equal importance is the MRI in evaluating the rotator cuff as well as the biceps preoperatively. In this age of miniarthrotomy and arthroscopic cuff repairs, it is important to know preoperatively the status of as many parts of the shoulder as possible. The obvious drawbacks are its cost and the potential for claustrophobia in some patients. Nevertheless, as the technology and our ability to use it increases, this will be the study of choice for the biceps and most shoulder problems.

Arthroscopy

The arthroscope may serve two roles in the treatment of biceps problems. The first is diagnostic. The care of many shoulder problems is often made confusing owing to the substantial differential diagnoses that can exist. For example, a patient with anterior shoulder pain and a diminished range of active motion may have a rotator cuff tear, adhesive capsulitis, biceps tendinitis, and even tendinitis due to instability. Preoparative testing may yield only a portion of the answer, hence the need to consider an arthroscopic inspection.

As we have learned, the optimal arthroscopic inspection of the shoulder entails a thorough inspection of the glenohumeral articulation, the ligamentous complex, the rotator cuff, the biceps, and the subacromial space. There are three components to the biceps examination: the root or origin of the tendon as it attaches to the superior aspect of the glenoid, the intra-articular portion, and the point of exit from the joint as it enters the bicipital groove.

The origin of the biceps varies from patient to patient, with its attachment to the superior glenoid labrum being both anterior as well as posterior to the apex of the glenoid. Furthermore, the rigidity of this attachment will also vary. Some patients will have a very mobile superior labrum whereas others will be firmly adherent to the underlying glenoid neck. The determination of a pathologic situation is made after considering these variables.

From the labrum, the tendon courses 2 to 3 cm before exiting the joint. An arthroscopic inspection, if properly performed, should reveal any abnormalities (other than pure intratendinous tears). Using the inflow cannula or a probe to pull the tendon back into the joint, the entire extent of the tendon may be viewed and probed and its integrity checked. Fiber failure will often result in partial-thickness tears and a "strip cheese" appearance. A debridement with a shaver will reveal the actual amount of tendon involved.

The final area of inspection is the exit point as the tendon dives in to the groove. A normal tendon will have a fine vascular network about the peritenon, which begins just as the tendon is exiting the joint. By pulling the tendon with the probe or inflow cannula, the first 1 to 1.5 cm of the tendon from the groove may be pulled in the joint for inspection. In cases of significant bicipital tendinitis, this portion of the tendon will evidence a synovitis with injected vessels.

The second application for arthroscopy is that of treatment. As discussed in the prior section on traction injuries, many problems as relate to the biceps may be addressed arthroscopically. Partial-thickness tears and fraying may be debrided, residual stumps from old long-head tears may be resected to prevent mechanical symptoms, superior avulsions may be repaired with tacks or suture, and in cases of recalcitrant tendinitis, the intra-articular attachment may be released after a limited tenodesis approach.

Injections

Typically, we consider injections as a therapeutic modality, reserved for recalcitrant cases of tendinitis and bursitis. The shoulder, due to its extensive soft tissue envelope and the many problems that may affect it, is often difficult to diagnose. The selective and judicious use of injections may serve as the surgeon's optimal diagnostic tool in many cases: the subacromial space in impingement and cuff tears; the glenohumeral joint in capsulitis and arthritis; the acromioclavicular joint in idiopathic osteolysis; and the biceps sheath in biceps tendinitis. Small-gauge needles, small amounts of local anesthetic, and sterile conditions can provide a wealth of information.

In differentiating bicipital problems from cuff and impingement problems, a sequential subacromial and then a bicipital injection may be helpful. In patients with purely inflammatory problems, an occasional dose of a corticosteroid may be beneficial for their treatment and your understanding of the pathology. Injections about the biceps must be properly placed to avoid intratendinous injections. With the patient sitting on the examination table, he or she is asked to flex the elbow 90 degrees and the arm is internally rotated 10 degrees. The groove is palpated and prepared and the injection placed about the sheath. If the sheath is entered, you should make certain that there is no resistance to the injection; this would imply an intratendinous injection. After 5 minutes the patient should be re-examined noting any changes.

PATHOLOGY

Impingement

As stated before, disorders of the biceps tendon seldom occur as an isolated entity but more commonly in conjunction with other disease processes. The most common is the impingement syndrome. A pathologic continuum, the impingement syndrome involves the rotator cuff, the acromioclavicular joint, the subacromial bursae, and in many cases, the biceps tendon. In overhead athletes, primary and secondary impingement (due to instability) may result in biceps problems. Any surgical procedure directed solely at the bicipital disease will often fail unless the inciting mechanical impingement or instability is also addressed. One is reminded that in this select group of patients, the basic disease process is not so much a degenerative one as a dysfunctional one.

In the adult population, we know that the biceps is not uncommonly involved in impingement problems. Its presence among athletes is probably greater than we think due in large part to the early age at which many youngsters begin to throw, their relative lack of strength, and our unwillingness to recognize impingement in this age group. The relative level of impingement is determined by several various factors such as acromial morphology, posterior capsular tightness, strength of the periscapular musculature, type of overhead sport, and mechanics of the throwing motion—full overhead, three-quarter, and side arm.

With the arm in a neutral rotation, such as the cocking phase of throwing, the biceps courses beneath the anterior aspect of the acromium. Most athletes participating in an overhead sport use a three-fourths motion, which in and of itself helps to decrease impingement. As the throwing motion is elevated to full overhead, there is greater chance for irritation of the biceps. This is potentiated if there is coexistent posterior capsular tightness, which will cause superior humeral migration, resulting in further impingement. If the periscapular muscles, specifically the serratus anterior, is weak and readily fatigues, there is also a greater degree of impingement because the scapula is unable to rotate out of the way of the humeral head during normal forward elevation.

The concept of acromial morphology as it affects the incidence of rotator cuff pathology has been well described.[25] Most authors agree that type III acromiums are associated with a higher incidence of tears, and in theory, bicipital lesions secondary to impingement may also be seen with the hooked acromium.

Clearly, within the younger athletic population, instability is one of if not the principal cause of rotator cuff and biceps impingement. With progressive increases in anterior laxity, the normal amount of anterosuperior humeral head migration during forward elevation is exaggerated, and the head abuts the anterior acromium. These patients represent one of the more difficult diagnostic dilemmas of the shoulder. Seldom is the extent of instability or impingement such that a clear diagnosis can be made. Instead, there is often a combination of primary instability with impingement superimposed. Careful examination with attention directed toward findings of instability (i.e., apprehension) and not just pain is important. Selective injections, both subacromial and intra-articular may help sort out the two diseases.

Instability

Several authors have addressed the issue of biceps subluxation. During the 1960s and 1970s, the concept of recurrent biceps instability was very popular and served as the diagnosis for which many biceps were tenodesed.[3,10] Some thought that transverse ligament integrity was the key to stability, and if lax, the biceps would sublux when an abduction, external rotation force, were applied. By contrast, three different studies have shown that rotator cuff tendon, in and about the region of the cuff interval, is the principal restraint. Petersons cadaveric study[27] mentioned previously found that subluxation only occurred when the supraspinatus and subscapularis tendons were torn. Studies by Meyer[22-24] and Paavolainen et al[26] further confirmed that true subluxation requires a defect in the rotator cuff interval. As such, most patients in whom the proposed diagnosis is that of subluxation will likely have a concomitant rotator cuff defect allowing the tendons medial translation. This clearly is more common in the older (older than 50 years) age group but may occasionally be encountered in younger athletes. The treatment is directed at the source of the instability, the rotator interval defect. If this is imbricated in the area of the biceps tendon's exit from the joint, stability should result.

Not all cases of biceps instability are due to a proximal cuff defect, however. Occasionally, one will encounter an isolated subscapularis tear, due to a forceful internal rotation motion against resistance. In this setting, with the medial restraint to subluxation disrupted, the biceps will sublux. An MRI will readily identify both lesions. If athroscopy is used diagnostically, one will find the biceps intact but exiting the joint not at its typical 2-o'clock position but much lower, due to the displacement about 3 or 4 o'clock. The intra-articular portion of the subscapularis tendon will also be altered if not absent. In such cases, the subscapularis should be repaired to its normal insertion in the lesser tuberosity. The biceps may be stable if the rotator cuff interval is repaired; however, should there be residual instability, then a tenodesis is warranted.

Primary (Intrinsic) Biceps Tendinitis

For years, the controversy regarding the existence of a primary intrinsic form of biceps tendinitis has raged on, with opponents to the concept stating this is merely a component of the impingement process. Proponents argue that there clearly are cases of isolated disease of the tendon that begin and remain within the bicipital groove. The macroscopic picture is one of gross tendon failure with fraying and attrition. The groove itself will often have developed a narrower breadth and osteophytic spurs along its margins. The peritenon vasculature is congested and the surrounding synovium inflamed and hypertrophic to the point of compromising the tendon's vascular supply. Microscopically, the collagen fibrils have lost much of their lamellar alignment, falling into disordered haphazard bundles. White cells and macrophages replace the normally acellular environment. And yet, despite all this pathology, the more proximal subacromial space will be pristine owing to the fact that, in this specific patient, the problem resides within the biceps tendon alone. The real question becomes one of whether it is this primary disease that then migrates proximally and involves the remaining tendon or if there truly is a primary impingement process of the biceps.

This argument continues within the literature. Dines et al[7] reported on 20 patients with a primary diagnosis of biceps tendinitis who underwent tenodesis. There were 6 failures of the 20 patients due to impingement and instability. Of these, four underwent a second procedure. Their conclusion was that biceps tenodesis, when indicated, should be accompanied by an acromioplasty and coracoacromial ligament release, believing the biceps disease to be secondary to an impingement problem.

Cofield and Becker[4] reported on the long-term follow-up of 51 patients undergoing tenodesis. Of the 54 shoulders in the series, results changed significantly over time. Early on, at the 6-month mark, 94 percent of the patients were satisfied. At long-term follow-up of 7 years, only 54 percent were still happy with the procedure. Their conclusion was that isolated biceps tenodesis was seldom effective or indicated as an isolated procedure.

DePalma and Callery[6] reported on the results of 86 biceps tenodeses for primary tenosynovitis. Although their follow-up was only on average 27 months, the results were reasonable, with 64 percent excellent, 16 percent good, 8 percent fair, and 10 percent poor. Eighty percent of their patients achieved a satisfactory result at 2 years, with no significant change over time. Given the proper indications, this would imply that an intrinsic disease process does exist and may be successfully treated with tenodesis alone.

Similarly, Post[28] reported on 17 patients in whom a biceps tenodesis or transfer had been performed for primary tendinitis. He was careful to exclude as many other factors such as impingement, instability, and rotator cuff tears to have a pure patient population. Of the patients having a tenodesis alone, 88 percent achieved satisfactory results, one requiring a subsequent acromiopasty and two manipulations. Like DePalma and Callery, Post thought that there does exist a primary intrinsic biceps tendinopathy that is amenable to an isolated tenodesis.

Intra-articular Pathology

Several various disorders of the biceps tendon have been presented. They include lesions secondary to an impingement process, subluxations, and primary attritional tendinitis. All these problems originate in or involve, mainly, that portion of the tendon within the bicipital groove. As with all tendons, many of the pathologic conditions may affect either the origin or insertion of the tendon. Such is the case with the biceps and its proximal intra-articular origin. This area of the tendon is exposed to a different group of mechanical forces, owing both to its location about the superior aspect of the humeral head and its varying insertion along the superior labrum.

In the late 1980s and early 1990s, Snyder et al[30] began to describe a lesion of the proximal glenolabral complex, which included the biceps attachment. They termed this pathologic finding the SLAP (*s*uperior *l*abrum *a*nterior to *p*osterior) lesion. In a retrospective review of more than 700 shoulder arthroscopies, they found 20 patients with varying degrees of this SLAP lesion. They found the most common mechanism to be a fall on an outstretched forward elevated arm, similar to that seen in posterior instability cases. The most common complaint was pain overhead and a ''popping'' or ''clicking'' sensation. Based on this, they thought many of these patients had experienced an overloading of the superior labral complex with a resultant shearing of the biceps attachment. They classified these tears into four categories, I to IV. The lower grades entail a vertical longitudinal labral tear beginning posteriorly, and as the grade increases, so does the anterior extent of the labrum and the amount of the biceps-labral detachment. A grade IV lesion has a bucket handle tear of the labrum and a hypermobile biceps attachment (see Ch. 22).

Andrews et al[1] reported on tears of the glenoid labrum in 73 baseball pitchers and other throwing athletes who underwent arthroscopic examination. Most of them were located over the anterosuperior portion of the glenoid labrum near the origin of the tendon of the long head of the biceps. Much like Synder et al, Andrews et al noted that the tendon of the biceps appeared to originate through and be continuous with the superior portion of the labrum. In many cases, the biceps seemed to have pulled the labrum off the glenoid. They confirmed this finding by directly observing the origin of the biceps as the muscle body of the biceps was electrically stimulated. With the stimulation, the biceps tightened and actually lifted the superior labrum off the glenoid. Thus, tensile as well as compressive forces would appear to contribute to these intra-articular problems. Those athletes participating in rigorous repetitive overhead throwing would be at risk for these injuries as might those sustaining marked abduction, external rotation injuries such as subluxations.

DIFFERENTIAL DIAGNOSIS

Instability

There are two principal differences between biceps tendinitis and anterior shoulder instability: sense of "miss trust" and episodic pain. In instability, the patient will relate a history of miss trust of the shoulder in positions of abduction and external rotation. The apprehension sign will be positive as will the relocation test. Although pain may accompany the instability, it is more a sense of the joint being unstable than hurting. Furthermore, any pain that does accompany an instability problem is usually very short-lived and resolves quickly within the first day of a subluxation. The pain of biceps tendinitis is more constant and exacerbated by certain positions such as external rotation and abduction, owing to the tension placed on the biceps. These patients will complain of anterior shoulder pain even in the resting position. As the arm is brought out away from the body, this pain will intensify and remain localized to the anterior shoulder. If the patient with instability does have pain on testing, it may be anterior or posterior joint line in location, seldom directly over the biceps.

Few tests short of arthroscopy will be helpful in differentiating instability from biceps problems. MRI and dual-contrast CT arthrography can demonstrate labral irregularities, yet the diagnosis will most likely be made in the office during the history and physical examination.

Impingement and Rotator Cuff Tears

The most common error in the diagnosis and treatment of biceps problems is that of omission. Most patients presenting with findings of bicipital pain will, after further examination, often have concomitant findings for impingement or rotator cuff tears. One is reminded that the spectrum of rotator cuff tears is representative of the impingement continuum, which originates with reversible inflammatory changes of the cuff and progresses, if unabated, to full-thickness cuff tears.

Patients with impingement or cuff disease will complain of pain not only anteriorly as with biceps problems but anterior superiorly and referred to the middeltoid laterally. Bicipital pain is worse with elbow flexion, forearm supination, and forward elevation, whereas cuff and impingement pain is mild with the arm below the horizontal and intensifies with overhead activities. The impingement sign is positive as is the empty can test of resisted forward elevation with the arm pronated.

More often than not, patients presenting with biceps findings will have an on-going problem with impingement and may well have reached stage 2 or 3 cuff damage. Thus, the patient who presents with a tear of the long head of the biceps must be thoroughly examined to rule out coexistent treatable cuff disease. Standard radiographic studies looking for abnormal acromial morphology and arthrography or MRI to determine cuff integrity are appropriate. Selective injections will help to sort out impingement from biceps. A subacromial injection with relief of the impingement sign yet persistent anterior bicipital pain would imply coexistent problems. However, if a subacromial injection fails to help the bicipital pain and a second injection, anteriorly about the biceps sheath, eliminates the anterior pain, then the diagnosis of primary biceps tendinitis is made.

Instability and SLAP Lesions

Patients with true recurrent anterior instability will complain of a sense of giving way with their shoulder in certain positions whereas those with SLAP tears complain more of pain with activities overhead and to the side. Typical of this are throwing athletes due in large part to the enormous force applied to the biceps during deceleration. They may well recall a traumatic episode, as will the instability patients. However, those with superior labral and biceps origin tears often complain of a "click or clunk" with certain motions, not so much a feeling of giving way. These patients are often mistaken as having a recurrent instability, and it is not until arthroscopy that the actual diagnosis is made.

TREATMENT

Primary Biceps Tendinitis

The treatment of this disorder depends on several variables. Assuming there is no coexistent cuff or impingement problems, the tendinitis is treated conservatively for an extended period of time. Rest, anti-inflammatories, phonophoresis, and judicious use of injections will usually resolve the problem. In the athlete, the specific throwing motion may need to be modified to decrease the trauma to the biceps.

Failing conservative measures, a tenodesis may be considered. We perform this with the assistance of the arthroscope. The patient is positioned on his or her side with the arm suspended at 30 degrees of abduction. Standard

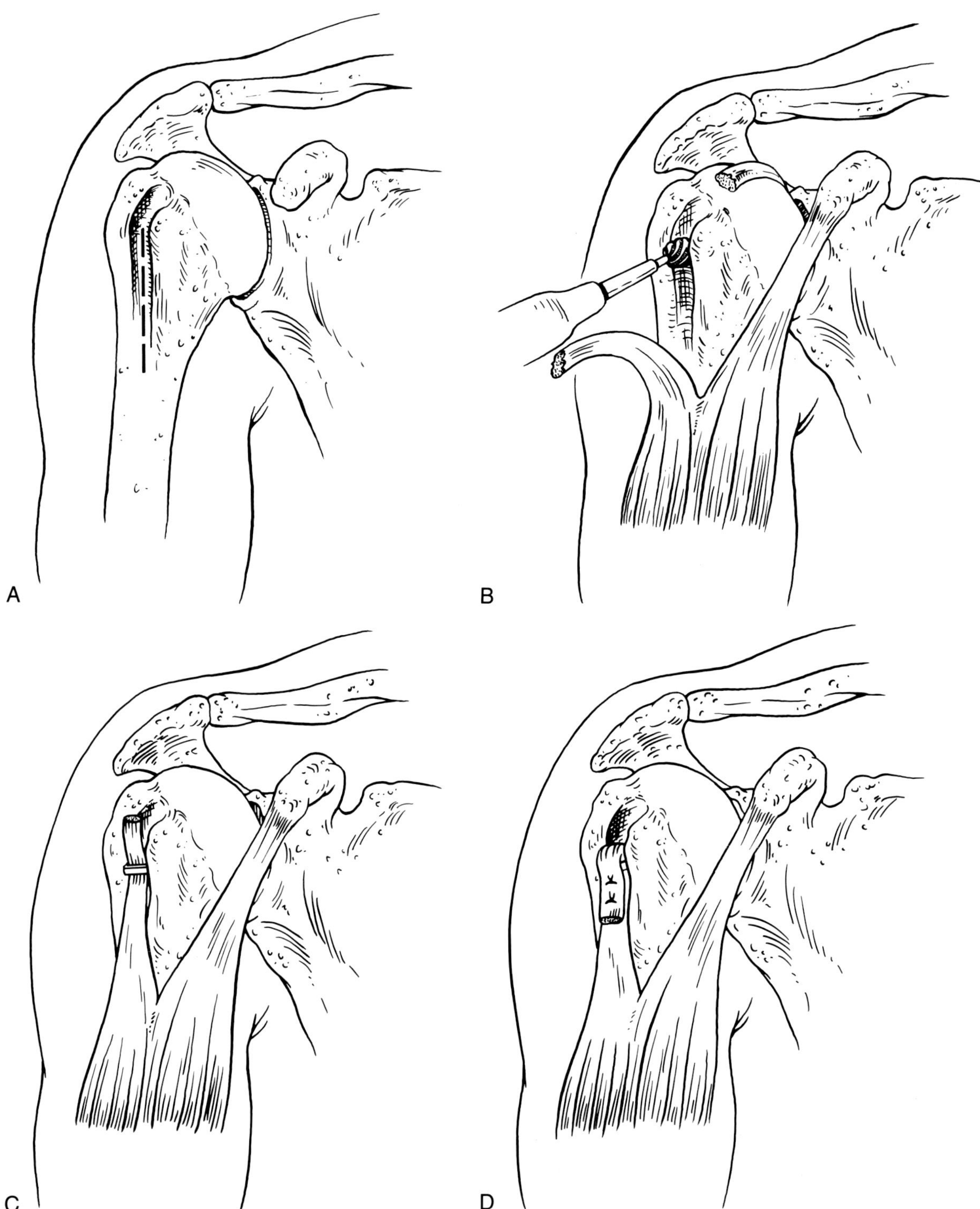

Figure 20-10. (**A**) The incision for biceps tenodesis is 3 to 4 cm long beginning 1 cm medial and 2 to 3 cm inferior to the anterolateral corner of the acromium. (**B**) The transverse ligament is released and the biceps delivered from the joint after which the groove is decorticated with a high-speed burr to prepare the site for attachment. (**C**) Staple technique for tenodesis. (**D**) Residual tendon is sutured back on itself. (*Figure continues.*)

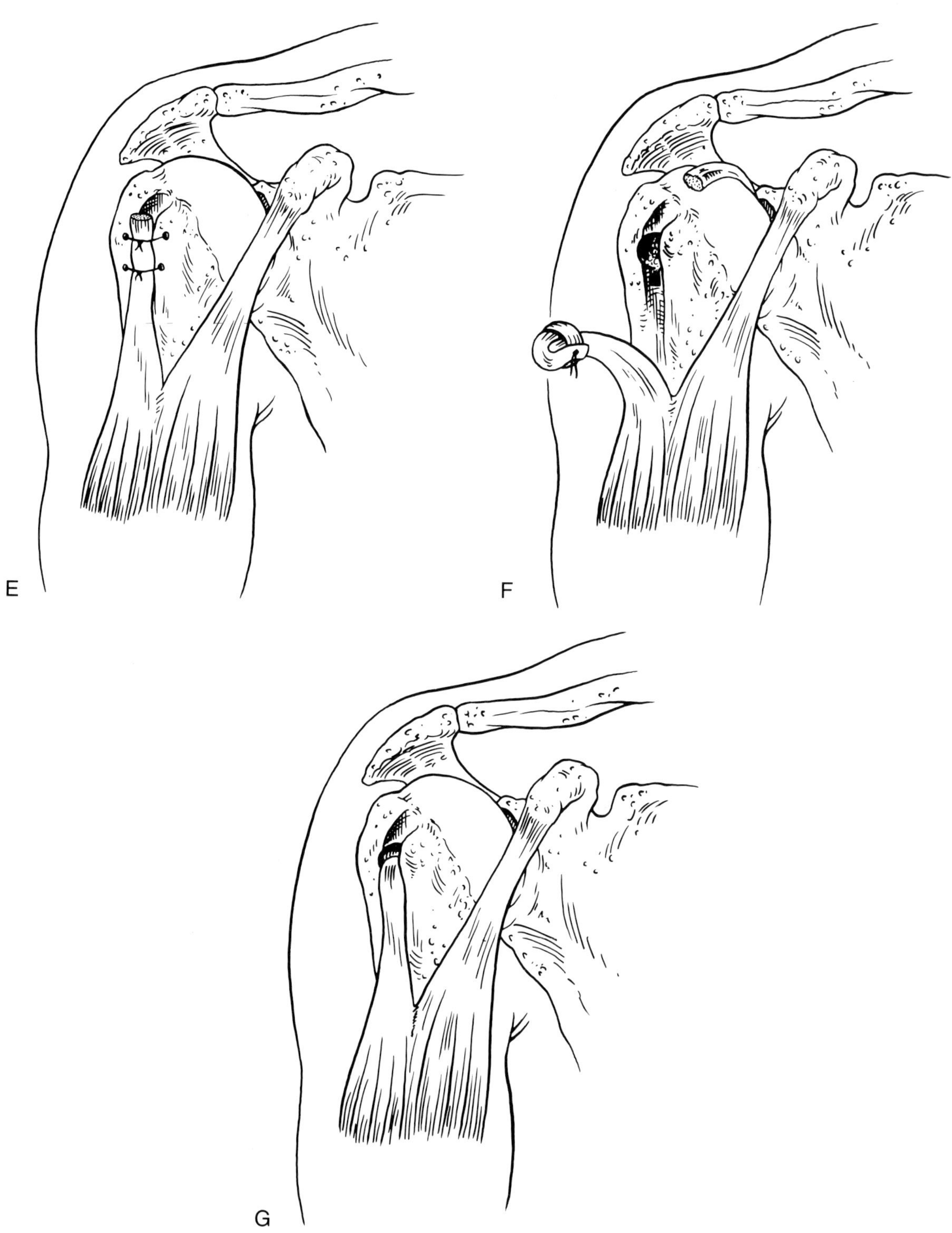

Figure 20-10 (*Continued*). (**E**) Simple suture technique for tenodesis. (**F & G**) Keyhole technique. The tendon is knotted and sutured back on itself and inserted under light tension back into the keyhole, thus locking it in place.

glenohumeral arthroscopy is performed to confirm the biceps disease and rule out other problems. After establishing an anterior working portal, an 18-gauge spinal needle is brought in from the anterosuperior position and placed through the biceps tendon. A single strand of size 0 PDS is passed through the needle and into the joint. The needle is withdrawn, leaving the suture through the tendon. The intra-articular end of the suture is grasped and brought out the anterior cannula. The two ends of the suture are held together with a hemostat. The biceps is then released from its attachment at the apex of the glenoid using a small basket.

At this point, a small 3- to 4-cm incision is made beginning 1 cm medial and 2 to 3 cm inferior to the anterolateral corner of the acromium (Fig. 20-10A). The deltoid is split in line with its fibers and the bicipital groove identified. The transverse ligament is released and the biceps delivered from the joint after which the groove is decorticated with a high-speed burr to prepare the site for attachment (Fig. 20-10B). At this point, any one of several different techniques may be used to tenodese the tendon. A simple approach is the use of a two-prong soft tissue staple, securing the tendon as in Figure 20-10C and D, with the residual stump of tendon sewn back on itself. Alternatively, the tendon may simply be sewn into the trough (Fig. 20-10E), or the keyhole technique may be used wherein the tendon is knotted and sutured back on itself (Fig. 20-10F) and inserted under light tension back into the keyhole, thus locking it in place (Fig. 20-10G). The inherent advantage of this technique is that it obvates the need for internal fixation and allows earlier active motion of the shoulder and biceps construct.

Subluxing Biceps

Subluxation of the biceps is a very rare occurrence, owing both to the bony groove within which it rests and the rotator cuff through which it passes exiting the joint. For there to be an actual subluxation or dislocation of the tendon, there must be an obligatory defect in one or both of these two structures. Several authors[20,22,23] have addressed the issue and agree that the necessary ingredient for subluxation is a defect proximally within the rotator cuff. Thus, should one make the diagnosis of a subluxing biceps tendon, the approach must entail attention to the rotator cuff interval and its status. If the interval is attenuated and allows for tendon medialization, then an imbrication of the subscapularis and the supraspinatus tendons as the biceps exits the joint will stabilize the tendon. If the tendon is badly damaged, a tenodesis may be needed. In all cases of rotator cuff disease, a concomitant acromioplasty is performed to decompress the subacromial space and prevent further cuff injury.

In some cases, the defect will be the subscapularis and anterior joint capsule, which has been avulsed from its normal attachment. Here, the biceps must be reduced and the subscapularis and capsule reattached near the lesser tuberosity. The rotator cuff interval is also repaired to stabilize the tendon from above.

Acute Tears of the Long Head of the Biceps

Two distinct groups of patients suffer from acute proximal biceps tears, and they are typically separated by age. Those with acute tears and only minimal antecedent problems are younger, usually younger than the age of 40. They may well have been involved in recreational lifting and recently increased their weight so much that they exceeded the tensile strength of their tendon. Their tear may be at the musculotendinous junction but will more likely be within the groove or off the glenoid. In both the latter cases, we recommend a primary tenodesis. Tenodesis gives them the best chance for a return to normal function, including lifting, and a cosmetic normal contour to the arm. The technique requires two short incisions. The first incision is made at the deltobicipital groove midarm. This measures 3 cm in length and is oriented vertically. The tendon is delivered from the wound, and a traction stitch is placed. The second incision is identical to that described for the biceps tenodesis and exposes the groove proximally. A tendon passer is used to pass the traction suture and tendon retrograde up to the proximal incision. The groove is then abraded and the tendon tenodesed with a single two-prong staple. Tears at the musculotendinous junction may be candidates for a primary repair and prolonged protection. All these patients with repairs or tenodesis are protected from any active elbow flexion for 3 to 4 weeks. Resistive work is started at 8 weeks.

The second group of patients are those older than the age of 50, many of whom have a prior history of shoulder problems and treatment. These are usually tears of attrition and occur within the groove. More often than not they will have findings for impingement or rotator cuff tears. If they have a prior history, then simple observation for 4 weeks is the treatment of choice. Most of the immediate pain of the tear will resolve, resulting in fairly normal strength and the residual deformity. If there is a strong prior history of shoulder problems, then diagnostic studies to determine cuff integrity are needed. If the cuff is intact and the patient has been suffering from impingement, then an option is to perform an arthroscopic subacromial decompression (ASD) and, for the younger active patient, also repair the torn biceps. After the ASD, the two-incision technique described above is used to tenodese the torn tendon.

If the patient has findings for a full-thickness rotator

cuff tear and has failed with prior treatment, then either a formal arthrotomy, acromioplasty, cuff repair, and biceps tenodesis or an ASD, miniarthrotomy, cuff repair, and biceps tenodesis are performed. The premise remains to address the cuff tear, the impingement process, and lastly, the biceps tendon.

SLAP Lesions

One will encounter a fair amount of variability in these lesions. Some may consist of only a vertical longitudinal tear of the superior labrum to the more complex disruptions of the entire labral-biceps complex. The treatment of the isolated tears of the labrum with no coexistent labral instability may be treated with an arthroscopic resection alone. If, however, the problem rests with not only a tear but also an unstable biceps attachment, then efforts should be directed toward its repair.

An arthroscopic approach is ideally suited to these problems: it provides a stable form of fixation to an otherwise inaccessible location and with far less morbidity than an open procedure. Although several different techniques exist for the arthroscopic treatment of these lesions, the one we prefer is the absorbable tack designed by Warren and produced by Linvatec. The system allows accurate placement of 6- or 8-mm bioabsorbable tacks at multiple locations about the superior margin of the glenoid. With the biceps anchor repaired, attention may be turned to the residual biceps tears.

CONCLUSION

It has been the intent of this chapter to present the many problems affecting the biceps tendon, with an emphasis on the recognition and differential diagnosis. It is hoped that the reader will come away with the understanding of the manner in which the biceps interacts with the other components of the shoulder girdle and its relationship to the various disease entities. As the surgeon approaches a suspected problem of the biceps, he or she is cautioned and reminded that this tendon is often affected by the other more common shoulder disorders, and these must be investigated and ruled out before any operative treatment.

REFERENCES

1. Andrews JR, Carson WG Jr, McLeod WD: Glenoid labrum tears related to the long head of the biceps. Am J Sports Med 13:337–41, 1985
2. Basmajian JV, Latif MA: Integrated actions and function of the chief flexors of the elbow. J Bone Joint Surg [Am] 39:1106–18, 1957
3. Clein LJ: Suprascapular entrapment neuropathy. J Neurosurg 43:337–42, 1975
4. Cofield RH, Becker D: Surgical tenodesis of the long head of the biceps brachii for chronic tendinitis. J Bone Joint Surg [Am] 71:376–81, 1989
5. Cone RO, Danzig L, Resnick D, Goldman AB: The bicipital groove: radiographic, anatomic, and pathologic study. AJR 41:781–8, 1983
6. DePalma AF, Callery GE: Bicipital tenosynovitis. Clin Orthop 3:69–85, 1954
7. Dines D, Warren RF, Inglis AE: Surgical treatment of lesions of the long head of the biceps. Clin Orthop 164:165–71, 1982
8. Furlani J: Electromyographic study of the m. biceps brachii in movements at the glenohumeral joint. Acta Anat (Basel) 96:270–84, 1976
9. Gilcreest EL, Albi P: Unusual lesions of muscles and tendons of the shoulder girdle and upper arm. Surg Gynecol Obstet 68:903–17, 1939
10. Giuliani P, Scarpa G, Marchini M, Nicoletti P: Development of scapulohumeral articulation in man, with special reference to its relation to the tendon of the long head of the biceps muscle of the arm. Arch Ital Anat Embriol 82:85–98, 1977
11. Glousman R, Jobe F, Tibone J et al: Dynamic electromyographic analysis of the throwing shoulder with glenohumeral instability. J Bone Joint Surg [Am] 70:220–6, 1988
12. Habermeyer P, Kaiser E, Knappe M et al: Functional anatomy and biomechanics of the long triceps tendon. Unfallchirurg 90:319–29, 1987
13. Hammond G, Torgerson W, Dotter W, Leach R: The painful shoulder. Inst Course Lect 83–90, 1971
14. Hitchcock HH, Bechtol CO: Painful shoulder. Observations on the role of the tendon of the long head of the biceps brachii in its causation. J Bone Joint Surg [Am] 30:263–73, 1948
15. Hueter C: Zur diagnose der verletzungen des m. biceps brachii. Arch Klin Chir 5:321–3, 1864
16. Itoi E, Kuechle DK, Newman SR et al: Stabilising function of the biceps in stable and unstable shoulders. J Bone Joint Surg [Br] 75:546–50, 1993
17. Kumar VP, Satku K, Balasubramaniam P: The role of the long head of the biceps brachii in the stabilization of the head of the humerus. Clin Orthop 244:172–5, 1989
18. Lippmann RK: Frozen shoulder, periarthritis, bicepital tenosynovitis. Arch Surg 47:283–96, 1943
19. Lippmann RK: Bicipital tenosynovitis. NY State J Med 44:2235–40, 1944
20. Ludington NA: Rupture of the long head of biceps flexor cubiti. Am J Surg 77:358–63, 1923
21. Metsen F, Kirby R: Office evaluation and management of shoulder pain. Orthop Clin North Am 13:45, 1982
22. Meyer AW: Spolia anatomica. Absence of the tendon of the long head of the biceps. J Anat 48:133–5, 1913–1914
23. Meyer AW: Spontaneous dislocation of the tendon of the long head of the biceps brachii. Arch Surg 13:109–19, 1926
24. Meyer AW: Spontaneous dislocation and distruction of the tendon of the long head of the biceps brachii. Arch Surg 17:493–506, 1928

25. Morrison AS, Biglianni LU, April EW: The morphology of the acromium and its relationship to rotator cuff tears. Orthop Trans 10:228, 1986
26. Paavolainen P, Bjorkenheim JM, Slatis P, Paulku P: Operative treatment of severe proximal humeral fractures. Acta Orthop Scand 54:374–9, 1983
27. Peterson CJ: Spontaneous medial dislocation of the tendon of the long biceps brachii. Clin Orthop 211:224–7, 1986
28. Post M: Primary tendinitis of the long head of the biceps. Clin Orthop 246:117–25, 1989
29. Rowe CR (ed): The Shoulder. Churchill Livingstone, New York, 1988
30. Snyder SJ, Karzel RP, Del Pizzo W et al: SLAP lesions of the shoulder. Arthroscopy 6:274–9, 1990
31. Ting A, Jobe FW, Barto P et al: An EMG analysis of the lateral biceps in shoulders with rotator cuff tears. Presented at the Third Open Meeting of the Society of American Shoulder and Elbow Surgeons, California, 1987
32. Yeargason RM: Rupture of biceps. J Bone Joint Surg 13:160, 1931

CHAPTER TWENTY-ONE

Pectoralis Ruptures

Jeffrey S. Noble
Robert H. Bell

Although once thought to be a rare occurrence, ruptures of the pectoralis major probably occur more frequently than originally thought. Most cases occur in a younger (ages 20 to 35 years), more athletic population. In view of the infrequency of this injury and possible functional deficits, this chapter provides an overview of ruptures of the pectoralis major and recommendations with regard to their diagnosis and treatment.

ANATOMY

The pectoralis major muscle is divided into clavicular, manubrial, sternal, and abdominal portions, taking origin from the midclavicular region, sternal ribs, and external oblique fascia. The clavicular head may extend as far laterally as the deltoid and actually be fused with it, or its origin may be confined solely to the upper sternum. The manubrial portion of the sternal head arises from the midportion of the sternum and the costal cartilages of the first through fifth ribs. The abdominal portion arises from the fifth and sixth ribs and the external oblique fascia and transversalis muscles. Tendinous fibers of the two origins coalesce into three lamina, twisting 90 degrees on each other, such that the sternal portion inserts just lateral to the bicipital groove, posterior to the clavicular portion on the intertubercular groove of the humerus. The anterior lamina courses directly into the humerus and consists of the clavicular portion of the muscle belly. The manubrial and abdominal portions, or middle and posterior laminae, respectively, twist on each other before insertion, such that the manubrial fibers insert inferior to those of the abdominal portion (Fig. 21-1). Some authors have attributed the infrequency of pectoralis major ruptures to its complex trilaminar structure.[19]

As reported by Wolfe et al, the tendinous insertion varies in length from 1.0 to 1.5 cm in length anteriorly. The undersurface of the tendon at its insertion into the humerus ranges from 2.5 to 3.0 cm in length, with the overall width of the tendon measuring 5 to 6 mm.

The innervation of the pectoralis major is via the lateral and medial pectoral nerves. The clavicular head of the pectoralis is innervated by the lateral pectoral nerve, which carries fibers from C5, C6, and C7. The lower two-thirds of the pectoralis muscle receives its innervation from the lateral and medial pectoral nerves, with the medial pectoral nerve carrying fibers from C8 and T1. Although the arterial supply is extensive to the musculature, the pectoral branch of the coracoacromial artery supplies most of the vascular supply.

HISTORICAL REVIEW

Rupture of the pectoralis muscle was originally described in France by Patissier in 1822.[22] Unfortunately, the patient died after developing overwhelming sepsis due to infection of a large associated hematoma. Codman,[5] in 1934, mentioned only two cases of pectoralis avulsion in his review of the Library of the Surgeon General. Since these early reports, more than 100 cases of partial and complete ruptures of the pectoralis have been reported in the literature.[1-7,11-30,33-35]

Pulaski and Martin[24] reported that nonoperative treatment can lead to restoration of function, but strength is

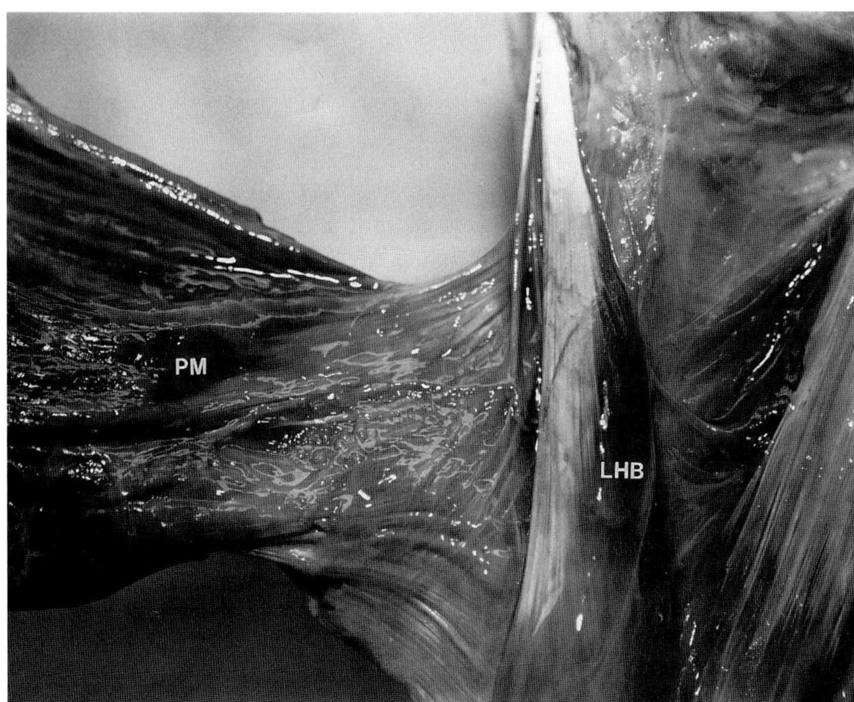

Figure 21-1. Cadaveric specimen illustrating the anatomic relationship of the insertion of the pectoralis major tendon (PM) lateral to the long head of the biceps (LHB). Note the extensive trilaminar structure of the undersurface of the pectoralis tendon.

never restored. Marmor and associates[18] concluded by muscle testing that although the pectoralis major is not necessary for daily shoulder function, it is extremely important during strenuous activities and athletics. DePalma,[8] although not encountering a case of pectoralis major rupture personally, recommended surgical repair as the treatment of choice in the younger patient. Zeman and associates,[35] reporting on a series of nine professional athletes, were able to return all those treated surgically to vigorous athletics. Those treated nonoperatively regained a normal range of motion but continued to demonstrate weakness and complain of mild pain. All these patients agreed that they could not return to their previous athletic level. Recent reports by Wolfe and others[34] have shown good results in athletes with surgical intervention, restoring preoperative strength and range of motion. It is therefore the consensus of most authors that early surgical repair is indicated in those patients who are engaged in strenuous activities and athletics requiring upper extremity strength.

INCIDENCE AND ETIOLOGY

The true incidence of pectoralis rupture is unknown. It occurs in most cases between the ages of 20 and 35 years (range, 2 to 72).[12,32] Almost exclusively reported in males, the injury occurs more commonly in the right extremity.[32] Attritional ruptures commonly associated with biceps and rotator cuff pathology are not typically seen with rupture of the pectoralis tendon. Rupture of the pectoralis tendon can either be related to direct trauma or, more commonly, indirectly, as in forced adduction against resistance.

Ruptures of the pectoralis major are classified as either partial or complete. Type 1 ruptures are considered contusions or sprains; type 2 are partial and incomplete in nature; and type 3 are considered complete.[30] Partial (type 2) ruptures probably occur more commonly and, at times, pose a diagnostic dilemma in differentiating partial from complete rupture. Complete ruptures (type 3) are rare and can be classified based on anatomic location of the tear (i.e., muscular origin, muscle belly, musculotendinous junction, or insertional tendon). Furthermore, correlation exists between the site of rupture and the mechanism of injury.[32] Tears of the muscular belly and musculotendinous junction are often caused by direct trauma, whereas avulsion of the tendon at its insertion commonly occurs indirectly, as seen in weight lifters, football players, and gymnasts.

DYNAMIC FUNCTION AND ARCHITECTURE

Portions of the pectoralis major exhibit differences in muscular activity according to the motions that are being carried out. The clavicular head is most active in forward flexion, reaching a peak at 75 degrees and again at 115 degrees.[31] During flexion, the manubrial and lower sternal portions are minimally active or inactive. No portion of the muscle is active during abduction. Elliot et al,[9] using electromyographic studies, have shown that the pectoralis major is maximally activated with the humerus in an extended position.

It is generally believed that muscular injury and tendon failure occur during the eccentric or lengthening phase of contraction. Such injuries may be a result of a violent contraction in conjunction with an excessively forceful stretch. Garrett et al[10] have shown that in a maximally contracted muscle, passive stretching produces rupture at an average of 26 percent of the resting fiber length. Although the pectoralis major is unusual in that it contains fibers of different lengths, one would expect it to act in a similar manner.

Wolfe et al[34] measured individual pectoralis muscle fiber lengths and expressed excursion as a percentage of resting fiber length during concentric and eccentric phases of bench lifting in a cadaveric model. They showed that compared with the cephalic fibers, the short inferior fibers, those of the lowest portion of the sternal head, became disproportionately stretched during the final 30 degrees of humeral extension. They concluded that the inferior fibers are at a mechanical disadvantage in the eccentric phase of the lifting. With the application of high external loads, maximal stretching of the fibers occurs with resultant rupture. Continued loading in this situation increases the tension in the remaining fibers, resulting in total rupture. They further calculated in one specimen that in the last 30 degrees of extension, the increase in the inferior fiber length exceeded 40 percent of the resting fiber length.

CLINICAL PRESENTATION

The clinical presentations are varied and depend on the extent of the injury, anatomic location, and its chronicity. Acute injuries involving rapid musculature contraction against resistance or direct blows are often associated with severe pain and a tearing sensation. Occasionally, an audible "pop" or "snap" is noticed by the patient. Extensive ecchymosis and swelling are common in the chest wall, axilla, and arm acutely. With muscular ruptures, extremely large hematomas may also develop. A minimal cosmetic defect may or may not be appreciated in the initial examination secondary to swelling. Weakness, especially in attempted adduction of the arm, is apparent and associated with pain.

Subacutely, as pain subsides, asymmetry of the muscle belly is prominent, causing a noticeable bulge and loss of the anterior axillary fold (Fig. 21-2). Localized tenderness and a palpable defect in the tendon aid in the diagnosis. Minimal deformity may not be noticed with the upper arm resting at the side (Fig. 21-3), but with attempted isometric contraction, the defect may be accentuated (Fig. 21-4). Pain and weakness with resisted adduction and internal rotation in the forward-flexed plane are present.

Patients with chronic complete tears will often have cosmetic defects with accentuation of the inferior border of the deltoid and a palpable loss of thickness of the anterior axillary fold. With contraction, the bulk of the retracted muscle belly is prominent. A full range of motion is usually present, with varying degrees of tenderness on palpation. Weakness with adduction and internal rotation is often detected. In certain situations, dynamometry can be useful

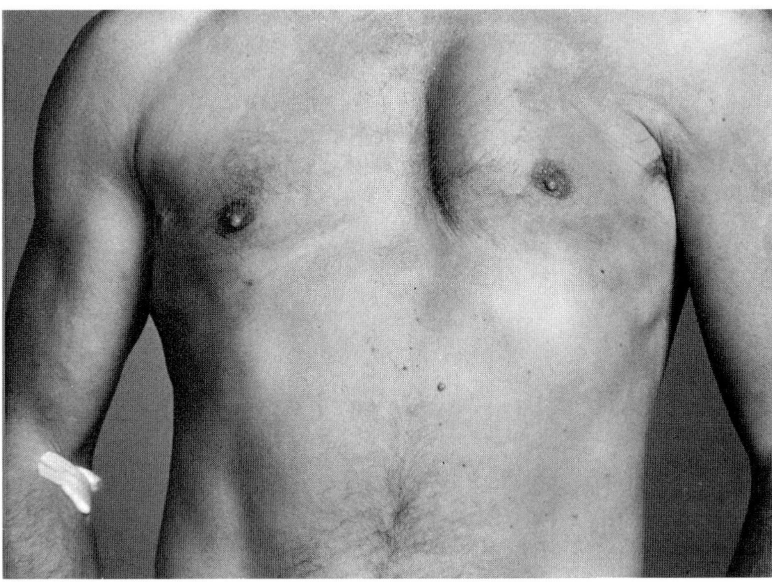

Figure 21-2. Patient presenting with subcute avulsion of the left pectoralis major tendon with noticeable asymmetry of the muscle belly and prominent bulge with loss of the anterior axillary fold.

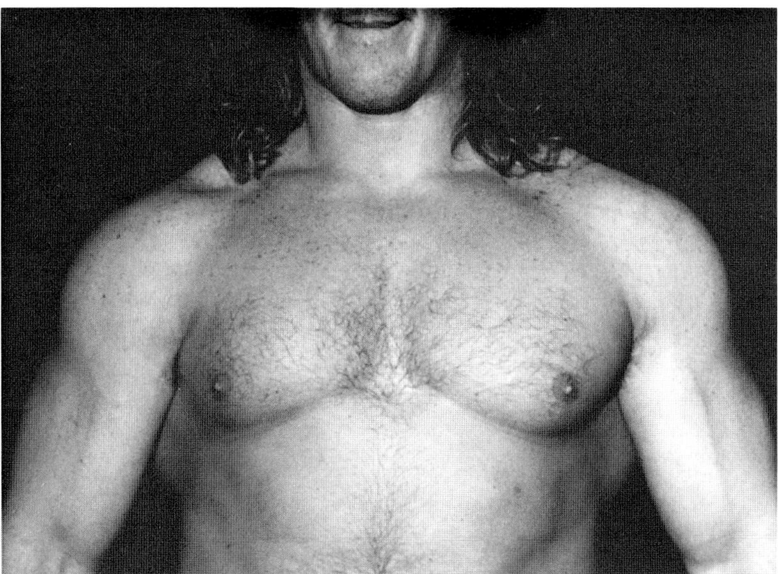

Figure 21-3. Professional weight lifter and body builder presenting with rupture of the right pectoralis major tendon, demonstrating minimal deformity with the upper arm resting at the side.

when minimal or no weakness is perceived on clinical manual muscle testing.[29]

TREATMENT RESULTS

Nonoperative management of complete pectoralis major muscle ruptures is indicated in many individuals, including the older and more inactive patients. Such individuals may not have a significant functional loss. However, Park and Espiniella,[21] in comparing a surgical versus a nonsurgical group of patients, found an 80 percent excellent and 10 percent good rating in those treated surgically. This was compared with a 17 percent excellent and 58 percent good rating in those treated nonoperatively. In the nonoperative group, varying degrees of adductive and internal rotation weakness were noted.

Athletes with complete pectoralis ruptures may lose 50 to 60 percent or more of their horizontal adduction strength.[14] Wolfe et al[34] have shown through Cybex testing in unilateral unrepaired complete tears a low-speed torque deficit of 26 percent and a work deficit of 39.9 percent. Such strength deficits are poorly tolerated in most athletic endeavors that require maximum power with adduction and internal rotation. Previous authors have stated that full return of strength cannot be achieved in complete ruptures

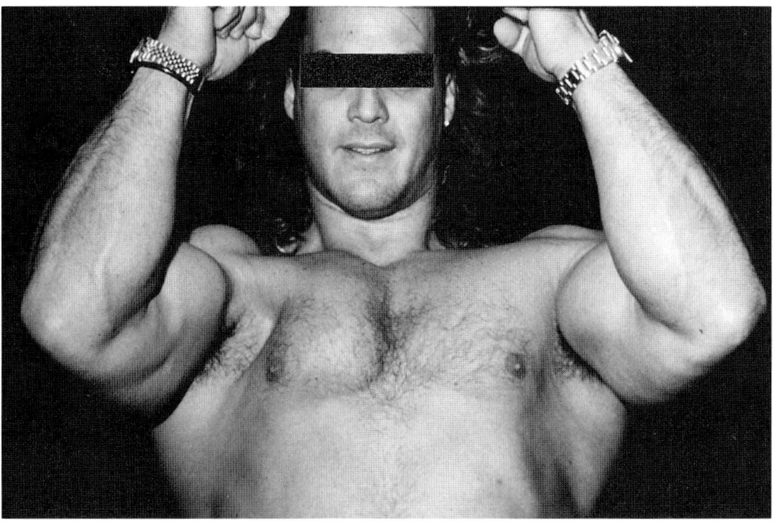

Figure 21-4. Same patient seen in Figure 21-3 during isometric contraction with accentuation of the defect of pectoralis major.

of the pectoralis through a nonoperative approach. It is thus recommended that surgical repair be undertaken in individuals and athletes who require significant upper extremity strength.

Understandably, ruptures of different portions of the pectoralis major carry a differing prognosis. McEntire et al[19] thought that rupture of the musculocutaneous junction resulted in a less favorable outcome than the more distal injuries, although both could be surgically addressed. It has been widely reported that an acute repair promises better results and is technically easier than late repairs more than 2 to 3 months after injury.

McEntire et al,[19] in 1972, in the review of the literature, found that 75 percent of all patients had a good or excellent result whether they were treated surgically or nonoperatively. However, several of these patients were not athletes, and a higher proportion of excellent results were found in the surgically treated group. Postoperatively, near-normal isokinetic strength can be attained as documented by Cybex testing. Wolfe et al,[34] for four patients with unilateral repaired pectoralis major ruptures who underwent Cybex testing, showed an average peak torque measuring 105.8 percent and a work/repetition of 109 percent as compared with their normal side. Zeman et al[35] reported on nine surgically treated athletes, all of whom returned to their previous level of performance.

DELAYED REPAIR

Delayed repair of complete pectoralis ruptures, more than 3 months from the initial injury, has been reported.[14,15,17,20,28,29,33,34] Schecter and Gristina[28] reported on the ease of delayed repair, but this was a partial rupture and the sternal portion was not fully retracted. Compared with acute repairs, those in chronic situations are technically more difficult secondary to adhesions, tendon retraction, and muscle atrophy.[13,15,20,29] It is the general consensus that the return of normal motion and strength is more predictable acutely.

Kretzler and Richardson[14,15] reported on two cases that were repaired an average of 5.5 years after the injury. Although repairable, their strength did not return to full but their horizontal adduction strength improved from 50 to 80 percent and from 60 to 84 percent, respectively. Although numbers are small, it appears that significant strength increase can be obtained despite a delayed repair of the pectoralis tendon.

IMAGING STUDIES

Routine plain radiographs are generally of little use in the diagnosis of pectoralis major ruptures. On our standard shoulder series, including a scapular anteroposterior, scapular lateral, and outlet view, usually no bony abnormality is seen, but radiographic absence of the pectoral shadow may be indicative of a potential tendon rupture. Ultrasonography for diagnostic purposes is low in cost and noninvasive in nature. However, it is extremely technician-dependent, limiting its use on a large-scale basis.

Magnetic resonance imaging has replaced computed tomography and ultrasonography in the detection of both the location and extent of tears of the pectoralis major tendon complex. Although limited by cost and the potential for claustrophobia in some patients, it remains an exceptionally accurate test in determining the location and extent of the rupture of the pectoralis tendon (Fig. 21-5).

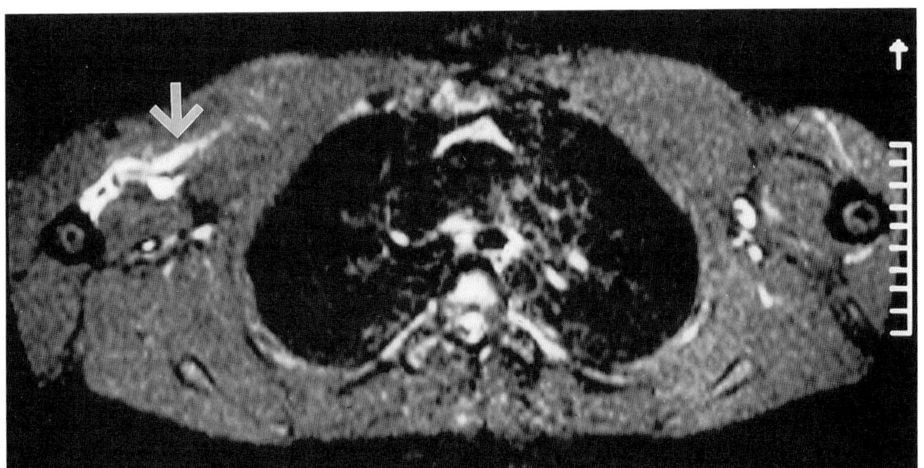

Figure 21-5. Magnetic resonance image (STIR axial image; TR, 2000; TE, 30) of the right shoulder and upper chest of an elite gymnast demonstrating detachment of the right pectoralis major tendon at its humeral insertion. The tendon is retracted approximately 2 cm medially from the humeral cortex, with an increase in the signal intensity in the fascial plane surrounding the retracted tendon.

COMPLICATIONS

Complications secondary to pectoralis major ruptures are uncommon. Sepsis and pseudocyst formation have been associated with the formation of large hematomas after rupture.[22,27] Post-traumatic myositis ossificans, causing swelling and pain, has also been reported.[25] Kawashima et al[12] described C6 to C8 and T1 hypoesthesias in a patient with a crush injury and musculotendinous rupture of the pectoralis major. Additional fractures of the humerus, clavicle, and scapula as well as associated muscular ruptures of the deltoid, latissimus dorsi, pectoralis minor, and rotator cuff have also been described.

SURGICAL RECONSTRUCTION

After routine preparation and draping, an anterior incision in the axillary line is made. The deltopectoral interval is deepened and a self-retaining retractor is placed. The avulsed pectoralis tendon is identified easily due to hemorrhage and retraction in acute cases (Plate 21-1). In the chronic situation, marked adhesions are occasionally encountered, and fibrous tissue may fill the gap between the humerus and the ruptured end of the pectoralis tendon, giving an illusion of an intact tendon. In this situation, the adhesions are taken down, and the original end of the tendon is then identified. Mobilization of the pectoralis can be extremely difficult in some of these chronic cases. Achieving enough slide of the muscle and tendon in these chronic cases so the tendon can be reapproximated to the humerus without excessive tension, even with the arm in an internally rotated position, can be challenging. The long head of the biceps tendon is identified as well as the pectoralis tendon insertional site on the humerus. Two rows of four holes are then fashioned in the humerus lateral to the long head of the biceps and separated approximately by one-quarter of an inch (Plate 21-2). Superficial decortication of the cortical bone to allow bleeding is performed. Alternatively, a groove can be fashioned in the cortical bone to allow the tendon to be pulled into the groove with the stitches exiting the second row of holes. Size 2 sutures are then passed after they are woven through the tendon remnant (Plate 21-3 and Fig. 21-6). With the arm position in adduction and internal rotation, the sutures are then tied (Fig. 21-7).

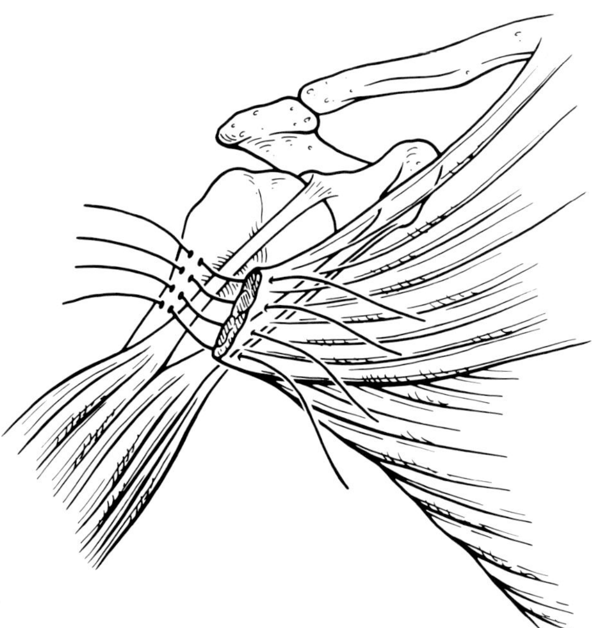

Figure 21-6. Surgical repair after passage of the sutures.

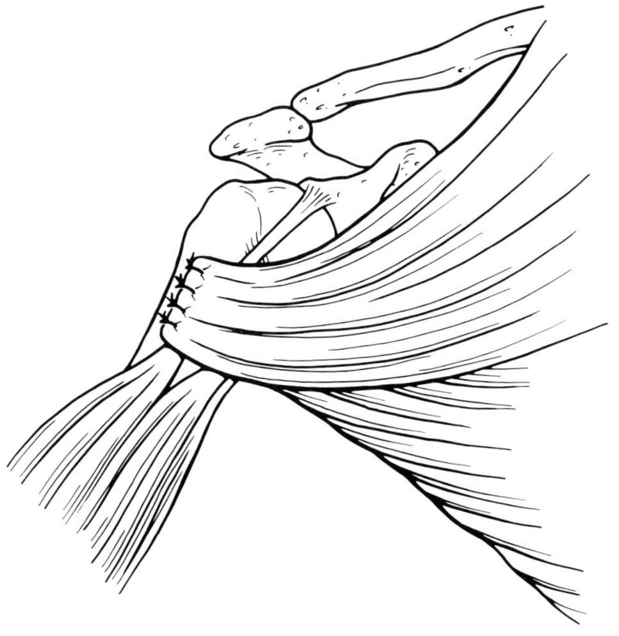

Figure 21-7. Final repair with the sutures tied and the arm positioned in adduction and internal rotation.

Another option for fixation can be the use of the interosseous anchors with attached sutures. Typically, it is easier to secure the suture to bone with these anchors than it is to pass the suture through drill holes. However, the weak link in most pectoralis repairs is the suture fixation in the tendon. Generally, a better and more secure weave with the sutures can be accomplished when the sutures are passed through the tendon first and then through drill holes in the bone. The use of suture anchors makes bone fixation of the sutures easier but makes tendon suturing more difficult.

After routine closure, the patient's arm is placed in a sling and swathe immobilization for 4 to 6 weeks. Gentle passive (phase I) exercises are begun at the 2-week mark. Active and passive range of motion with terminal stretching (phase II) is started at 4 to 6 weeks. Resistive exercises commence at 12 weeks. Full activity, including contact sports, gymnastics, and weight lifting, is not allowed until the 6- to 8-month mark, depending on the individual's progress.

SUMMARY

Ruptures of the pectoralis major, although once thought to be relatively rare, occur in a more athletic population. Although partial tears may be treated nonoperatively with uniformly good results, it is, at times, extremely difficult to acutely rule out whether the tear is complete and to determine its anatomic location.[26] In those individuals who are athletically inclined and wish to return to a high level of athletic participation, surgical repair, either at the distal insertional site or at the musculotendinous junction, should be performed. Nonoperative management of pectoralis major ruptures must be individualized, taking into consideration the patient's age, functional level, activities, and desires. Obviously, selective repair, especially in the athletic population, can have excellent results acutely with restoration of normal range of motion and strength. In chronic situations, surgical repair, although less predictable, can likewise offer excellent results.

ACKNOWLEDGMENT

We thank Jamie Huffman for her expertise and assistance with the illustrations.

REFERENCES

1. Bakalim G: Rupture of the pectoralis major muscle. A case report. Acta Orthop Scand 36:274–9, 1965
2. Berson BL: Surgical repair of pectoralis major rupture in an athlete. Case report of an unusual injury in a wrestler. Am J Sports Med 7:348–51, 1979
3. Buck JE: Rupture of the sternal head of the pectoralis major. J Bone Joint Surg [Br] 45:224, 1963
4. Butters AG: Traumatic rupture of the pectoralis major. BMJ 2:652–3, 1941
5. Codman EA: Rupture of the supraspinatus tendon and other lesions in or about the subcromial bursa. p. 502. In The Shoulder. 1st Ed. Thomas Todd Co., Boston, 1934
6. Coues WP: Rupture of pectoralis major muscle. Boston Med J 182:200, 1920
7. Delport HP, Piper MS: Pectoralis major rupture in athletes. Arch Orthop Trauma Surg 100:135–7, 1982
8. DePalma AF (ed): Surgery of the Shoulder. 3rd Ed. JB Lippincott, Philadelphia, 1983
9. Elliot BC, Wilson GJ, Kerr GK: A biomechanical analysis of the sticking region in the bench press. Med Sci Sports Exerc 21:450–62, 1989
10. Garrett WE, Safran MR, Seaber AV et al: Biomechanical comparison of stimulated and nonstimulated skeletal muscle pulled to failure. Am J Sports Med 15:448–54, 1987
11. Gudmundsson B: A case of agenesis and a case of rupture of the pectoralis major muscle. Acta Orthop Scand 44:213–8, 1973
12. Kawashima M, Sato M, Torisu T et al: Rupture of the pectoralis major. Report of two cases. Clin Orthop 109:115–9, 1975
13. Kingsley DM: Rupture of the pectoralis major. J Bone Joint Surg [Am] 28:644–5, 1946
14. Kretzler HH: Pectoralis major rupture. p. 317–20. In Post M, Murrey BF, Hawkins RJ (eds): Surgery of the Shoulder. Mosby Year Book, Chicago, 1990
15. Kretzler HH, Richardson AB: Rupture of the pectoralis major muscle. Am J Sports Med 17:453–8, 1989
16. Law WB: Closed incomplete rupture of pectoralis major. BMJ 2:499, 1954
17. Lindenbaum BL: Delayed repair of a ruptured pectoralis major muscle. Clin Orthop 109:120–1, 1975
18. Marmor L, Bechtol CO, Hall CB: Pectoralis major muscle. Function of sternal portion and mechanism of rupture of normal muscle. Case reports. J Bone Joint Surg [Am] 43:81–7, 1961
19. McEntire JE, Hess WE, Coleman SS: Rupture of the pectoralis major muscle. J Bone Joint Surg [Am] 54:1040–6, 1972
20. Orava S, Sorasto A, Aalto K et al: Total rupture of pectoralis major muscle in athletes. Int J Sports Med 5:272–4, 1984
21. Park JY, Espiniella JL: Rupture of pectoralis major muscle. A case report and review of literature. J Bone Joint Surg [Am] 52:577–81, 1970
22. Petissier P: Traite des Maladies des Artisans. p. 163. Paris, 1822
23. Pulaski EJ, Chandlee BH: Ruptures of the pectoralis major muscle. Surgery 10:309–12, 1941
24. Pulaski EJ, Martin GW: Rupture of the left pectoralis major muscle. Surgery 25:110–1, 1949
25. Purnell R: Rupture of the pectoralis major muscle: a complication. Br J Accident Surg 19:284, 1988
26. Roi GS, Rospizzi S, Dworzak F: Partial rupture of the pectoralis major muscle in athletes. Int J Sports Med (Germany) 11:85–7, 1990
27. Ronchetti G: Rottura sotto cutanea parziale del muscolo grand pettorale con formazione di pseudocistie ematica. Minerva Chir 14:22–8, 1959
28. Schecter LR, Gristina AG: Surgical repair of rupture of pectoralis major muscle. JAMA 188:1009, 1964
29. Scott BW, Wallace WA, Barton MA: Diagnosis and assessment of pectoralis major rupture by dynamometry. J Bone Joint Surg [Br] 74:111–3, 1992
30. Smart A: Rupture of pectoralis major. Guy's Hosp. Gaz 2:61, 1873
31. Spear KP, Garrett WE: Muscular control of motion and stability about the pectoral girdle. p. 159–72. In Matsen FA, Fu FH, Hawkins RJ (eds): The Shoulder: A Balance of Mobility and Stability. American Academy of Orthopaedic Surgeons, Rosemont, IL, 1993

32. Tietjen R: Closed injuries of the pectoralis major muscle. J Trauma 20:262–4, 1980
33. Urs NDK, Jani DM: Surgical repair of rupture of the pectoralis major muscle: a case report. J Trauma 16:749–50, 1976
34. Wolfe SW, Wickiewicz TL, Cavanaugh JT: Rupture of the pectoralis major muscle: an anatomic and clinical analysis. Am J Sports Med 20:587–93, 1992
35. Zeman SC, Rosenfeld RT, Lipscomb PR: Tears of the pectoralis major muscle. Am J Sports Med 7:343–7, 1979

TWENTY-TWO

Labral Disorders

Mark M. Williams
Ronald P. Karzel
Stephen J. Snyder

The subject of labral disorders has been an area of controversy for shoulder surgeons and has been traditionally difficult to diagnose and treat. The increased use of the arthroscope as both a diagnostic and surgical tool has advanced our understanding of the labrum. Recent studies of both cadaveric and human subjects have helped to clarify labral function and to distinguish normal anatomic variations from pathologic findings. This has been especially important for the overhead athlete in whom unique labral lesions have been identified. Advances in radiologic imaging studies have also been beneficial in facilitating the preoperative diagnosis of labral pathology. This chapter briefly reviews normal and pathologic labral anatomy and biomechanical considerations and discusses the assessment and management of labral lesions, including SLAP lesions.

NORMAL LABRAL ANATOMY

Histologic sections of the labrum reveal a ring of fibrous tissue with interposed elastic fibers that encircle the articular surface of the glenoid (Fig. 22-1). The typical attachment of the labrum blends centrally with the articular hyaline cartilage surface, whereas peripherally it is joined by the fibrous tissue of the capsule and ligaments forming the ''labroligamentous'' or ''capsulolabral complex.'' The superior labrum is noted to be confluent with the biceps tendon insertion. A fibrocartilaginous interzone has been described, and our dissections confirm this variably in the posterior, superior, and anterior labrum but rarely in the inferior labrum. A free inner or central edge of the labrum, which may or may not be present, may give it a ''meniscoid'' appearance, which can be confused with a pathologic detachment (Plate 22-1). This meniscus-like labral appearance is most often observed superiorly but may also be seen anteriorly or posteriorly, although less often along the inferior labrum. A meniscoid-type labrum is thought to be normal unless there are splits or fragmentation of the overhanging labral tissue, which can cause mechanical symptoms with catching and joint irritation. Also, in the normal shoulder, there is usually a smooth transition between the articular hyaline cartilage and the capsular attachment to the bone beneath the meniscoid labrum. Unless this smooth transition is interrupted, this is a normal variant.

In describing the normal labrum, Detrisac and Johnson[14] reported on a series of cadaveric dissections and classified the various normal labral shapes. They described five variations of normal labral anatomy that were based on whether the labrum is meniscoid or wedge-shaped: superior wedge, posterior wedge, anterior wedge, superior/anterior wedge, and circumferentially meniscoid labra. Detrisac (personal communication) has simplified this scheme into two types. In the first group, the labrum is attached peripherally but there is a free central edge. This free central edge occurs most often in the superior labral segment. This is known as the ''meniscoid''-type labrum. The other pattern of labral attachment is where the labrum is firmly anchored, both centrally and peripherally. There is no free inner edge in these patients.

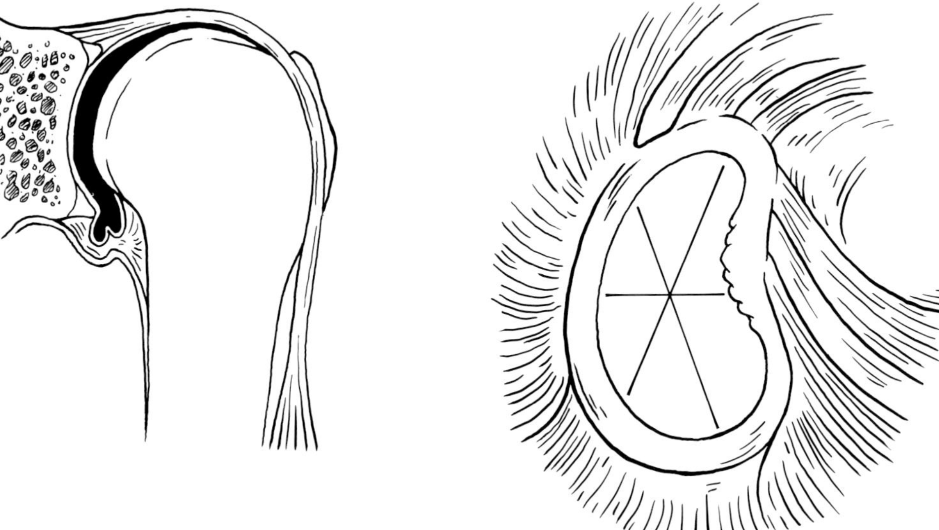

Figure 22-1. The glenoid labrum encircles the glenoid cavity and is attached peripherally to the rim. The capsule and ligaments attach directly to the labrum, thus forming a ''labroligamentous complex.'' The middle glenohumeral ligament may occasionally attach more medially, below the glenoid rim on the scapular neck.

We performed our own cadaveric dissections on 21 fresh-frozen specimens to assess cross-sectional anatomy.[39] The inferior labrum was most consistently triangular in shape with an attached central edge. The posterior labrum was similarly triangular but occasionally had an unattached medial surface. The anterior labrum lacked the triangular appearance but was attached both centrally and peripherally. It was indistinguishable from the capsule on both microscopic and macroscopic examination. Finally, the superior labrum had a consistent peripheral attachment that was often not on the glenoid facc but around the corner on the scapular neck. If often had a free central edge or meniscoid appearance.

ANATOMIC VARIANTS OF NORMAL

Other normal variants must be appreciated by the shoulder surgeon when evaluating labral anatomy. An elegant cadaveric study reported by Cooper et al[10] in 1992 also found the superior and anterosuperior labral segments to be loosely attached. They noted that in many specimens, the anterosuperior labrum inserted into the fibers of the inferior or middle glenohumeral ligament, instead of the actual glenoid margin. These investigators were the first to describe the presence of a sublabral hole or foramen in the region of the hourglass indentation of the anterior glenoid (the midglenoid notch) as a normal variant (Fig. 22-2). They found a sublabral foramen present in 17 percent

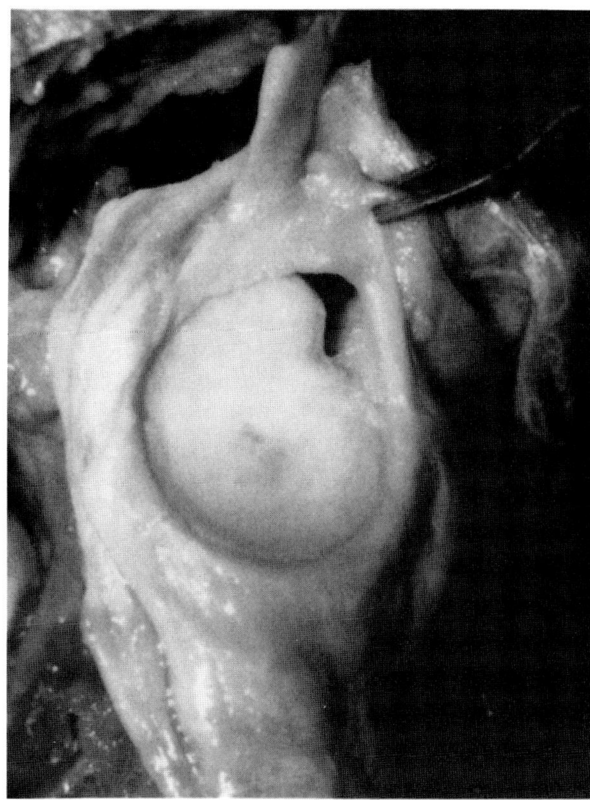

Figure 22-2. The labrum was not attached to the glenoid at the 2-o'clock position in this specimen. This represented a recess that communicated with the subscapularis recess. (From Cooper et al,[10] with permission.)

of their specimens. Sublabral foramina had free communication with the subscapularis recess beneath the unattached labral edge. It is important for the shoulder surgeon to recognize the sublabral foramen as a normal labral variant and not to confuse it with a Bankart lesion.

Although this chapter does not discuss labral lesions associated with glenohumeral instability, there is a labral lesion that our institution has described that is another normal variant in a stable shoulder that may also be confused with a Bankart lesion. We retrospectively reviewed 200 shoulder arthroscopy videotapes with specific attention to the anatomy of the anterosuperior glenoid quadrant and especially the labroligamentous complex.[41] There was a 12 percent incidence of a sublabral hole between the anterosuperior glenoid quadrant and the articular surface of the glenoid. When there was a sublabral hole present, there was a 75 percent incidence of a ''cord-like'' middle glenohumeral ligament attached directly to the labrum (Plate 22-2). Also, there was a separate subgroup of patients that demonstrated the three elements of a Buford complex, which occurred in 1.5 percent of this study population. The Buford complex is a convenient term for the cord-like middle glenohumeral ligament and absent anterosuperior labral complex (Plate 22-3). The three elements of the Buford complex are (1) a cordlike middle glenohumeral ligament, continuous with the anterosuperior labrum; (2) the combined structure attached to the superior labrum at the base of the biceps anchor; and (3) no additional anterosuperior labral tissue noted, which appears as a void beneath or posteromedial to the middle ligament cord, and this void could be mistaken for a sublabral hole or a Bankart lesion. Recognition of this unusual complex is important to avoid inadvertent ''treatment'' of this normal lesion.

BIOMECHANICAL CONSIDERATIONS OF THE LABRUM

The glenohumeral joint has more freedom of movement than any other joint in the body. The stability of the joint is dependent on the soft tissue structures because the bony anatomy does not provide inherent stability due to a hemispheric humeral head articulating with a shallow glenoid socket. Glenohumeral stability is dependent on the integrity of the surrounding soft tissues, including the labrum, the capsular ligaments, and the muscle tendon units. The labrum encircling the glenoid socket increases its depth and therefore increases the stability of the hemispheric humeral head.

Howell and Galinat[18] documented in a cadaveric study that the glenoid labrum contributes approximately 50 percent of the total depth of the socket. The diameters of the glenoid surface are increased in the vertical plane to 75 percent of the humeral head and to 57 percent in the transverse direction. Both Reeves[32] and Perry[30] have demonstrated that the bonding strength of the fibrous labrum to the glenoid neck increases with skeletal maturity. At a younger age (younger than 25 years), the bonding strength of the labrum to the glenoid is less than that of the capsule and the subscapularis tendon. As this represents the weak link in soft tissue stability, dislocations tend to disrupt the labral-glenoid bond. As the tissue matures with age, the bonding strength increases, making failure at the labrum (Bankart lesion) less likely.

Two studies have evaluated the contact areas of the labrum during glenohumeral motion. Karzel et al[21] demonstrated in a cadaveric shoulder model that in 90 degrees abduction with a compressive load applied, the labrum affected the distribution of the contact stresses. The posteroinferior labrum was observed to absorb most of the load in this position, in an analogous manner as a meniscus in the knee joint. Perhaps this is why the posterior labrum is uniformly strong and triangular in shape as opposed to the anterior labrum. Another cadaveric study by Jobe[20] demonstrated impingement of the superior labrum. Cadaver specimens positioned in 70 degrees of abduction and maximum external rotation were fixed with formalin. Fixation in this position caused a permanent impression on both sides of the joint where the bone contacted the labrum (Plate 22-4). The glenoid side revealed that the posterior superior labrum was compressed and distorted by the tuberosity and the interposed rotator cuff. When there was concomitant anterior instability, the posterior labrum impingement appeared to worsen. These observations may explain the posterior labrum lesions observed in throwers, along with articular side rotator cuff tearing.

Also, two studies have evaluated the vascularity of the glenoid labrum. Burkhead (personal communication) showed that the vascular supply to the labrum was very rich and abundant around the entire glenoid, with the exception of the superior labrum. Similarly, Cooper et al[10] found the superior and anterosuperior labrum segments to have less vascularity than the posterosuperior and inferior segments. These studies may also help to explain superior labral deterioration observed with advanced age.[12] The limited vascularity of the superior labrum may contribute to the development of the SLAP lesion (injury to the *s*uperior *l*abrum from *a*nterior to *p*osterior). The presence of a poor healing environment in this area could impede tissue healing after repetitive microtrauma or an isolated traumatic event. Detachment of the superior labrum and biceps anchor with failure to heal would result in the pathologic entity referred to as a SLAP lesion.[11,39]

DIAGNOSTIC GLENOHUMERAL ARTHROSCOPY—ROUTINE ARTHROSCOPIC EVALUATION

The importance of sequential systematic review of the anatomy of the glenohumeral joint cannot be overemphasized. The following routine examination has been previously described and is reviewed briefly.[36] Our routine 15-point arthroscopic examination includes 10 viewing positions from the posterior viewing portal and 5 from the anterior viewing portal. The 10 posterior viewing positions allow the visualization of the biceps tendon and anchor, posterior labrum and capsule, inferior recess, glenoid articular surface, rotator cuff insertion, posterior cuff, humeral bare spot, humeral articular surface, subscapularis recess, middle glenohumeral ligament, anterosuperior labrum, inferior glenohumeral ligament, and inferior labrum. The arthroscope is then switched to the anterior portal, and the five viewing positions from this portal allow the visualization of the posterior capsule and labrum, the posterior rotator cuff, the anterior glenoid labrum and glenohumeral ligaments, the subscapularis tendon and recess, and the attachment of the subscapularis tendon to the humeral head. If this routine examination is performed consistently, all intra-articular anatomy will be visualized by the surgeon. We emphasize this for completeness as well as for the surgeon to develop an appreciation of normal anatomy and its variants.

PATTERNS OF LABRAL INJURY

The labrum functions not only as a load-sharing structure with the glenoid but also as a structure for ligamentous attachment around the shoulder (i.e., it is an intricate component of the labroligamentous complex). From a biomechanical standpoint, there are several potential mechanisms of injury caused by overload. These overload mechanisms include compression, avulsion, sheer, traction, and chronic attritional changes. The preceding mechanisms of injury can occur either alone or in combinations, resulting in complex patterns of labral pathology. The overhead athlete is especially at risk for labral injury due to repetitive overload of the glenohumeral joint. For convenience in the description of labral injuries and patterns, the labrum is arbitrarily divided into six areas: (1) the superior labrum; (2) the anterosuperior labrum (above the midglenoid notch); (3) the anteroinferior labrum (below the midglenoid notch); (4) the inferior labrum; (5) the posteroinferior labrum; and (6) the posterosuperior labrum.

Labral tear patterns can be described according to their arthroscopic appearance, with descriptive terminology similar to a meniscal tear in the knee. As in the knee, the tear pattern noted by the arthroscopic surgeon can be described

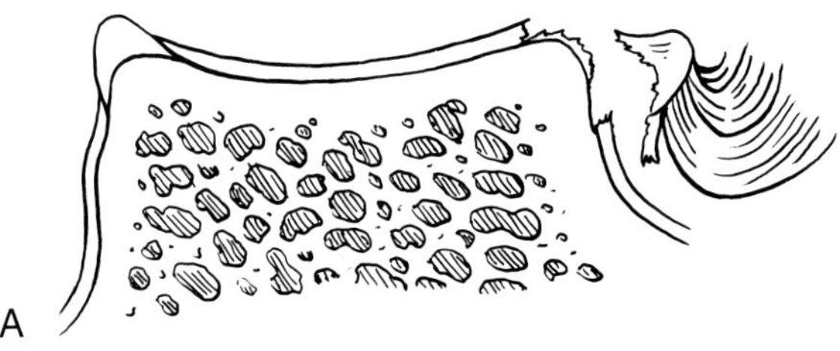

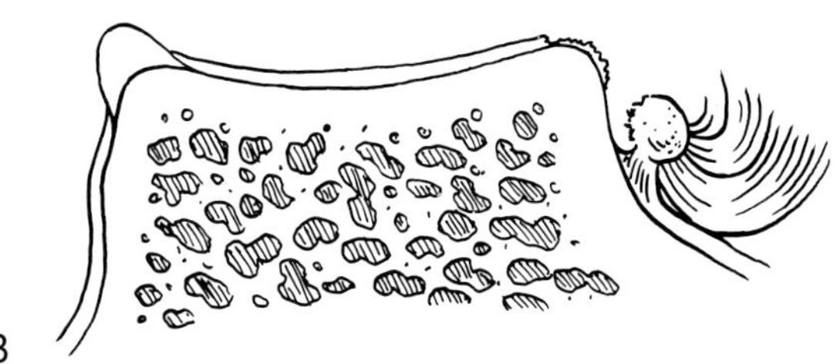

Figure 22-3. (**A**) Bankart lesion. (**B**) Acute anterior ligamentous periosteal sleeve avulsion (ALPSA) lesion. Note that the labrum has been avulsed and displaced down along the denuded anterior glenoid neck. (Adapted from Neviaser,[26] with permission.)

as follows: degenerative lesions, flap tears, split (vertical) nondetached tears, bucket handle tears, and SLAP lesions. The following sections illustrate specific examples of these entities and discuss specific management of these lesions. There is a separate category of labral tears associated with instability. These include the classic Bankart lesion[6] with anterior capsulolabral separation or Neviaser's[26] ALPSA (*a*nterior *l*abral *p*eriosteal *s*leeve *a*vulsion) lesion, in which the capsulolabral complex is disrupted in a periosteal sleeve-type fashion. The ALPSA lesion differs from the Bankart lesion in that the anterior scapular periosteum remains intact and attached to the labroligamentous complex, which allows the labroligamentous periosteum sleeve to retract inferiorly and medially on the scapular neck (Fig. 22-3).

Degenerative Lesions

A degenerative labrum appears frayed and represents a breakdown of the fibrous glenoid labrum. This lesion may represent part of the continuum of degenerative joint disease. DePalma[12] suggests that particularly in the superior labrum, this is a normal finding associated with the natural aging process of the shoulder. DePalma and colleagues[13] demonstrated in a prospective study that the incidence of degenerative tears was approximately 50 percent in 50-

year-olds and 60 percent of all 60-year-olds, although only a small percentage of patients had pain. This low incidence of symptomatic lesions has not been found by other authors.[1,4] Joint degeneration may be accelerated with chronic joint abuse and especially with repetitive compression overload. In this situation, when the smooth gliding surfaces of the uninjured labrum degenerate to roughened irregular fibrous elements, an abrasive articular interface may occur. The humeral head articular cartilage may be damaged secondarily, causing a chondromalacic "kissing lesion" (Plate 22-5). Similarly, humeral head degenerative changes may accelerate adjacent labral breakdown and cause progressive intra-articular degeneration. Degenerative labral tears are readily managed with arthroscopic resection of the damaged labral tissue.

Flap Tears

Flap tears of the labrum are the most common pattern of acute or subacute injury noted. Most flap tears are seen in the posterosuperior segment of the labrum but may be found in any location. A flap tear, like its meniscal counterpart, typically has a fairly broad base with a free edge corresponding to a radial tear (Plate 22-6). The etiology of flap tears is uncertain, but it seems to be associated with chronic sheer stress on the shoulder.[35] An example of this would include repetitive subluxation, which can occur in the throwing or overhead athlete. Perhaps the impingement of the posterosuperior labrum by the greater tuberosity as noted by Jobe[20] causes the typical posterior labral flap tears and fraying seen in throwers. When a flap tear has a significant unstable fragment, this may catch in the joint and may become symptomatic with particular activities. Patients may present with mechanical symptoms of clicking, catching, and popping that may mimic instability. Flap tears, like degenerative tears, are managed by arthroscopic resection of the unstable tissue.

A specific type of flap tear has been described by Neviaser.[27] He identified five cases of anterior shoulder pain with similar lesions in which a superficial anteroinferior labral flap tear was observed in association with inferior glenoid articular cartilage damage (Plate 22-7). This glenolabral articular disruption lesion was treated with combined labral debridement and glenoid chondroplasty or abrasion arthroplasty. All symptoms were reportedly eliminated within 3 months after debridement.

Vertical Split Labral Tears (Including Bucket Handle Lesions)

Vertical split labral tears are probably the most dramatic, although the least common, type of anterior or posterior labral lesions. These lesions may demonstrate a complete vertical disruption of labral tissue, creating a displaceable fragment or incomplete rent as seen in a meniscus (Plate 22-8). When a vertical split labral lesion is identified, a meniscoid-type labrum must be present, overlying the glenoid surface. As meniscoid labra are observed most often in the superior quadrant, a SLAP lesion (described later in this chapter) is commonly associated with vertical tears. Occasionally, anterior and posterior vertical labral splits may be observed, whereas a vertical labral tear is seldom found in the inferior segment of the labrum.

The etiology of vertical tears is thought to occur from an intra-articular compression injury that pinches the labral tissue between the articular surfaces of the humeral head and the glenoid. The mechanism of injury may occur from a fall on the outstretched arm or perhaps from episodic humeral hyper-rotation, causing compression of the anterior or posterior labrum. Vertical tears may produce a symptom complex that presents as "pseudo-instability,"[28] with locking, catching, and popping. When the labral fragment is not displaced, patients may demonstrate joint irritation symptoms that are activity-related. Pain seldom occurs at rest.

Clinical examination reveals remarkably few findings. If there is a displaceable fragment, then it may be trapped with a rotation-compression test of the shoulder. This maneuver is best performed in the supine position with the arm held in 90 degrees of abduction while a compressive load is applied to the glenohumeral joint and combined with humeral rotation. This maneuver, as in the McMurray's test for the knee, tends to accentuate pain and popping when the extremity is taken through a range of motion while maintaining compression. As in any shoulder examination, glenohumeral stability should be specifically assessed using tests for apprehension, suppression, anterior and posterior translation (drawer testing), and the sulcus sign of inferior instability. Although a bucket handle tear of the anterior, superior, or posterior labrum may be associated with clinical instability, this is an uncommon occurrence.

Imaging of the shoulder with a possible vertical labral tear is best accomplished using either a computed tomography (CT) arthrogram or a magnetic resonance imaging (MRI) scan with gadolinium enhancement[11,31] (Fig. 22-4). The images must be carefully evaluated because they are frequently confused with those of anterior instability. The pattern of capsular insertion into the labrum should be carefully assessed.

Treatment of Vertical Labral Tears

The management of isolated vertical labral tears is straightforward when they are not associated with glenohumeral instability. An anterior lesion is best visualized from the standard posterior portal. A small labral tear can be

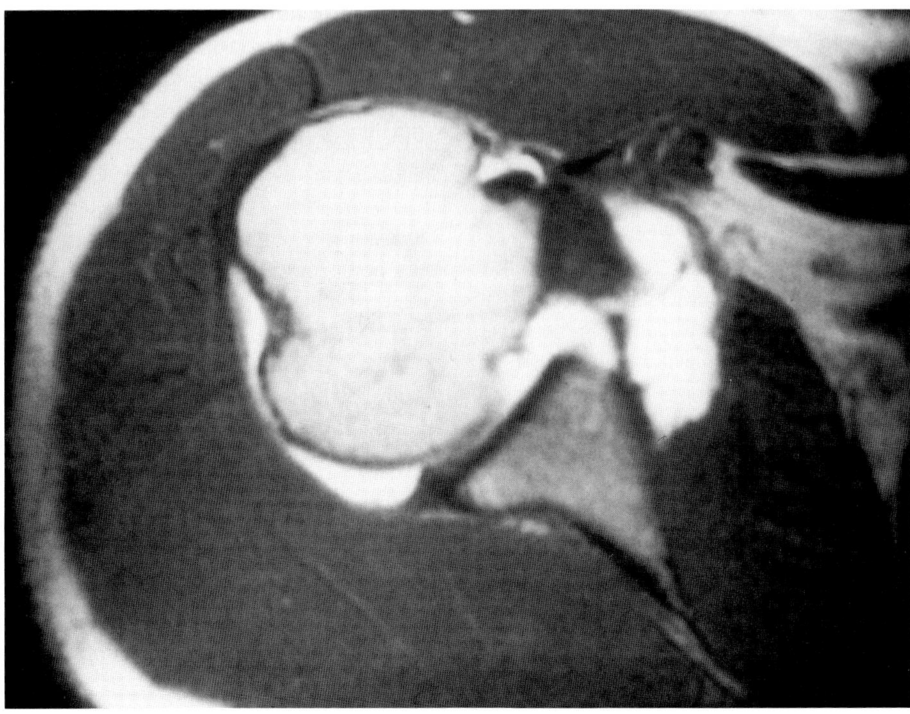

Figure 22-4. MRI scan with intra-articular gadolinium enhancement is often a valuable imaging modality in cases of labral pathology.

resected using a 4.5-mm motorized shaver or an arthroscopic basket punch through the anterior portal. Larger fragments can be treated with resection techniques similar to those used for meniscal surgery. A small basket punch inserted through the anterior operating cannula can resect the inferior attachment first. The superior attachment can then be grasped with a clamp and, when rotated while maintaining a firm grasp, will usually avulse cleanly. The motorized shaver is then used to complete the debridement and smooth the edges. The goal of treatment, as for the meniscus, is a stable peripheral rim. Posterior lesions can be managed in a similar fashion while using an anterior visualization portal and a posterior instrumentation portal. An alternative method is to use a suction punch to sequentially resect the labral tear back to a stable rim. The surgeon must be aware of normal anatomic variants previously described to avoid resecting Buford complexes[41] or creating iatrogenic Bankart-type lesions.

A management dilemma arises when a vertical tear is incomplete. If a vertical tear is incomplete and relatively small, then the surfaces may be debrided to stimulate healing, and partial labral resection may not be required. When contemplating excision of more complete or larger lesions, the surgeon must determine if an instability problem will occur after removal of an incomplete central labral fragment. This is a rare problem in our experience if the labrum is meniscoid-type. In this case, the torn portion is redundant and is not the true capsuloligamentous attachment. The best assurance of capsulolabral integrity is careful probing of the capsuloligamentous attachment while visualizing from the ipsilateral portal. Video documentation in this situation is recommended for future reference.

Glasgow et al[16] reported in 1992 the results of arthroscopic partial glenoid labral resection in 28 overhead athletes (29 shoulders). These athletes developed a sudden inability to perform their sports activities due to pain. With a 2-year minimum follow-up, they reported 91 percent good or excellent functional outcome in those with normal stability versus only a 25 percent good functional outcome and a 75 percent fair or poor functional outcome in those with unstable joints. They concluded that in patients with anterior instability and labral tears, labral debridement was not a successful alternative to formal stabilization. Similarly, Altchek et al[2] recently reviewed a group of 40 athletes at a minimum of 2 years after labral debridement. Forty percent of their group had instability on examination at surgery, but still 72 percent reported relief during the first postoperative year. Nevertheless, only 7 percent of the patients had significant long-term relief, and they also concluded that debridement was not an effective treatment for symptomatic relief in the overhead athlete. In 1993, Payne and Jokl[29] reported an average of 2-year follow-up of 14 patients with labral debridement who were classified based on the location of the labral tear. All patients had shoulder pain with overhead activity and were found to have stable glenohumeral joints on preoperative examination. Overall results were found to deteriorate with time, from 93 percent excellent or good at 6 months to 71 percent excellent or good at greater than 1 year (average, 2 years). Best results were noted in the superior and anteroinferior labral segments. Anterosuperior lesions were most at risk for delayed glenohumeral instability. These studies emphasize the point that the surgeon must maintain a high index of suspicion for glenohumeral instability with labral tears. Andrews stated that in his experience with high-level overhead athletes, glenohumeral instability should be considered present until proved otherwise.

Superior Labral Tears

Andrews et al[3] described a lesion of the shoulder in high-level throwing athletes that occurs in the anterosuperior labrum associated with avulsion and fraying of the labral tissues. This lesion was noted in 73 elite throwing athletes and sometimes involved a portion of the biceps tendon. The possible related mechanism of injury in these patients was traction to the anterosuperior labrum by the long head of the biceps tendon during the deceleration phase of throwing. Partial rotator cuff tears were also noted in some patients in addition to their labral injuries. Arthroscopic debridement of the loose labral fragments as well as the frayed cuff and biceps tendon was followed by a vigorous rotator cuff and throwing rehabilitation program. Eighty-eight percent of these athletes returned to a high level of throwing for at least one additional season after their rehabilitation. In a similar report, these authors maintain that when a superior labral detachment extends down to or inferior to the middle glenohumeral ligament, repair or shoulder stabilization is indicated primarily.

SLAP Lesions of the Shoulder

The superior labrum is defined as the segment between the 10-o'clock and 2-o'clock positions in the glenoid. It is replete with anatomic variations and has been the subject of extensive study and documentation to determine which elements of the anatomy were normal variants and which were truly pathologic. This segment of the labrum is functionally important as an integral component of the biceps tendon anchor to the superior glenoid. Careful review of many diagnostic arthroscopy videotapes revealed four distinct but related lesions that have been classified as SLAP lesions.[38] Although uncommon, these lesions may be a source of significant disability and are difficult to diagnose without arthroscopy, and they are often successfully managed arthroscopically.

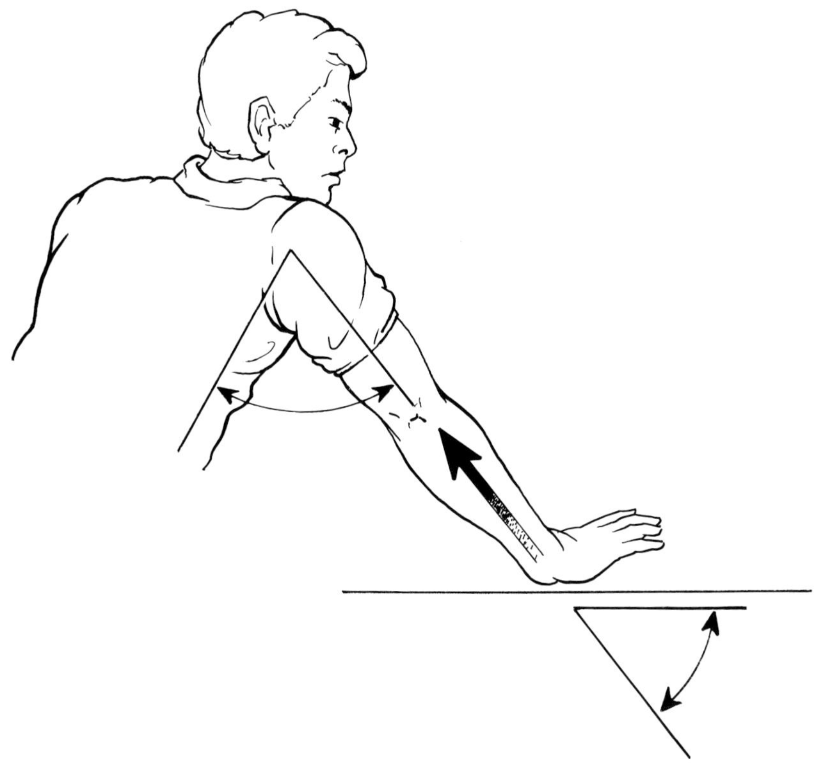

Figure 22-5. Proposed mechanism of injury for SLAP lesions.

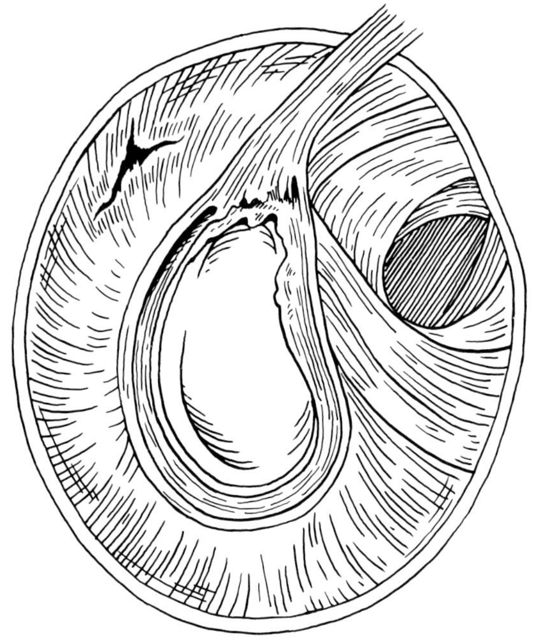

Figure 22-6. SLAP type I lesion with superior labral degeneration (see also Plate 22-9).

Definition and Proposed Etiology

A SLAP lesion is defined as an injury of the *s*uperior *l*abrum from *a*nterior to *p*osterior in relation to the biceps tendon anchor. Although there is no biomechanical proof to support the etiology of SLAP lesions, it is proposed, based on clinical evidence, that one mechanism of injury is a fall on the outstretched abducted arm that causes superior joint compression with a proximal subluxation force[38,39] (Fig. 22-5). Other lesions appear to be due to a sudden contraction of the biceps tendon, which avulses the superior labrum from the glenoid, or to smaller repetitive stresses transmitted through the biceps tendon. Glenohumeral instability and subluxation of the humeral head may also be associated with SLAP lesions.

Classification

Type I lesion	Superior labrum appears frayed and degenerative. The biceps tendon anchor is normal (Fig. 22-6 and Plate 22-9).
Type II lesion	Pathologic detachment of the superior labrum and biceps anchor. The superior labrum may also be frayed (Fig. 22-7 and Plate 22-10).
Type III lesion	Vertical tear through a meniscoid-like superior labrum, producing a bucket handle lesion that may displace into the glenohumeral joint. The biceps anchor and remaining labrum remain intact (Fig. 22-8).
Type IV lesion	Vertical tear of the superior meniscoid-like labrum, which also extends to a variable amount into the biceps tendon. As in a type III SLAP lesion, the biceps anchor and the remainder of the superior labrum are well attached (Fig. 22-9).
Complex lesion	Combination of two or more of the other SLAP lesions. This usually consists of a type II and type IV combination lesion (Fig. 22-10).

Diagnosis

Diagnosing SLAP lesions clinically, as in the case for most labral tears, is often difficult. Because labral tears are frequently associated with other pathology such as instability and rotator cuff tears, these entities need to be ruled out. The history of injury may be suggestive, particularly a history of a fall onto an abducted and forward flexed arm. The patient may complain of pain associated with locking, snapping, and pseudosubluxation. These symptoms are nonspecific, however, and the history may be more consistent with a diagnosis of impingement syndrome, biceps tendinitis, or glenohumeral instability.

Physical examination findings are also typically nonspecific. Irritation of the biceps or anchor tendon may be demonstrated with a biceps tension test. In this test, patients complain of pain with resisted forward flexion of the supi-

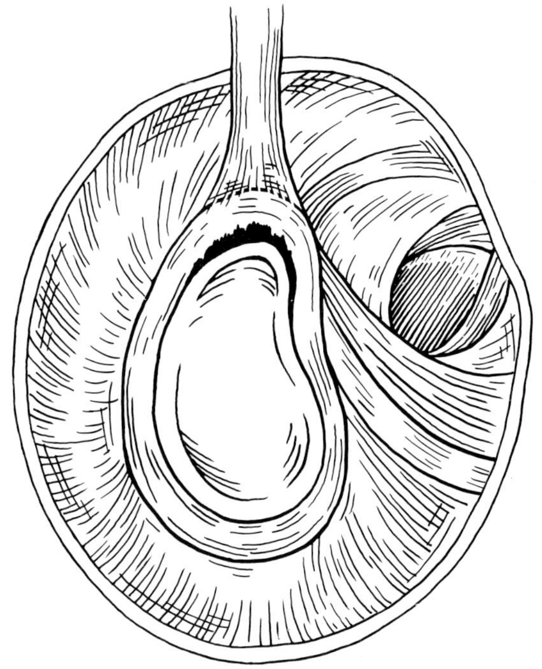

Figure 22-7. SLAP type II lesion, avulsion of labrum, and biceps anchor (see also Plate 22-10).

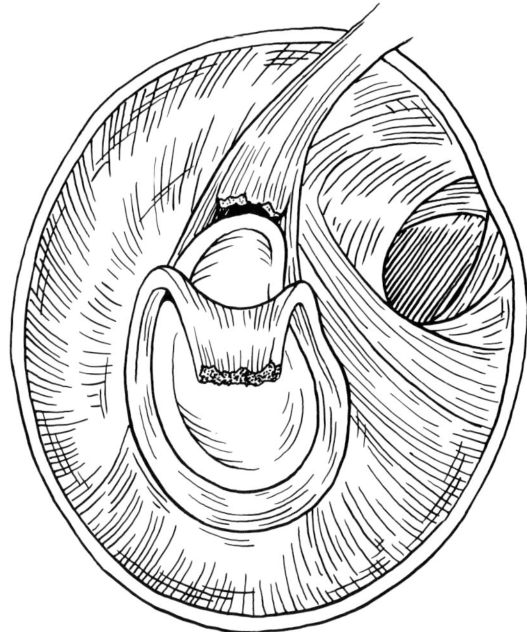

Figure 22-8. SLAP type III lesion, which may be seen with anterior glenohumeral instability.

nated arm. Similarly, the compression-rotation test, which has been previously described, may be useful. Loose labral tissue may become trapped with this maneuver, and pain or clicking may be reproduced, especially if the labrum is subluxed into the joint.

Diagnostic imaging techniques are likewise often nonspecific in diagnosing SLAP lesions. Plain radiographic films are unlikely to be helpful. Iannotti and Wang[19] have described a rare variation of SLAP lesions in which a fracture of the superior glenoid tubercle is present with a SLAP lesion. CT arthrography and, more recently, MRI have been helpful in many cases in diagnosing labral pathology including SLAP lesions.[11,23,24] Unfortunately, the difficulty with advanced imaging studies is related to the normal variation of the labrum and its radiographic appearance, and the danger with these imaging techniques is often the overdiagnosis of labral pathology.[9,25] Recently, a magnetic contrast agent, gadolinium, has been injected intra-articularly into shoulders in an attempt to increase the accuracy of MRI evaluation[22] (Fig. 22-4). This technique, called magnetic resonance arthrography (MRA), was able to detect SLAP lesions in instances in which conventional MRI scanning was not. The technique was also helpful for detecting isolated labral tears. Others have reported that saline MRA is useful in the evaluation of the anterior labrum in cases in which unenhanced MRI is equivocal.[40] Although early results are encouraging, these studies still tend to overdiagnose labral pathology, and yet in other cases, may also give a false-negative result. Therefore, the surgeon is cautioned to avoid reliance on an MRI scan as the primary indication for surgical management of a SLAP lesion. The limitations of the history, physical examination, and diagnostic studies require the maintenance of a high degree of suspicion for labral pathology. Many patients with persistent shoulder pain whose symptoms do not fit readily into one of the more commonly recognized etiologies of shoulder pain will be found at the time of surgery to have labral pathology. Therefore, the ultimate diagnosis of labral pathology depends on performing accurate diagnostic arthroscopy.

Treatment

The treatment of SLAP lesions depends on the type of labral pathology as previously classified. A type I SLAP lesion is the most benign subtype (Fig. 22-6). This may be seen as a component of an early degenerative glenohumeral joint process in a middle-aged or older individual. When the superior labrum is degenerative in a younger individual, then it may be considered the primary pathology and may contribute to the symptom complex. The treatment of a type I lesion is arthroscopic debridement of the degenerative tissue. The treatment goal is to obtain an intact stable labrum to remove any source of joint irritation and possible catching. Debridement is best performed with a motorized shaver through the standard anterior and posterior arthroscopic portals. Debridement must be performed carefully to avoid damage to the remaining superior labrum and the biceps anchor.

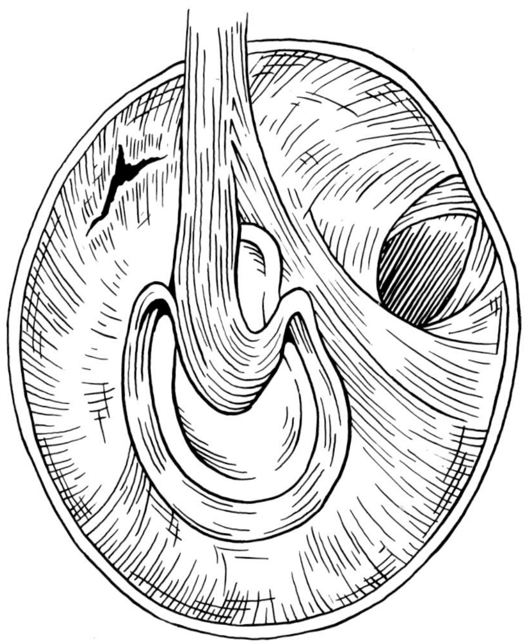

Figure 22-9. SLAP type IV lesion, with vertical tear of superior labrum extending into the biceps tendon.

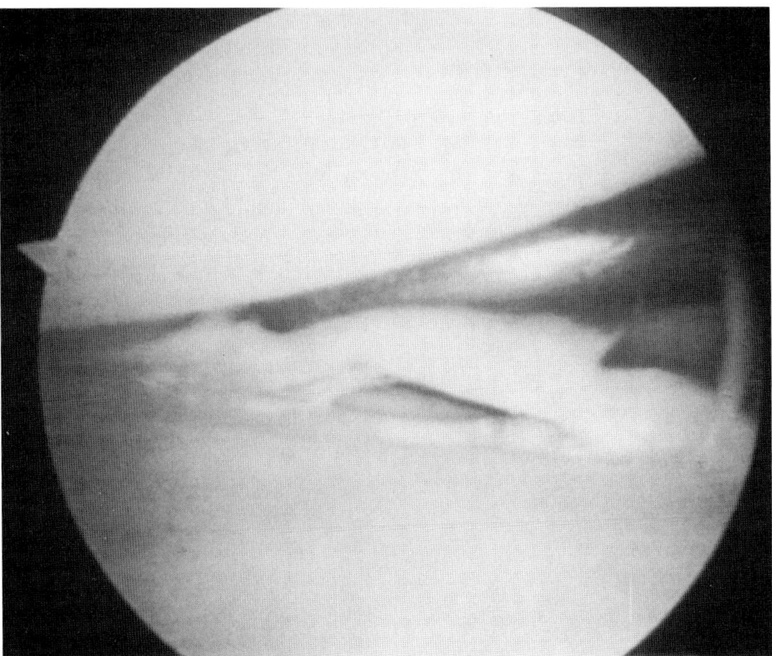

Figure 22-10. Complex SLAP lesion. (From Snyder et al,[41] with permission.)

A type II lesion is often overdiagnosed in our opinion. The frequent meniscoid-like appearance of the superior labrum with a correspondingly free inner edge may give the appearance of pathologic detachment (Plate 22-11). In the case of acute trauma, the diagnosis is fairly evident because hemorrhagic labral tissue is easily identified. Chronic lesions, however, may represent a more challenging diagnosis because the natural healing process may conceal the pathologic detachment of the avulsed soft tissues. In a chronic type II SLAP lesion, as in a chronic Bankart lesion of the anterior labrum, the denuded bone below the avulsed labrum may appear smooth and be covered with fibrous scar tissue. Several observations may help to differentiate normal glenolabral attachment from pathologic detachment. First, in a normal shoulder, the articular cartilage of the superior glenoid extends to the labral attachment. A SLAP lesion will usually have a space between the glenoid articular cartilage margin and the attachments of the labrum and biceps anchor. Second, if the superior labrum tissue is noted to arch away from the underlying bone (more than 3 to 4 mm), then the integrity of the superior labrum and biceps anchor attachment should be questioned (Plate 22-12). Finally, a somewhat lax labral attachment in its "normal" position is generally not considered to be a SLAP lesion but rather a normal variation.

Type II SLAP lesions are often noted in conjunction with an anterior glenohumeral dislocation. An explanation of this phenomenon was reported by Rodosky et al,[34] who stated that the disruption of the superior biceps and labral attachment mechanism (i.e., a type II SLAP lesion) leads to increased stress on the anteroinferior capsular and labral attachments, which may contribute to the anterior instability pattern.

For type II SLAP lesions, surgical treatment must be directed not only at the torn labral tissue but also toward reattachment of the biceps anchor to the superior glenoid neck. The technique is similar to that used for arthroscopic capsulolabral reconstruction in instability surgery. Our method of surgical management has progressed as our surgical techniques and instrumentation have improved. Initially, type II lesions were simply debrided of interposed fibrous material, and the superior glenoid neck was decorticated in an attempt to incite an inflammatory fibrovascular response to restore the integrity of the detached anchor. Postoperatively, the arm was immobilized in a sling for several weeks, with the arm maintained in internal rotation and the elbow flexed in an attempt to promote the healing of soft tissue to bone. Several of these patients underwent second-look procedures and were noted to have healed. Nevertheless, in many cases, early motion is desirable, especially when a SLAP lesion is found with additional pathology such as rotator cuff impingement. It seems evident that more secure juxtaposition of the superior labrum to the glenoid would be important for more consistent healing while allowing for early motion.

Several series of successful SLAP lesion repairs have been reported. These series have used various arthroscopic repair techniques. Field and Savoie[15] used a transglenoid suture fixation technique on 20 patients with type II and type IV injuries. They used absorbable monofilament sutures and found that at an average of 21 months, all 20 patients were rated as good or excellent. Yoneda et al[42] reported on 10 young athletes with type II SLAP lesions that were arthroscopically managed with abrasion and arthroscopic staple fixation. A second-look arthroscopic evaluation was performed at 3 to 6 months for hardware removal and demonstrated that all 10 lesions had healed. Although this was a small series, 88 percent good and excellent results were reported at 2 years. They thought that those patients with unsatisfactory results had problems due to unrelated pathology. Resch and his Austrian colleagues[33] have described two other methods for SLAP repair that they performed on a small series of 14 patients: in six cases, they used 2.7-mm titanium cannulated screws and in the eight others, they used absorbable tacks (Suretac, Acufex Microsurgical, Inc., Mansfield, MA). At 6 months minimum follow-up, they evaluated their results as a combined group and found eight patients were able to return to their overhead sport, four patients were improved, and two were unimproved.[33]

At the Southern California Orthopedic Institute, we initially attempted to repair a type II SLAP lesion with an absorbable polylactide BioTak (Concept, Inc., Largo, FL). This procedure is difficult because of the acute angle of insertion and frequent fracturing of the tack. Our present technique is technically simpler and uses an implantable suture anchor with a strong nonabsorbable braided suture, which may be secured with a mattress suture technique. The anchors that we currently prefer are the absorbable BioTak suture anchor, the 4-mm Revo titanium suture anchor screw (Concept Inc., Largo, FL), or the GII suture anchor (Mitek Inc., Norwood, MA) (Fig. 22-11) (Note that at the time of this writing, the BioTak suture anchor is experimental.)

Technique for Arthroscopic Fixation of Type II SLAP Lesions

After a routine 15-point diagnostic glenohumeral arthroscopic evaluation is performed, the arthroscope is maintained in the standard posterior portal for viewing throughout the procedure. Two anterior portals are required to perform the repair. The first anterior portal developed is the *anterosuperior portal* and is easily accomplished using a transarticular rod technique. This portal is located directly anterior to the biceps tendon. This position is ideal for inserting anchors and suture needles through the anterior surface of the biceps tendon and the adjoining superior labrum. A plastic operating cannula with a flow-restricting diaphragm is useful to control fluid while allowing for instrument passage. The other anterior operating portal developed is the *anterior midglenoid portal.* It is created approximately 2 cm inferior to the first portal (lateral to the coracoid process). For this portal, an outside-in technique is used to place a second plastic operating cannula with a blunt-tipped obturator at the level of the superior edge of the subscapularis tendon. It is extremely important to maintain these two portals with their respective intra-articular cannulas throughout the procedure. If the cannulas inadvertently back out of the joint during the process of

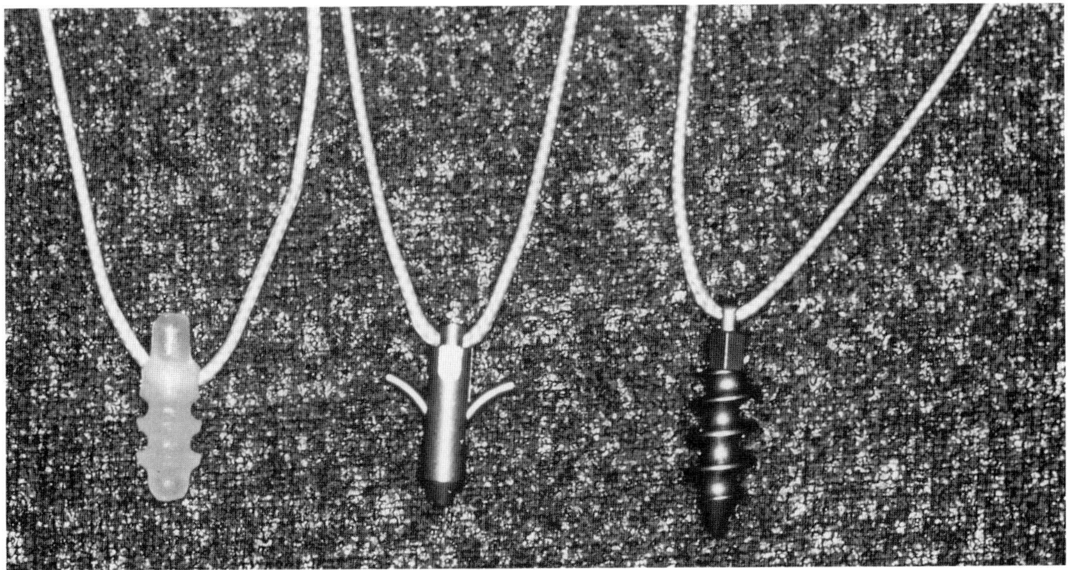

Figure 22-11. A BioTak suture anchor (Linvatec Inc., Largo, FL) is seen on the left. A Mitek GII Suture Anchor (Mitek, Inc., Norwood, MA) is seen in the center. A Revo 4-mm titanium suture anchor screw (Linvatec Inc., Largo, FL) is seen on the right.

arthroscopic suture placement, they may be difficult to re-establish precisely, and unwanted soft tissue may be captured when arthroscopic knot tying is attempted.

Debridement of the fibrous membrane over the superior glenoid neck is performed with the soft tissue shaver inserted through the anterior superior cannula. At this time, frayed and fragmented portions of the labrum and biceps anchor may also be debrided conservatively. Next, a 4.0-mm ball-shaped burr is used to decorticate the exposed bone beneath the superior labrum and the biceps anchor (Plate 22-13). Care should be taken when abrading to avoid any damage to the articular cartilage. A pilot hole can be made with the burr at the precise location where the suture anchor is to be implanted, and this should be directly below the biceps tendon. This hole serves as a target to ensure reliable positioning of the drill hole and also prevents skiving when drilling at this acute angle. An arthroscopic drill bit or Revo (Linvatec Corp., Largo, FL) bone punch is then inserted through the anterosuperior cannula, and the drill point is placed in the pilot hole, adjacent to the articular cartilage and just below the biceps tendon anchor point. The drill or punch is maintained at a 45 degree angle to the articular surface while the drill is inserted to its hub (Plate 22-14). A suture anchor loaded with a size 1 or 2 braided permanent suture is then passed through the anterosuperior cannula into the predrilled anchor hole below the biceps anchor and impacted or screwed into place under direct visualization (Plate 22-15). Once the anchor with its accompanying permanent suture is implanted securely, a crochet hook is inserted through the anterior midglenoid portal, and one or both limbs of the suture are retrieved through that cannula (Plate 22-16). (Note that there is less possibility for the suture to become twisted if one limb at a time is retrieved through the anterior midglenoid cannula.) Again, it is important at this stage to maintain both anterior cannulas intra-articularly to prevent capturing unwanted soft tissue when passing sutures. A 6-in. 17-gauge epidural needle is inserted through the anterosuperior cannula to pierce the labrum and biceps anchor near the anterior edge. The stylet is removed, and a Suture Shuttle Relay (Concept, Inc., Largo, FL) is inserted into the needle, passing through the tissues and into the joint. A grasper is placed through the anterior midglenoid cannula to hold the shuttle as the needle is extracted from the joint (Plate 22-17). Next, the shuttle with its central eyelet is pulled through the anterior midglenoid cannula. One limb of the suture is threaded through the eyelet of the shuttle, and this first stitch is carried with the shuttle retrograde through the labrum and biceps anchor and out the anterosuperior cannula.

To place a mattress stitch, the epidural needle is reinserted through the anterosuperior cannula, piercing the labrum and biceps anchor approximately 5 mm away from the first puncture site. A second Suture Shuttle Relay is passed in a similar manner, retrieved anteriorly through the midglenoid cannula, and the second limb of the permanent suture is passed retrograde through the biceps/labral tissues and out the anterosuperior cannula. The two limbs of the suture are then tied together using a knot pushing device through the anterosuperior cannula (Plate 22-18). Care should be taken to maintain the superior labrum in a reduced position and observe that the knot seats snugly on the anterior surface of the biceps tendon so that the labrum and biceps anchor are held firmly opposed to the underlying bone (Plate 22-19). A minimum of five single knots is recommended for security before the suture tails are cut and removed. A palpating probe should test the integrity of the repair (Plate 22-20).

In cases in which the superior labral detachment is large, additional anchors may be used either anterior or posterior to the biceps anchor. At times when an anterosuperior sublabral hole is present along with a type II SLAP lesion, it is best to use at least two bone anchors for security.

Our postoperative protocol is immobilization in an Ultra Sling (DonJoy, Carlsbad, CA) for 3 weeks. Patients are encouraged to perform gentle elbow, wrist, and hand exercises for the first week. After the first week, patients are allowed to remove the sling but are instructed to avoid external rotation beyond neutral and extension of the arm behind the body with the elbow extended for an additional 4 weeks. At 4 to 5 weeks, therapy is progressed with protected biceps strengthening. No stressful biceps activity is allowed for 3 to 4 months, however.

We have had the opportunity to perform a second-look arthroscopic evaluation on two patients at approximately 3.5 months after this type of suture anchor repair for type II SLAP lesions. Both patients demonstrated excellent secure reattachment of the avulsed labrum and biceps anchor, with no signs of soft tissue irritation from the braided suture material. The shoulder surgeon must be aware that there are no long-term clinical follow-ups to document the efficacy of this technique. Therefore, the surgeon should use his or her best clinical judgment in each case and, as in any informed consent, should discuss with the patient the potential benefits and risks before performing this or any type of arthroscopic labral repair.

Treatment of Type III SLAP Lesions

A type III SLAP lesion is a bucket handle tear that occurs only with a meniscoid-type superior labrum; the biceps tendon is not involved by definition (Fig. 22-8). Therefore, it is adequate to simply excise the loose labral fragment to prevent symptomatic catching and snapping. This debridement can be performed routinely using standard arthroscopic basket punches and motorized shaving devices using standard anterior and posterior portals. Our preference is to use an electrosurgical tool with a Subacromial Electrode (Concept, Inc., Largo, FL) tip via an insulated operating cannula to transect the torn labrum.

By using a nonconductive surgical irrigant and the lowest possible power setting, a very clean and safe tissue debridement can be performed. After resection of the loose labral tissue, a palpating probe should examine the labrum and biceps anchor to be certain that it is indeed stable.

Treatment of Type IV SLAP Lesions

A type IV SLAP lesion is a bucket handle tear that involves the biceps tendon and, as in a type III SLAP lesion, must be associated with a meniscoid-type labrum in the superior quadrant (Fig. 22-9). By definition, the biceps tendon is partially torn, and the torn tendon tends to displace with the labral flap into the joint. Usually, the remaining biceps tendon is firmly anchored to the superior glenoid, but in other cases, the anchor itself may be detached (the reader is referred to Treatment of Combined Type II and IV Lesions, below). A type IV SLAP lesion represents an especially difficult problem, particularly in a young person. If the segment of damaged biceps tendon is small and less than 10 to 15 percent of the diameter of the biceps tendon, simple resection of the torn tissue should be sufficient. When the superior labrum bucket handle tear is associated with a tear encompassing 30 percent or more of the biceps tendon, then consideration should be given to suture repair of the torn segment (Plate 22-21). In an older individual with a normal rotator cuff, primary biceps tenodesis should be considered, particularly if the remaining biceps tendon appears degenerative. As previously mentioned, we have encountered type IV lesions in which, after debridement of the loose soft tissues (labrum and biceps anchor), the remaining biceps stump is poorly attached to bone. This situation necessitates either fixation as described for a type II lesion or excision with primary biceps tenodesis.[37]

Repair of a type IV lesion consists of inserting multiple sutures through the labrum and biceps stump to repair the detached segments. As in a type II lesion, our preference is to use permanent sutures placed in a mattress fashion with knots that are tied away from the articular surface above the labral rim. To secure this repair, usually three or four mattress sutures are required. Obviously, suture anchors are not typically required due to stability of the remaining labral tissue.

Our technique for repair of a type IV SLAP lesion is performed with a standard posterior viewing portal and an anterosuperior operating portal established with an outside-in technique. The repair is initiated with a 6-in. 17-gauge epidural needle percutaneously inserted inferior to the lateral acromion edge and passed through the biceps tendon and across its split portion. A Suture Shuttle Relay is passed through the needle and is retrieved with a grasping clamp from the anterior cannula. The needle is withdrawn, the shuttle is loaded from the percutaneous side, and the first stitch is passed through the tendon and its split component as the shuttle is pulled through the anterosuperior portal. The epidural needle is reinserted to once again puncture the biceps tendon and labrum 3 to 4 mm away from the first suture site. The shuttle is similarly passed through the needle and retrieved from the anterosuperior cannula. The suture limb, which had been previously carried out the anterior cannula by the first shuttle, is rethreaded into the eyelet of this second shuttle and passed retrograde back through the biceps and labrum by withdrawing or pulling the shuttle by its opposite or percutaneous end. Both suture limbs will be percutaneous at this point, and a crochet hook inserted through the anterior cannula is used to retrieve both limbs out the anterior cannula to be tied. An arthroscopic knot pushing device is used to tie the suture limbs together, closing the tear in the biceps and labrum. This suturing procedure is repeated anterior and posterior to the biceps tendon until the labral tear is adequately repaired. If the tear extends a considerable distance posteriorly, the arthroscope is changed to the anterior portal to allow for insertion of instruments through a posterior operating cannula.

A case report by Burkhart and Fox[8] described a triad of lesions including a type IV SLAP lesion in association with a Bankart lesion and a full-thickness rotator cuff tear. They sequentially performed arthroscopic transglenoid Bankart reconstruction, then arthroscopic repair of the SLAP lesion (size 2-0 PDS suture), followed by open rotator cuff repair. The patient apparently did well at 1-year follow-up. They noted that the biceps-labral complex was torn as a result of anterior glenohumeral dislocation. Burkhart and Fox[7] have also reported two cases in which SLAP lesions were associated with complete tears of the long head of the biceps tendon.

Treatment of Combined Type II and IV (Complex) SLAP Lesions

On occasion, a type IV SLAP lesion may be associated with a type II detachment of the remaining biceps stump (complex lesion). In this situation, it is suggested that the torn segment of the superior labrum and biceps anchor be debrided. If an adequate portion of the biceps remains, then it may be reattached to the superior glenoid neck using the suture anchor technique as described previously for the type II SLAP lesion. If the remaining biceps tendon appears to be fragmented or degenerative, then a biceps tenodesis should be considered.

SUMMARY

Labral tears have become increasingly recognized as a cause of shoulder pathology, and arthroscopic techniques have allowed effective treatment in many cases. Associated pathology, particularly glenohumeral instability, should also be treated as necessary. Long-term follow-up studies are still needed to determine the effectiveness of our present techniques.

REFERENCES

1. Albright J, El Khoury G: Shoulder arthrotomography in the evaluation of the injured throwing arm. In Zarins B, Andrews JR, Carson WG (eds): Injuries to the Throwing Arm. WB Saunders, Philadelphia, 1985
2. Altchek DW, Warren RF, Wickiewicz TL, Ortiz G: Arthroscopic labral debridement: a three year follow-up study. Am J Sports Med 20:702–6, 1992
3. Andrews JR, Carson WG, McLeod WD: Glenoid labrum tears related to the long head of the biceps. Am J Sports Med 13:337–41, 1985
4. Andrews JR, Gidumal RH: Shoulder arthroscopy in the throwing athlete: perspectives and prognosis. Clin Sports Med 6:565–71, 1987
5. Andrews JR, Kupterman SP, Dillman CJ: Labral tears in throwing and racquet sports. Clin Sports Med 10:901–11, 1991
6. Bankart ASB: The pathology and treatment of recurrent dislocation of the shoulder joint. Br J Surg 26:23–90, 1938
7. Burkhart SS, Fox DL: SLAP lesions in association with complete tears of the long head of the biceps tendon: a report of two cases. Arthroscopy 8:31–35, 1992
8. Burkhart SS, Fox DL: Arthroscopic repair of a type IV SLAP lesion—the red-on-white lesion as a component of anterior instability. Arthroscopy 9:488–92, 1993
9. Chandrani V, Ho C, Gerharter J et al: MR findings in asymptomatic shoulders: a blind analysis using symptomatic shoulders as controls. Clin Imaging 16:25–30, 1992
10. Cooper DE, Arnoczky SP, O'Brien SJ et al: Anatomy, histology, and vascularity of the glenoid labrum: an anatomical study. J Bone Joint Surg [Am] 74:46–52, 1992
11. Coumas JM, Waite RJ, Goss TP et al: CT and MR evaluation of the labral capsular ligamentous complex of the shoulder. AJR 158:591–7, 1992
12. DePalma AJ: Surgery of the Shoulder. 3rd Ed. JB Lippincott, Philadelphia, 1983
13. DePalma AJ, White JB, Callery G: Degenerative lesions of the shoulder joint at various age groups which are compatible with good function. Instr Course Lect 7:168–80, 1950
14. Detrisac DA, Johnson LL: Arthroscopic Shoulder Anatomy; Pathologic and Surgical Implications. Slack, Thorofare, NJ, 1986
15. Field LD, Savoie FA: Arthroscopic suture repair of superior labral detachment lesions of the shoulder. Am J Sports Med 21:783–90, 1993
16. Glasgow SG, Bruce RA, Yacobucci GN, Torg JS: Arthroscopic resection of glenoid labral tears in the athlete: a report of 29 cases. Arthroscopy 8:48–54, 1992
17. Hodler J, Kursunoglu-Brahme S, Snyder SJ et al: The SLAP (superior labrum anterior and posterior) lesion: standard and MR arthrography. Presented at Radiol Soc North Am, Chicago, 1990
18. Howell SM, Galinat BJ: The glenoid-labral socket. A constrained articular surface. Clin Orthop 243:122–5, 1989
19. Iannotti JP, Wang ED: Avulsion fracture of the supraglenoid tubercle: a variation of the SLAP lesion. J Shoulder Elbow Surg 1:26–30, 1992
20. Jobe CM: Evidence linking posterior superior labral impingement and shoulder instability. Paper presented at the American Shoulder and Elbow Surgeons Meeting, Seattle, Washington, 1991
21. Karzel R, Nuber G, Lautenschlager E: Contact stresses during compression loading of the glenohumeral joint: the role of the glenoid labrum. Proc Inst Med Chicago 42:64, 1989
22. Karzel RP, Snyder SJ: Magnetic resonance arthrography of the shoulder: a new technique of shoulder imaging. Clin Sports Med 1:123–36, 1993
23. McCauley TR, Pope LF, Jokl P: Normal and abnormal glenoid labrum: assessment with multiplanar gradient-echo MR imaging. Radiology 183:335–7, 1992
24. Nelson ML, Leather GP, Nirschl RP et al: Evaluation of the painful shoulder. A prospective comparison of magnetic resonance imaging, computerized tomographic arthrography, ultrasonography and operative findings. J Bone Joint Surg [Am] 73:707–16, 1991
25. Neumann CH, Petersen SA, Jahnke AH: MR imaging of the labral-capsular complex: normal variations. AJR 157: 1015–21, 1991
26. Neviaser TJ: The anterior labroligamentous periosteal sleeve avulsion lesion: a cause of anterior instability of the shoulder. Arthroscopy 9:17–21, 1993
27. Neviaser TJ: The GLAD lesion: another cause of anterior shoulder pain. Arthroscopy 9:22–23, 1993
28. Pappas AM, Goss TP, Klemmen PK: Symptomatic shoulder instability due to lesions of the glenoid labrum. Am J Sports Med 11:279–88, 1983
29. Payne LZ, Jokl P: The results of arthroscopic debridement of glenoid labral tears based on tear location. Arthroscopy 9:560–5, 1993
30. Perry J: Anatomy and biomechanics of the shoulder in throwing, swimming, gymnastics and tennis. Clin Sports Med 2:247, 1983
31. Rafii M, Firooznia H, Golimbu C et al: CT arthrography of the capsular structures of the shoulder. AJR 146:361, 1986
32. Reeves B: Experiments on the tensile strengths of the anterior capsular structures of the shoulder in man. J Bone Joint Surg [Br] 50:858, 1968
33. Resch H, Golser K, Thoeni H, Spencer G: Arthroscopic repair of superior glenoid labral detachment (the SLAP lesion). J Shoulder Elbow Surg 2:147–55, 1993
34. Rodosky MW, Harner CD, Rudert et al: The role of the biceps-superior labrum complex in anterior stability of the shoulder. Pittsburgh Orthop J 1:57–68, 1990
35. Scarpinato DF, Bramhall JP, Andrews JR: Arthroscopic management of the throwing athlete's shoulder: indications, techniques and results. Clin Sports Med 10:913–27, 1991
36. Snyder SJ: A complete system for arthroscopy and bursoscopy of the shoulder. Surg Rounds Orthop 3:57–65, 1989
37. Snyder SJ: Review of "case report: arthroscopic repair of a type IV SLAP lesion—the red-on-white lesion as a component of anterior instability." Arthroscopy 9:494–6, 1993
38. Snyder SJ, Karzel RP, Del Pizzo W et al: SLAP lesions of the shoulder. Arthroscopy 6:274–9, 1990
39. Snyder SJ, Rames R, Wolbert E: Labral lesions. p. 491–9.

In McGinty JB (ed): Operative Arthroscopy. Raven Press, New York, 1991

40. Tirman PFJ, Stauffer AE, Crues JV et al: Saline magnetic resonance arthrography in the evaluation of glenohumeral instability. Arthroscopy 9:550–9, 1993
41. Williams MM, Buford D, Snyder SJ: The Buford complex—the "cord-like" middle glenohumeral ligament and absent anterosuperior labrum complex: a normal anatomic capsulolabral variant. Arthroscopy 10:241–7, 1994
42. Yoneda M, Hirouka A, Saito S et al: Arthroscopic stapling for detached superior glenoid labrum. J Bone Joint Surg [Br] 73:746–50, 1991

CHAPTER TWENTY-THREE

Arthritis and Arthroplasty

Steven A. Petersen

Arthritic conditions afflicting the shoulder most commonly involve the acromioclavicular joint and rarely the glenohumeral joint. Although primary arthrosis of the glenohumeral joint is uncommon, arthritis associated with dislocation may be more frequently encountered in an athletic population. Return to athletic activities after treatment for acromioclavicular joint arthritic conditions is often expected. Functional outcomes after treatment for glenohumeral arthritis are more unpredictable, and therefore prevention or early recognition is favored in the treatment of this condition. This chapter reviews the causes of shoulder arthritis, its clinical presentation, and required diagnostic testing, discusses the various treatment options and indications for surgery, and relates the expected outcomes of such treatment to the abilities of the athlete to return to sport participation.

DEGENERATIVE CONDITIONS AFFECTING THE ACROMIOCLAVICULAR JOINT

Arthritis of the acromioclavicular joint can result from joint incongruity caused by type 3 intra-articular distal clavicle fractures or grades I and II acromioclavicular joint separations. Degenerative arthritis of the acromioclavicular joint has also been related to excessive sporting activities and heavy manual work.[78] Age-related degenerative changes involving the acromioclavicular joint are common and have been described by DePalma et al[27] and Petersson[68] (Fig. 23-1).

DePalma et al demonstrated degenerative changes involving the acromioclavicular disc as early as the second decade of life, with similar changes involving the articular surface of the joint. Petersson described similar age-related changes occurring within the acromioclavicular disc and observed that the more complete the disc the more normal the articular surface. He found that after age 60 years, meniscal disc and articular surface degeneration were common, although on one occasion, a normal-appearing disc in a 78-year-old patient was associated with a normal joint. It would appear that the articular disc has a protective function for the acromioclavicular joint, separating the joint surfaces and dampening forces between the articular surfaces. An incomplete disc has been described by DePalma et al as a meniscoid form, likely resulting from regressive changes in a complete disc and associated with articular surface degeneration of the acromioclavicular joint. Degenerative changes and inferiorly directed osteophyte formation are most often pronounced on the clavicular joint surface, the frequency of osteophytes increasing with the severity of joint space narrowing. Inferiorly directed osteophytes from the acromioclavicular joint have also been associated with bursal surface impingement of the rotator cuff, and clinically these two conditions are often coexistent.[70]

Osteolysis of the distal clavicle often presents as isolated acromioclavicular joint pain and may be confused with degenerative changes of the joint. This disorder has been associated with acute trauma resulting from intra-articular distal clavicle fractures and acromioclavicular joint separation as well as the repetitive microtrauma caused by excessive athletic training[11,57,75] (Fig. 23-2). Weight lifting exercises to include bench pressing and overhead sterngth training have been related to this disorder, as have gymnastics, rugby, football, and hockey. Microscopically, it has been demonstrated that demineralization, subchondral cyst formation, and erosion of thc distal clavicle describe the pathology of osteolysis, which infrequently involves the acromion and is well demonstrated by technetium scintigra-

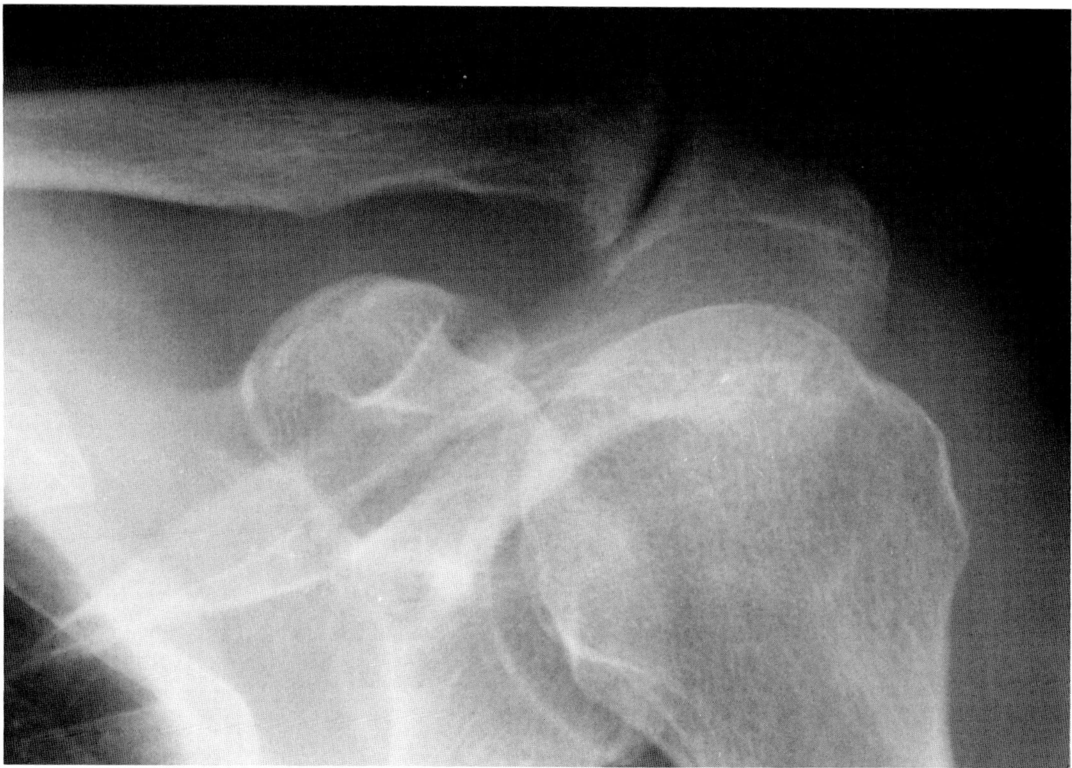

Figure 23-1. Age-related degenerative changes involving the acromioclavicular joint include joint space narrowing and an inferiorly directed distal clavicle osteophyte as illustrated in the anteroposterior radiograph of this symptomatic 62-year-old factory worker who eventually required distal clavicle excision.

phy. Osteolysis of the distal clavicle most commonly is unilateral, the differential diagnosis including gout, neoplasm, infection, or Gorrham's disease. Osteolysis involving both shoulders is less common, and rheumatoid arthritis, hyperparathyroidism, and scleroderma should be considered in the differential diagnosis.

GLENOHUMERAL JOINT ARTHRITIS

Glenohumeral joint arthritic disorders may be secondary to severe trauma, avascular necrosis, crystalline disorders such as pseudogout or gout, rotator cuff insufficiency, arthritis of dislocation, or inflammatory arthropathies.[64] Primary osteoarthritis of the shoulder is uncommon in the general population, usually affecting the older age group with a prevalence approximating 0.1 percent.[73]

Arthritic changes of the shoulder in an athletic population are more likely to be the result of the repetitive trauma from contact sports or related to the treatment of dislocation. Anecdotal experience in treating professional athletes would suggest that violent contact sports such as football or excessive strength training and conditioning in weight lifters and other professional athletes may predispose this population to arthritic changes of the shoulder (Fig. 23-3). Epidemiologic studies have supported the association between repetitive microtrauma or overhead work and its association with glenohumeral arthropathy.[48]

Atraumatic avascular necrosis of the humeral head frequently occurs in younger active individuals with a common history of corticosteroid use as adjuvant treatment for medical conditions such as sickle cell anemia, Gaucher's disease, lupus erythematosus, caisson disease, or organ transplantation.[16,65] Multiple lower extremity joint involvement often places excessive loads on the shoulder as they assume weightbearing responsibilities. Anabolic steroids have been incriminated in the causation of avascular necrosis of the femoral head, and perhaps this could be extrapolated to the shoulder.[72] Cruess[26] has staged the progression of disease from stages I to V: stages I to III maintaining concentricity of the head, stage IV representing subchondral collapse with head deformity, and stage V a progression to glenohumeral arthritis. Pain management and avoidance of glenoid arthritic changes are the goals of treatment, as the rapid progression to glenoid arthritis is common after subchondral collapse of the humeral head has occurred.

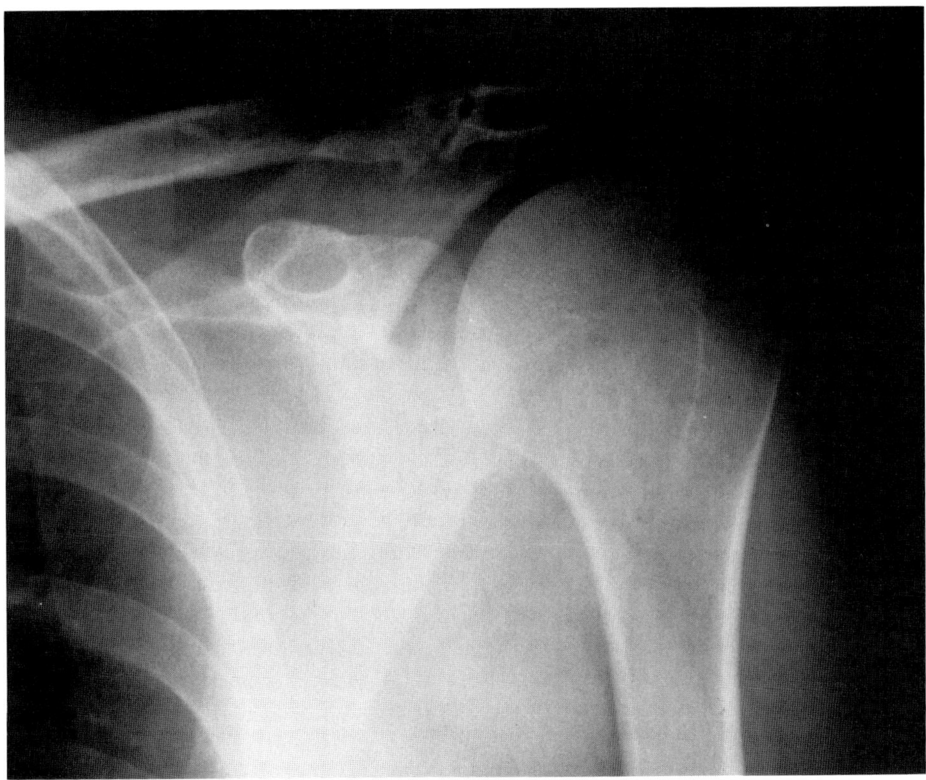

Figure 23-2. Osteoarthritic changes involving the distal clavicle of a 35-year-old female body builder. Note subchondral cystic change with irregularity of the distal clavicle. Her symptoms improved after modification of her training program.

Arthritis of dislocation deserves special attention in the context of arthritic disorders in the athletic population.[6] Limitation of external rotation after dislocation, or resulting from the treatment for dislocation, often results in glenohumeral arthritis[77] (Fig. 23-4). Alterations in glenohumeral joint kinematics in patients with anterior shoulder instability have been described by Howell et al,[44] likely the result of an incompetent anterior capsule. Interruption of the normal translatory pattern of the humeral head on the glenoid by injury or excessive stabilization of the capsule could result in abnormal joint contact stresses resulting in arthritis.[5,38,39,80] It is through these disordered mechanics that degenerative arthritis may arise, as changes in normal joint contact areas have been shown to cause articular surface changes and may be a factor in the genesis of "dislocation arthropathy."[53,61] Janevic and associates[45] have demonstrated experimentally that glenohumeral translation after a Bankart repair did not reproduce the normal joint mechanics with or without excessive tightening of the capsule. Their study revealed changes in the kinematics of the glenohumeral joint when stressing the anterior capsule in abduction and external rotation after a Bankart repair, resulting in a posterior shift in the glenohumeral contact area, thereby reproducing what is thought to occur clinically with an excessively overtightened anterior capsule.

Clinical experience supports the notion that an overtightened anterior repair often results in osteoarthrosis of the glenohumeral joint[40,41,54,55,63,66] Severe loss of external rotation after Putti-Platt, Magnuson-Stack, Bristow, dutoit, and Bankart procedures has been related to glenohumeral arthritis. Hawkins and Angelo[41] have reported on osteoarthritis of the glenohumeral joint as a late complication of Putti-Platt capsulorrhaphy in anterior dislocators. In their series, symptoms related to glenohumeral arthritis occurred on average 13.2 years after capsular repair, and all patients had significant limitation in external rotation, averaging −5 degrees (range, −30 to +25 degrees). Hawkins and Hawkins,[40] MacDonald et al,[55] and Lusardi et al[54] have all described similar experiences occurring after excessively tight anterior capsular repairs, resulting in the limitation of external rotation and disabling glenohumeral arthritis. Neer et al[63] have described the pathologic changes associated with arthritis of recurrent dislocation to include marked shortening of the subscapularis and anterior capsule and posterior erosion of the glenoid.

Glenohumeral arthritis resulting as a complication from the surgical treatment of shoulder instability has also been

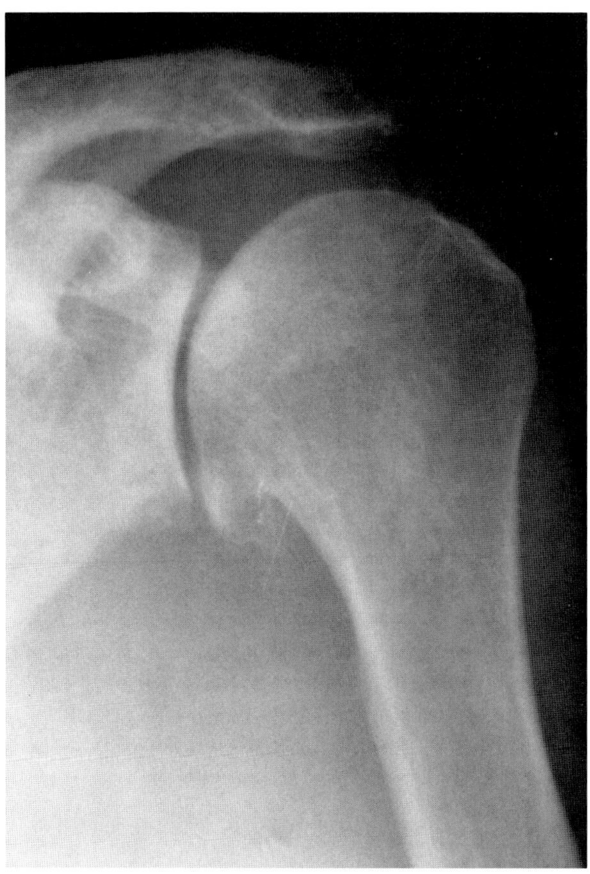

Figure 23-3. Atraumatic osteoarthritis of the glenohumeral joint in a competitive 34-year-old weight lifter. Interestingly, he has a past history of anabolic steroid use.

reported to occur after intra-articular fracture during glenoid osteotomy, intra-articular penetration of hardware, and joint injury from bone block procedures[46,87,88] (Fig. 23-5).

CLINICAL PRESENTATION

Acromioclavicular Joint Arthritis

Pain and deformity involving the acromioclavicular joint are characteristic of isolated acromioclavicular joint arthritis. Trapezial spasm and pain may be associated with a painful acromioclavicular joint due to the relationship of the deltotrapezial fascia with the superior joint capsule of the acromioclavicular joint. Difficulty in sleeping on the affected side and pain with overhead activity, crossed-arm adduction, and activities performed behind the back are associated with acromioclavicular joint discomfort.

Local joint tenderness with swelling or enlargement of the acromioclavicular joint are typical physical findings. Subacromial impingement of the rotator cuff can occur in association with acromioclavicular joint arthritis and may confuse the clinician. Provocative maneuvers for producing acromioclavicular joint pain include horizontal adduction with internal rotation and crossed-arm adduction. Unfortunately, these tests are relatively nonspecific and can be symptomatic from rotator cuff tendinitis or posterior capsular tightness. A painful arc of motion above 150 degrees of abduction has also been associated with acromioclavicular joint pathology.[51] Direct injection of the acromioclavicular joint with lidocaine is the most direct method in diagnosing the acromioclavicular joint as the source of shoulder pain.

Radiographic evaluation of the acromioclavicular joint has been described by Zanca, as reported by Rockwood and Young,[75] as an anteroposterior radiograph with a 10 degree cephalic tilt. This allows an unobstructed view of the acromioclavicular joint and distal clavicle, which may otherwise be overlapped by the spine of the scapula. A soft tissue technique is preferred to avoid overpenetration of the radiograph and allow for accurate detail of joint pathology as well as demonstrate the inclination of the joint surface geometry. Petersson and Redlund-Johnell[71] have described age-related radiographic changes in normal

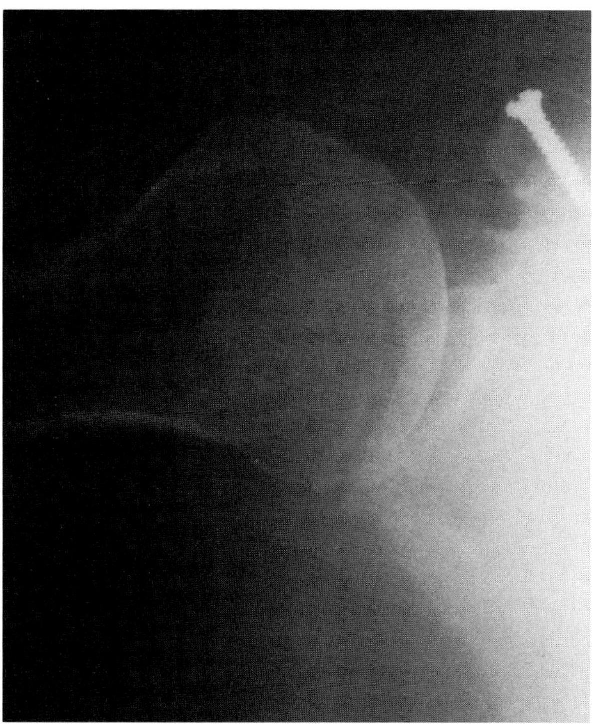

Figure 23-4. Axillary radiograph in a 62-year-old right-handed dentist demonstrating arthritic changes occurring 21 years after an anterior capsulorrhaphy had been performed for recurrent dislocation of his left shoulder. He retired from his dental practice because of painful limited range of motion.

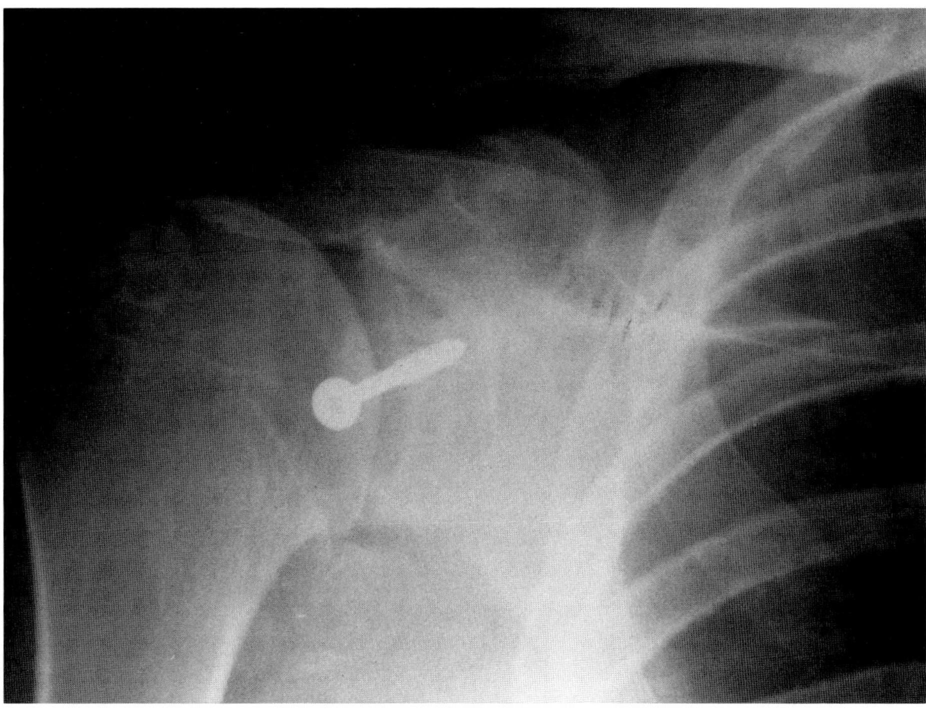

Figure 23-5. Severe degenerative glenohumeral arthritis in a 26-year-old businessman, 10 years after intra-articular placement of a coracoid screw during a Bristow repair for a recurrent anterior dislocation. Note the large loose body in the axillary pouch.

acromioclavicular joints, suggesting that a joint space of 0.5 mm or less is a normal finding in patients older than 60 years of age. Although they found that the joint space is usually wider in men, a joint space greater than 7 mm in men and greater than 6 mm in women is an abnormal finding regardless of the patient's age. Subchondral sclerosis with inferiorly directed clavicular osteophytes is characteristic of acromioclavicular joint arthritis.

Radiographic findings in osteolysis of the distal clavicle include loss of subchondral bone detail, cystic resorption of the distal clavicle, and generalized osteopenia of the distal clavicle with or without associated osteophyte formation or tapering of the distal clavicle.[11,57] On occasion, technetium scintigraphy may be used in diagnosing osteolysis of the distal clavicle.

Glenohumeral Joint Arthritis

Glenohumeral arthritis is associated with gradual loss of motion and pain often referred to the deltoid tuberosity. Concurrent afflictions involving the acromioclavicular joint, rotator cuff, and cervical spine can occur. Ellman et al[29] have described early degenerative glenohumeral arthritis that initially presented as impingement tendinitis, with the correct diagnosis made during arthroscopy. They have developed a compression-rotation test that may be of value in discriminating arthritis from subacromial bursitis or rotator cuff tendinitis (Fig. 23-6). The diagnosis of arthritis of the glenohumeral may also be facilitated by diagnostic lidocaine injection into the glenohumeral joint.

Restricted painful elevation with excessive scapulothoracic motion characterizes glenohumeral arthritis. Limitation of external rotation is a common finding in the arthritis of dislocation with internal rotation contractures often present. Diffuse atrophy of the involved shoulder is common, reflecting shoulder disuse and deconditioning.

Radiographic evaluation of glenohumeral arthritis includes a true anteroposterior radiograph of glenohumeral joint (40 degree posterior oblique or Grashe view), a lateral scapular view, and an axillary view, allowing assessment of the joint space, subchondral joint changes, and periarticular osteophytes. A true anteroposterior radiograph in external rotation may help to define small inferior humeral neck osteophytes that would otherwise be missed.[50] Arthritis of dislocation is frequently associated with marked posterior glenoid wear that may require computed tomography for accurate assessment and preoperative planning.[33] Petersson and Rodlund-Johnell[71] were unable to demonstrate joint space narrowing of the glenohumeral joint in normal shoulders as they had done with acromioclavicular joints, and joint space narrowing should not be accepted as a normal finding regardless of the patient's age. Inferior glenoid and humeral head osteophytes are the most frequently noted

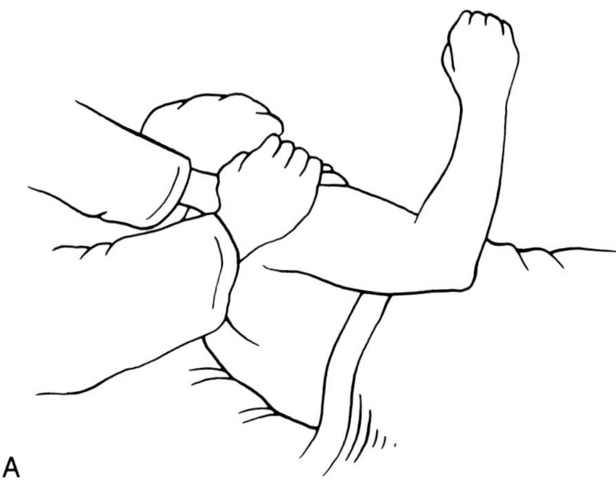

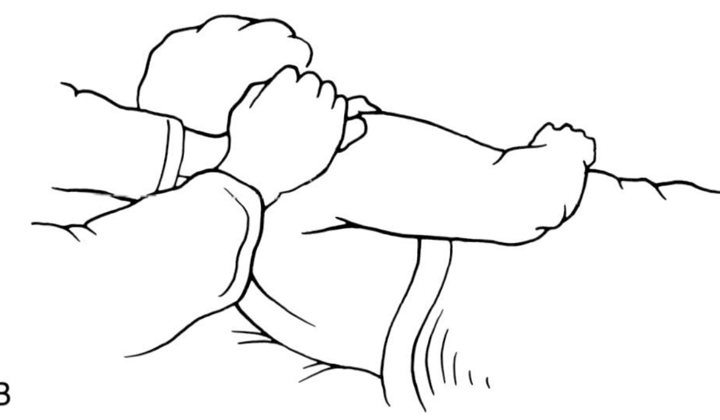

Figure 23-6. (**A & B**) Ellman's compression-rotation test may help to discriminate glenohumeral arthritis from impingement tendinitis. With the patient lying on their unaffected side, compression is applied to the patient's affected shoulder while rotating the shoulder in internal and external rotation. Glenohumeral arthritis is suspected if the patient's symptoms are reproduced.

radiographic findings, with joint space narrowing a relatively late finding in glenohumeral arthritis.

Full-thickness rotator cuff tears are associated with glenohumeral osteoarthritis only 5 percent of the time. Age-related changes involving the rotator cuff have been associated with more advanced arthritic glenohumeral joint changes and are commonly described as ''cuff arthropathy.''[50] Loss of the normal humeral-acromial distance on an anteroposterior radiograph (less than 9 mm) implies associated rotator cuff disease, the extent of which can be confirmed by clinical examination. Rotator cuff insufficiency adversely affects the prognosis of treatment for glenohumeral arthritis. Shoulder weakness during elevation and external rotation implies a large, if not massive, rotator cuff tear and is usually associated with loss of active range of motion, with preservation of passive motion. An intra-articular injection of lidocaine may be required to assess accurately the strength of the shoulder if a rotator cuff tear is present. If, after injection, weakness persists, compromise of the rotator cuff has occurred and is unlikely to be dramatically changed by surgical reconstruction.

TREATMENT ALTERNATIVES

Acromioclavicular Joint Arthritis

Nonoperative management of acromioclavicular joint arthritis provides acceptable symptomatic relief on most occasions. The use of nonsteroidal anti-inflammatory medications, activity modification, and symptomatic measures to include heat or ice massage, comprise the conservative management of this condition. On occasion, a local steroid injection into the acromioclavicular joint is appropriate; however, multiple injections should be avoided. Adjunctive physical therapy may be helpful in the treatment of acromioclavicular joint arthropathy, maintaining joint flexibility and preserving periscapular and rotator cuff strength. Similarly, pain resulting from osteolysis of the distal clavicle will usually respond to modification of activity combined with the above symptomatic measures. Persistent pain is an indication for surgical treatment after failing to respond to a 6-month trial of aggressive nonoperative management.

Excision of the distal clavicle has been successfully performed since first described by Gurd[37] and Mumford[62] in 1941. Success in treating acromioclavicular joint arthritis by open techniques has since been reported to range from 75 to 91 percent.[23,31,69,75] The success of this procedure in athletes has been specifically addressed by Cook and Tibone.[23] They objectively evaluated the postoperative return of strength after distal clavicle excision performed in athletes, all of whom had sustained a type 1 or 2 acromioclavicular joint injury and, after failing aggressive management, had open resection of the distal 1.9 cm of the clavicle. All but one patient were satisfied with their surgery, and five of six professional athletes returned to their level of sport. Slow-speed Cybex testing demonstrated shoulder flexion and extension strength loss at slower speeeds that were not demonstrated with faster speed testing, refuting claims of general fatigue after this procedure. The most common complaint among those who did not return to their previous performance level was a loss of bench press strength. As this exercise involves scapular protraction against a fixed clavicle, it was theorized that the loss of the posterior acromioclavicular ligament affected clavicular stability, which became apparent only during maximal muscular effort, confirmed by slow-speed Cybex testing.

An alternative to open resection of the distal clavicle is arthroscopic excision through either a subacromial approach or a direct superior approach. Gartsman et al[35] have demonstrated the ability to reproducibly perform a subacromial excision of the distal clavicle, approximating the technical success of open excision. By following strict criteria assuring complete distal clavicle excision, they have had clinical success in 17 of 20 patients, the three failures requiring open surgery for retained superior or anterior portions of the distal clavicle, all of which were successfully excised at reoperation.[34] Excellent results of this technique have also been reported by Tolin and Synder[82] and Kay et al,[49] obtaining results comparible with open techniques with the additional benefit of earlier return to activities of daily living.

Flatow and Bigliani have enjoyed considerable success in approaching the acromioclavicular joint directly through a superior approach, as initially described by Johnson.[4,31,47] The advantage of this technique is the direct approach to the distal clavicle, thus avoiding injury to the anterior and posterior acromioclavicular ligaments. The direct superior technique may be favored over a subacromial approach for tight osteoarthritic joints or in those joints that are medially inclined and not easily displaced into the subacromial space for excision via the subacromial approach. It has been observed that minimal resection (5 to 6 mm) of the distal clavicle, accomplished by the superior approach, allows for adequate joint decompression. Preservation of the acromioclavicular ligaments by this technique prevents clavicular stump impingement against the acromion during shoulder elevation and may allow for more conservative, yet successful distal clavicle excision. In a series of patients treated by this technique for arthritis or osteolysis of the acromioclavicular joint, 91 percent had resolution of their symptoms with return to full activity.[4] Failures resulted from incomplete resection of posterior cortical ridges and in acromioclavicular joints treated for painful degenerative changes associated with unstable grade II acromioclavicular joint injury.

Surgical Technique of Distal Clavicle Excision—Tips, Quips, and Pearls

Open Excision of Outer Clavicle

The decision to perform open versus arthroscopic excision for symptomatic arthritis or osteolysis of the acromioclavicular joint is the surgeon's preference. Flatow et al[31] have prospectively compared arthroscopic with open surgery with comparable results at final follow-up. Arthroscopic benefits include shorter hospitalizations, quicker return to work and activities of daily living, and earlier relief of their pain. Open excision can also be performed in an outpatient setting, and attention to the details of surgical technique may avoid pitfalls previously identified in the literature, namely, posterior clavicular instability.

Open excision of the distal clavicle is routinely performed under general or regional interscaline anesthesia in a beach chair position (Fig. 23-7). A short oblique incision, placed immediately lateral to the acromioclavicular joint along Langer's line, allows for a cosmetic, yet practical approach to the acromioclavicular joint. Dissection is carried down to the deltotrapezial fascia, which is incised horizontally, over the acromioclavicular joint, and for a distance of 1.5 to 2 cm medial to the joint along the distal clavicle. Subperiosteal dissection of the distal 1.5 cm of the distal clavicle is performed with careful perservation of anterior and posterior subperiosteal flaps. This dissection is carreid laterally to the anterior acromion, preserving the anterior and posterior acromioclavicular ligaments during the dissection. Hypertrophic superior joint osteophytes can be removed to a smooth surface, contouring the joint to a normal appearance. Residual disc material can be sharply excised and the distal 10 to 15 mm of the clavicle removed. This allows a finger to be inserted and adequate decompression can be tested with crossed-arm adduction. If a large anteroinferior osteophyte is present along the clavicular surface, the excision of the distal clavicle can be slightly beveled in a medial direction, allowing for complete excision of the osteophyte (Fig. 23-8). A Darrach elevator, placed anteriorly and posteriorly, facilitates excision of the distal clavicle with protection of the anterior and posterior subperiosteal envelope. The inferior border of the clavicle can be rasped smooth and the periosteal envelope closed securely with size 2 nonabsorbable suture, approximating the deltotrapezial fascial envelope in an anatomic fashion and preserving the integrity of the anterior and posterior acromioclavicular ligaments. The subcutaneous tissues are closed with interrupted absorbable suture and the skin in a routine fashion. A sterile dressing is applied, and the patient is placed in a sling for comfort. Postoperative management may be improved with the use of ice therapy as well as nonsteroidal anti-inflammatory drugs for pain management. The patient is started on immediate pendulum exercises and allowed passive range of motion without restriction, advancing to active motion at 5 to 7 days and resistive exercises at 3 to 4 weeks.

Arthroscopic Excision of Distal Clavicle

Arthroscopic resection of the distal clavicle can be accomplished by subacromial or direct superior approaches. When performed subacromially, it is usually in combination with an anterior acromioplasty. Regardless of the technique used, it is important to localized the acromioclavicular joint position and inclination using several 22-gauge needles. Gartsman et al[35] have validated the reproducibility and accuracy of acromioclavicular joint resection through

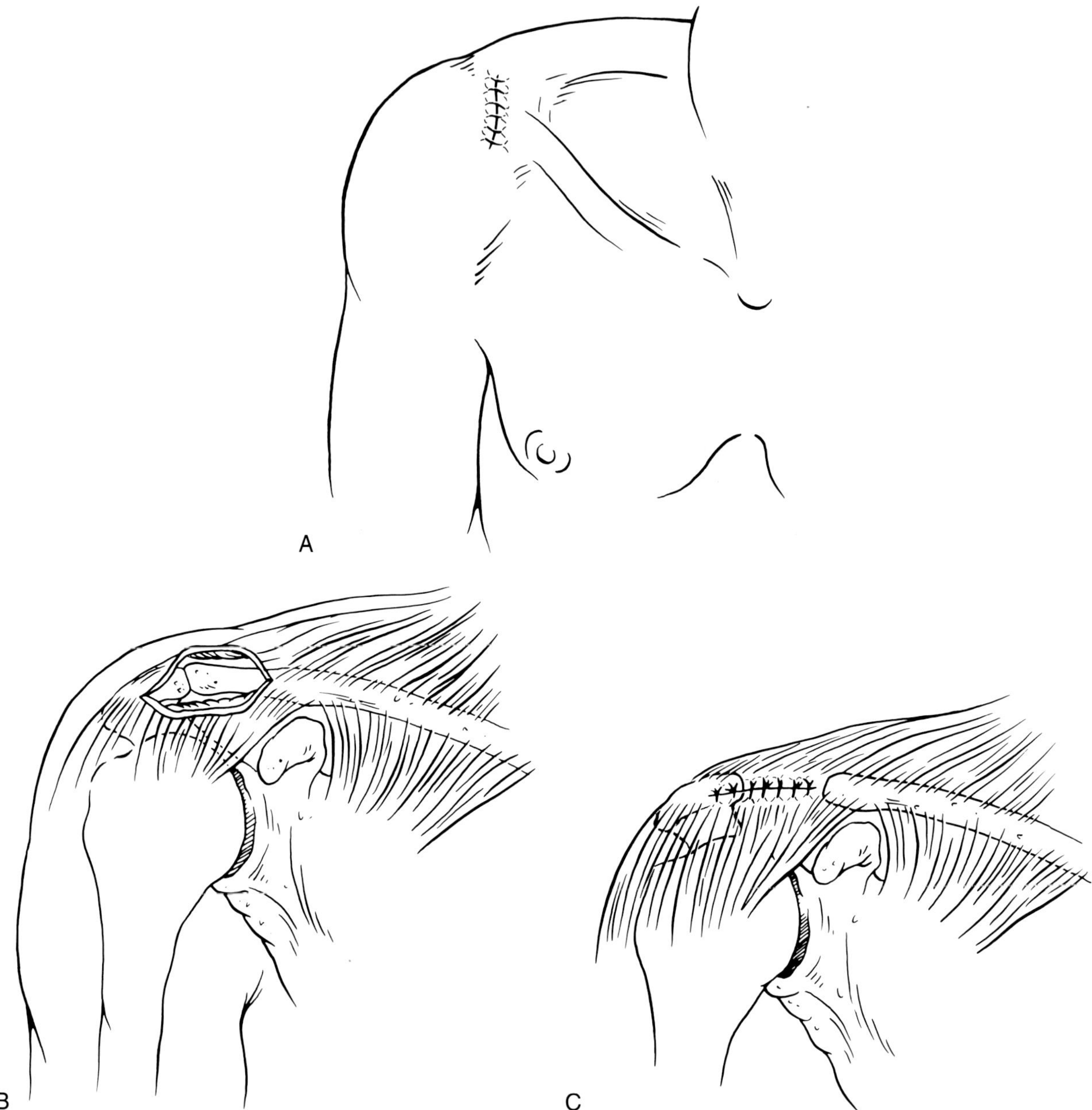

Figure 23-7. (**A–C**) Open distal clavicle excision for symptomatic acromioclavicular joint arthritis. Careful subperiosteal dissection and repair of the deltotrapezial fascia perserves the acromioclavicular ligaments and enhances postoperative function.

the subacromial approach. A distal clavicle excision is performed using a 5.5-mm burr placed either in the anterior portal immediately adjacent to the acromioclavicular joint or the lateral portal. If soft tissue swelling increases during the procedure or the patient is large (greater than 100 kg), the arthroscope is often moved from the posterior to the lateral portal, the clavicle then seen end-on and bone resection more easily performed. After excising the soft tissue from the joint with an aggressive soft tissue resecter, the distal clavicle is pushed downward to facilitate the resection. The anterior border of the distal clavicle is removed from its inferior to superior cortex and then resection continued from an anterior-to-posterior direction, generally removing 10 to 15 mm of bone from the distal clavicle and 5 mm from the medial acromion. Gartsman[34] has suggested that success is achieved when (1) all inferior projections of the distal clavical have been removed; (2) sharp edges have been tapered from the anterior, posterior, infe-

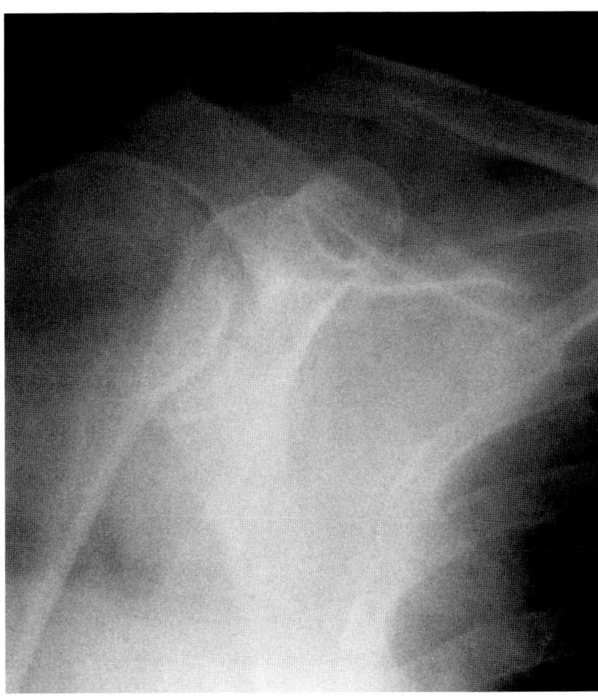

Figure 23-8. Successful distal clavicle excision. A biplanar osteotomy was performed, preserving clavicular length while removing a prominent inferior distal clavicular osteophyte.

rior, or superior surface; (3) the superior surface of the capsule is clearly visualized, and joint fibers identified but not excised; (4) the distal clavicle appears to have more bone removed anteriorly than posteriorly and superiorly than inferiorly; and (5) impingement of the distal clavicle against the acromion is avoided after resection when the arm is guided through its full range of motion.

The superior arthroscopic approach is usually performed in the beach chair position, the joint insufflated with several millimeters of normal saline and the anterosuperior and posterosuperior portals localized after the position and angle of the acromioclavicular joint are confirmed by needle placement.[31] A 2.7-mm arthroscopy unit is placed posterior for visualization and a motorized 2.0-mm resecter directed anteriorly, debriding the meniscal remnants and any debris within the joint. After the articular surfaces are exposed, small burrs are used, advancing from a 2-mm burr, widening the joint to accommodate a standard 4-mm arthroscopic unit. The capsular ligaments are subperiosteally dissected from the distal clavicle, and a large tapered burr is used to resect the distal clavicle, alternatively switched from anterior to posterior. Uniform bone resection is achieved in this manner and the bone surface beveled with a rasp inserted through the arthroscopic portals if necessary. At the conclusion of the operation, the edges of the distal clavicle are probed, and all overhanging ridges excised and loose fragments removed. With either arthroscopic technique, the patient is placed in a sling for comfort, with motion started immediately and resistive exercises added within the first 10 days. As with the open procedure, cold therapy and aggressive anti-inflammatory medication may help with postoperative pain management.

Glenohumeral Joint Arthritis

Nonoperative management for the treatment of glenohumeral arthritis strives to maintain or enhance shoulder motion and provide for general shoulder conditioning and strength through the use of nonsteroidal anti-inflammatories and aggressive physical therapy. Judicious use of intra-articular steroid injections may provide for dramatic relief of shoulder pain, allowing immediate benefits from an aggressive therapy program and potentiation of the nonsteroidal anti-inflammatory drug effect. The exact number of intra-articular cortisone injections that should be administered has not been accurately quantified, although there does not seem to be any benefit in giving more than three to four injections in a lifetime. Corticosteroids appear to impede the inflammatory cycle by inhibition of phospholipidase A enzyme, interrupting the arachidonic acid chain cycle earlier than the aspirin or nonsteroidal medications.[74] Intra-articular administration of steroids temporarily reduces the synthesis of articular cartilage matrix in a dose-related fashion.[56] Arthropathy related to intra-articular steroid injections has been reported, although any association remains anecdotal, and it would be safe to say that for selective use, it remains beneficial.[52]

The surgical management of glenohumeral arthritis is indicated if pain persists despite an aggressive trial of nonoperative treatment. The surgical management of glenohumeral arthritis ranges from arthroscopic debridement and extensive soft tissue releases to joint arthroplasty. Specific treatment is based on patient diagnosis and concomitant pathology, with the integrity of the rotator cuff an important prognostic factor in predicting the restoration of shoulder function.

Shoulder arthroscopy has become an important tool in defining the diagnosis as well as providing treatment for mild-to-moderate degenerative changes of the shoulder.[12,29,47,58] Arthroscopy defines the extent of intra- and extra-articular pathology and has been found successful in relieving symptoms of mild-to-moderate arthritis two-thrids of the time.[67] Removal of loose bodies, debridement of degenerative labral and unstable chondral flaps, and treatment and definition of rotator cuff pathology or concomitant subacromial bursal inflammation, stenosis, or adhesive capsulitis are the many benefits of arthroscopic treatment. The success of arthroscopic debridement in treating shoulder arthritis is related to the severity of the disease and the integrity of the rotator cuff and is discouraged in patients with degenerative subluxation, marked joint space narrowing, large osteophytes, or the presence of a full-thickness rotator cuff tear. The return of shoulder function and motion remains unpredictable after arthroscopy and may relate to the elimination of mechanical irregularities by debridement of unstable labral or chondral flaps. Gentle manipulation and release of capsular adhesions at the time of arthroscopy may also allow for improved motion. Although long-term benefits of this technique have not been reported, arthroscopic debridement would appear to be indicated in patients with mild-to-moderate arthritic disease with an intact rotator cuff who have failed nonoperative treatment and wish to remain active. Complications are rare, and future treatment options would not seem to be compromised.

Surgical release of an internal rotation contracture in patients with arthritis after anterior capsulorrhaphy of the shoulder offers predictable relief of pain and improvement in shoulder function and often delays the need for shoulder arthroplasty.[54,55,66] Marked loss of external rotation after an overly tightened anterior capsule characterizes this disorder. The pain-free interval after the capsular repair may last for 13 years, and patients are usually seen for treatment on average from 10 to 17 years after capsulorrhaphy. Symptomatic arthritis can develop quickly after excessively tightened anterior repairs, with some patients having arthritic changes noted within the first year after capsulorrhaphy. The severity of arthritis is directly related to the limitation of external rotation, with patients often having posterior subluxation of the humeral head and concomitant posterior glenoid erosion. In a series by Lusardi and associates,[54] patients who had severe osteoarthritis averaged −17 degrees of external rotation compared to −6 degrees in those patients with less severe degenerative changes. In addition to external rotation, flexion is also usually limited, with associated tightness of the inferior capsule. Release of the capsular contracture and subscapularis lengthening is recommended in patients with osteoarthritis that has failed nonoperative management. Combining soft tissue releases with total shoulder arthroplasty is usually indicated in those patients who have severe arthritic changes with marked posterior subluxation of the shoulder and posterior glenoid erosion.

The degree of soft tissue release is related to the amount of internal contracture present. Lusardi and associates[54] were often able to correct the internal rotation contracture by a medial transfer of the subscapularis tendon in patients who had external rotation limited to 0 degrees. Severe loss of external rotation (−10 to −50 degrees) required subscapularis and capsular release. In their experience, after soft tissue release, all shoulders had marked pain relief, with improvement in external rotation averaging 43 degrees. MacDonald and associates[55] have reported their experience with 10 patients having an internal rotation contracture after anterior capsulorrhaphy, most of the patients having had a Putti-Platt repair. All patients in their series had a subscapularis lengthening averaging 2 cm, noting average improvement in external rotation measuring 38 degrees (from an average of −8 degrees preoperatively to 30 degrees postoperatively). None of their patients lost motion, and there were no complications reported in their series. All patients had improvement in their preoperative symptoms, usually within the first 2 months after soft tissue release. Norris and Evans[66] also have experience with 38 patients who underwent subscapularis lengthening to treat internal rotation contractures, most of the patients having failed instability repair. They noted improvement in external rotation averaging 42 degrees (from 4 degrees preoperatively, 46 degrees postoperatively) and elevation improving an average of 27 degrees (96 degrees preoperatively, 123 degrees postoperatively). An average of 21 degrees of external rotation was gained with every centimeter of subscapularis lengthening that they achieved. Eighteen of their 20 patients noted symptomatic improvement after surgery.

Reconstructive options for avascular necrosis are varied and depend on the stage of the disease and whether the sphericity of the head has been compromised by subchondral collapse. Encouraging early results with core decompression have been obtained in early-stage disease (I to III), although long-term studies are lacking.[84] The combination of core decompression and vascularized bone grafting has been reported for osteonecrosis of the hip and may offer a treatment option for the shoulder.[83] Loss of joint congruity after subchondral collapse of the humeral head has been successfully treated by hemiarthroplasty. Rutherford and Cofield[76] have reported encouraging results in treating patients with stage III and IV and early stage V disease with hemiarthroplasty for severe shoulder pain. In six shoulders with significant glenoid arthritis, total shoulders were performed. No pain or slight pain was experienced in 94 percent of their patients, and motion approached normal, as the rotator cuff was usually unaffected and periarticular contracture was uncommon. They found in their series that symptom progression was unlikely to occur with early stage I to III disease, and nonoperative treatment for tolerable symptoms in these patients was advised.

Post-traumatic arthropathy after fracture-dislocation of the proximal humerus is rare in the young athletic population. Unstable comminuted fractures may require arthroplasty, with hemiarthroplasty favored if glenoid involvement is limited. Success of arthroplasty is contingent on the integrity of the periarticular tissues and rotator cuff.[22,60] Reasonable results can be expected if there is union of the tuberosities without fracture deformity and if there is an intact rotator cuff.[28]

Reconstructive options in treating osteoarthritis have historically included arthrodesis as a consideration, along with hemiarthroplasty or total shoulder arthroplasty. Although pain relief is predictably achieved by arthrodesis, functional limitations after arthrodesis have been well documented, and the indications of arthrodesis are usually reseved for severe sepsis, failed arthroplasty, and brachial plexus lesions.[18,43] Hemiarthroplasty for the treatment of osteoarthritis with minimal glenoid involvement remains an attractive option, avoiding the complications associated with glenoid replacement. Burkhead[10] has developed a technique including hemiarthroplasty and glenoid debridement with interposition of capsular or fascial tissue over the glenoid as an option to total shoulder arthroplasty. His early results have favored this technique over hemiarthroplasty alone. Cofield and associates[20] have reported on 35 patients with osteoarthritis, treated by humeral hemiarthroplasty and averaging 8.7 years follow-up. Postoperatively, 13 patients had persistent severe or intermittently severe pain, and seven shoulders had undergone revision. Bonutti and Hawkins[6] have noted variable results after revision of failed humeral hemiarthroplasty, with only 54 percent of their patients satisfied with their revision surgery, and patients often requiring additional surgical procedures. Whether hemiarthroplasty in osteoarthritic patients remains a conservative procedure has yet to be proved, and selection of patients for this procedure requires careful consideration of the patient's lifestyle demands and the degree of glenoid arthritis noted at the time of surgery.

The success of total shoulder arthroplasty in treating arthritic conditions of the shoulder is largely dependent on the status of the rotator cuff, severity of periarticular contractures, and the extent of glenoid bone loss. Survivorship of nonconstrained total shoulder arthroplasty has been 90 percent at 5 years and 71 percent at 11 years, 85.7 percent of the patients with osteoarthritis having good-to-excellent results.[2,9,13,14,32,36,63,81] The average gain in elevation in patients with osteoarthritis approximates 60 degrees, with 33 degrees gained in external rotation.[85] Hawkins and associates[42] have reported their results on osteoarthritic shoulders with intact rotator cuffs, 26 of 29 shoulders (89.6 percent) obtaining satisfactory pain relief. Forward elevation increased on average from 74 degrees to 151 degrees, external rotation from 17 degrees to 49 degrees, and internal rotation from the superior gluteal fold to T9. They had no complications in patients with osteoarthritis, although, on average, the incidence of component revision for nonconstrained implants has been reported to be between 0 and 13 percent.[1-3,7,14,25,36,42,59,63,79,85,86]

Both Neer et al[63,65] and Lusardi et al[54] have reported on their experience in treating arthritis related to dislocation. In the series of Neer et al,[63] 22 of 26 shoulders had previous surgery for recurrent dislocation with preoperative soft tissue contracture of the deltoid and subscapularis as well as deep erosion of the glenoid noted as common occurrences. The clinical ratings of 17 of the patients after 2 years demonstrated that 13 achieved excellent results, 3 satisfactory, and 1 unsatisfactory. Their average gain in active elevation was 51 degrees, with improvement of 66 degrees in external rotation. Their only failure was a shoulder with recurrent posterior subluxation due to excessive glenoid component retroversion. Lusardi et al[54] retrospectively followed eight shoulders requiring total shoulder arthroplasty and one requiring hemiarthroplasty for arthritis after anterior capsulorrhaphy of the shoulder. All nine patients had erosion of the posterior glenoid, one requiring bone grafting. A subscapularis lengthening was performed on all occasions. All patients had improvement in their pain, with eight of nine having mild discomfort, their pain only occurring with strenuous activity and not requiring analgesics. One patient had no pain after the procedure. Elevation improved in all patients, averaging a gain of 38 degrees (range, 10 to 80 degrees), with flexion averaging 134 degrees overall. Improvement in external rotation averaged 47 degrees (range, 25 to 65 degrees), with overall external rotation measuring 30 degrees (range, 0 to 60 degrees) in this group. Internal rotation averaged to the level of the eleventh thoracic vertebra (range, sacrum to T4), with an average improvement of three vertebral levels. There were no complications encountered in their retrospective review.

Neer and Brems[65] have advised that return to sporting activities after total shoulder replacement is possible. They have had experience in patients returning to farming, carpentry, semiprofessional basketball, golf, and tennis without complication. Provided that a secure and properly performed arthroplasty has been accomplished, noncontact sports, tennis, and golf may be encouraged. Contact sports and heavy weight lifting are not advised, as they carelessly extend limits of the procedure and its component materials.

Surgical Technique—Tips, Quips, and Pearls

Subscapularis and Capsular Release for Internal Rotation Contracture of the Shoulder

The patient is placed in the beach chair position with the involved shoulder draped free over the side of the surgical table and the patient's head and body carefully secured with all extremities carefully padded. Anesthetic choices include general anesthesia or regional interscaline block. Soft tissue release of the subscapularis and anterior capsule can be performed through an anteromedial or modified axillary skin incision, using the deltopectoral interval for the surgical approach. If present, the cephalic vein should be preserved and subdeltoid scarring carefully released from the subdeltoid and subacromial spaces. The lateral border of the conjoint tendon is an important landmark and frequently scarred to the surrounding tissues from previous surgery. This margin is carefully dissected free, being aware of the neurovascular structures medial to the coracoid, a retractor carefully placed under the conjoint tendon, providing medial retraction. Deep to the conjoint tendon is the subscapularis, and by slipping one's finger inferiorly between the subscapularis and conjoint tendon, the axillary nerve can be palpated and carefully protected throughout the procedure. Subacromial and subdeltoid scar should be incised, and this can usually be accomplished by blunt dissection or the use of a Darrach elevator. On occasion, contracture of the coracohumeral ligament may be found to limit external rotation, and this can be released at its insertion along the lateral aspect of the coracoid. The superior insertion of the pectoralis can be released to enhance exposure, releasing the proximal 1 to 1.5 cm. External rotation of the humerus is often difficult because of the internal rotation contracture, and protection of the axillary nerve is essential. Palpation of its proximal portion, as described above, and distal insertion into the deltoid, which can be accomplished by palpation around the humeral neck, can allow the surgeon to assess its integrity during the procedure by carefully placing tension on one portion and feeling a gentle tug on the other.[30] I have found that during the release of the subscapularis and capsule that a Darrach retractor carefully placed under the subscapularis margin and over the axillary nerve affords protection of this important neurologic structure. In shoulders with a mild internal rotation contracture (external rotation, 0 degrees), a subscapularis release may be achieved by medial transfer of the tendon to the anterior humeral neck. This procedure has been described by Lusardi et al,[54] in which the tendon is released at its insertion and repaired through transosseous holes drilled into the neck of the humerus, medial to the biceps tendon.

In most situations, a coronal lengthening of the subscapularis tendon is required along with an anterior capsulotomy (Fig. 23-9). The long head of the biceps tendon is an important landmark in planning the lateral vertical incision through the subscapularis tendon. The incision is made 1.5 cm medial to the long head of the biceps tendon and extended through the superficial fibers of the subscapularis proceeding from the rotator interval to the tendon's inferior edge. The junction between the capsule and the subscapularis is best identified inferiorly, and it is perferred to leave a portion of the subscapulari behind rather than risk perforation of the capsule. A coronal dissection is completed medially, creating an anterior layer continuous with the subscapularis muscle medially, and a posterior layer attached to the lesser tuberosity laterally. This requires dissection through the posterior fascia of the subscapularis at the level of the glenoid. The subscapularis tendon should be free of any adhesions from the back of the coracoid or capsule to facilitate this maneuver. If at least 20 degrees of external rotation cannot be achieved, the anterior capsule is divided vertically at the level of the glenoid from the rotator interval to the 6-o'clock position. The humerus is then externally rotated, and the subscapularis tendon is sutured to the underlying free margin of the incised anterior capsule. One centimeter of lengthening approximates an improvement in 20 degrees of external rotation. If an unrepaired Bankart lesion is discovered, the medial flap of the capsule is sutured back to the glenoid through drill holes or the use of suture anchors, and the suture passed anteriorly through the subscapularis at the level of the glenoid, thus providing a buttress against anterior instability. If forward elevation remains restricted, the inferior capsule can be released along the humeral neck. The deltopectoral interval may be loosely approximated and tagged with nonabsorbable suture for future identification of the interval. The patient is placed in a sling for comfort, and the use of ice has proved very helpful in pain management and control of swelling.

Postoperatively, motion is started immediately with passive range of motion through the arc of motion achieved at the time of surgery, advancing to active motion at 4 to 6 weeks, depending on the security of the repair. Resistive exercises are usually started between 8 and 12 weeks, allowing contact activities no earlier than 9 months. Overhead sports can be cautiously advanced after 6 months, with overhead plyometric activities preceding throwing or serving activities.

Total Shoulder Replacement

Several considerations need to be addressed in treating soft tissue contractures and glenoid bone deficiencies in osteoarthritis and arthritis of dislocation by glenohumeral arthroplasty.[15,24] Anterior soft tissue releases for contracted subscapularis and anteroinferior capsular tissue are performed as described above. Biologic fixation of the component remains an attractive option in young active patients (Fig. 23-10).[17,19] If posterior subluxation is encountered, the humeral component retrotorsion is decreased from 40 degrees to approximately 20 degrees. Glenoid deficiency can be addressed by several options, to include (1) glenoid preparation with concentric spherical reaming; (2) removal of the "proud glenoid rim" to match the deficient side; (3) asymmetric surface preparation with the use of an augmented or custom component; or (4) autogenous bone graft reconstruction. Concentric reaming ensures the stability of the glenoid component even if the posterior third of the glenoid is deficient, and bone grafting is rarely required.[21]

Postoperatively, the patient is protected in a sling for

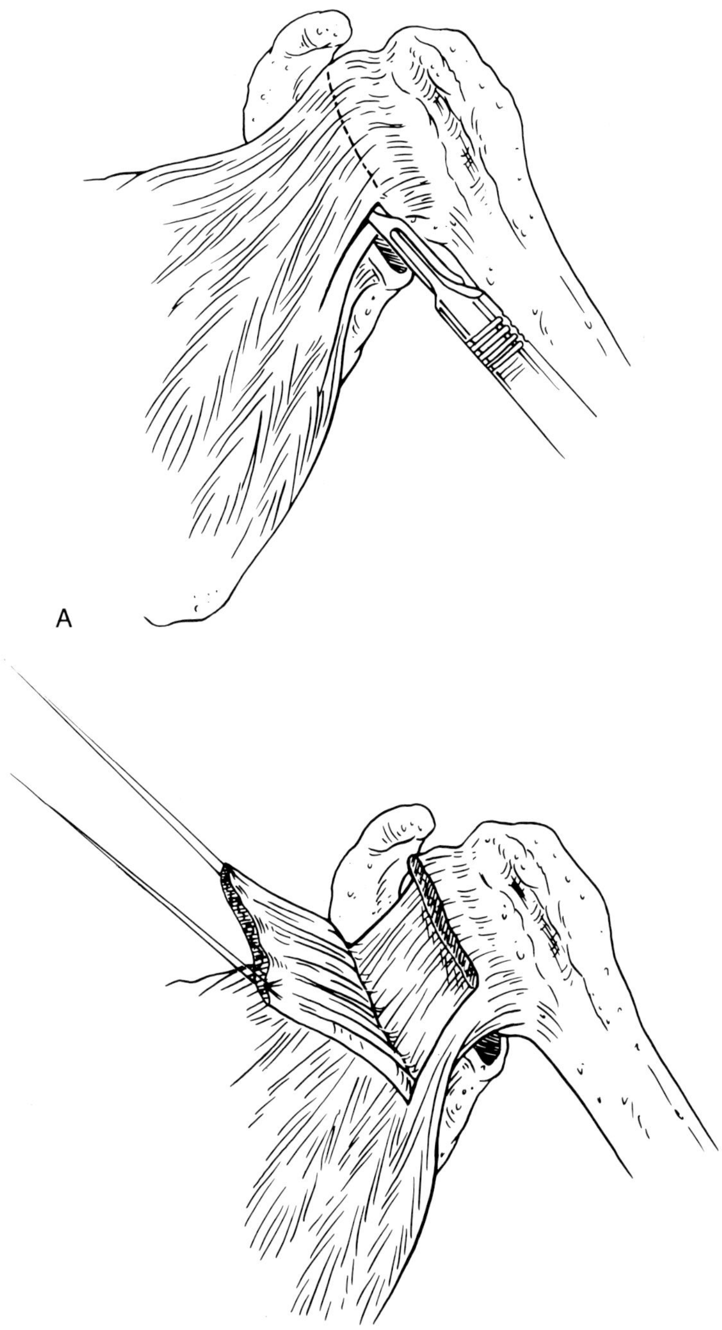

Figure 23-9. (**A–C**) Subscapularis and anterior capsular lengthening for fixed internal rotation of contracture of the glenohumeral joint. The axillary nerve is carefully protected during the procedure. (**D**) Inferior capsular release may be required for marked loss of elevation, the release performed along the humeral neck either by subperiosteal release or capsular incision. (*Figure continues.*)

protection, with passive motion initiated during the first 2 weeks and usually advanced to active motion by week 4 to 8. Progression of therapy is carefully balanced between protecting the integrity of soft tissue repairs and restoring motion in often chronically scarred periarticular tissues.[8]

An abductor brace may be necessary during the first 6 weeks to avoid excessive tension on fragile soft tissue repairs, with passive motion started at the level of the brace. Resistive strengthening usually starts between week 8 and 12.

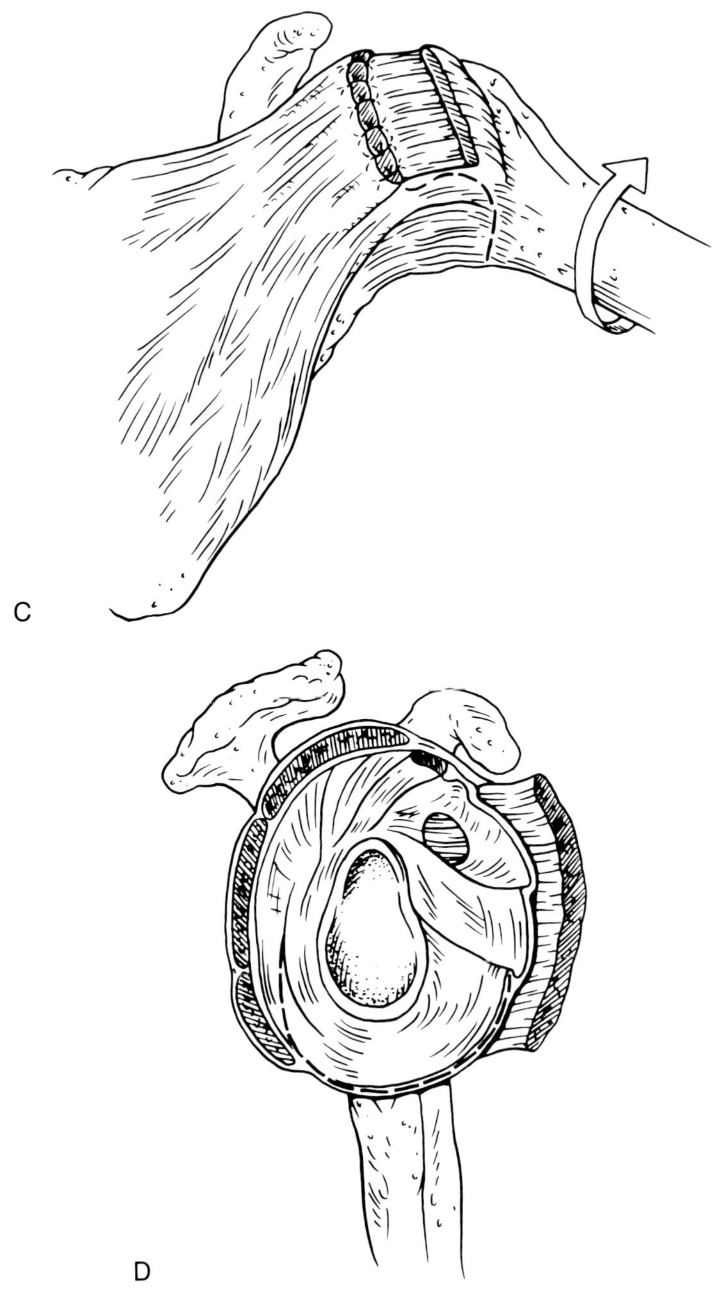

Figure 23-9. *(Continued).*

SUMMARY

Arthritic conditions of the shoulder commonly respond to nonoperative management, limiting the athlete because of pain and loss of motion. Surgical treatment for acromioclavicular joint arthritis allows for excellent restoration of function and return to sporting activities as well as relief of pain. Preservation of the acromioclavicular ligaments may allow for optimal results of this otherwise straightforward procedure.

Glenohumeral arthritis in the athlete is usually the result of excessive loss of external rotation after surgical management of shoulder instability. This complication can be avoided by attention to technique at the time of capsular repair, allowing at least 25 degrees of external rotation and avoiding the intra-articular placement of staples, screws,

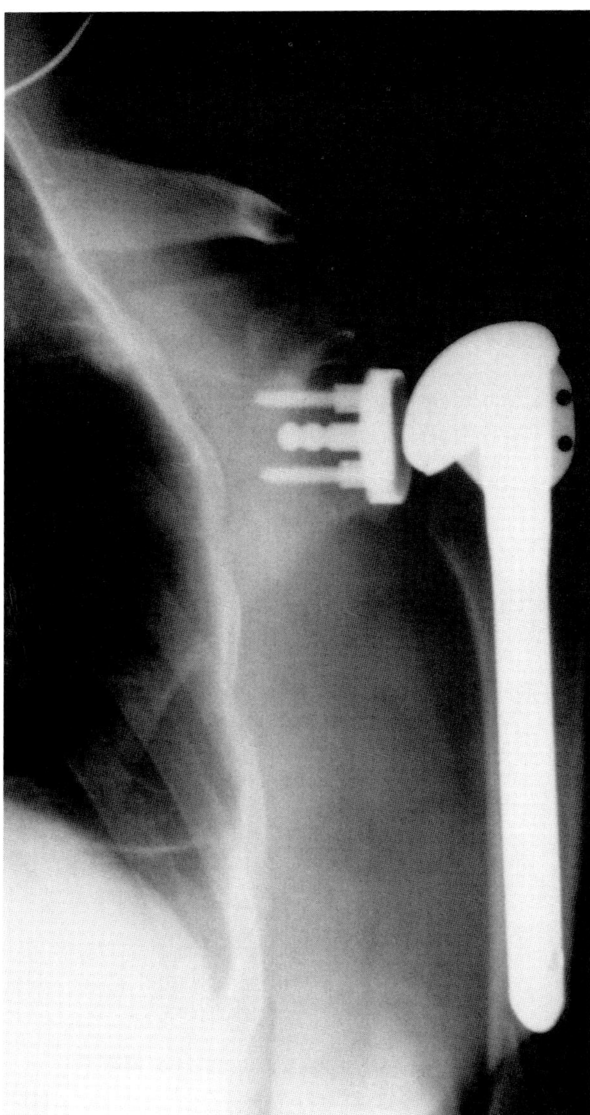

Figure 23-10. Porous coated total shoulder arthroplasty provides for biologic fixation of both the humeral and glenoid components. Although glenoid fixation is more secure with this technique, polyethylene wear may be increased.

or suture anchors. The inability to achieve more than 0 degrees of external rotation 6 to 9 months after a capsular repair should alert the surgeon to consider early soft tissue release, thereby avoiding arthritic change. When confronted by an established arthritis and an internal rotation contracture, anterior soft tissue release with subscapularis lengthening may provide for enough pain relief, restoration of function, and elimination of posterior subluxation of the humerus on the glenoid, delaying the need for shoulder arthroplasty and, perhaps, arresting the progression of arthritis. If shoulder arthroplasty has been performed, noncontact sports are often allowed. Appropriate care after arthroplasty would include avoidance of heavy weight lifting, laboring, or contact activities, otherwise for excellent pain relief and functional restoration.

REFERENCES

1. Amstutz HC, Thomas BJ, Kaho M et al: The DANA total shoulder arthroplasty. J Bone Joint Surg [Am] 70:1174, 1988
2. Barrett WP, Franklin JL, Jackins SE et al: Total shoulder arthroplasty. J Bone Joint Surg [Am]69:865, 1987
3. Barrett WP, Thornhill TS, Thomas WH et al: Nonconstrained total shoulder arthroplasty in patients with polyarticular rheumatoid arthritis. J Arthroplasty 4:91, 1989
4. Bigliani LU, Nicholson GP, Flatow EL: Arthroscopic resection of the distal clavicle. Orthop Clin North Am 24:133, 1993
5. Black KP, Lim TH, McGrady L et al: In vitro evaluation of shoulder external rotation following a Bankart reconstruction. Trans Orthop Res Soc 19:227, 1994
6. Bonutti PM, Hawkins RJ: Revision hemiarthroplasty of the shoulder. Orthop Trans 14:598, 1990
7. Boyd AD, Thomas WH, Sledge CB, Thornhill TS: Failed shoulder arthroplasty. Orthop Trans 14:255, 1990
8. Brems JJ: Arthritis of dislocation. p. 194. In Friedman RJ (ed): Arthroplasty of the Shoulder. Thieme Medical Publications, New York, 1994
9. Brenner BC, Ferlic DC, Clayton ML, Dennis DA: Survivorship of unconstrained total shoulder arthroplasty. J Bone Joint Surg [Am] 71:1289, 1989
10. Burkhead WZ: Hemiarthroplasty with biologic resurfacing of the glenoid for glenohumeral arthritis, abstracted. J Shoulder Elbow Surg, suppl. 2:29, 1993
11. Cahill BR: Osteolysis of the distal port of the clavicle in male athletes. J Bone Joint Surg [Am]64:1053, 1982
12. Cofield RH: Arthroscopy of the shoulder. Mayo Clin Proc 58:501, 1983
13. Cofield RH: Unconstrained total shoulder prosthesis. Clin Orthop 173:97, 1983
14. Cofield RH: Total shoulder arthroplasty with the Neer prosthesis. J Bone Joint Surg [Am] 66:899, 1984
15. Cofield RH: Integral surgical maneuvers in prosthetic shoulder arthroplasty. Semin Arthroplasty 1:112, 1990
16. Cofield RH: Osteonecrosis. p. 170. In Friedman RJ (ed): Arthroplasty of the Shoulder. Thieme Medical Publications, New York, 1994
17. Cofield RH: Uncemented total shoulder arthroplasty. Clin Orthop 307:86, 1994
18. Cofield RH, Briggs BT: Glenohumeral arthritis. J Bone Joint Surg [Am] 61:668, 1979
19. Cofield RH, Daly PJ: Total shoulder arthroplasty with a tissue-ingrowth glenoid component. J Shoulder Elbow Surg 1:77, 1992
20. Cofield RH, Frankel MA, Zuckerman JD: Humeral head replacement in glenohumeral arthritis, abstracted. J Shoulder Elbow Surg, suppl. 2:13, 1993
21. Collins D, Tencer A, Sidles J, Matsen FA III: Edge displacement and deformation of glenoid components in response to eccentric loading. The effect of preparation of the glenoid bone. J Bone Joint Surg [Am] 74:501, 1992

22. Compito CA, Self EB, Bigliani LU: Arthroplasty and acute shoulder trauma. Reasons for success and failure. Clin Orthop 307:27, 1994
23. Cook FF, Tibone JE: The Mumford procedure in athletes. An objective analysis of function. Am J Sports Med 16:97, 1988
24. Criag EV: Total shoulder arthroplasty. p. 757. In Chapman MW (ed): Operative Orthopaedics. JB Lippincott, Philadelphia, 1988
25. Cruess RL: Shoulder resurfacing according to the method of Neer. J. Bone Joint Surg [Br] 62:116, 1980
26. Cruess RL: Osteonecrosis of bone. Current concepts as to etiology and pathogenesis. Clin Orthhop 208:30, 1986
27. DePalma AF, Callery G, Bennett GA: Variation anatomy and degenerative lesions of the shoulder joint. AAOS Instr Course Lect 6:225, 1949
28. Dines DM, Warren RF, Altchek DW, Moeckel B: Posttraumatic changes of the proximal humerus: malunion, nonunion, and osteonecrosis. Treatment with modular hemiarthroplasty or total shoulder arthroplasty. J. Shoulder Elbow Surg 2:11, 1993
29. Ellman H, Harris E, Kay SP: Early degenerative joint disease simulating impingement syndrome: arthroscopic findings. Arthroscopy 8:482, 1992
30. Flatow EL, Bigliani LU: Locating and protecting the axillary nerve in shoulder surgery: the tug test. Orthop Rev 21:503, 1992
31. Flatow EL, Cordasco FA, Bigliani LU: Arthroscopic resection of the outer end of the clavicle from a superior approach: a critical, quantitative, radiographic assessment of bone removal. Arthroscopy 8:55, 1992
32. Frich LH, Moller BN, Sneppen O: Shoulder arthroplasty with the Neer Mark II prosthesis. Arch Orthop Trauma Surg 107:110, 1988
33. Friedman RJ, Hawthorne K, Genez BM: Evaluation of glenoid bone loss with computerized tomography for total shoulder arthroplasty. Orthop Trans 15:749, 1991
34. Gartsman GM: Arthroscopic resection of the acromioclavicular joint. Am J Sports Med 21:71, 1993
35. Gartsman GM, Combs AH, Davis PF, Tullos HS: Arthroscopic acromioclavicular joint resection: an anatomic study. Am J Sports Med 19:2, 1991
36. Gristina AG, Romano RL, Kammire GC et al: Total shoulder replacement. Orthop Clin North Am 18:4455, 1987
37. Gurd FB: The treatment of complete dislocation of the outer end of the clavicle: a hitherto undescribed operation. Ann Surg 113:1094, 1941
38. Harryman DT II, Sidles JA, Clark JM et al: Translation of the humeral head on the glenoid with passive glenohumeral motion. J Bone Joint Surg [Am] 72:1334, 1990
39. Harryman DT II, Sidles JA, Harris SL et al: The role of the rotator interval capsule in passive motion and stability of the shoulder. J Bone Joint Surg [Am] 74:53, 1992
40. Hawkins RH, Hawkins RJ: Failed anterior reconstruction for shoulder instability. J. Bone Joint Surg [Br] 67:709, 1985
41. Hawkins RJ, Angelo RL: Glenohumeral osteoarthritis. A late complication of the Putti-Platt repair. J Bone Joint Surg [Am] 72:1193, 1990
42. Hawkins RJ, Bell RH, Jallay B: Total shoulder arthroplasty. Clin Orthop 242:188, 1989
43. Hawkins RJ, Neer CS III: A functional analysis of shoulder fusions. Clin Orthop 223:65, 1987
44. Howell SM, Galinat BJ, Renzi AJ et al: Normal and abnormal mechanics of the glenohumeral joint in the horizontal plane. J Bone Joint Surg [Am] 70:227, 1988
45. Janevic J, Craig EV, Hsu K-C et al: Biomechanics of repair of anterior glenohumeral instability. Trans Orthop Res Soc 17:4955, 1992
46. Johnson GH, Hawkins RJ, Haddad R, Fowler PJ: A complication of posterior glenoid osteotomy for recurrent posterior shoulder instability. Clin Orthop 187:147, 1984
47. Johnson LL: The shoulder joint: an arthroscopic perspective of anatomy and pathology. Clin Orthop 223:113, 1987
48. Katevuo K, Aitasalo K, Lehtinen R, Pietilai J: Skeletal changes in dentists and farmers in Finland. Community Dent Oral Epidemiol 13:23, 1985
49. Kay SP, Ellman H, Harris E: Arthroscopic distal clavicle excision: technique and early results. Clin Orthop 301:181, 1994
50. Kerr R, Resnick D, Pineda C, Haghighi P: Osteoarthritis of the glenohumeral joint: a radiographic-pathologic study. Am J Radiol 144:967, 1985
51. Kessel L: The shoulder. p. 389. In Rob C, Smith R (eds): Clinical Surgery. Vol 13. Butterworths, London, 1967
52. Leadbetter WB: Injection therapy in sports injuries. p. 527. In Leadbetter WB, Buckwalter JA, Gordon SL (eds): Sports-Induced Inflammation. AAOS, Rosemont, IL, 1989
53. Lew WD, Lewis JL, Craig EV: Stabilization by capsule, ligaments, and labrum: stability at the extremes of motion. p. 69. In Matsen FA III, Fu FH, Hawkins RH (eds): The Shoulder: A Balance of Mobility and Stability. AAOS, Rosemont, IL, 1993
54. Lusardi DA, Wirth MA, Wurtz D, Rockwood CA Jr: Loss of external rotation following anterior capsulorrhaphy of the shoulder. J Bone Joint Surg [Am] 75:1185, 1993
55. MacDonald PB, Hawkins RJ, Fowler PJ, Miniaci A: Release of the subscapularis for internal rotation contracture and pain after anterior repair for recurrent anterior dislocation of the shoulder. J Bone Joint Surg [Am] 74:734, 1992
56. Mankin JH, Conger KA: The acute effects of intra-articular hydrocortisone on articular cartilage in rabbits. J Bone Joint Surg [Am] 48:1383, 1966
57. Matthews LS, Simonson BG, Wolock BS: Osteolysis of the distal clavicle in a female body builder. A case report. Am J Sports Med 21:150, 1993
58. Matthews LS, Wolock BS, Martin DC: Arthroscopic management of degenerative arthritis of the shoulder. p. 567. In McGinty JB, Caspowi RB, Jackson RW, Poehling GG (eds): Operative Arthroscopy. Raven Press, New York, 1991
59. McCoy SR, Warren RF, Bade HA et al: Total shoulder arthroplasty in rheumatoid arthritis. J Arthroplasty 4:105, 1989
60. Moeckel BH, Dines DM, Warren RF, Altchek DW: Modular hemiarthroplasty for fractures of the proximal humerus. J Bone Joint Surg [Am] 74:884, 1992
61. Mow VC, Bigliani LU, Flatow EL et al: The role of joint instability in joint inflammation and cartilage deterioration: a study of the glenohumeral joint. p. 337. In Leadbetter WB, Buckwalter JA, Gordon SL (eds): Sports-Induced Inflammation. AAOS, Rosemont, IL, 1989

62. Mumford EB: Acromioclavicular dislocation. A new operative treatment. J Bone Joint Surg 23:799, 1941
63. Neer CS, Watson KC, Stanton FJ: Recent experience in total shoulder replacement. J Bone Joint Surg [Am] 64:319, 1982
64. Neer CS III: Degenerative lesions of the proximal humeral articular surface. Clin Orthop 20:116, 1961
65. Neer CS III, Brems JJ: Shoulder replacement in the athletic and active patient. p. 93. In Jackson DW (ed): Shoulder Surgery in the Athlete. Aspen, Rockville, IL, 1985
66. Norris TR, Evans J: Internal rotation contracture of the shoulder abstracted. J Shoulder Elbow Surg, suppl. 2:7, 1993
67. Olgivie-Harris DJ, Wiley AM: Arthroscopic surgery of the shoulder. J. Bone Joint Surg [Br] 60:201, 1986
68. Petersson CJ: Degeneration of the acromioclavicular joint: a morphological study. Acta Orthop Scand 54:434, 1983
69. Petersson CJ: Resection of the lateral end of the clavicle: a 3 to 30-year followup. Acta Orthop Scand 54:94, 1983
70. Petersson CJ, Gentz CF: Ruptures of the supraspinatus tendon. The significance of distally pointing acromioclavicular osteophyte. Clin Orthop 174:143, 1983
71. Petersson CJ, Redlund-Johnell I: Radiographic joint space in normal acromioclavicular joints. Acta Orthop Scand 54:431, 1983
72. Pettine KA: Association of anabolic steroids and avascular necrosis of femoral heads. Am J Sports Med 19:96, 1991
73. Phillips WC Jr, Kattapuran SV: Osteoarthritis with emphasis on primary osteoarthritis of the shoulder. Del Med J 63:609, 1991
74. Roach JE, Tomblin W, Eyring EJ: Comparison of the effects of steroid, aspirin and sodium salicylate on articular cartilage. Clin Orthop 106:350, 1975
75. Rockwood CA Jr, Young DC: Disorders of the acromioclavicular joint. p. 413. In Rockwood CA Jr, Matsen FA III (eds): The Shoulder. WB Saunders Co, Philadelphia, 1990
76. Rutherford CS, Cofield RH: Osteonecrosis of the shoulder. Orthop Trans 11:239, 1987
77. Samilson RL, Prieto V: Dislocation arthropathy of the shoulder. J Bone Joint Surg [Am] 65:456, 1983
78. Stenlund B: Shoulder tendinitis and osteoarthritis of the acromioclavicular joint and their relation to sports. Br J Sports Med 27:125, 1993
79. Swanson AB, Swanson Degroot G, Sattel AB et al: Bipolar implant shoulder arthroplasty. Clin Orthop 249:227, 1989
80. Terry GC, Hammon D, France P et al: The stabilizing function of passive shoulder restraints. Am J Sports Meu 19:26, 1991
81. Thornhill TS, Karr MJ, Averill RM et al: Total shoulder arthroplasty: the Brigham experience. Orthop Trans 7:497, 1983
82. Tolin BS, Snyder SJ: Our technique for the arthroscopic Mumford procedure. Orthop Clin North Am 24:143, 1993
83. Urbaniak JR: Aseptic necrosis of the femoral head treated by vascularized fibular graft. p. 178. In Urbaniak JR (ed): Microsurgery for Major Limb Reconstruction. CV Mosby, St. Louis, 1987
84. Urquhart MW, Mont MA, Maar DC et al: Results of core decompression for avascular necrosis of the humeral head. Orthop Trans 16:780, 1992
85. Wilde AH: Shoulder arthroplasty: what is it good for and how good is it? p. 459. In Matsen FA III, Fu FH, Hawkins RJ (eds): The Shoulder: A Balance of Mobility and Stability. AAOS, Rosemont, IL, 1993
86. Wilde AH, Borden LS, Brems JJ: Experience with the Neer total shoulder replacement. p. 224. In Bateman JF, Welsh RP (eds): Surgery of the Shoulder. BC Decker, Philadelphia, 1984
87. Wildner M, Terreri S, Reichelt A: The x-ray appearance of the shoulder 10–23 years after the Eden-Hybbinette procedure, abstracted. J Shoulder Elbow Surg, suppl. 2:16, 1993
88. Zuckerman JD, Matsen FA III: Complications about the glenohumeral joint related to the use of screws and staples. J Bone Joint Surg [Am] 66:175, 1984

CHAPTER TWENTY-FOUR

Rehabilitation Exercises and Return to Sports

Robert Litchfield
Richard J. Hawkins
Gene Hagerman
John Atkins

Athletes involved in repetitive overhead activities place unique demands on the shoulder girdle. Rehabilitation to avoid injury, after injury, or in the painful shoulder of an overhead athlete creates a challenge for the athlete, trainer, and physician. The shoulder complex is particularly prone to injury, as it maintains a precarious balance between motion and stability. The complex interaction of muscle fatigue, eccentric overload, instability, and impingement can cause disability in such athletes. The act of throwing can involve angular velocities during the acceleration phase in excess of 7,000 degrees per second. After ball release, the muscles above the shoulder must absorb this enormous kinetic energy during the deceleration phase, during which the muscles are firing eccentrically.[1]

The athlete can present with a single traumatic injury to the shoulder, or more commonly, a chronic overuse type of syndrome. In either situation, the athlete must follow along a carefully sequenced program to restore motion, strength, and functional kinematics to eventually allow a return to the preinjury performance level.

This chapter briefly discusses problems unique to overhead athletes, basic principles of shoulder rehabilitation, the specific components of the rehabilitation process, and the steps leading to a return to sports. We discuss the recovery from acute shoulder trauma, from chronic overuse syndromes, and after operative intervention.

PROBLEMS UNIQUE TO OVERHEAD ATHLETES

Repetitive overhead activities, such as throwing, tennis, or volleyball, place the athlete at considerable risk for overuse injuries. The glenohumeral joint is inherently unstable, and stability is provided predominantly by the capsular, ligamentous, and muscular structures. Dynamic stability provided by the musculotendinous units of the rotator cuff are of primary importance in the midrange of motion. At the extremes of motion, the capsuloligamentous restraints play a more prominent role.[21] The repetitive high-velocity nature of throwing can lead to microtrauma in the musculotendinous stabilizers. The mode of failure is almost always eccentric in nature. This leads to decreased or asynchronous firing of these injured muscles and consequently less dynamic joint stability. This places a larger burden on the static stabilizers to maintain stability. In time, these static restraints may also fail, leading to subtle or frank glenohumeral instability. Altered biomechanics due to instability can lead to secondary impingement in the coracoacromial arch as the humeral head rides anteriorly and superiorly.[9,12,15] The chronic sequela can be a rotator cuff tear. It is therefore common for the overhead athlete, especially throwers and tennis players, to present with subtle anterior subluxation and secondary impingement tendinitis.

Scapular stabilizers, such as the trapezius, serratus anterior, rhomboids, and levator scapulae, can also be subjected to eccentric overload and fiber failure. Injury occurs during the deceleration phase of throwing, during which an enormous amount of kinetic energy must be absorbed by these muscles,[11] and may be clinically apparent as a winging scapula or as altered scapulothoracic rhythm. It is common for throwers with a painful shoulder to demonstrate scapular abnormalities on physical examination. A temporal lag in scapular protraction or lateral rotation during overhead activities can contribute to coracoacromial arch impingement. It is undetermined whether the role of the scapular musculature in impingement and instability is primary or secondary, although most believe it is secondary. In either case, the role of the scapula in normal function and in the painful shoulder needs to be emphasized and studied.

Many studies have documented asymmetry, particularly in hypertrophy of the shoulder musculature including the forearm flexor mass, of overhead athletes.[2,3,14] Also, these studies found increased external rotation and loss of internal rotation. Most overhead athletes demonstrate diminished internal rotation of the dominant arm on physical examination. These differences were even greater in competitive pitchers than in position baseball players. Similar adaptive changes have been found in the dominant arm of competitive tennis players.[3]

Capsular tightness likely has a significant role in problems about the athlete's shoulder. The work of Harryman et al[8] has illustrated that posterior capsular tightness can lead to increased anterior translation in an experimental model. Also, posterior tightness causes an increase in proximal migration of the humeral head during shoulder elevation. Abnormal biomechanics such as this can contribute to subacromial impingement. These factors may make a posterior capsular stretching program an important part of rehabilitation of the overhead athlete with instability and secondary impingement.

Intra-articular pathology is often found in the thrower's shoulder with subtle or obvious instability. The arthroscope has helped to identify attenuated inferior glenohumeral ligaments,[12] labral pathology,[1,12] partial undersurface rotator cuff tears,[17] and "kissing lesions" (an area of chondromalacia on the posterior aspect of the humeral head). The kissing lesion is produced by impingement of the humeral head on the posterior glenoid rim during abduction and external rotation in a shoulder with anterior subluxation.[12]

Shoulder arthroscopists have recently identified undersurface rotator cuff abrasions above the superior glenoid labrum in throwing athletes that have been interpreted as a form of "intrinsic impingement" of the rotator cuff.[10,22]

The role of the biceps brachii in throwing has been considered minimal by some authors,[7] but more recent publications suggest that the biceps plays an integral role in overhead function. Superior labral pathology is a common arthroscopic finding in the throwing athlete.[1] The most common lesion is a superior labral avulsion at the biceps insertion, the so-called SLAP (superior labral anterior to posterior) lesion.[19] Biomechanical studies have shown that the elbow and humerus undergo enormous torsion forces during baseball pitching.[7] Also, electromyographic (EMG) analysis has shown that the biceps has tremendous activity in the final 30 degrees of elbow extension during the deceleration phase of the throw.[11] The biceps is the only muscle involved in arm deceleration that crosses both the elbow and shoulder.

Recent work by Rodosky et al[18] using a dynamic cadaveric model has illustrated the biceps contribution to anterior stability of the glenohumeral joint by increasing the shoulder's resistance to torsional forces in the abducted and externally rotated position.[18] Also, they demonstrated that the biceps helps to diminish the stress placed on the inferior glenohumeral ligament.

It would appear that the biceps brachii plays a significant role in deceleration of the pitching arm and also in anterior stability of the glenohumeral joint.

BASIC PRINCIPLES OF SHOULDER REHABILITATION

The objective in any shoulder rehabilitation program is to return the athlete to pain-free function in the shortest time, allowing the athlete to maximize performance and avoid future problems. In most settings, a shoulder rehabilitation program is directed toward the athlete who presents with a painful shoulder. This may be the result of an acute injury or from chronic overuse of the shoulder. The athlete may also require rehabilitation after surgery. A program may be instituted for an athlete who has no shoulder problem but simply wants to have an effective functioning shoulder for maximum performance. Conditioning programs for the asymptomatic athlete are outlined in Chapter 25.

The first principle is to rehabilitate the shoulder in functional planes of motion. Most exercises are performed anterior to the scapular plane or in the scapular plane, which is generally a pain-free range. Exercises in the coronal plane, for example, should be avoided because this is a nonfunctional motion, often creating impingement and excessive load on the rotator cuff tendons.

The second principle is to use short lever arms to strengthen the shoulder. Early in the rehabilitation program, particularly in the painful athlete, passive and active movements are initiated with the elbow flexed to decrease the moment arm about the shoulder. During the resisted and strengthening phases of rehabilitation, loads are applied with the arms close to the body, with flexion of the elbows. EMG analysis has documented high levels of activity in the supraspinatus, with straight arm resisted exercises with scapular plane elevation.[20] Due to the long lever arm, these exercises may be pain-inducing and, if so, should be avoided. Sometimes, these exercises are effective in the painless shoulder, but most athletes who present with a painful shoulder find this exercise debilitating.

The third principle is to gain muscular control of the arm in the deceleration phase of overhead activities, particularly the throw. In this phase, enormous stresses occur, making the shoulder more prone to injury. Therefore, it is important to include in the conditioning a rehabilitation program with exercises that strengthen muscles (e.g., the latissimus dorsi and biceps brachii) that play a prominent role in this phase of the throwing motion.[1,11] During deceleration, muscles are contracting as they are elongating and are therefore working eccentrically. During a fast eccentric contraction, muscle and tendon stretch receptors cause an increased muscle contraction through recruitment. It is in this phase of activity in which the muscle tendon unit is at greatest risk for injury. Because most injury appears to occur during eccentric loading of the muscle, it seems important to strengthen eccentrically to more effectively control deceleration.

The fourth principle is to obtain a stable scapular platform, which is essential to success in any shoulder rehabilitation or conditioning program. This is the concept of proximal stability for distal mobility. Subtle degrees of scapular winging and dysrhythmia are observed in almost all types of shoulder disorders and are particularly associated with instability, anterior, posterior, or multidirectional in nature.

The fifth principle is to progress the exercise program in the overhead athlete to reproduce forces and loading rates that will approach the athlete's functional demands. This phase of conditioning is controversial and can be counterproductive if the progression is not cautiously and carefully followed. This phase of rehabilitation helps the athlete re-establish kinesthesia and proprioception of the upper extremity. Muscle and joint afferents need to be retrained to allow the athlete to discriminate joint position and movement including direction, amplitude, speed.[16] For muscles and soft tissues to adapt to increased loads, they must undergo progressive and controlled overload.

The sixth principle is to individualize rehabilitation based on the athletes needs. Many sports involve primarily open-chain activity whereas others have a larger component of closed-chain kinetics. By definition, open-chain activity involves movement of the distal segment in relation to a fixed proximal segment, and closed-chain activity involves movement of the proximal segments in relation to a fixed distal segment. An example of an open-chain activity would be the throwing of a baseball, in which the body is fixed and the arm is moving freely in space. By contrast, a closed-chain activity would be exemplified by a chin-up or handstand, in which the distal segment is fixed and the proximal segment is mobile. Athletes should be rehabilitated with a combination of open- and closed-chain exercises, depending on the specific demands of their sport.

In summary, a shoulder rehabilitation program should address the unique demands placed on the athlete's shoulder and the resultant pathologic entities.

Specific Shoulder Conditioning and Therapy

The following program would be applied to the athlete who presents with a painful shoulder. We must implement strategies to restore motion, strength, and functional kinematics to the shoulder. Having described the various problems that are unique to the overhead athlete and the various principles of rehabilitation, we can now move on to specifically apply these to the exercise program. The patient who has a painful shoulder must achieve motion and strength without further compromising the underlying pathology or disrupting reconstructed tissues.

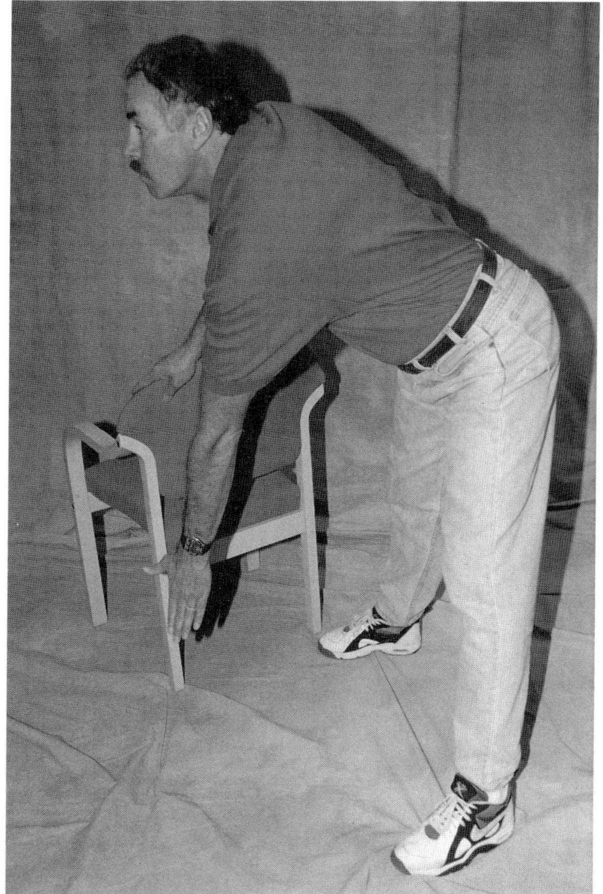

Figure 24-1. Pendulum exercise.

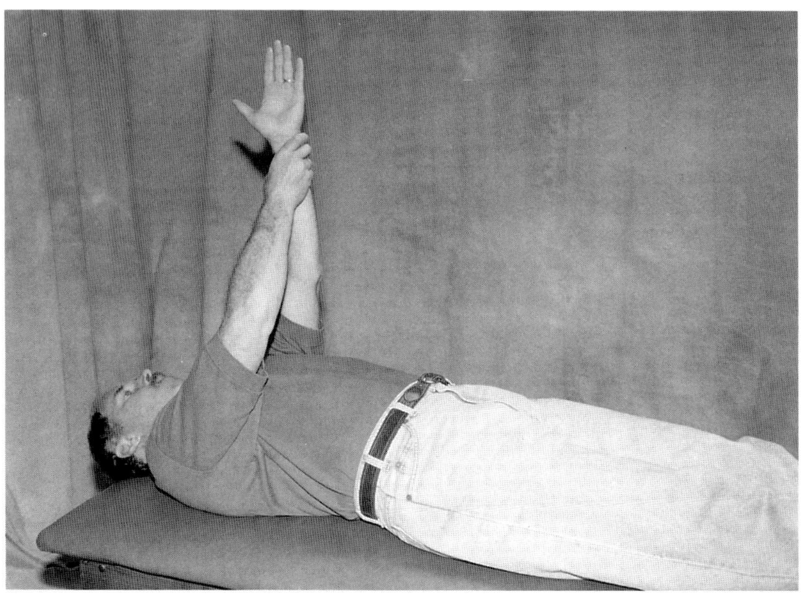

Figure 24-2. Supine active assisted forward elevation.

Rehabilitation After an Acute Injury

The overhead athlete may sustain an acute injury, such as an acromioclavicular separation, rotator cuff contusion, clavicle or proximal humeral fracture, or even a full-thickness rotator cuff tear. After an appropriate decision regarding management of these patients, rehabilitation becomes an important component for restoring motion, strength, and function to the shoulder. After an acute injury, the initial program should be to restore motion to the shoulder as pain-free as possible. This may often be initiated with simple pendulum exercises and passive assisted motion (Figs. 24-1 to 24-3). Passive motion can most easily be accomplished supine with the elbow flexed to minimize the length of the lever arm on the shoulder. Similarly, external rotation and internal rotation need to be passively obtained after an injury. This passive program can be progressed to an active exercise program with terminal stretching in the planes of elevation, external rotation and internal rotation, and eventually an appropriate strengthening program focusing on the short rotators of the glenohumeral joint and the scapular musculature. Once motion and strength have been restored, athletes then resume sport-specific motions such as plyometrics incorporating a resistance cord or plyometric ball (Figs. 24-4 and 24-5). This phase needs to be closely monitored by an experienced

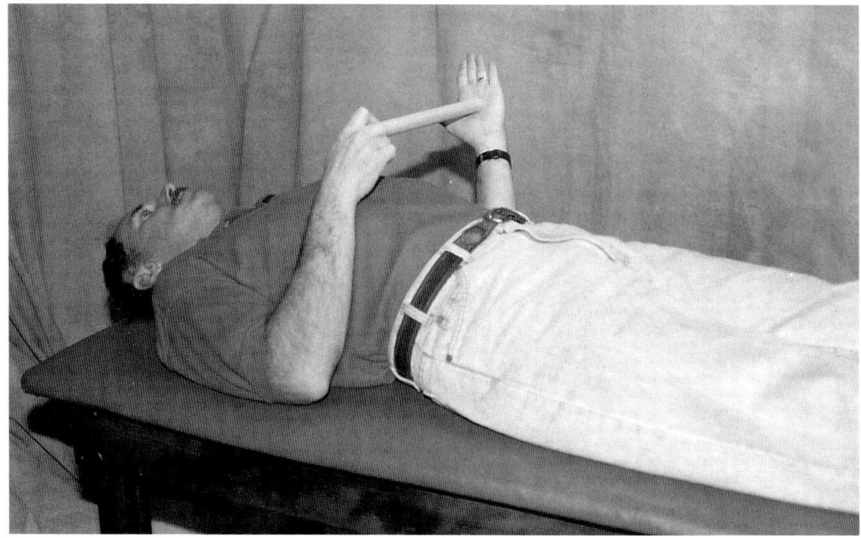

Figure 24-3. Supine active assisted external rotation.

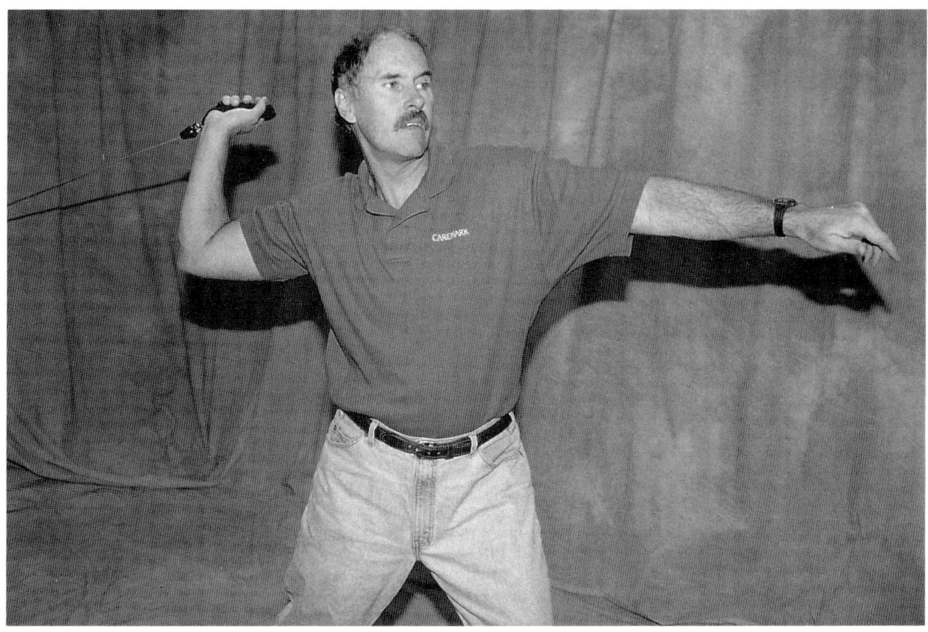

Figure 24-4. Plyometric strengthening with Body Lines.

trainer to avoid reinjury. In addition to range of motion and strengthening exercises, various modalities can be important in alleviating the pain of an acutely injured shoulder.

Rehabilitation of the Painful Shoulder

Rehabilitation design for the painful shoulder follows the description of the problems unique to the overhead athlete and the principles of shoulder rehabilitation previously described in this chapter. The diagnosis as to the cause of the shoulder pain is fundamental to the appropriate rehabilitation program.

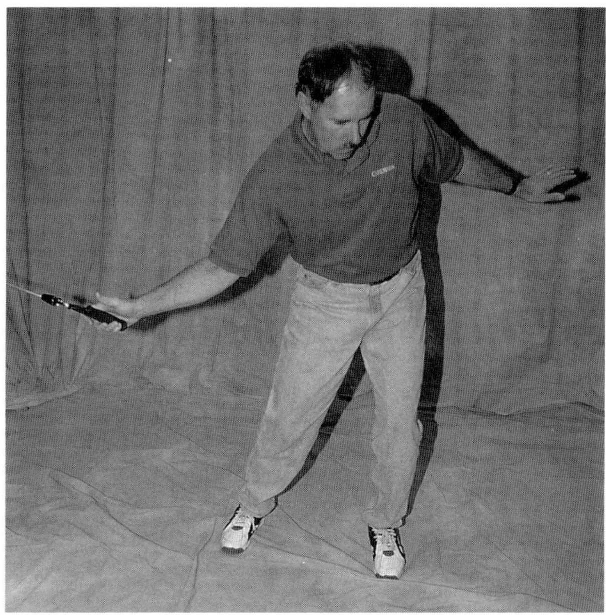

Figure 24-5. Forehand tennis stroke with Body Lines.

Rehabilitation After Shoulder Surgery

Occasionally, the athlete will have a shoulder problem unresponsive to nonoperative management. Common procedures performed on the athlete include arthroscopic or open stabilization, subacromial decompression, and management of partial or complete rotator cuff tears. After operative intervention, rehabilitation of the shoulder becomes of paramount importance in restoring the athlete's function. The specific rehabilitation program is determined by the extent of the operative procedure and the loads that can be placed on the reconstructed tissues. The sequence of events, however, is essentially the same. Initial treatment is directed at minimizing surgical pain and inflammation while re-establishing full passive and active range of motion, followed by a strengthening program directed at the glenohumeral and scapular musculature. The final phase involves sport-specific motions and loads.

Range of Motion

After surgical or traumatic injury to the shoulder, a program of passive assisted range of motion is commenced. In the initial stages, these are best performed supine to minimize the gravitational forces acting on the extremity (Figs. 24-2 and 24-3). Occasionally, limits are placed on the extent of motion allowed (e.g., after anterior stabilization frequently external rotation is limited, and after rotator cuff repairs frequently internal rotation is avoided). Once passive motion has been restored, an active program is initiated. In conjunction with the active program, each repetition incorporates a terminal stretch to maximize the range of motion. If the situation dictates, introduce proprioceptive neuromuscular facilitation (PNF) stretching to the patient for enchancing range of motion and neuromuscular education.[6] PNF patterns may vary from rotational to diagonal.

Mobilization techniques may also be incorporated by an appropriately trained therapist to aid in re-establishing normal joint motion mechanics. Various techniques including directional glides and distraction of both the glenohumeral scapulothoracic articulations may be useful. Details of these techniques are beyond the scope of this chapter.

Stretching of the Shoulder

Most overhead athletes present with limited internal rotation and a tight posterior capsule, manifested by limitation of crossed-arm adduction. Stretching historically has been in many directions about the shoulder, and we now appreciate in the overhead athlete that many of these stretches are detrimental, either worsening underlying pathology or initiating problems. For example, stretching the painful shoulder in the overhead position in forward flexion is probably unwise due to the exacerbation of an impingement process. Similarly, stretching the abducted, extended, and externally rotated arm may be harmful in the overhead athlete for fear of exacerbating anterior subluxation. Therefore, these stretches should seldom be performed in the painful shoulder. In the throwing and overhead athlete, we prefer to emphasize a rigorous posterior capsular stretching program (Figs. 24-6 to 24-8). In asymptomatic athletes, it is beneficial to have maximum external rotation, allowing a greater force generation capability for power. However, too much repetitive external rotation in the abducted position leads to anterior subluxation. Such stretching must be carefully implemented and only performed in situations in which anterior subluxation is not a problem. It has been shown that increasing internal rotation and eliminating posterior capsular tightness increases the ability of the overhead athlete to perform.[13]

Modalities

Modalities can be an integral part of a shoulder rehabilitation program. The methods or equipment used can assist in reducing inflammation, pain, and swelling. The use of modalities may alter physiologic responses including metabolism, muscle spasm, and neuromuscular feedback.

Pain management, relief of muscle spasms, and anti-inflammatory effect can be achieved using cryotherapy.[5] Ice bags, ice massage, and cold packs are examples of cold application. Cryotherapy should be routinely used immediately after injury or surgical intervention. Thermotherapy or heat application can be incorporated to increase local blood flow, as well as to reduce muscle spasms, just to name a few of its physiologic functions.[5] Thermotherapy

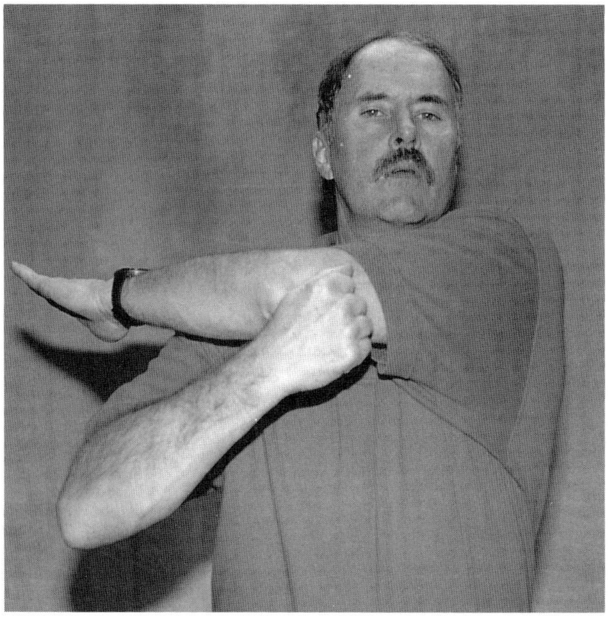

Figure 24-6. Posterior capsular stretching.

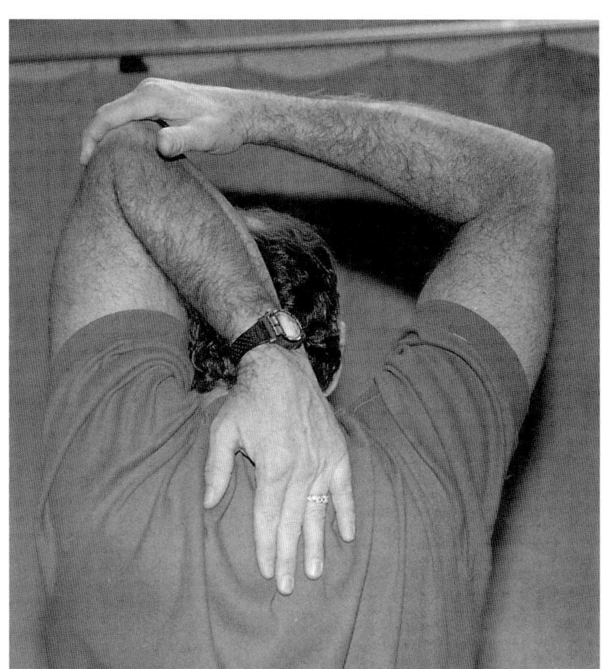

Figure 24-7. Posterior inferior stretching.

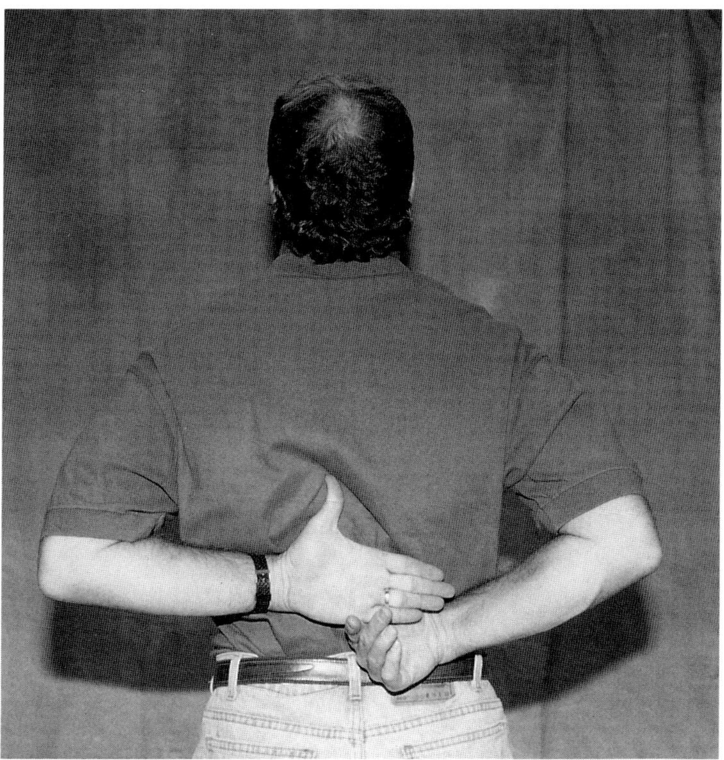

Figure 24-8. Posterior capsular stretching, internal rotation.

includes warm water, showers or mini-baths, moist packs, and ultrasound. Often times, ultrasound can be delivered with a medication (i.e., cortical steroid) to enhance its effectiveness. The clinician must determine the appropriate timing for heat application. This method is often used before the patient's stretching or warming up program. Ice or cold usually follows the stretching/exercising regimen. In some instances, a contrast of using heat (3 to 5 minutes) followed by cold (1 to 2 minutes) can be appropriate when increased blood flow to the local area is the goal.

Electrical muscle stimulation is another modality being used by clinicians. This modality appears to be most useful in neuromuscular re-education as opposed to inducing muscle hypertrophy.

Strengthening Program

A strengthening program is fundamental to rehabilitate the injured athlete and to prevent injury in the healthy thrower. Strengthening a pitcher's shoulder has long been considered taboo by many minor and major league pitching coaches. The biomechanical demands placed on the throwing shoulder as illustrated by Dillman et al[4] and Jobe et al[12] certainly give strong support for a strengthening training program, especially in eccentric modes. It is extremely difficult, if not impossible, to replicate the muscle forces and loading rates encountered during the baseball throw in a strength training program. We have incorporated a variable resistance rubberized bungy cord (Body Lines, Innovation Sports, Irvine, CA) as the mainstay in our strengthening program. The benefits of this apparatus include portability, leading to increased compliance, and a variable length-tension relationship, allowing use during all stages of the conditioning process. Very high loading rates can be achieved with highly sport-specific actions. The resistance cord can be used both concentrically and, more important, eccentrically. During the terminal stages of rehabilitation, the resistance cord can be used as a plyometric device.

The strengthening program starts with internal and external rotational exercises with the elbow flexed 90 degrees and the arm placed comfortably at the side (Figs. 24-9 and 24-10). The emphasis during these exercises is slow controlled motion in a pain-free range. Muscles are worked both concentrically and eccentrically. Our preliminary EMG evidence suggests a greater subscapularis firing with increasing abduction during an eccentric contraction. During deceleration of the throwing arm, the infraspinatus must contract eccentrically to help control the humeral head. With this in mind, we have devised an exercise to eccentrically strengthen the infraspinatus while minimizing concentric loads on the muscle (Figs. 24-11 and 24-12). In athletes with anterior glenohumeral instability, the trainer

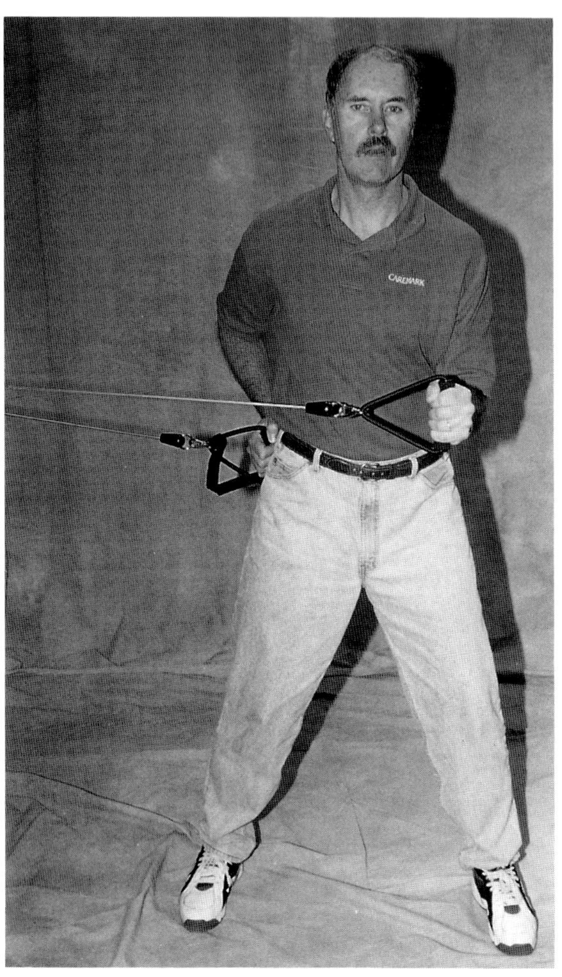

Figure 24-9. External rotation.

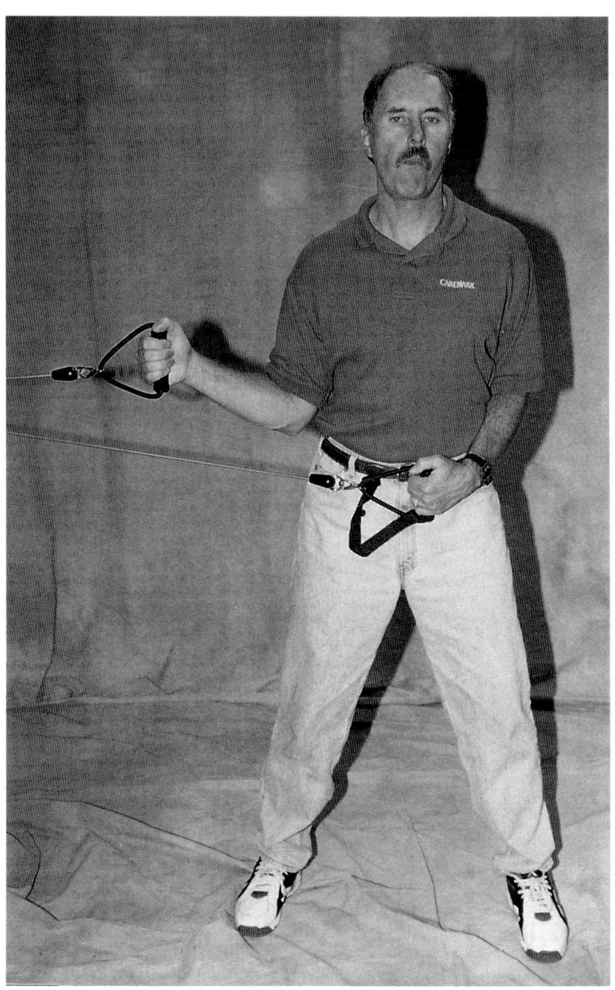

Figure 24-10. Internal rotation.

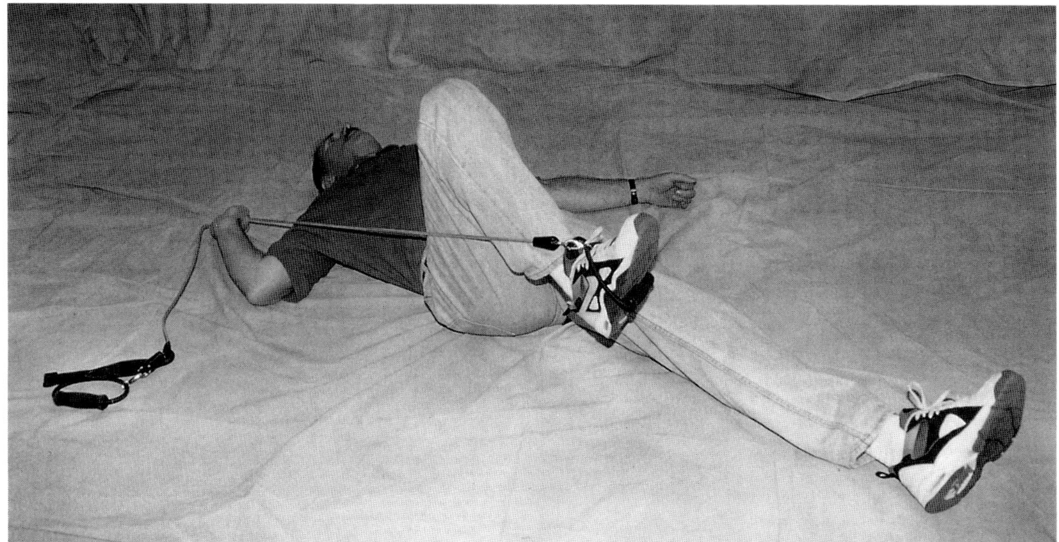

Figure 24-11. Load released during concentric external rotation.

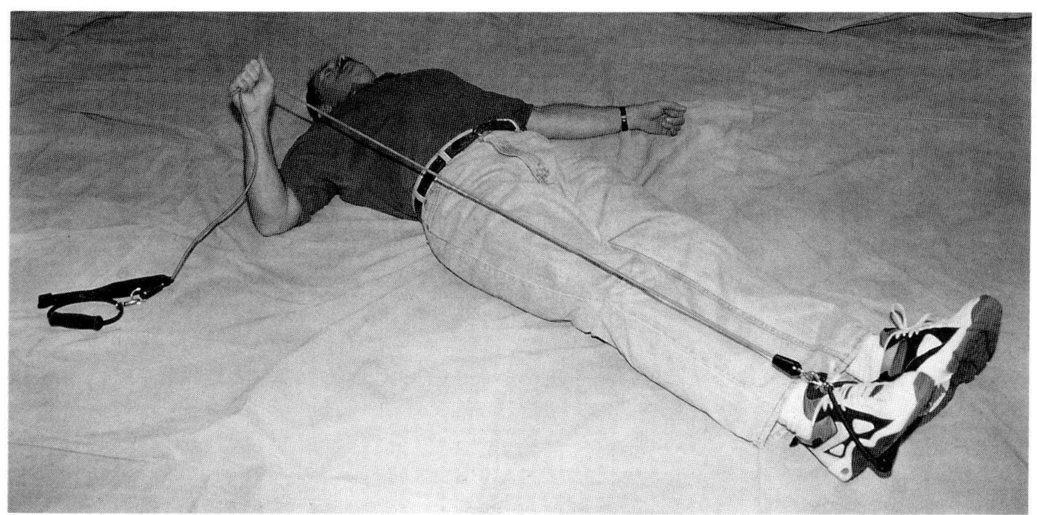

Figure 24-12. Eccentric infraspinatus strengthening.

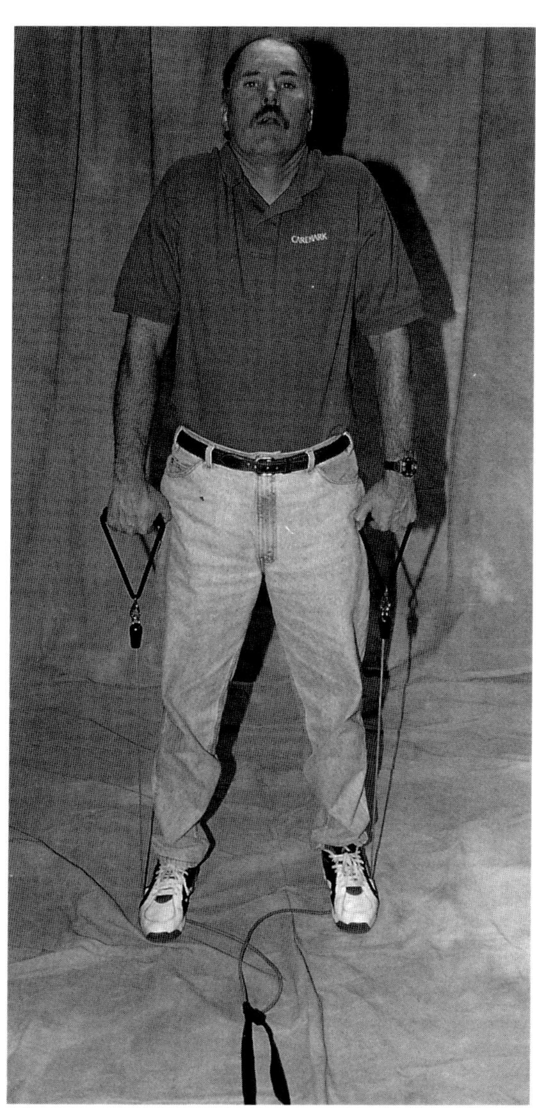

Figure 24-13. Shoulder shrugs.

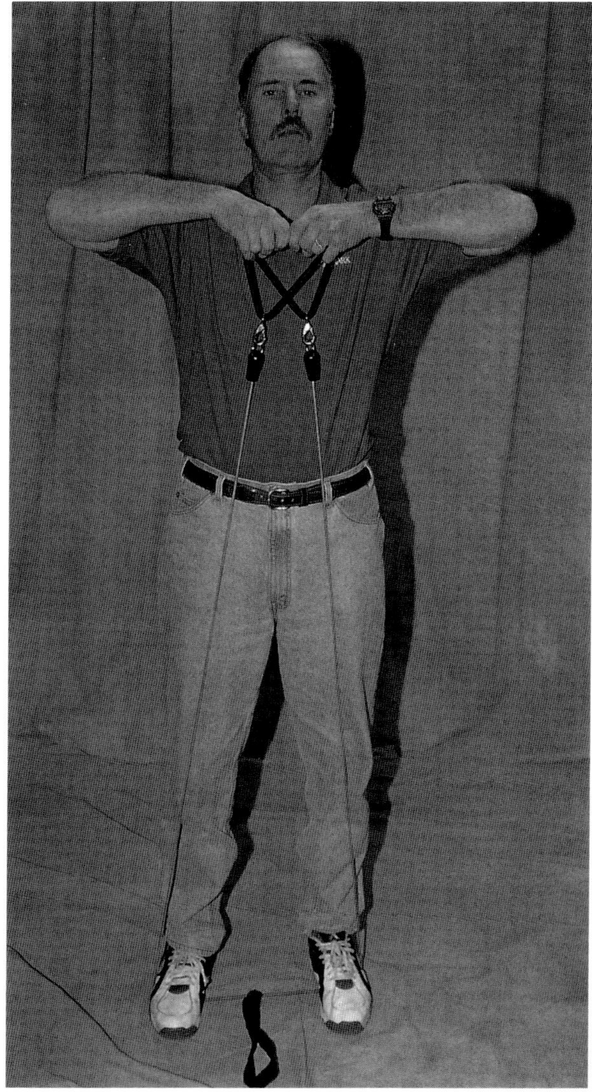

Figure 24-14. Upright row.

must be careful to avoid the abducted position during the rehabilitation process. The amount of resistance depends on the athlete's level of conditioning and discomfort. If an exercise is painful, an attempt is made to find a portion of the range of motion that is painless.

Three specific exercises have been selected to strengthen the scapular musculature. The first is the shoulder shrug, which works the trapezius, levator scapulae, and the rhomboids. The shoulder girdle is rotated slowly in posteriorly oriented circles, with an emphasis on upright posture, slow rotation, and full scapular retraction (Fig. 24-13). The second exercise is the upright row, which works the trapezius, deltoid, biceps, and serratus anterior (Fig. 24-14). Athletes are instructed to bring the hands up only as far as shoulder level because further elevation can cause impingement. The final scapular strengthening exercise is the wide-grip seated row, which emphasizes the lower trapezius, rhomboids, and the serratus anterior (Fig. 24-15).

The latissimus dorsi has been shown to have a significant role in deceleration of the pitching arm during the follow-through phase.[4] With this in mind, we incorporate latissimus pull-downs as part of our routine conditioning and therapy program for the throwing athlete (Fig. 24-16).

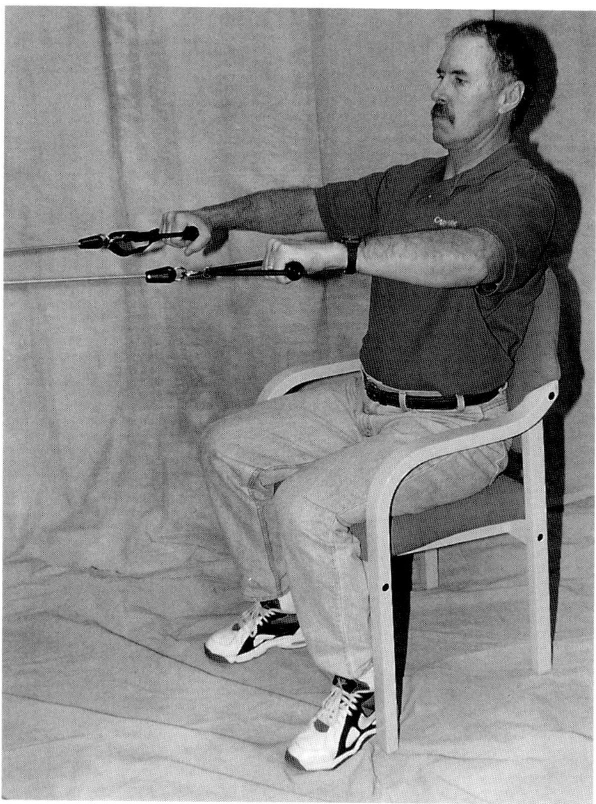

Figure 24-15. Wide-grip seated row.

Recently, we have added biceps curls to the program in response to the increasing body of evidence that the biceps is important in glenohumeral stability and deceleration of the pitching arm.

The strengthening program using the Body Lines resistance cord takes only 15 to 30 minutes for most athletes to complete, which leads to high compliance. During the first 3 weeks, the athlete performs each exercise using three sets of 10 repetitions with a 30-second rest between sets. At the 3-week mark, each set is lengthened to 25 to 30 repetitions. We have been recommending the program continue on a daily basis so it can be incorporated into the athlete's daily routine, even after resolution of the injury.

Sport-specific exercises are gradually introduced as the athlete progresses. A variable resistance cord can be attached to a baseball, football, or tennis racquet to help mimic the loads encountered during an actual throw. The athlete can gradually alter the loading rates and can start to reproduce the complex biomechanics of the sport. This component of the rehabilitation program is not initiated until the athlete is pain-free in all exercises, and normal strengthening and motion have been achieved. This phase of the program needs to be carefully supervised to ensure proper mechanics and to avoid injury. In addition to the shoulder-specific exercises outlined above, the athlete should continue with lower extremity and trunk strengthening and an aerobic program.

Many exercises have been described and implemented to rehabilitate the painful shoulder At our clinic, we see many overhead athletes, particularly throwers, who had been on programs that do not help eliminate their pain. Probably the most common problem we see in these athletes is that they have been exercising in a long lever arm position. For example, they are performing resisted abduction exercises in the coronal plane, which frequently exacerbates an impingement process. Similarly, we have found that thumbs-down supraspinatus-resistant exercises often increase shoulder pain in the overhead athlete. Many athletes insist on continuing heavy weight training with long lever arms in the abducted and forward elevated position and in the military position, often precluding them from eliminating the shoulder pain. Exercises such as flys have been known to cause rotator cuff tears, particularly on the isokinetic machinery.

As mentioned previously, the shoulder can be exercised with either open- or closed-chain activities. In the latter phases of the strengthening program, it is good to add additional closed-chain exercises. Open-chain exercises, as described earlier, using the Body Lines resistance cord facilitates dynamic control and kinesthetic awarness in the extremity. Closed-chain exercises, for example, a push-up or chin-up, stimulates glenohumeral capsular receptors to enhance static control. Closed-chain exercises may also mimic sport-specific actions such as those encountered in gymnastics.

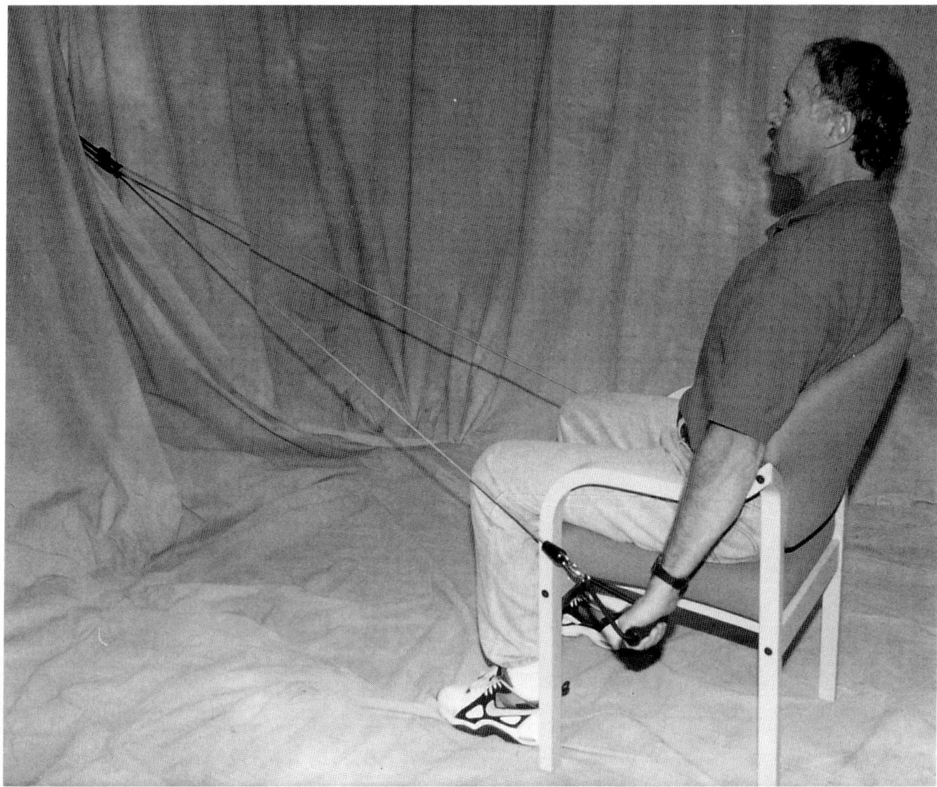

Figure 24-16. Lat pull-down.

RESISTANCE TRAINING AFTER SHOULDER REHABILITATION

Many traditional free weight and machine strengthening programs place excessive demands on the shoulder, especially in an athlete recovering from injury. We have identified several especially problematic exercises. These exercises frequently put the shoulder in a position of impingement against the coracoacromial arch and can be a source of pain and disability. Other weight training exercises place undo stress on the anterior capsular and ligamentous structures that are so commonly injured in this group of athletes. Exercises of concern in producing or exacerbating existing shoulder problems are listed in Table 24-1. We have suggested modifications or alternate exercises to avoid these problems.

The ultimate goal of a resistance training program is to produce strength, power and endurance. Generally, the athlete should begin with a low-load and a low-volume program. Emphasis is on regaining muscle endurance, along with beginning strength development. Once endurance has been achieved, more focus on strength can be incorporated. To develop the strength component, load should be increased and the number of repetitions reduced. Power is achieved by shortening the duration of the repetition. Power development is the final phase of resistance training and must be carefully monitored to avoid reinjury.

The use of isokinetic machines for rehabilitation and objective testing is somewhat controversial. Isokinetic measurement is based on a lever arm that moves at a preset speed that remains static throughout the prescribed range of motion. In skilled hands, isokinetic machines can be valuable in assessment of the athlete's progress and possibly as a rehabilitation tool itself.[24]

Table 24-1. Modifications of Strength Training

Exercise	Problem	Alternate Exercise
Wide-grip bench press	Anterior shoulder stress	Narrow-grip press
Chest flys supine	Anterior shoulder stress	Standing flys, hands in view
Military press	Impingement	Incline press, narrow grip
Triceps pull-overs	Impingement	Triceps press-downs
Lateral pull-downs— behind neck	Impingement	Lateral pull-downs— to chest
Pull-ups, behind neck	Impingement	Front Pull-ups

RETURN TO SPORT

Returning a high-performance athlete to the pre-injury level of function is the final challenge. Despite re-establishing full motion, strength, and kinematics to the shoulder, it is often difficult to take the final step to full athletic performance. Timing and determination of return to sport are critical in the overhead athlete. Throwing athletes who present with shoulder pain and go through a rehabilitation program need to be very gradually returned to their challenging endeavor so that they do not overload the shoulder and retard their ability to return to competition. The muscles and ligaments of the arm must be able to safely accommodate the stresses of throwing. This takes time and a gradual progression of the program. It is in this phase of the recovery process that plyometrics may have an important role. The plyometric program can incorporate the use of a resistance cord or a plyoball. The primary purpose of plyometric training is to increase the excitability of the muscle and joint receptors for improved response of the neuromuscular system. There is a fine line between stressing the periarticular tissues to initiate positive adaptive changes and overstressing them leading to re-injury.

Several ''interval programs'' have been devised to systematically stress the shoulder complex while the athlete is performing sport-specific activities.[23] These programs dictate the length, frequency, and intensity of the overhead throw. Interval programs can also be designed for non-throwing sports such as tennis or golf. The final criteria for return to competitive play includes full pain-free motion and strength and pain-free graduation through the interval program.

SUMMARY

The unique demands on the shoulder particularly by the throwing athlete place him or her at high risk for overuse and overloading of the soft tissues about the shoulder. The overhead throw or tennis serve produces enormous angular velocities about the shoulder joint. The manager, trainer, and physician need to have a good understanding of the basic biomechanics of the sport. This knowledge will aid in recognition, prevention, and treatment of injury. Team physicians need to familiarize themselves with the spectrum of pathology inherent to the shoulder in the overhead athlete.

This chapter has discussed problems unique to overhead athletes, basic principles of shoulder rehabilitation. A rehabilitation and return-to-sport program based on these principles has been described.

REFERENCES

1. Andrews JR, Carson WG, McLeod WD: Glenoid labrum tears related to the long head of the biceps. Am J Sports Med 13:337, 1985
2. Brown LP, Niehues SSL, Harrah A et al: Upper extremity range of motion and isokinetic strength of the internal and external rotators in major league baseball pitchers. Am J Sports Med 16:577, 1988
3. Chinn JC, Priest JD, Kent BE: Upper extremity range of motion, grip strength and girth in highly skilled tennis players. Phys Ther 54:474, 1988
4. Dillman CJ, Fleisig GS, Werner SL, Andrews JR: Biomechanics of the shoulder in sports: throwing activities. In Postgraduate Advances in Sports Medicine. Forum Medicum, Inc., 1991
5. Drez D: Therapeutic Modalities for Sports Injuries. Mosby Year Book, St. Louis, 1989
6. Engle RP: Proprioceptive neuromuscular facilitation for the shoulder. p. 451. In Andrews JR, Wilk KE (eds): The Athlete's Shoulder. Churchill Livingstone, New York, 1994
7. Gainor BJ, Piotrowski G, Puhl J et al: The throw: biomechanics and acute injury. Am J Sports Med 8:114, 1980
8. Harryman DT II, Sidles JA, Clark JM et al: Translation of the humeral head on the glenoid with passive glenohumeral motion. J Bone Joint Surg [Am] 72:1334, 1990
9. Hawkins RJ, Kennedy JC: Impingement syndrome in athletes. Am J Sports Med 8:151, 1980
10. Jobe CM, Sidles J: Evidence for a superior glenoid impingement upon the rotator cuff, abstracted. J Shoulder Elbow Surg 2:64, 1993
11. Jobe FW, Moynes DR, Tibone JE, Perry J: An EMG analysis of the shoulder in pitching: a second report. Am J Sports Med 12:218, 1984
12. Jobe FW, Tibone JE, Jobe CM, Kvitne RS: The shoulder in sports. p. 961–90. In Rockwood CA, Matsen FA III (eds): The Shoulder. WB Saunders, Philadelphia, 1990
13. Kibler BW, McQueen C, Uhl T: Fitness evaluations and fitness findings in competitive junior tennis players. Clin Sports Med 7:403, 1988
14. King JW, Brelsford HJ, Tullos HS: Analysis of the pitching arm of the professional baseball pitcher. Clin Orthop 67:16, 1969
15. Neer CS, Walsh RP: The shoulder in sports. Orthop Clin North Am 8:583, 1977
16. Newton R: Joint receptor contributions to reflexive and kinesthetic response. Phys Ther 62:22, 1982
17. Pappas AM, Zawacki RM, McCarthy CF: Rehabilitation of the pitching shoulder. Am J Sports Med 13:223, 1985
18. Rodosky MW, Harner CD, Fu FH: The role of the long head of the biceps muscle and superior glenoid labrum in anterior stability of the shoulder. Am J Sports Med 22:121, 1994
19. Snyder SJ: SLAP lesions of the shoulder. Arthroscopy 6:274, 1990
20. Townsend H, Jobe FW, Pink M, Perry J: Electromyographic analysis of the glenohumeral muscles during a baseball rehabilitation program. Am J Sports Med 19:264, 1991.
21. Turkel SJ, Panio MW, Marshall JL, Girgis FG: Stabilizing

mechanisms preventing anterior dislocation of the glenohumeral joint. J Bone Joint Surg [Am] 63:1208, 1981

22. Walch G, Liotard JP, Boileau P, Noel E: Postero-superior glenoid impingement in the throwing athlete. Paper presented at the 5th International Conference on Surgery of the Shoulder, Paris, 1992
23. Wilk KE, Arrigo CA: Interval sport programs for the shoulder. p. 669. In Andrews JR, Wilk KE (eds): The Athlete's Shoulder. Churchill Livingstone, New York, 1994
24. Wilk KE, Arrigo CA, Andrews JR: Standardized isokinetic testing protocol for the throwing shoulder: the thrower's series. Isokinetics Exerc Sci 1:63, 1991

TWENTY-FIVE

Conditioning and Training Techniques

Kevin E. Wilk

Conditioning exercises and drills have been an accepted form of training in preparation for sporting events since the ancient Greek Olympics. In fact, thousands of years ago, Milo of Croton began his daily routine of lifting a baby bull until it was fully grown.[13] This was the earliest description of progressive resistance exercise. It has long been believed that athletes who have superior training and conditioning are stronger, better skilled, and less prone to injury. Conditioning drills have played a significant role in sports, particularly in track and field, long-distance running, and swimming. Much of the impetus for improved conditioning techniques and enhanced performance emerged during the 1950s.[16] During that time interval, training was introduced.[16] Roger Bannister broke the 4-minute-mile barrier; also, several other performance barriers were cracked. Bannister's accomplishment came as a result of a careful and scientific approach to conditioning. Thus, strength training became a part of the preparation and conditioning of several amateur and professional athletes. In the early 1960s, conditioning coaches were added to the professional football coaching staffs.[12] But not until more recently (mid-1980s) was conditioning appreciated by the baseball community as a whole.[12] This chapter discusses the basic elements and principles of a conditioning program for the overhead athlete, particularly the baseball player. Also, the concepts of performance, periodization, and specific conditioning drills are thoroughly described.

Optimum athletic performance requires two complementary abilities: skill and power.[6,7] All sports from basketball to baseball share these two elements. Skill is derived from the individual's own attributes (natural ability) and learned technical skill as well as expertise. The learned portion of the skill equation takes years of training to develop. It requires hard work, determination, and guidance/direction from a qualified coach. One of the cornerstones of conditioning is the law of specificity, or the SAID principle, which states the body will make specific adaptations to imposed demands.

Muscular power is derived from both natural ability and developed muscular characteristics. Power is a component of muscular strength but adds the additional element of time. Thus, power is defined as total work divided by time. Therefore, power combines both strength and speed. In athletes, explosive strength is often used synonymously with the term *power*. Traditional weight training can develop strength, but another form of training is required to develop explosiveness or speed. *Speed* refers to the ability of the athlete to rapidly contract a muscle or muscle group. One component of speed is *acceleration,* which describes how quickly the golf club accelerates as it approaches the ball or how rapidly the arm moves during the throwing motion. The importance of speed and acceleration in athletics is obvious. Plyometrics or stretch-shortening exercises are one form of conditioning drills that can develop this type of explosive power and speed. Plyometrics is defined and thoroughly discussed later in this chapter.

Before discussing the conditioning program for the overhead athlete, first we need to define and discuss some commonly used terms that are components of a conditioning program. Each of these components can be developed in a different manner and with a varying degree of emphasis, depending on the sport, position, and physical abilities of the athlete relative to the demands of the sport. Each of these components is a dependent variable and cannot be considered as an isolated independent variable.[12]

Strength is the ability to exert force during a maximum voluntary contraction. Strength enhancement can occur by either increasing the cross-sectional area of the muscle or by enhancing neuromuscular recruitment. Strength can be measured by many types of muscular contractions, including isometric, isotonic concentric, isotonic eccentric, and isokinetic contractions. It appears that there is no positive correlation between these types of contractions.[2] The upper extremity athlete in most cases cannot afford excessive muscular hypertrophy (size) due to loss of flexibility and motion. Therefore, the overhead athlete must be strong but not bulky. Strength can be also subdivided into two components: (1) static strength, meaning muscular tension can be applied without movement or little movement, and (2) dynamic strength, referring to the application of force through a range of motion. The overhead athlete must exhibit strength components, static for joint stability and dynamic to produce powerful movements.

Endurance is work capacity. The equation for work is force times distance. More practically, it is the capacity to resist fatigue. This is a cumulative process of training that incorporates the ability to recover adequately before performing the next training session or competition. Because the shoulder complex relies greatly on muscle to provide stability through static muscular strength, endurance for the overhead athlete is critical in maintaining dynamic joint stability.

Muscular power is the ability to perform work divided by time. Power is dependent on the central nervous system to ensure a high frequency of firing through the motor neurons and a high degree of motor unit recruitment.[12] Power is a key element to any athlete, particularly the thrower, tennis player, or swimmer.

Plyometrics are exercise drills that use a stretch (eccentric contraction) before a concentric contraction (shortening) to enhance explosive power.[24] Plyometrics are specific drills for the enhancement of power, motor unit recruitment, and dynamic flexibility. The key for most sporting activities is power, explosiveness power, and not strength. For example, while pitching a baseball, the delivery phase takes approximately 0.143 seconds.[10] Therefore, it is imperative for the thrower to generate the highest possible force in the shortest possible time. This is a classic example of power. The tennis player during a serve cocks the arm back to create a stretch on the shoulder adductor/internal rotator muscle groups. This type of activity stimulates the muscle spindle (stretch) and thus produces an enhanced concentric shortening contraction that is explosive and powerful.[24] Plyometric training can be used to produce this effect. All sport movements evolve this stretch-shortening muscular cycle to produce muscular power.

Speed is the ability for the body or body part to more through space in the least amount of time. Speed is an important element in many sports; however, in the overhead athlete speed is also important, but deceleration is even more critical to prevent arm injuries. The relationship between strength and speed is not fully understood at this time, particularly when there is little resistance applied to the limb.

Flexibility is the ability to move a joint or muscle through its entire range of motion while maintaining continuity of the joint/muscle. Adequate flexibility is vital for the overhead athlete. The overhead athlete must be loose enough to perform the dynamic motions required while exhibiting dynamic joint stability. The overhead athlete exhibits tremendous shoulder motion; this may contribute to many muscular and joint injuries.

Neuromuscular control is the ability to move through space and function within the environment while maintaining dynamic joint stability.[21] Thus, it is the athlete/patient's ability to recognize joint position (proprioception/kinesthesia), maintain shoulder stability through the cocontraction of various shoulder muscles, and dynamically move the limb through space.[21] In the case of the baseball pitcher, arm acceleration occurs at 7,000 degrees per second and with large forces; therefore, the glenohumeral joint muscles must function to propel the arm while stabilizing the shoulder to prevent subluxation.

BASIC CONDITIONING PRINCIPLES

Several basic principles are used when designing the conditioning program for the overhead athlete. These principles should be adhered to by the athlete and conditioning specialist.

1. *The entire body should be conditioned, not just the arm.* Over 52 percent of the kinetic energy in the baseball throw is generated by the legs and trunk.[17] The athlete must train the trunk and legs to produce axial rotation and energy and transfer this explosive power to the arm.
2. *The large muscles propel and small muscles decelerate/stabilize.* The large muscles (latissimus dorsi and pectoralis major) are the acceleration muscles during the throwing act whereas the smaller muscles (infraspinatus/teres minor) decelerate the arm. The rotator cuffs and the deltoid form several force couples and act to stabilize the glenohumeral joint.[20,22] The exercise program should train each of these muscles specifically in the fashion they must function, thus utilizing the SAID principle of conditioning.
3. *The arm should be trained through the hips/legs.* The legs and hips drive the arm through the trunk. The energy is generated in the legs and hips and transferred up to the shoulders. Thus, training a rotational component at the hips can serve to enhance arm speed. This concept is true for golf and tennis, as well as baseball.
4. *An athlete should train for performance—not work capacity.* Quality of effort, intensity, and correct execution of every drill should be emphasized to maximize the effects of the exercise. An athlete should not train to merely fatigue the muscle or to get stronger.[12]
5. *Proximal stability must be established for distal mobility.* The core of the body must provide a stable base and correct postural alignment.[21] The core of the body includes the hips, waist, abdominal area, and scapula. Weak core stability will predispose the athlete to shoulder injury because greater stresses will be applied to the shoulder in an attempt to stabilize it during functional activities. Core stability and dynamic joint stability must be established before incorporat-

ing sport-specific training drills. Also, adequate scapular stability allows a normal length-tension relationship of the glenohumeral musculature, which enhances muscular performance and may diminish musculotendinous injuries.

6. *An athlete should train for muscular balance.* Muscular balance entails bilateral, antagonist to agonist, and proximal to distal balance.[12] In the overhead athlete, it is common to emphasize merely the throwing arm or the posterior rotator cuff muscles. The nonthrowing arm acts to generate axial rotation to create throwing arm speed; therefore, bilateral arm strength is vital. Also, balance between the posterior and anterior cuff muscles is imperative to both prevent injury and provide adequate joint stability.[20]
7. *Strength training is emphasized before power or endurance.* A base level of strength must be achieved before power drills or muscular endurance exercises can be successfully initiated. I emphasize static muscular strength before dynamic strength, then the development of endurance speed and power.
8. *Isolated movement patterns strengthen weak muscles; combined movement patterns re-establish functional activities.* Isolated movement patterns, such as resisted shoulder abduction or resisted external rotation, are used to strengthen a particular muscle that is weak. Combined movement patterns, such as simulating the throwing motion, strengthen the overall pattern; however, strong muscles can substitute for weak ones. Therefore, if the clinician identifies a weak muscle or muscle group, isolated movements should be performed first to strengthen it before proceeding to combined movement patterns to reinforce/establish an overall functional movement pattern.
9. *Fundamental movement skills should be established before specific sport skills.* The athlete must possess a degree of fundamental movement skills, locomotion, stability, and coordination before very specific sport skills are performed. The athlete who grows up specializing in one sport has a tendency to be very limited in other movement skills.[12] Athletes who participate in other sports or other conditioning drills (cross-train) tend to be "better athletes."[12] Therefore, it is preferred to establish fundamental movement skills before the development and implementation of a sport-specific conditioning program.
10. *The program should be sport-specific but should use cross-training principles.* Many athletes make the mistake of merely skill training for one particular sport. Often these athletes find themselves peaking out, unable to advance to the next level, and may, in fact, be prone to injury or tissue breakdown. Thus, one technique to counteract this training mistake is to cross-train. By using the participation of other sports that emphasize similar desirable goals, such as speed or agility, the athlete may obtain peak performance without the boredom of continuous training.
11. *Conditioning is year-round but must be periodized.* The conditioning program for the athlete must be a year-round commitment. The conditioning program should not be initiated just 4 weeks before the season starts; this will lead to injury, tissue breakdown, and diminished performance. The program should use the concept of periodization.[14] This concept is thoroughly discussed later in this chapter.
12. *Basic conditioning principles are the building blocks to the highly skilled athlete.* The athlete should condition to participate in sports but not play to condition. These basic conditioning principles should be used to enhance performance and prevent injury.

The major objectives of the conditioning program for the overhead athlete are injury prevention and performance enhancement. These two objectives are closely related to each other. A thorough, well-designed conditioning program will prevent injuries; a healthy athlete who trains properly should improve athletic performance and experience a long productive career. The conditioning program for the overhead athlete (baseball pitcher, tennis) should include the previously discussed components: strength, endurance, power, plyometrics, speed, flexibility, and skill training. The athlete who trains or overemphasizes one component more than another, such as strength or power, is prone to injury or diminished performance. Also, the athlete cannot train at the same level throughout the year; rather, the program must be specifically adjusted over the course of a year. Therefore, the conditioning program should exhibit in-season and off-season goals and guidelines. The adjustment of the program throughout the year is referred to as "periodization of training."[14]

The concept of periodization refers to the year-round sequence and progression of weight resistance training and skill training of the athlete. The periodization model specifies various phases during the year; most often, the program will use four specific and different training seasons existing during the calendar year (Table 25-1). These four seasons are the competition phase, postcompetition (second-transition) phase, preparation phase, and first-transition phase. Also, the program is based on controlling and adjust-

Table 25-1. Conditioning Program

Phase I
In-season training
Competitive season
6 months
April–October
Phase II
Postseason training
6–8 weeks
October, November
Phase III
Preparation phase
Off-season
12–14 weeks
December, January, February
Phase IV
First-transition phase
4–6 weeks
March, April

ing three variables: volume of work, intensity of effort, and skill technique training.[14] As illustrated in Figure 25-1, volume and technique are inversely related, whereas intensity and technique are directly related. In some year-round sports such as professional tennis, golf, or swimming, this concept is difficult to use. In these sports, often the athletes are expected to perform at a high level for 10 to 11 months. This is not realistic and cannot be accomplished for a long period of time or over a career. Usually, these athletes exhibit peaks and valleys during the year and their careers.

The conditioning program and sport-specific drills should change based on the time of the year. The objectives of using the periodization model are to (1) control peaking of athletic abilities at the proper time, (2) prevent the athlete from being untrained or under trained at the beginning of the season, and (3) prevent the athlete from overtraining (i.e., training at a high intensity for a long duration). All three of these scenarios can and often do lead to injuries. Also, they may all be reasons for diminished athletic performance.

We have modified the original concept of periodization and applied it to the baseball pitcher. Table 25-2 illustrates a typical program for the throwing athlete. The program is subdivided into four seasons (phases), each possessing it own goals as well as conditioning and skill exercises. This program is discussed as it relates to the throwing athlete.

There are four phases in the baseball pitcher's periodization model, which we have arbitrarily labeled 1 to 4. The 11- to 12-month program is described.

During the off-season, there are three phases: two phases before the season and one postseason phase. The first phase before the season is considered the preparation phase. For most professional baseball players, the competitive season usually ends the first week of October. Immediately after the season, this phase is referred to as the postseason training phase (second transition) and lasts approximately 6 to 8 weeks. The goals during this phase are mental and physical recuperation, soft tissue healing, and remaining physically active without baseball-related activities. During this phase, cardiovascular conditioning is emphasized with aerobic capacity training, and no skill training related to the athlete's particular sport is performed. We encourage athletes to perform low-intensity/long-duration conditioning activities, such as bicycling, swimming, and jogging, along with participation in recreational sports such as golf or tennis. The emphasis of this phase is aerobic capacity, general fitness, and body weight maintenance.

The first preparation phase begins approximately the day after Thanksgiving or December 1 and lasts 12 to 14 weeks. During this phase, the athlete begins to condition and prepare for sport-specific drills. The volume/quantity of exercise is high while intensity is moderate and skill training is relatively low. The goals of this phase are to increase the exercise demands gradually and progressively, beginning with light isotonic concentric work and progressing to isotonic eccentric, and eventually plyometrics. Baseball-

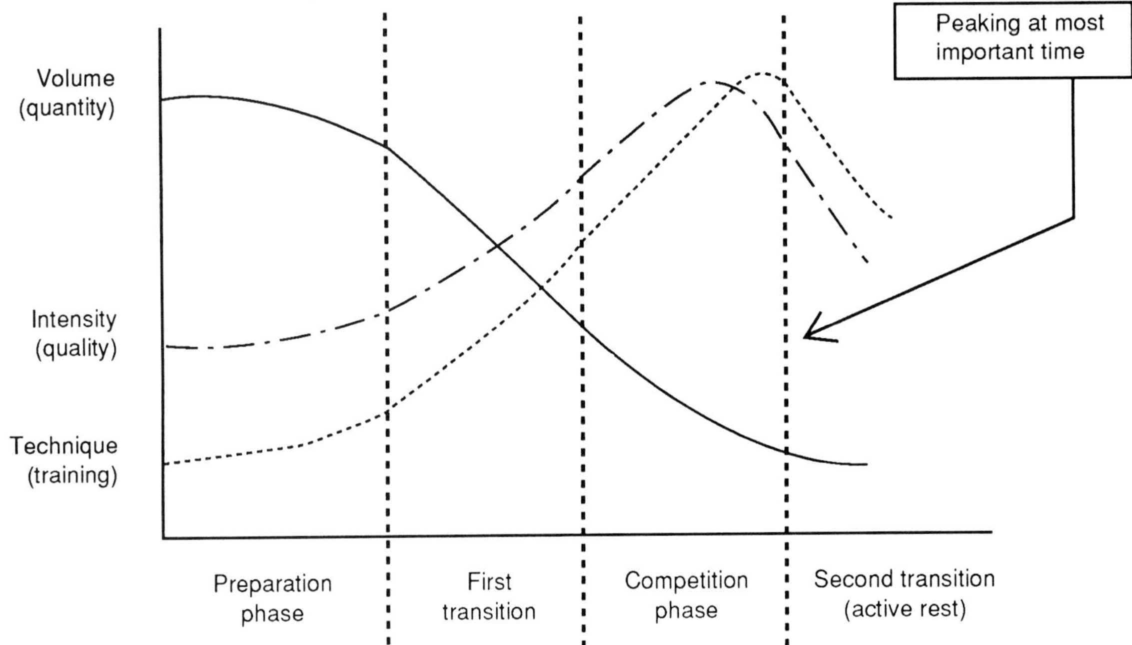

Figure 25-1. Relationship between volume, intensity, and technique. Volume refers to the amount of work performed (sets, reps, etc.); intensity, to the quality of effort; and technique, to the activity or skill.

Table 25-2. Concept of Periodization in Baseball

	Goals	Conditioning Exercises	Skill Training Activities
In season training "Competitive season" (6 months)	Maintain strength, power, endurance to prevent arm injuries Prevent the breakdown of tissue Maintain cardiovascular endurance	Low weight/moderate number of repetitions per exercise: thrower's 10 exercise program Cardiovascular endurance 20–30 minutes daily to maintain fitness level/stamina training	Continue throwing activities to maintain proper throwing mechanics and refinement of pitches Throwing program is designed to emphasize the player's position Throwing/batting activities (volume) regulated by player's health status
Postseason training "Active-rest" (2 months)	Mental and physical recuperation period Physical activity, but not baseball-type activities Allow tissues to heal Relaxation sports participation	Light conditioning program—bicycle, swimming, walking, jogging, aerobics Conditioning low intensity/long duration	No baseball-related drills Relaxation sports, such as golf, tennis, racquetball
Preparation phase "Off-season" (10–12 weeks)	Gradually and progressively increase exercise demands—throwing exercises and drills Begin with light isotonic program; progress to eccentric and plyometric exercises Skill training is low to start with and throwing begins halfway through this phase *Ultimate goal* is be *in condition* for spring training reporting date	Total body exercise program with emphasis on large muscle groups Moderate weight/moderate repetitive numbers to start with; isotonic concentric Progress program to eccentric program; progress to moderate weight/increase repetitions Cardiovascular training is emphasized—30 minutes/daily to enhance fitness level Plyometric training drills initiated 2–3 weeks before spring training	Initially no skill training 4–5 weeks into program, throwing program is initiated; interval long-toss program Batting practice initiated 4–5 weeks into phase
First transitional phase "Spring training" (4–6 weeks)	Enhance conditioning level and enhance skill training (razor sharp) Initially high-volume conditioning, moderate-level skill training Then moderate-level conditioning, high-level skill training	Volume of conditioning drills is high at start of phase and sharply decreases halfway through Intensity of training and quality of movements is fine-tuned Plyometrics early phase, then discontinued Thrower's 10 program	Skill technique training is emphasized Throwing/batting activities are emphasized; these skill activities are fine-tuned

related drills (skill training) are low at the start but gradually increase halfway through the program. The ultimate goal of this phase is to obtain an optimal level of fitness when the athlete reports to spring training.

We subdivide this first preparation phase into two stages of 6 to 7 weeks. During the first stage, the emphasis is placed on total body conditioning and strengthening of the larger muscle groups, such as the latissimus dorsi, pectoralis major, subscapularis, deltoid, gluteal, quadriceps, hamstrings, and biceps/triceps brachii. The athlete will perform exercises such as rowing, pull-downs, push-ups, bench press, military press, half squats, and lunges. Also, if the athlete has exhibited rotator cuff weakness during the preconditioning program or isokinetic testing, specific cuff strengthening exercises will also be used. Rhythmic stabilization (RS) drills will be performed against manual resistance to enhance dynamic stabilization of the glenohumeral and scapula-thoracic musculature. The stabilization exercises performed include proprioceptive neuromuscular facilitation D_2 flexion/extension patterns (Fig. 25-2), external/internal rotation RS in both the scapular plane and 90/90 position (Fig. 25-3), and scapula-thoracic RS drills (Fig. 25-4). Also, during this phase, the athlete stretches to maintain flexibility and performs some type of cardiovas-

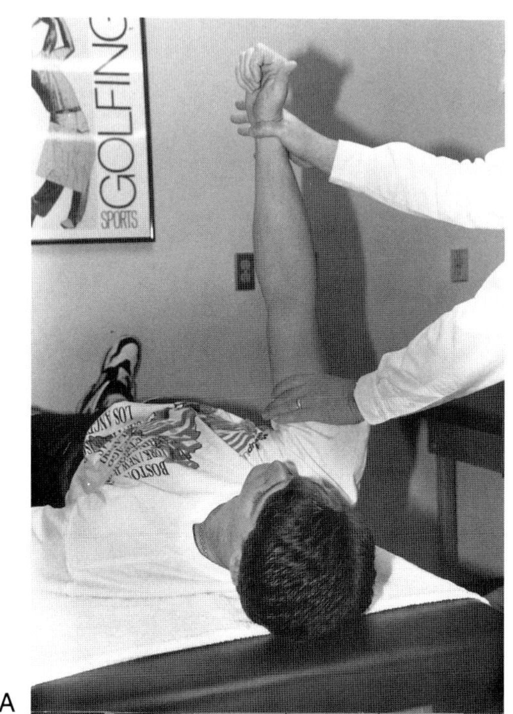

A

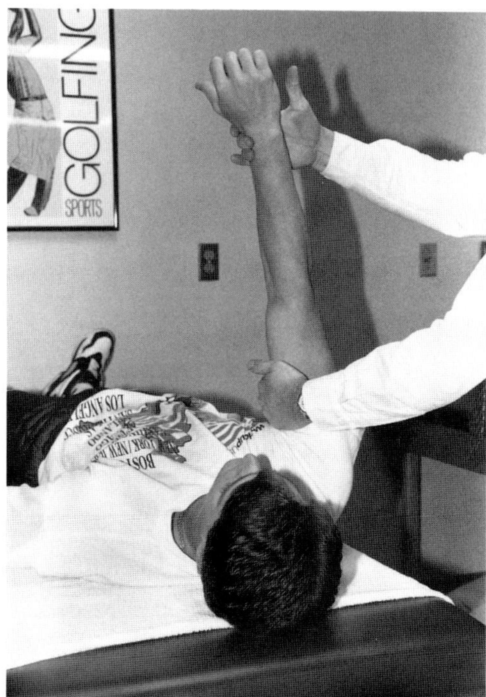

B

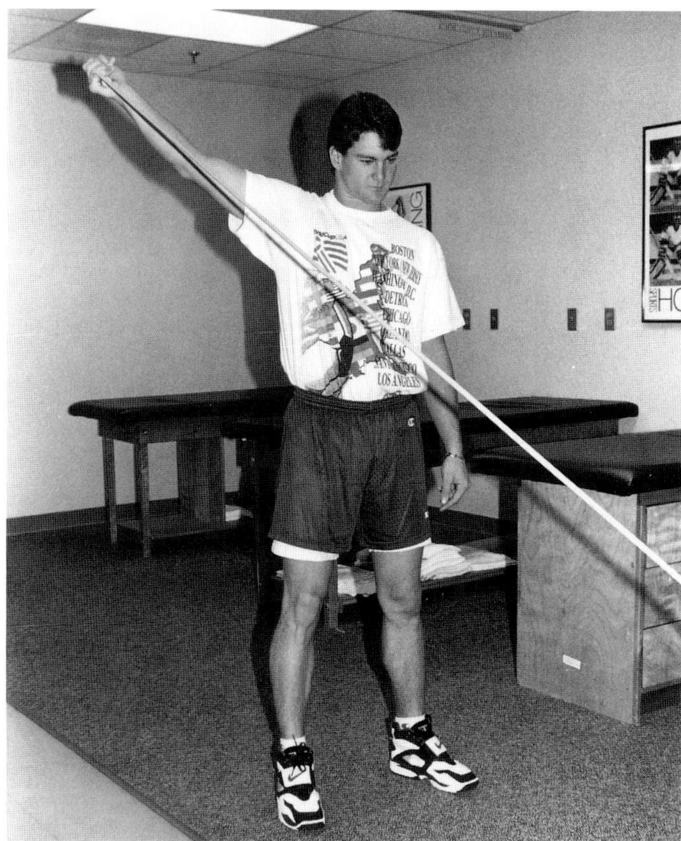

C

Figure 25-2. Exercises to promote dynamic shoulder stability: rhythmic stabilization drills during D_2 flexion/extension proprioceptive neuromuscular facilitation (PNF) exercises. (**A**) The patient statically holds arm at 90 degrees flexion as he externally rotates and (**B**) internally rotates against manual resistance. These static holds are performed at 30, 60, and 90 degrees of flexion. (**C**) PNF drills with exercise tubing.

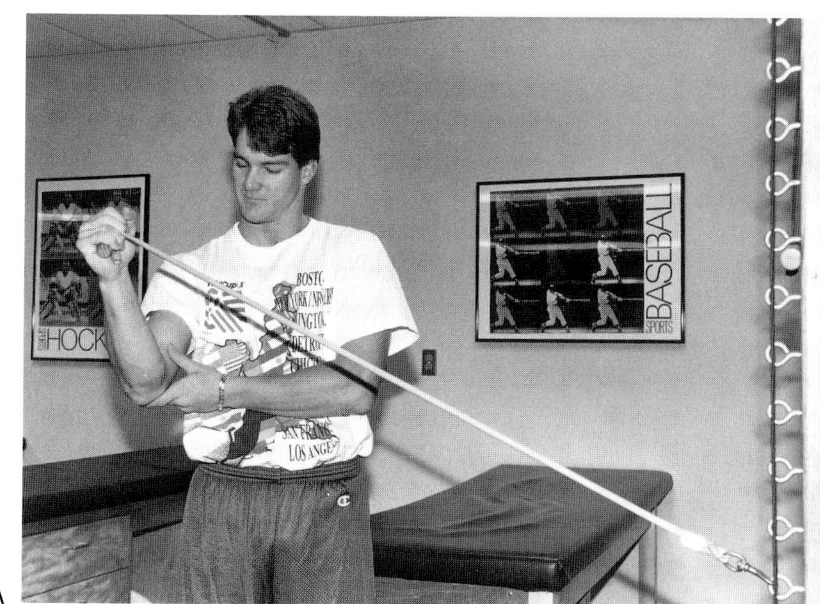

A

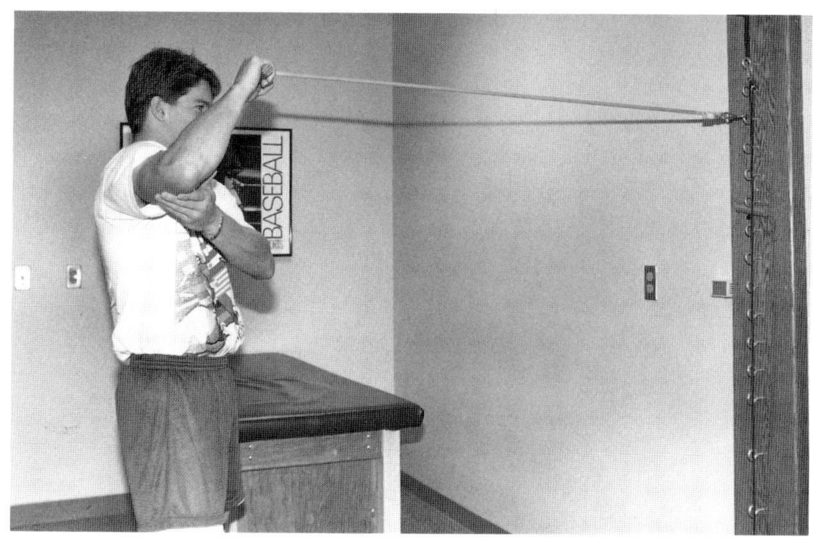

B

Figure 25-3. External rotation strengthening exercises using exercise tubing. (**A**) Performed in the scapular plane of shoulder and at (**B**) 90 degrees of shoulder abduction and 90 degrees of elbow flexion (90/90 position).

A

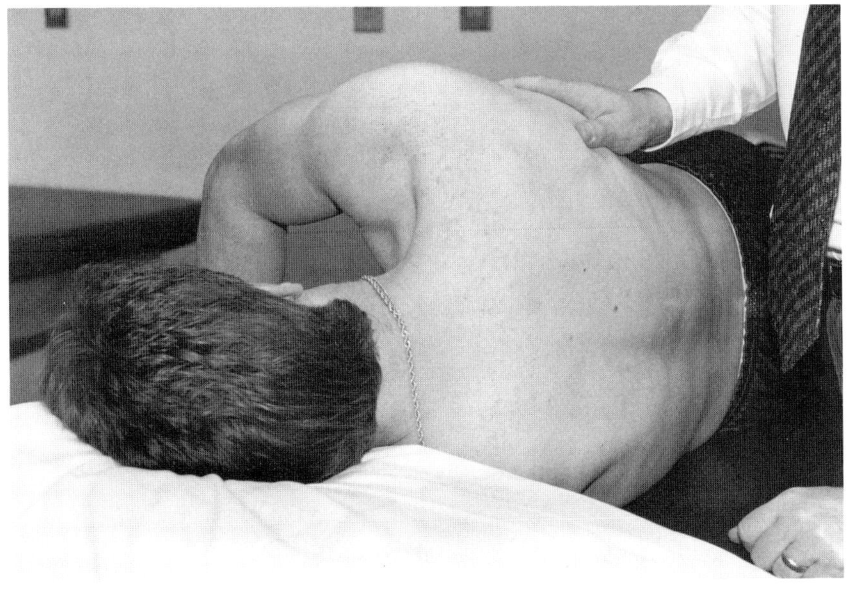

B

Figure 25-4. (**A & B**) Neuromuscular control drills for the scapulothoracic joint. These drills are performed against manual resistance, and the patient is asked to slowly elevate/depress the scapula, then to slowly retract/protract the scapula. The purpose of this exercise drill is to isolate the scapulothoracic musculature and enhance the patient's proprioceptive ability of this joint.

cular exercise for 25 to 30 minutes. Core stability and balance are emphasized through balance drills on a balance board and beam. The pitcher is asked to maintain the balance position of windup on the balance beam or board (Fig. 25-5). Also, the thrower may practice lateral movements, side stepping, throws to first base in this balance position, and other balance drills to enhance core stability (Fig. 25-6).

During the second stage of the first preparation phase, the goals are to improve rotator cuff strength, initiate eccentric/plyometric drills, and initiate light throwing and hitting drills. During this 6 to 7-week phase, the throwing athlete is established on our throwers' 10 exercise program (Fig. 25-7). Plyometric drills specific for the thrower (Figs. 25-8 to 25-12 and a throwing program are also implemented. The throwing program begins with our long-toss program progressing to 120 to 150 feet, then initiates a throwing program from the mound[19] (Table 25-3 and Fig. 25-13). A complete plyometric program for both pitching and hitting is outlined in Tables 25-4 and 25-5. During this second stage, the intensity and skill-specific training aspects are increasing as the volume of exercise is decreasing (Table 25-2).

The next preparation is often referred to as the first transitional phase, and in baseball this is spring training. This phase consists of 4 to 6 weeks of conditioning and skill training, preparing the player for the competitive season. The goals of this phase are to enhance the conditioning level and skill level of the athlete, along with sport-specific training to become mentally and physically prepared for the upcoming season. During this conditioning phase, the level of conditioning exercises is gradually decreased while the quality of work performed and the amount of skill training is rapidly increased, maintaining the inverse relationship between volume and technique. Plyometrics drills can be used early in this phase, but as the competitive season approaches, these drills should decrease. During spring training, the goal is not to achieve peak performance;

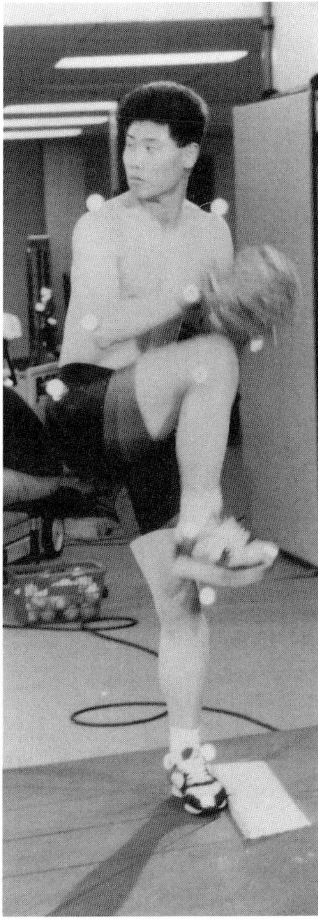

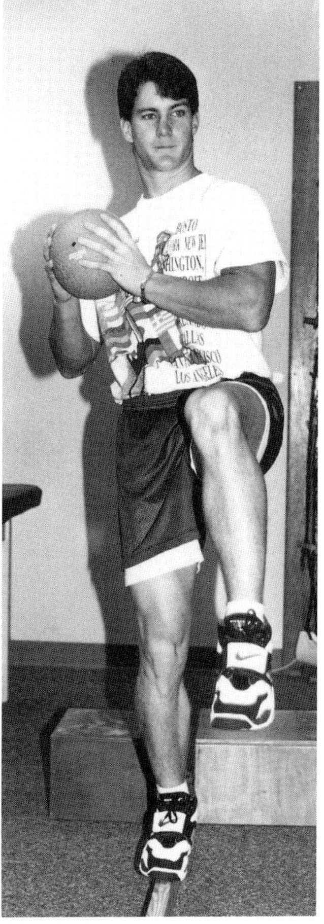

Figure 25-5. (**A**) The balance position during the windup phase in baseball throwing. (**B**) The patient performs a balance drill on a 1½-inch balance beam. The patient is asked to repeatedly balance on one foot/leg as he brings the other leg up in the balance position and holds a 5-to 7-lb ball.

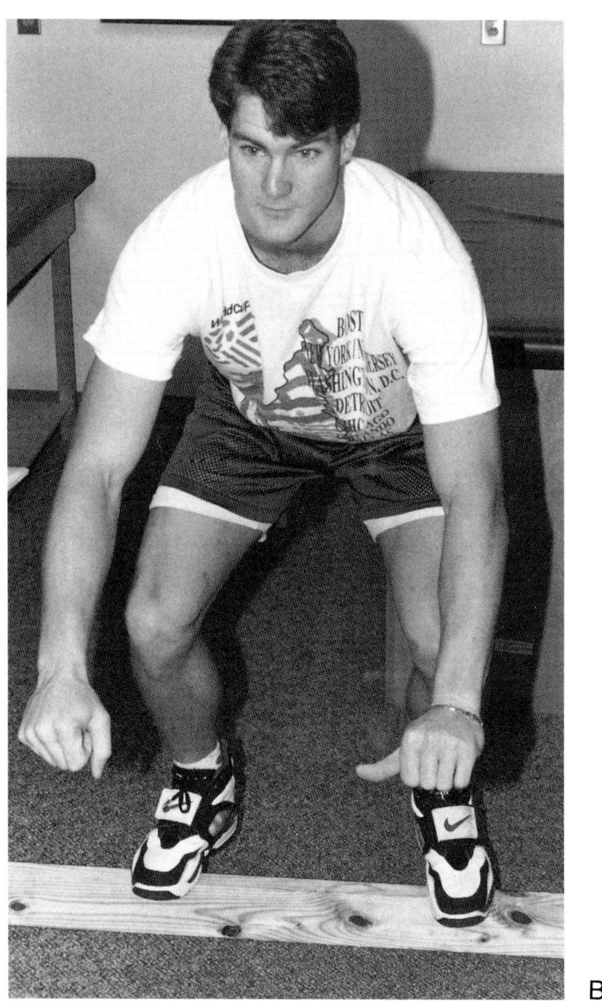

A

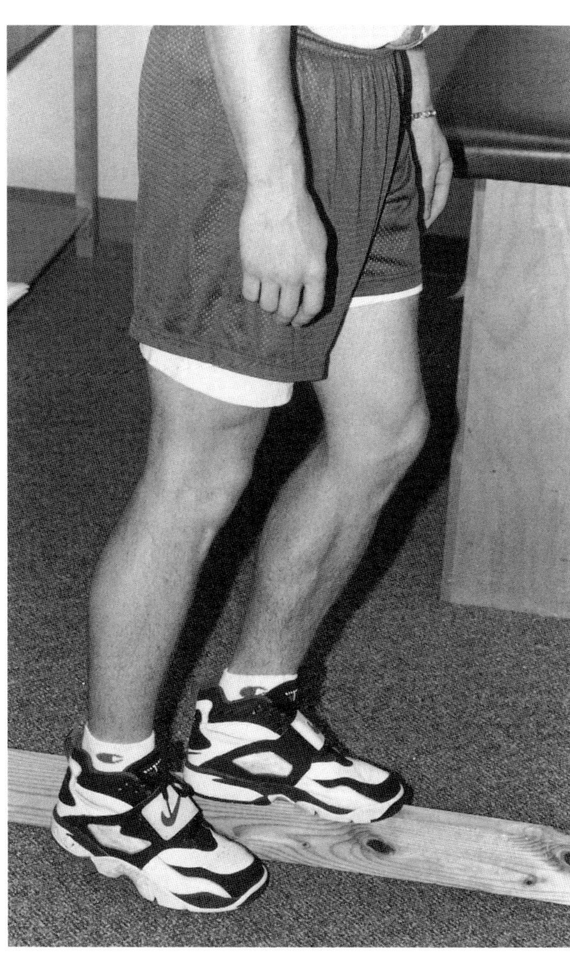

B

Figure 25-6. Core stability and balance drills. (**A**) Squats performed on a balance beam. (**B**) Lateral step-up and heel to toe. The patient is asked to balance on one foot, perform a lateral step, and then place heel to opposite foot toe and perform step-up. This is performed reciprocally along an 8-foot balance beam. (*Figure continues.*)

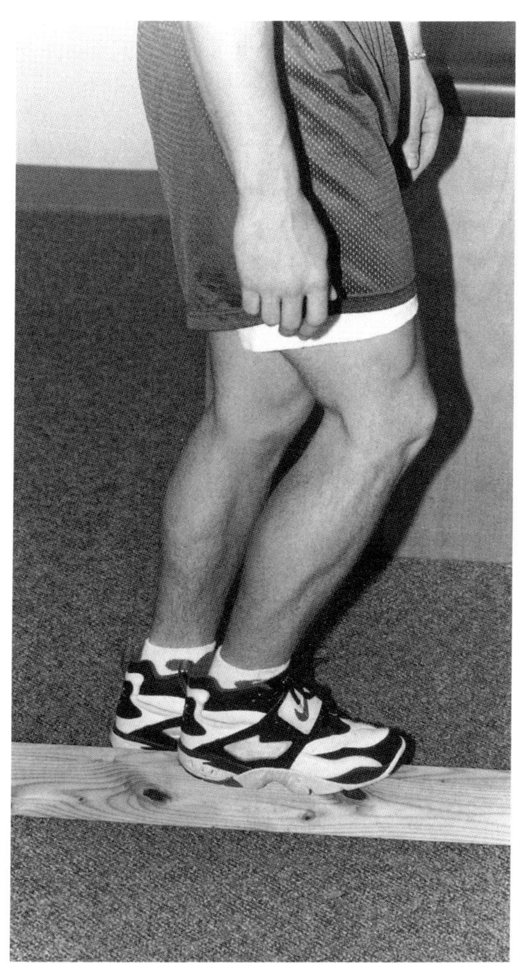

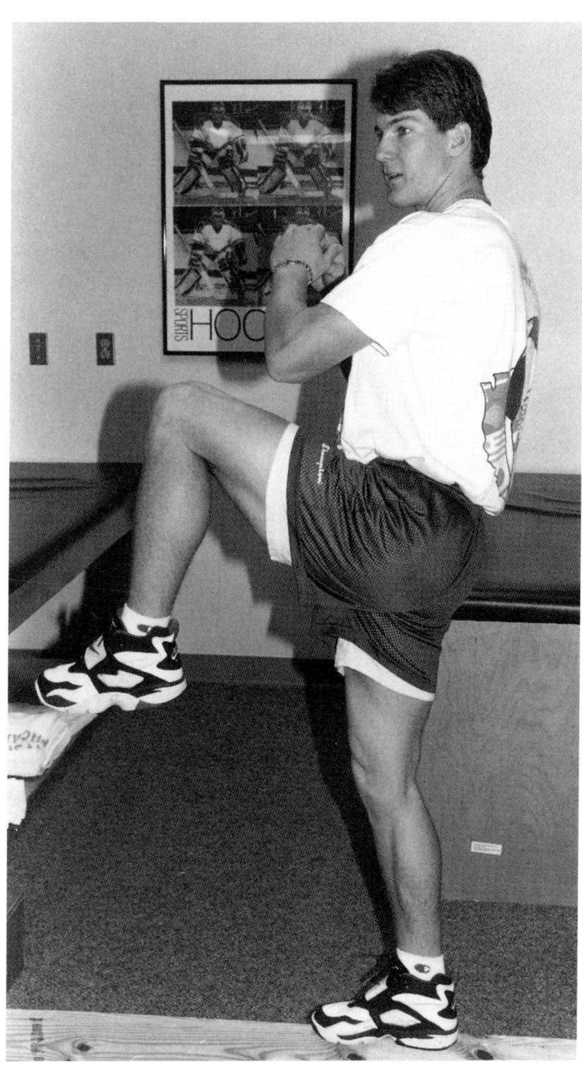

Figure 25-6 (*Continued*). (**C & D**) Balance position drill. Patient performs a 5-second hold, then is instructed to perform throw to first base on home plate through verbal command.

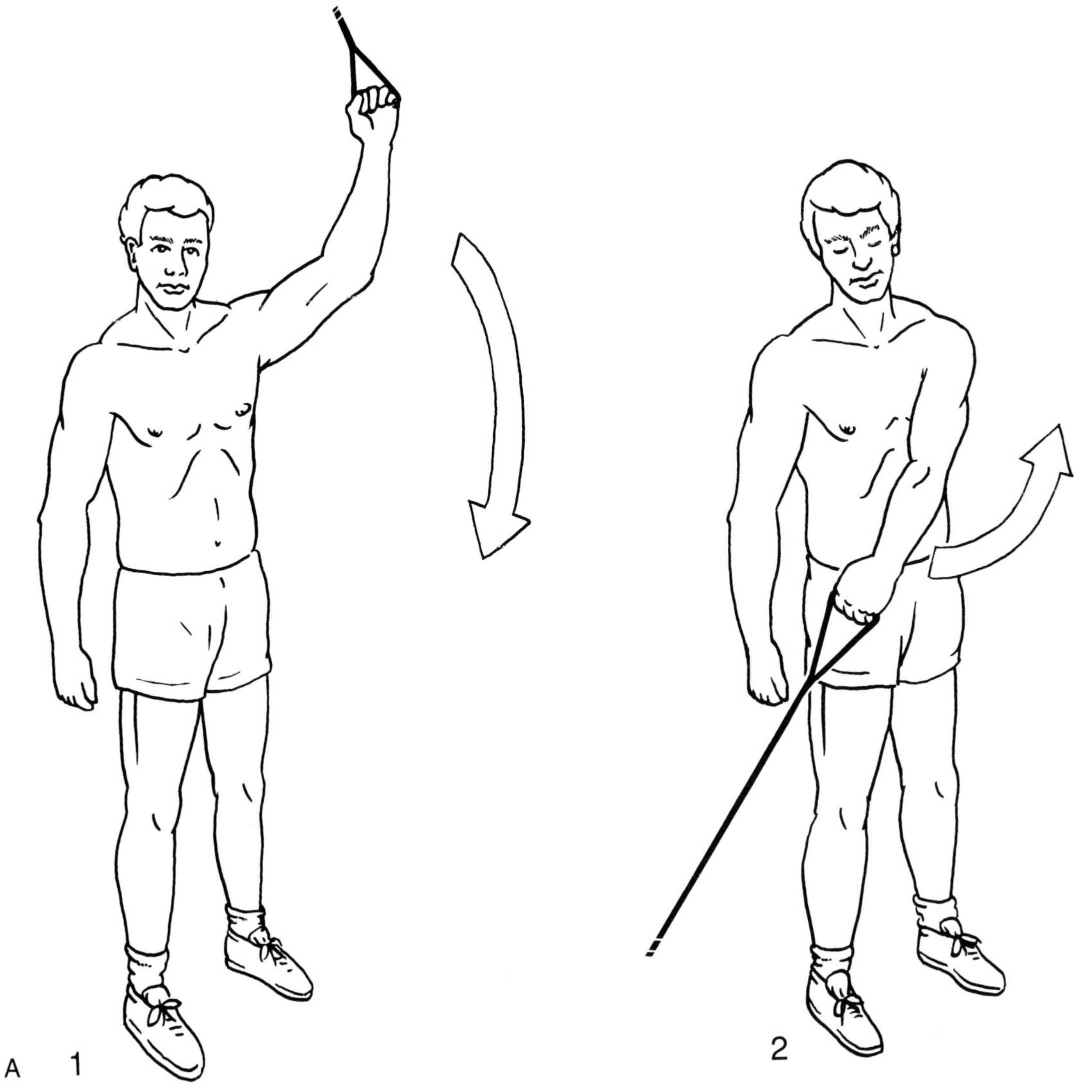

Figure 25-7. The thrower's 10-exercise program is designed to exercise the major muscles necessary for throwing. The program's goal is to be an organized and concise exercise program. Also, all exercises, including number of sets and repetitions to be performed daily, are specific to the thrower and are designed to improve strength, power, and endurance of the shoulder complex musculature. (**A**) (*1*) *Diagnonal pattern D_2 extension:* thrower involved hand to grip tubing handle overhead and out to the side, pulling tubing down and across the body to the opposite side of leg. During the motion, the thrower leads with the thumb. (*2*) *Diagonal pattern D_2 flexion:* gripping tubing handle in hand of involved arm, the thrower begins with arm out from side 45 degrees and palm facing backward. After turning palm forward, the thrower proceeds to flex elbow and bring arm up and over univolved shoulder. Turning palm down, the thrower reverses to take the arm to the starting position. Exercise should be performed in controlled manner. (*Figure continues.*)

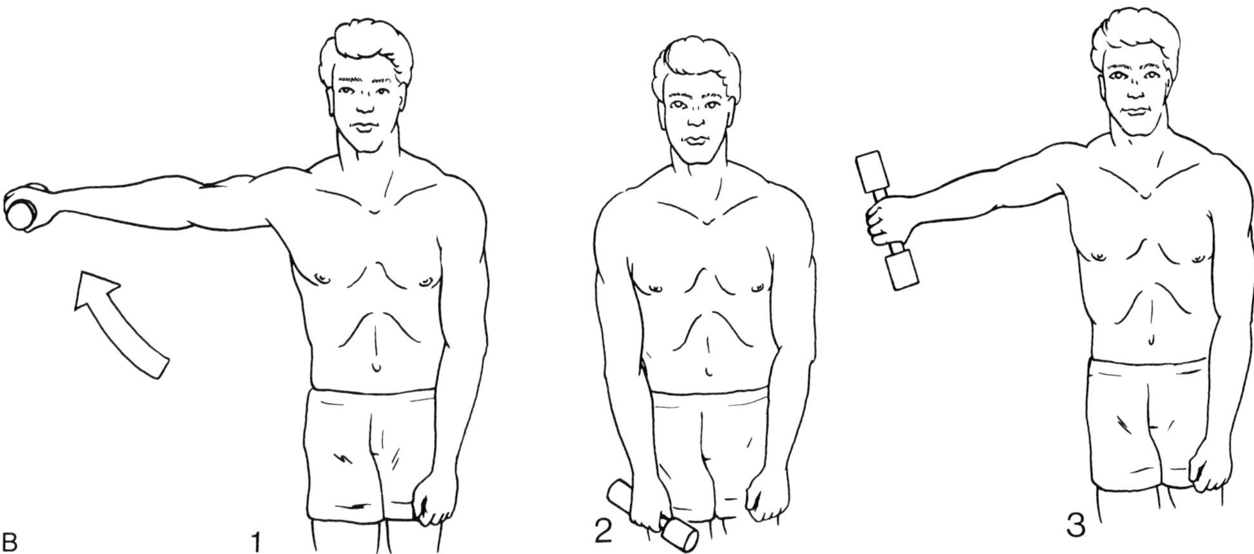

Figure 25-7. (*Continued*). (**B**) Dumbbell exercises for deltoid and supraspinatus. (1) *Deltoid strengthening:* thrower stands with arm at side, elbow straight, and palm against side. The arm is then raised to the side, palm down, until arm reaches 90 degrees. (*2*) *Supraspinatus strengthening:* thrower stands with elbow straight and thumb down. (*3*) The arm is raised to shoulder level at 30 degrees angle in front of body but not above shoulder height. This is held 2 seconds and lowered slowly. (*Figure continues.*)

the peak should occur in the middle to the latter half of competition phase. Peaking during spring training will result in a decrease in performance during the season. Many of the drills performed in spring training vary from team to team based on the philosophies of the organization, coaches, and players. The types of exercises and drills performed in baseball have changed dramatically in the past 5 years. In the past, plyometrics drills were not performed, but because of continued work by Gambetta,[11,12] Chu,[6,7] and others,[20,22] these drills have proved effective and safe for the overhead athlete.

The competitive season in baseball is long and demanding. The season lasts approximately 6 months (from April to October). During the season, I believe it is imperative to perform strengthening exercises to enhance and maintain tissue strength. The goals of this phase are to (1) reach peak performance, (2) maintain and possibly increase power, endurance, and strength to prevent arm injuries, (3) prevent tissue breakdown, and (4) maintain cardiovascular endurance. The exercises we recommend are the throwers' 10 program, neuromuscular control drills, stretching exercises, and cardiovascular exercise for 20 to 30 minutes. It must be explained to athletes that sport participation does not condition; rather, the athlete conditions to participate. During the season, due to tissue breakdown, the athlete becomes susceptible to injury and diminishing performance if conditioning exercises are not performed to counteract this effect.

Much of the discussion thus far has centered around the overhead thrower. This is in part due to the tremendously dynamic and violent nature of throwing. However, every movement in sports involves a stretch-shortening cycle to produce explosive power and speed. When one considers jumping, before beginning the jump the individual will slightly squat to produce a stretch on the gastrocsoleus, quadriceps, and gluteal muscles to activate the quick stretch on the muscle spindle. Once the quick stretch is elicited, then an explosive concentric (shortening) contraction can occur. Many researchers have stated that if an eccentric contraction precedes a concentric contraction, the resultant concentric contraction will be enhanced by 25 to 40 percent.[1,4,5] Other sports, such as throwing, golf, and tennis, use a similar stretch-shortening couple for power. Plyometrics uses a similar series of contractions to produce explosive power.

The golf swing is a dynamic activity that requires significant skill and physical condition. The professional golfer is an exceptional athlete. During the golf swing, and in particular the back swing, the purpose is to produce a stretch on the legs, hips, trunk, and shoulders. Then once a sufficient level of stretch has been accomplished, the body begins to recoil and produce an explosive powerful concentric contraction to accelerate the club to about 2,200 degrees per second. During the acceleration phase of the golf swing, it is the legs and hips that produce energy, which is transferred up through the trunk into the shoulders

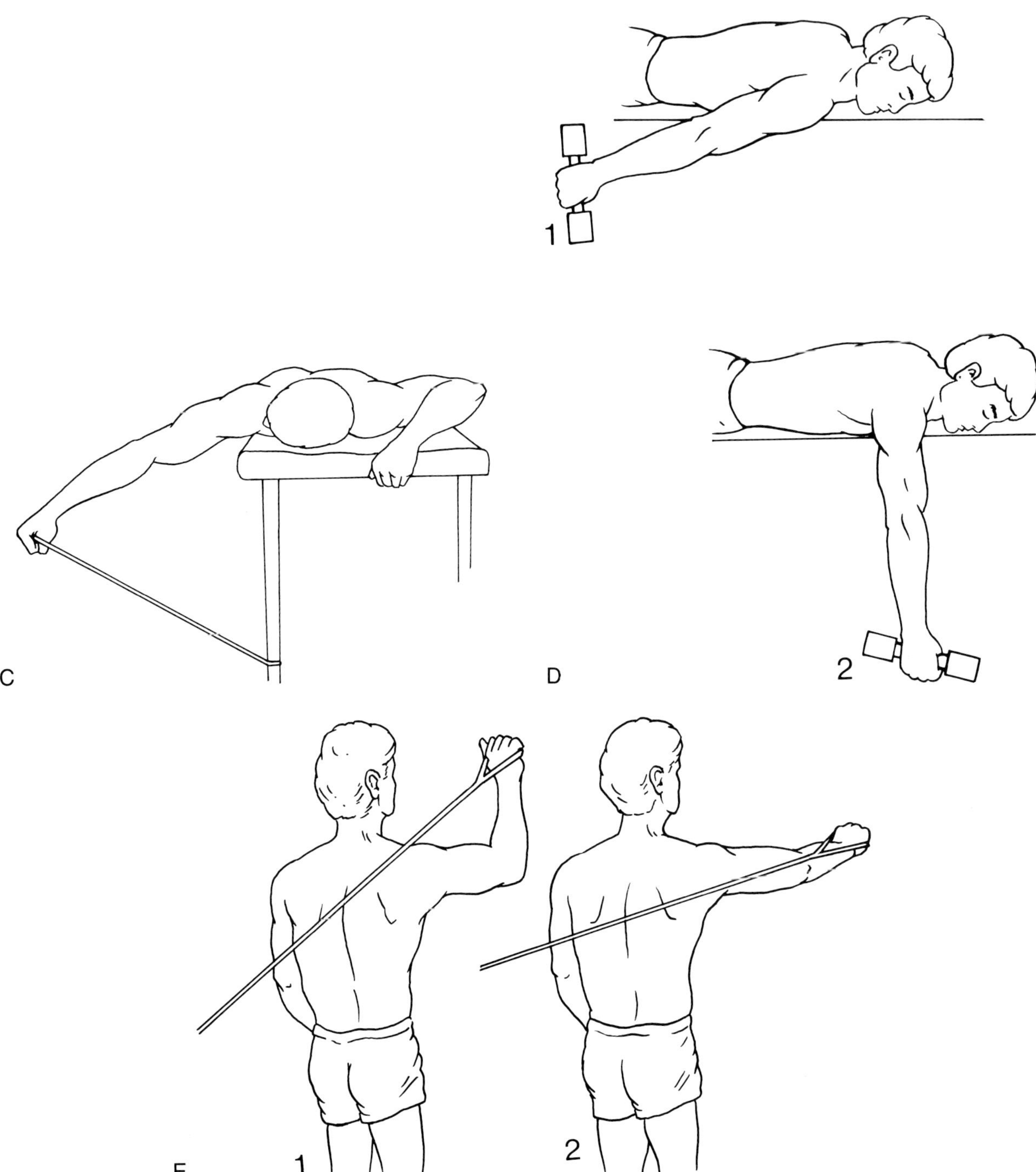

Figure 25-7. (*Continued*). (**C**) *Prone shoulder abduction for rhomboids.* Diagonal pattern D_2 flexion: thrower uses involved hand to grip tubing handle across body and against thigh of opposite side leg. Starting with palm down, the patient rotates palm up to begin, Proceeding to flex elbow and bring arm up and over involved shoulder with palm facing inward. The palm is ten turned down and reversed to take arm to starting position. Exercises should be performed in a controlled manner. (**D**) *Prone shoulder extension for latissimus dorsi.* (*1*) Thrower lies on table, face down, with involved arm hanging straight to the floor, and palm facing down. (*2*) The arm is raised straight back as far as possible, held 2 seconds, and lowered slowly. (**E**) *Internal rotation at 90 degree abduction.* (*1*) Thrower stands with shoulder abducted to 90 degrees, externally rotated 90 degrees and elbow bent to 90 degrees. (*2*) Keeping shoulder abducted, thrower rotates shoulder forward keeping elbow bent at 90 degrees. Tubing and hand are returned to start position slowly and controlled. (*Figure continues.*)

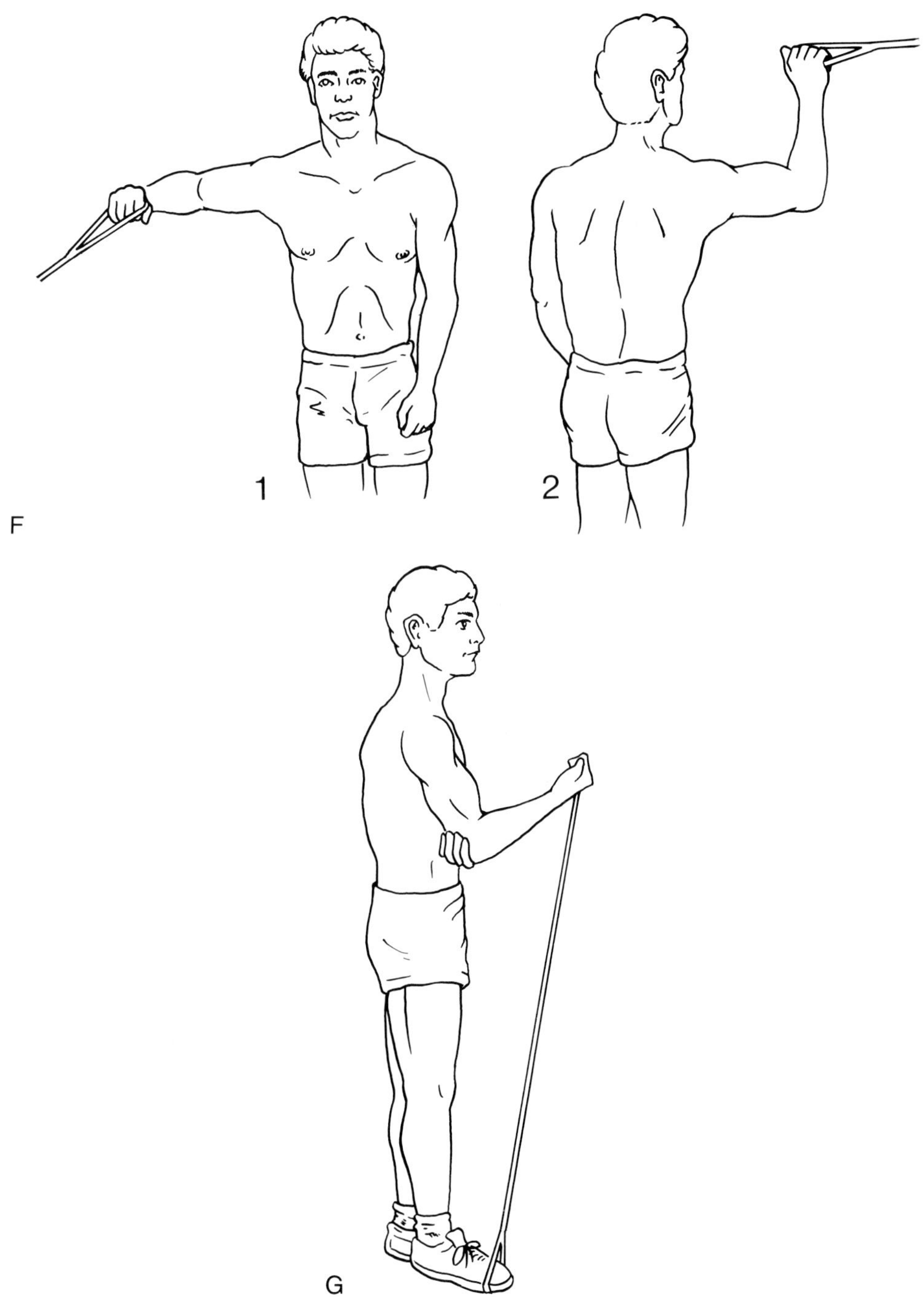

Figure 25-7. (*Continued*). (**F**) *External rotation at 90 degrees abduction.* (*1*) Thrower stands with shoulder abducted 90 degrees and elbow flexed 90 degrees. Thrower grips tubing handle while the other end is fixed straight ahead. (*2*) Keeping shoulder abducted, the shoulder is rotated back, keeping elbow at 90 degrees. Tubing and hand are returned to start position slowly and with controlled. (**G**) *Biceps strengthening with tubing:* thrower stands with tubing securely in hand and opposite end under the same foot of the involved side, controlling tension. Assisting with opposite hand, the arm is flexed through full range of motion. Thrower returns to starting position within a slow 5 count. (*Figure continues.*)

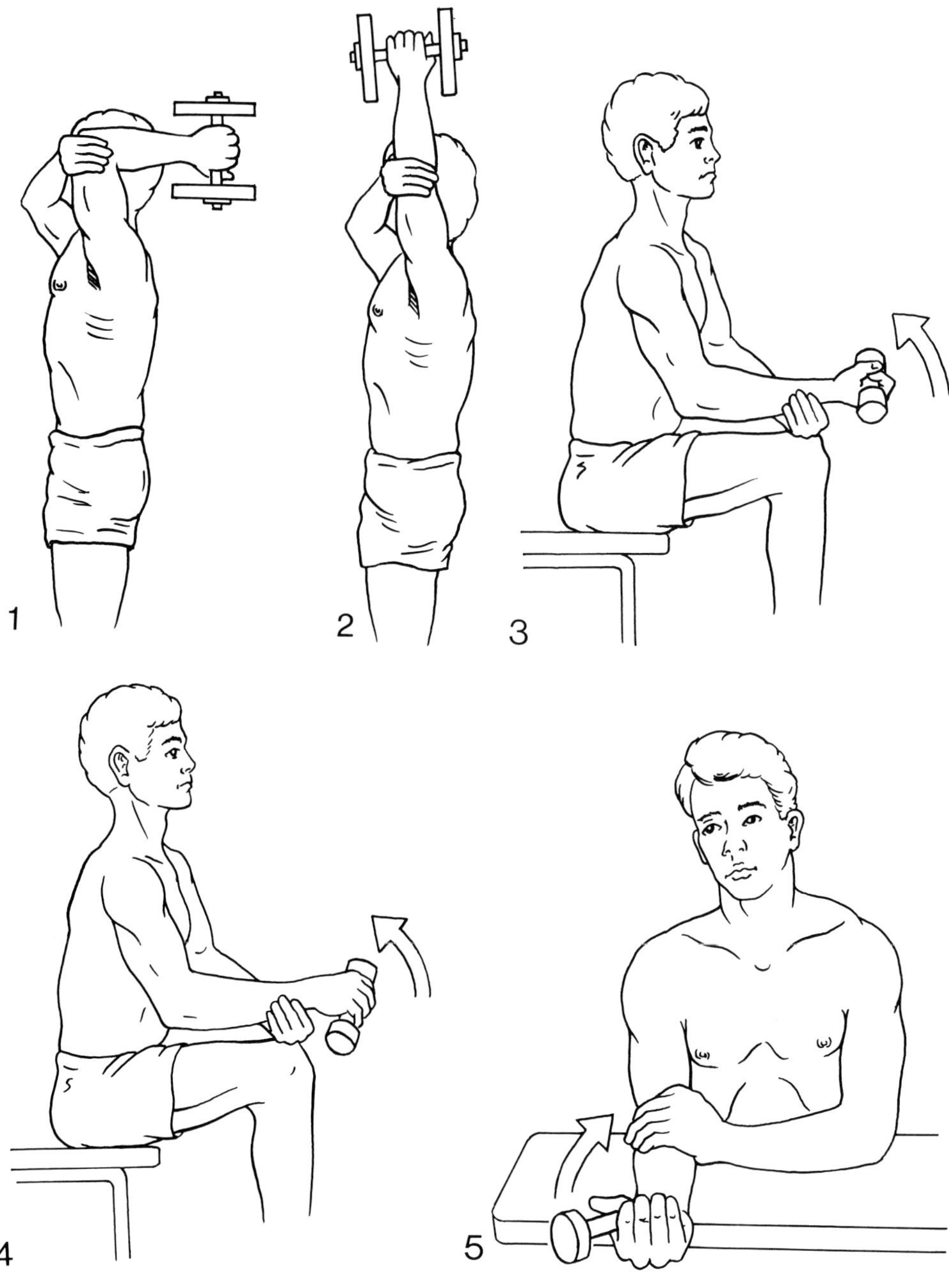

Figure 25-7. (*Continued*). (**H**) *Dumbell exercises for triceps and wrist extensors/flexors. (1 & 2) Triceps curls:* thrower, raises involved arm overhead. Support is provided at elbow from uninvolved hand. Thrower straightens arm overhead, holds 2 seconds, and lowers slowly. (*3*) *Wrist flexion:* the forearm should be supported on a table with hand off edge: palm should face upward. Using a weight or hammer, thrower lowers that hand as far as possible and then curls it up as high as possible. This is held for a 2 count. (*4*) *Wrist extension:* the forearm should be supported on a table with hand off edge; palm should face downward. Using a weight or hammer. Thrower lowers the hand as far as possible and then curls wrist up as high as possible. This is held for a 2 count. (*5*) *Forearm supination:* forearm should be supported on table with wrist in neutral position. Using a weight or hammer held in a normal hammering position. Thrower rolls wrist, bringing hammer into full supination. This is held for a 2 count. Patient raises back to starting position. (*Figure continues.*)

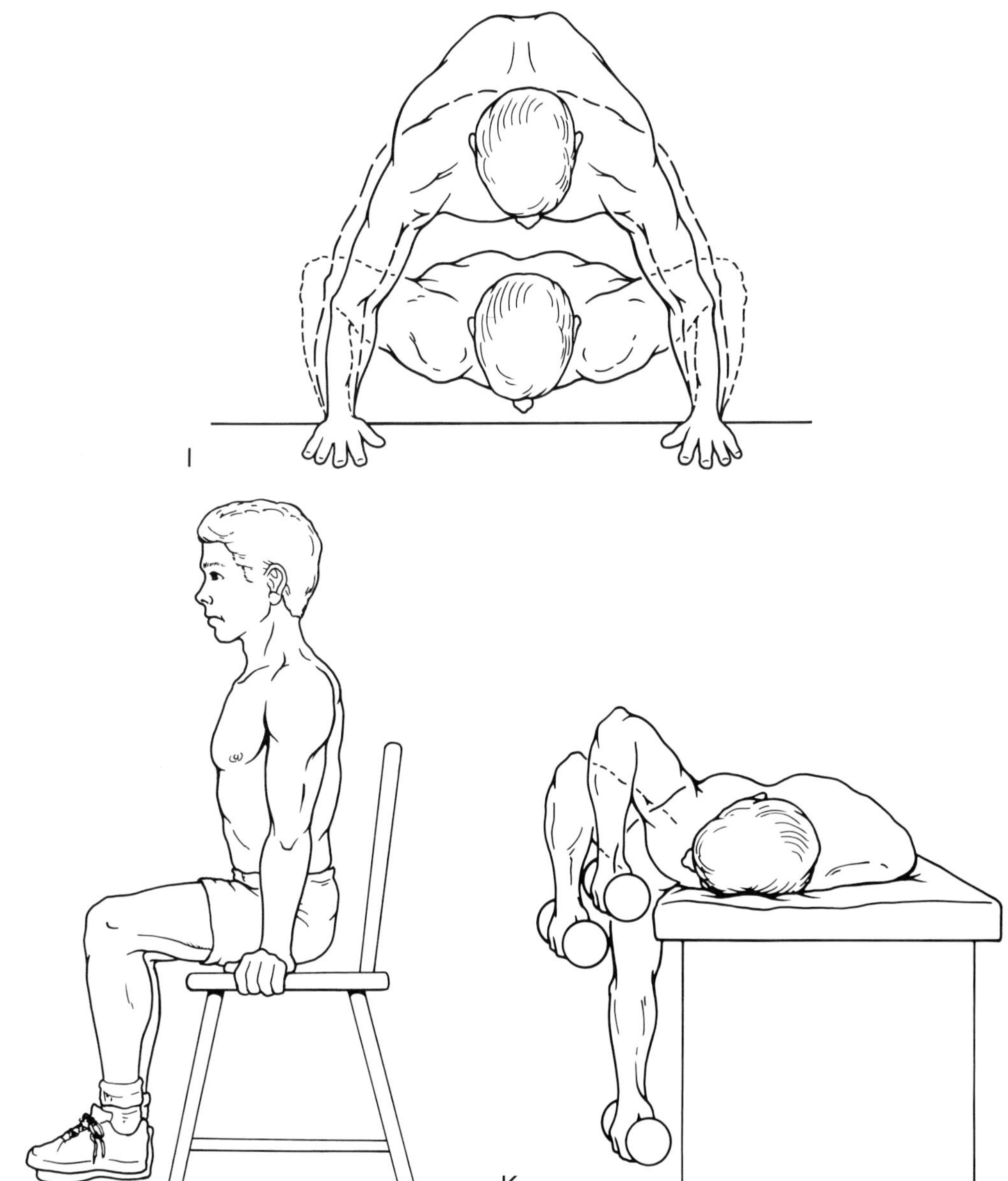

Figure 25-7. (*Continued*). (**I**) *Serratus anterior strengthening program:* thrower starts with push-up into wall and gradually progresses to table top and eventually to floor as tolerable. (**J**) *Press-ups:* seated on a chair or on a table, thrower places both hands firmly on the sides of the chair or table, palm down and fingers pointed outward. hands should be placed equal with shoulders Thrower slowly pushes downward through the hands to elevate the body, holding the elevated position for 2 seconds. This is then repeated. (**K**) *Rowing:* thrower lies on stomach with involved arm hanging over side of the table, dumbbell in hand and elbow straight. Thrower slowly raises arm, bending elbow, and brings dumbbell as high as possible, holding at the top for 2 seconds, then slowly lowering. This is then repeated.

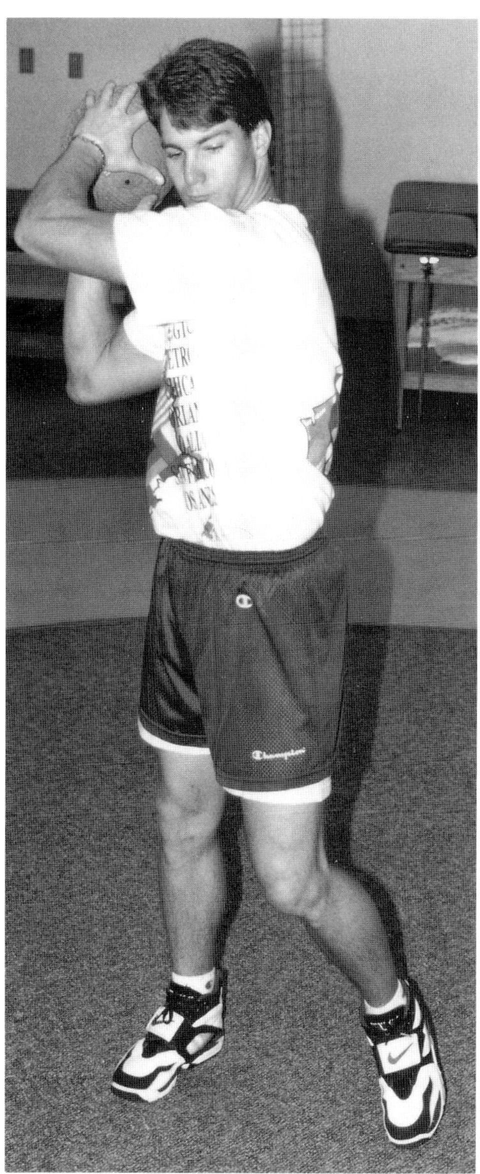

A

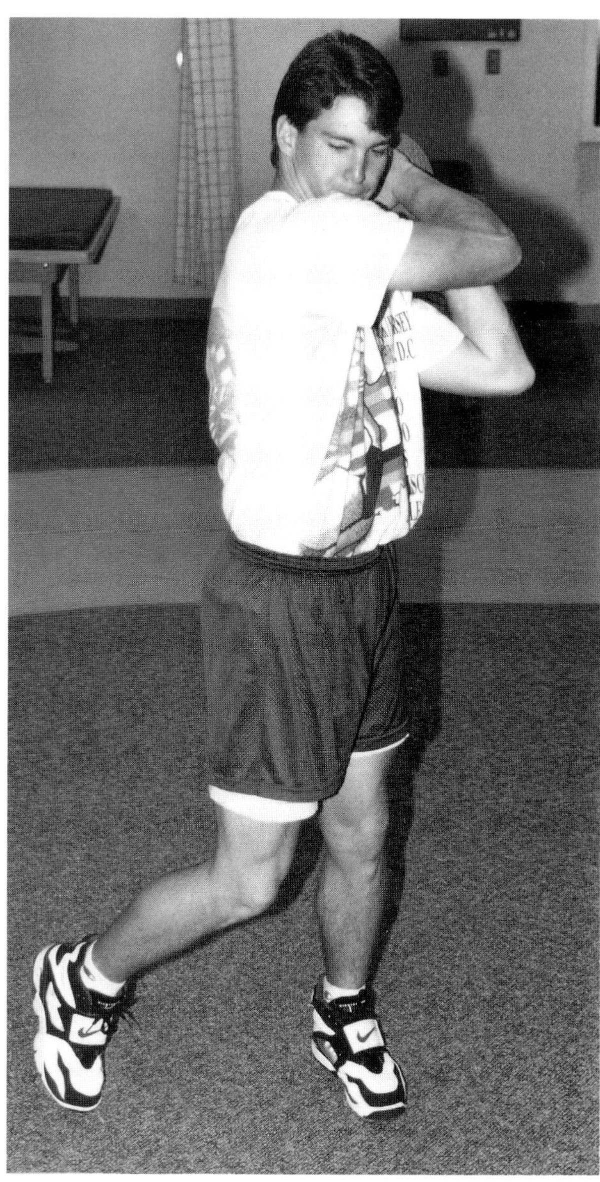

B

Figure 25-8. (**A & B**) Side-to-side throw using a 7-lb plyoball. The patient throws the plyoball into a bounce-back device (plyoback) as he rotates from side to side.

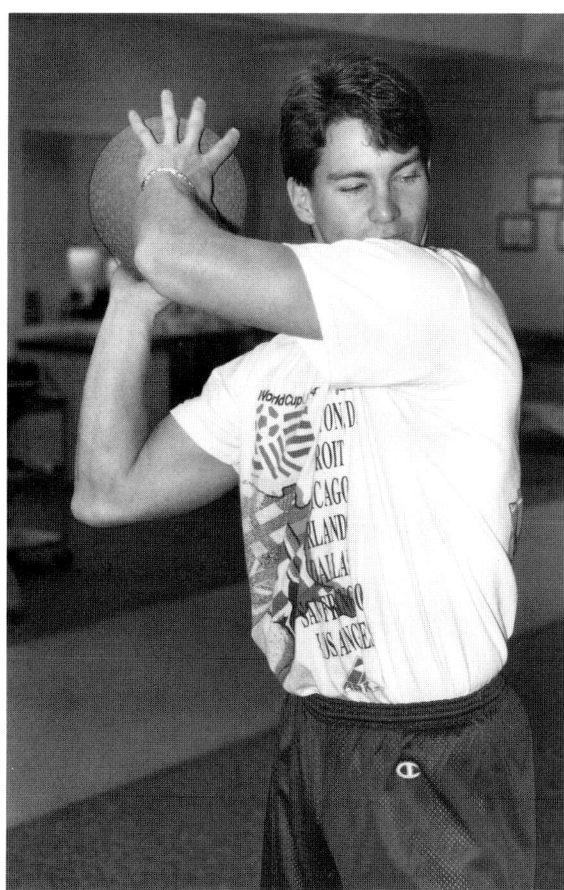

Figure 25-9. Two-hand side throw using a 7-lb plyoball. The patient stands sideways to the plyoback and throws it into the plyoback. This drill promotes trunk rotation and hip movement.

and arms, which eventually produces a powerful swing (Fig. 25-14). The trunk rotates approximately 45 to 50 degrees, occurring at an angular velocity of approximately 525 degrees per second. G. S. Fleisig, S. Ballentine, R. Escamilla, and J. R. Andrews, unpublished data). Wilk, et al[23] have established strengthening exercises and explosive plyometric drills specific to the golfer in an attempt to train and enhance this explosive power (Fig. 25-15). Golf, similar to baseball throwing, couples skill and power to produce a highly skilled athlete.

The same principles can be applied to the tennis player. The tennis serve, forehand and backhand stroke, involves a cocking phase to produce a stretch before the acceleration phase prior to the ball contact (Fig. 25-16). During the acceleration phase of the tennis serve, the shoulder is internally rotating at an angular velocity of 1,500 to 2,300 degrees per second.[9,15] Thus, exercise and conditioning drills for tennis players should incorporate techniques specific to the sport. These drills and exercises should incorporate the concepts of strength, speed, power, and skill previously discussed.

In conclusion, conditioning exercises and drills play a significant role in the athlete's performance level and assist in prevention of injury. Optimum sports performance requires skill and power. The conditioning program should address the development of both entities. There are many elements that promote the development of skill and power. When designing a conditioning program, it should use the

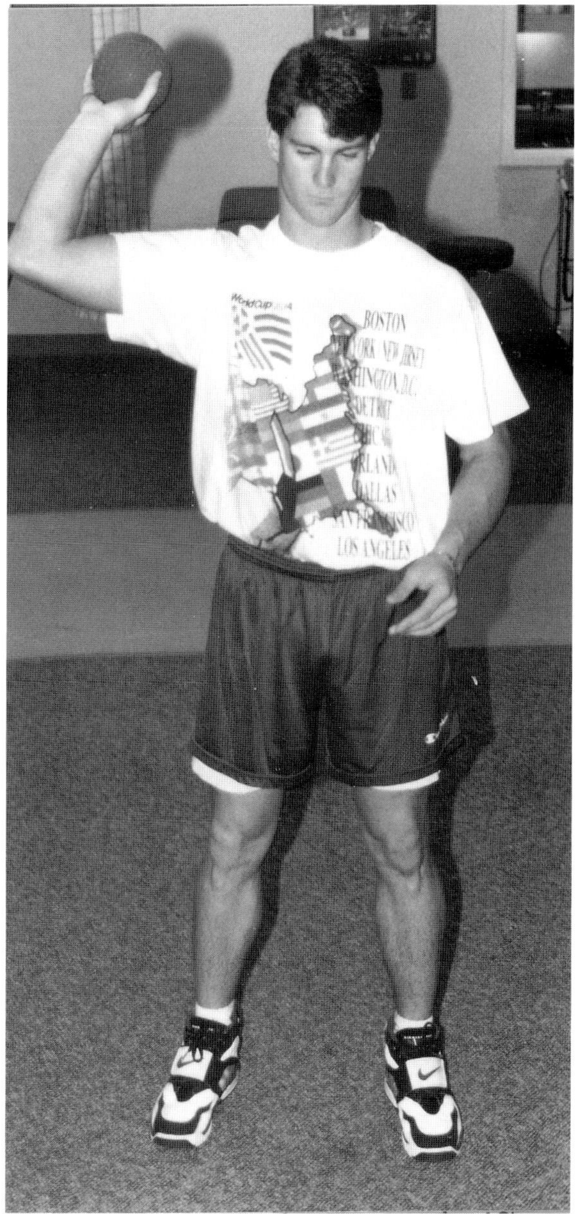

Figure 25-10. One-hand overhead baseball throw using a 2-lb plyoball.

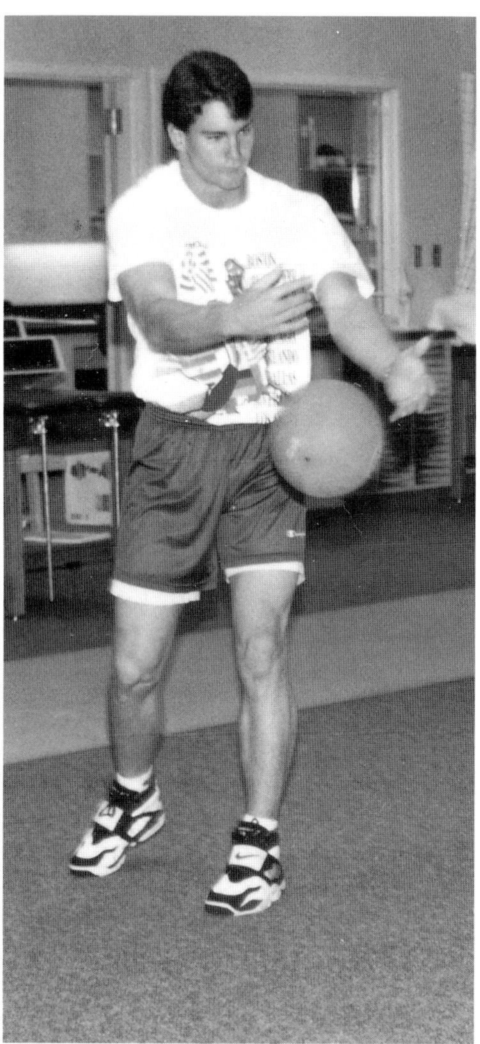

Figure 25-11. Two-hand underhand side throw performed with a 12-lb plyoball.

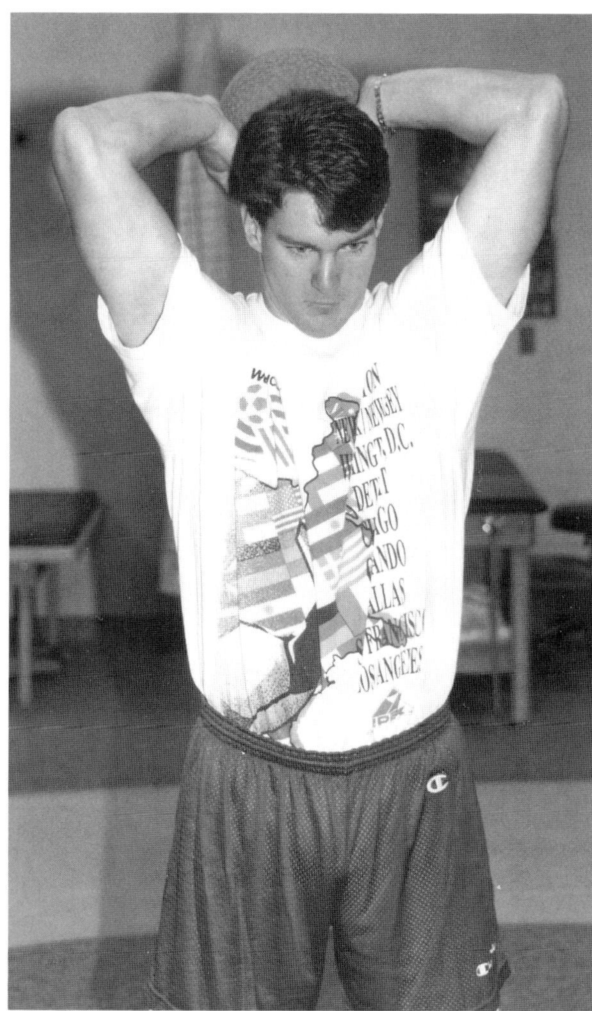

Figure 25-12. Two-hand overhead soccer throw. This drill promotes abdominal strength and flexibility as well as shoulder strength.

Table 25-3. Interval Throwing Program Starting Off the Mound, Phase II

Stage one: fastball only	
Step 1. Interval throwing 15 throws off mound 50%	Use interval throwing to 120 phases as warm-up.
Step2. Interval throwing 30 throws off mound 50%	
Step3. Interval throwing 45 throws off mound 50%	All throwing off the mound should be done in the presence of the pitching coach to stress proper throwing mechanics.
Step 4. Interval throwing 60 throws off mound 50%	
Step 5. Interval throwing 30 throws off mound 75%	Use speed gun to aid in effort control.
Step 6. 30 throws off mound 75% 45 throws off mound 50%	
Step 7. 45 throws off mound 75% 15 throws off mound 50%	
Step 8. 60 throws off mound 75%	
Stage two: fastball only	
Step 9. 45 Throws off mound 15 Throws in batting practice	
Step 10. 45 Throws off mound 75% 30 Throws in batting practice	
Step 11. 45 Throws off mound 75% 45 Throws in batting practice	
Stage three	
Step 12. 30 Throws off mound 75% warm-up 15 Throws off mound 50% breaking balls 45–60 Throws in batting practice (fastball only)	
Step 13. 30 Throws off mound 75% 30 Breaking balls 75% 30 throws in batting practice	
Step 14. 30 Throws off mound 75% 60–90 Throws in batting practice 25% breaking balls	
Step 15. Simulated game: progressing by 15 throws per work-out.	

principles discussed in this chapter, such as periodization, specificity, power, endurance, flexibility, and core stability, but it is imperative to design a program tailor-made for each athlete. It is critical to establish dynamic joint stability and core stability first, before plyometrics or skill training. There are three elements of establishing a conditioning program: (1) programming, (2) organization and implementation, and (3) the management of the program.[18] The management of the program is critical; the athlete must stay motivated and challenged and must see improvement. Gambetta[11] refers to the three M's of a conditioning program: manageable, measurable, and motivational. Another concept of a conditioning program not discussed in this chapter but that is vitally essential is nutrition. The athlete must eat properly, to fuel the body, providing energy through complex carbohydrates and proteins for muscle

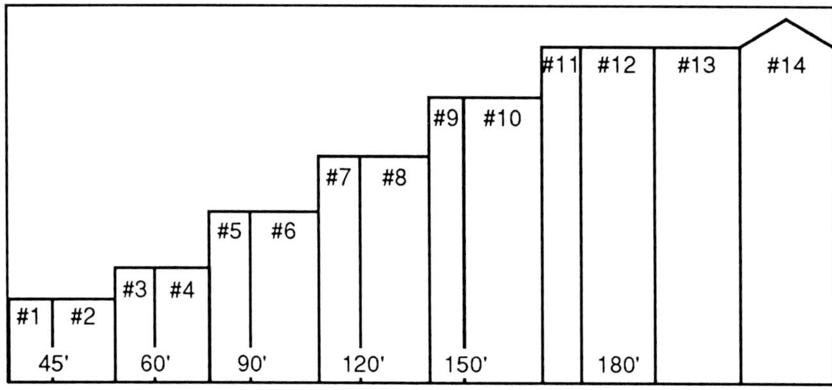

45' Phase

Step 1: A) Warm-up throwing
B) 45' (25 throws)
C) Rest 15 minutes
D) Warm-up throwing
E) 45' (25 throws)

Step 2: A) Warm-up throwing
B) 45' (25 throws)
C) Rest 10 minutes
D) Warm-up throwing
E) 45' (25 throws)
F) Rest 10 minutes
G) Warm-up throwing
H) 45' (25 throws)

60' Phase

Step 3: A) Warm-up throwing
B) 60' (25 throws)
C) Rest 15 minutes
D) Warm-up throwing
E) 60' (25 throws)

Step 4: A) Warm-up throwing
B) 60' (25 throws)
C) Rest 10 minutes
D) Warm-up throwing
E) 60' (25 throws)
F) Rest 10 minutes
G) Warm-up throwing
H) 60' (25 throws)

90' Phase

Step 5: A) Warm-up throwing
B) 90' (25 throws)
C) Rest 15 minutes
D) Warm-up throwing
E) 90' (25 throws)

Step 6: A) Warm-up throwing
B) 90' (25 throws)
C) Rest 10 minutes
D) Warm-up throwing
E) 90' (25 throws)
F) Rest 10 minutes
G) Warm-up throwing
H) 90' (25 throws)

120' Phase

Step 7: A) Warm-up throwing
B) 120' (25 throws)
C) Rest 15 minutes
D) Warm-up throwing
E) 120' (25 throws)

Step 8: A) Warm-up throwing
B) 120' (25 throws)
C) Rest 10 minutes
D) Warm-up throwing
E) 120' (25 throws)
F) Rest 10 minutes
G) Warm-up throwing
H) 120' (25 throws)

150' Phase

Step 9: A) Warm-up throwing
B) 150' (25 throws)
C) Rest 15 minutes
D) Warm-up throwing
E) 150' (25 throws)

Step 10: A) Warm-up throwing
B) 150' (25 throws)
C) Rest 10 minutes
D) Warm-up throwing
E) 150' (25 throws)
F) Rest 10 minutes
G) Warm-up throwing
H) 150' (25 throws)

180' Phase

Step 11: A) Warm-up throwing
B) 180' (25 throws)
C) Rest 15 minutes
D) Warm-up throwing
E) 180' (25 throws)

Step 12: A) Warm-up throwing
B) 180' (25 throws)
C) Rest 15 minutes
D) Warm-up throwing
E) 180' (25 throws)
F) Rest 10 minutes
G) Warm-up throwing
H) 180' (25 throws)

180' Phase (continued)

Step 13: A) Warm-up throwing
B) 180' (25 throws)
C) Rest 10 minutes
D) Warm-up throwing
E) 180' (25 throws)
F) Rest 10 minutes
G) Warm-up throwing
H) 180' (50 throws)

Step 14: Begin throwing off the mound or return to respective position

Figure 25-13. Interval throwing program.

Table 25-4. Plyometrics for the Pitcher

Warm-up drills
Two-hand side-to-side twists
Two-hand wood chops
Two-hand side bends
IR/ER strengthening exercise tubing
Push-ups
Throwing drills
Two-hand overhead soccer throw
Two-hand chest press
Two-hand side-to-side throw
Two-hand overhead side throw
Two-hand underhand side throw
One-hand baseball throw
Trunk drills
Plyo push-ups
Plyoball sit-ups
Plyoball sit-ups and throw
Wall drills
Wall plyoball dribble
Two-hand between throw
Two-hand side-to-side throw
Two-hand overhead throw
One-hand baseball throw

Table 25-5. Plyometrics for the Hitter

Warm-up drills
Two-hand side bends
Two-hand wood chops
Two-hand side-to-side twists
Push-ups
IR/ER strengthening with exercise tubing
Hitting drills
Supine chest pass throws (two hands)
Two-hand overhead throws
Two-hand standing chest pass
Two-hand overhead side throw
Two-hand underhand side throw
One-hand backhand side throw (ER)
One-hand side throw (IR)
Trunk drills
Plyo push-ups
Plyoball sit-ups
Plyoball sit-up and throw

regeneration, as well as being low in fats.[3,8] Conditioning principles have changed dramatically, and they will continue to change as new techniques and drills are designed and tested. All sport movements require the interaction of two critical components, skill and power. Power is developed through the attainment of strength first, as a baseline, then trained more specifically through stretch-shortening drills, referred to as plyometrics. It is essential for athletes, as well as medical individuals, to realize that they must obtain a sufficient level of physical condition before sports participation and not to expect to play themselves into shape; this often leads to injury and diminished sports performance.

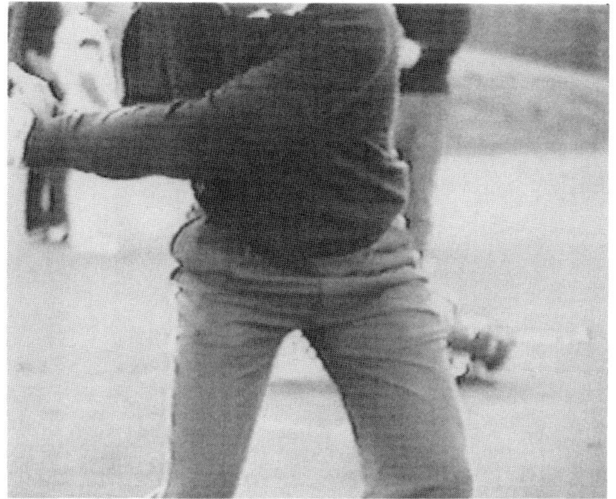

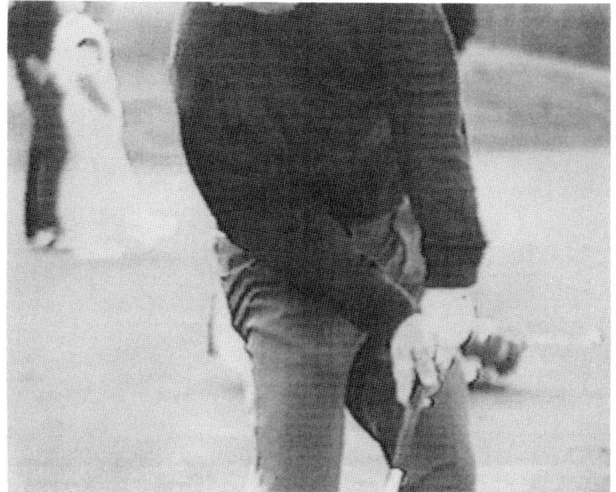

Figure 25-14. (**A & B**) Motion analysis of a golf swing. This figure illustrates the amount of hip and trunk rotation during the acceleration phase of the golf swing. This rapid and explosive hip/trunk rotation generates energy, which accelerates the shoulder and arm and promotes golf club speed.

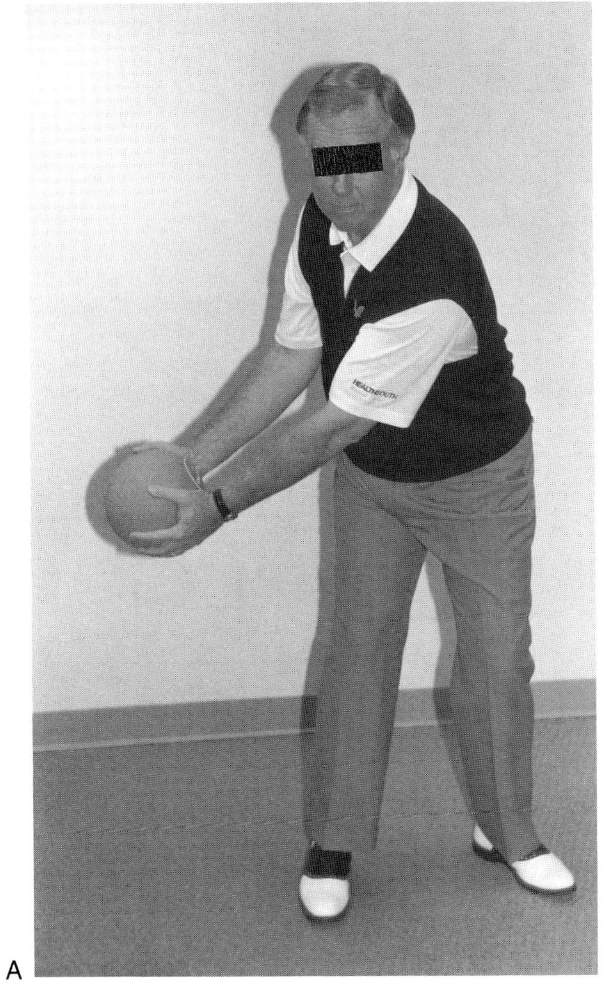

A

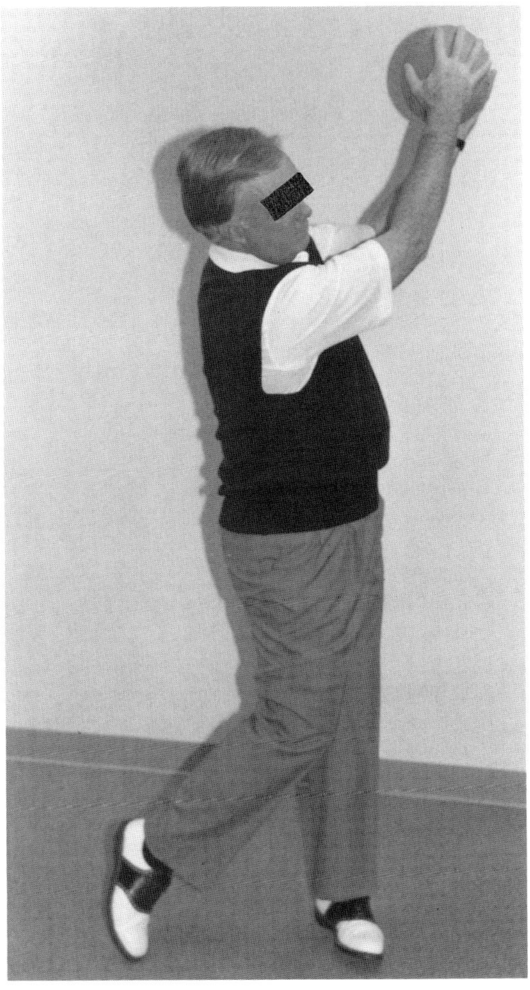

B

Figure 25-15. Plyometric exercise drills for the golfer. (**A**) Side-to-side trunk rotation; (**B**) two-hand underhand side throw.

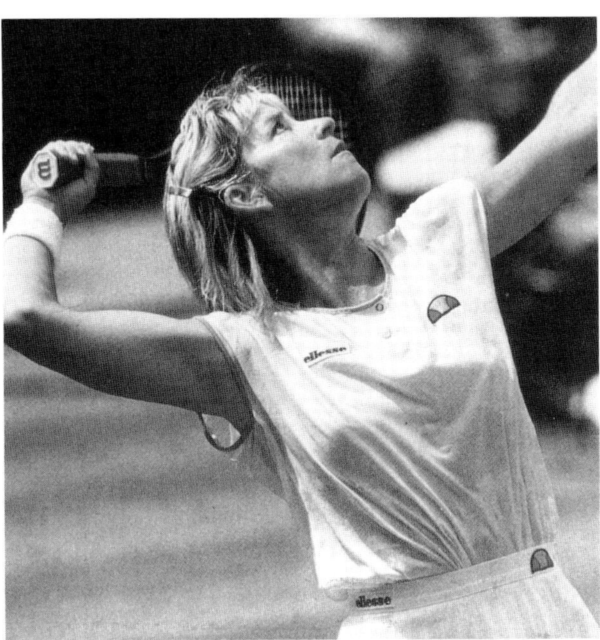

Figure 25-16. During the tennis serve, the cocking phase produces a stretch on the shoulder's adductor/internal rotators, thus producing an explosive, powerful acceleration phase.

REFERENCES

1. Assmussen E, Bonde-Peterson F: Storage of elastic energy in skeletal muscle in man. Acta Physiol Scand 91:385–92, 1974
2. Bennett JG, Stauber WT: Evaluation and treatment of anterior knee pain using eccentric exercise. Med Sci Sports Exerc 15:461–8, 1983
3. Berning JR, Steen SN: Sports Nutrition for the 90's. Aspen Publishers, Gaithersburg, MD, 1991
4. Bosco C, Komi P: Potentiation of the mechanical behavior of the human skeletal muscle through prestretching. Acta Physiol Scand 106:467–72, 1979
5. Cavanga G, Disman B, Margarai R: Positive work done by a previously stretched muscle. J Appl Physiol 24:21–32, 1968
6. Chu D; Plyometric Exercises with a Medicine Ball. Bittersweet Publishing Co., Livermore, CA, 1989
7. Chu D, Parariello RA: Sport specific plyometrics; baseball pitchers. J Natl Strength Conditioning Assoc 11:81–84
8. Clark N: Nancy Clark's Sports Nutrition Guidebook. Leisure Press, Champaign, IL, 1990
9. Dillman CJ: The upper extremity in tennis and throwing sports. Paper presented at the United States Tennis Association National Meeting, Tucson, Arizona, 1991
10. Fleisig CS, Dillman CJ, Andrews JR: Biomechanics of the shoulder during throwing. p. 355–68. In Andrews JR, Wilk KE (eds): The Athletic Shoulder. Churchill Livingstone, New York, 1994
11. Gambetta V: Conditioning of the shoulder complex. p. 643–51. In Andrews JR, Wilk KE (eds): The Athletic Shoulder. Churchill Livingstone, New York, 1994
12. Gambetta V, Odgers S: The Complete Guide to Medicine Ball Training. Optimum Sports Training, Sarasota, FL, 1991
13. Hunter-Griffin LY (ed): Athletic Training and Sports Medicine. 2nd Ed. American Academy of Orthopaedic Surgeons, Chicago, IL, 1984
14. Marveyev L: Fundamentals of Sports Training. Progress Publishing, Moscow, 1977
15. Shapiro R, Stine RL: Shoulder rotation velocities. Technical report submitted to the Lexington Clinic, Lexington, KY, 1992
16. Stone WJ, Kroll WA: Sports Conditioning and Weight Training. 2nd Ed. WC Brown Publishers, Dubuque, IA, 1988
17. Toyoshima S, Hoshikawa T, Miyashita M: contribution of the body parts to throwing performance. p. 169–74. In Nelson RC, Morehouse CA (eds): Biomechanics IV. University Park Press, Baltimore, MD 1974
18. Verhoshansky YV: Programming and Organization of Training. Sportiuny Press, Livonia, MI, 1988
19. Wilk KE, Andrews JR, Arrigo CA et al: Preventive and Rehabilitative Exercises for the Shoulder and Elbow. American Sports Medicine Institute, Birmingham, AL, 1992
20. Wilk KE, Andrews JR, Arrigo CA, et al: The strength characteristics of internal and external rotator muscles in professional baseball pitchers. Am J Sports Med 21:61–6, 1993
21. Wilk KE, Arrigo CA: An integrated approach to upper extremity exercise. Orthop Phys Ther Clin North Am 9:337–49, 1992
22. Wilk KE, Arrigo CA: Current concepts in the rehabilitation of the athletic shoulder. J Orthop Sports Phys Ther 18:365–78, 1993
23. Wilk KE, Johnson H, Andrews JR: The golfers power and skill training program. In Andrews JR, Wilk KE (eds): Golf. Odysseus Publishers, Birmingham, AL, in press
24. Wilk KE, Voight ML, Keirns MA et al: Stretchshortening drills for the upper extremity: theory and clinical application. J Orthop Sports Phys Ther 17:225–39, 1993

CHAPTER TWENTY-SIX

Protective Devices for the Shoulder Complex

Mark DeCarlo
Kathy Malone

The goal of rehabilitation after athletic injury involves returning the injured individual to safe sports participation. The physician caring for an athlete with a shoulder injury should have a basic understanding of the protective equipment available for use, including custom-made and commercially purchased devices. It is also imperative that the clinician have a clear understanding of the rules governing the sport. By recognizing the specific needs of the athlete and understanding the functions of different protective devices for the shoulder, the physician can make informed decisions and practical recommendations to athletes, parents, and coaches.

PROTECTIVE PADDING AND TAPING

Shoulder Pads

Shoulder pads are an essential component of the required equipment for participation in competitive football, ice hockey, and men's lacrosse. The basic shell and padding design of shoulder devices serves to decrease injury to the shoulder girdle by absorbing and dispersing impact forces. Shoulder pads, which have evolved over time into highly technical protective devices, are designed to cover the clavicle, acromion, scapula, and proximal humerus. An improper fit or lack of cushion will not adequately protect these areas and may predispose an athlete to injury.

Types

The selection and fit of shoulder pads should be considered part of the comprehensive approach to preventing and treating injuries to the shoulder. Size and configuration of pads are dictated by the sport and the demands of the position. Fitting shoulder pads is generally left to the discretion of the coach, certified athletic trainer, or equipment manager. Athletes themselves should be made aware of the basic guidelines to use when fitting shoulder pads because their equipment sizes will likely change during the course of their scholastic career.

There are generally two types of shoulder pads: flat and cantilevered. Both types are made of a polyethylene plastic shell that covers open-cell foam encased in nylon. Flat pads lie close to the shoulder girdle and are worn by athletes who require extensive glenohumeral mobility, including quarterbacks, receivers, and punters. These pads are often the choice of lacrosse players because they provide protection while allowing adequate motion (Fig. 26-1). Cantilevered pads are named for the bridge that extends over the pad (Fig. 26-2). The cantilever is made from spring steel or hard plastic and is placed under the arch of the shoulder pad. It serves to absorb and disperse force away from the shoulder girdle to the torso. These pads provide more bulk and are often used by players who consistently use their shoulders as a contact point. Football players and ice hockey players typically use the cantilevered shoulder pad (Fig. 26-3). High-quality shoulder pads can range in cost

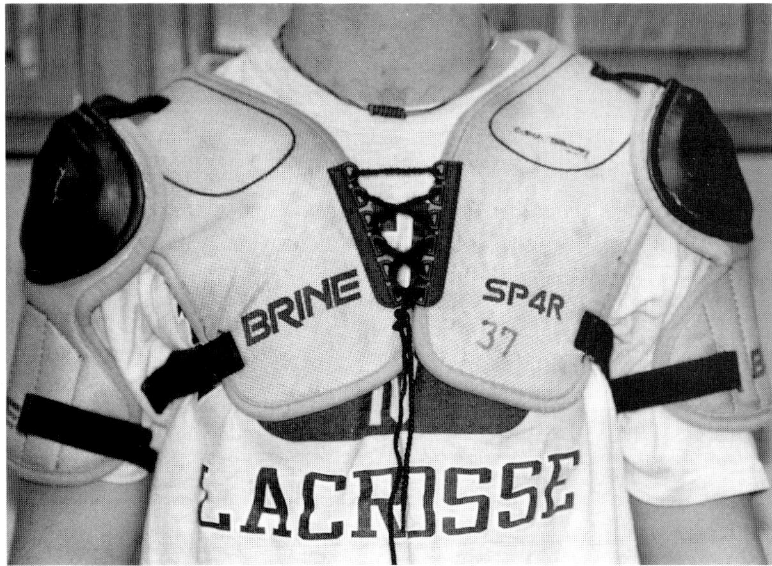

Figure 26-1. Flat shoulder pads that lie close to the shoulder girdle.

from $180.00 to $240.00. With a presciption from an attending physician, some insurance companies will reimburse up to 80 percent of the cost of the shoulder pad.

Proper Fitting

Well-fitting pads protect the proximal shoulder and permit unrestricted glenohumeral and cervical motion. Preliminary measurements may be required to ensure proper sizing and may vary among manufacturers. Common sites for measurements include the distance across the back between acromioclavicular (AC) joints or between the outer deltoid of each arm.

The neck opening should be wide enough to allow for overhead arm motion without pinching or sliding. The lateral aspect of the acromion should be covered by the lateral edge of the pads, and the flaps should fit comfortably over the deltoid area. A tight jersey will help keep the flaps in place. Straps from the back that pass under the arms and hook in the front should be pulled tight but not restrict normal breathing.

Helmet fitting should also be a consideration when choosing proper shoulder pads. Large pads may restrict cervical motion and predispose the athlete to cervical spine injury.

Important guidelines when fitting shoulder pads include the following[3]:

Inner padding should cover the tips of the shoulders.

Neck opening should not be constrictive, yet should minimize the area exposed to injury.

Epaulets (or flaps) and cups should cover the deltoid muscle and allow movements required by the athlete's specific position.

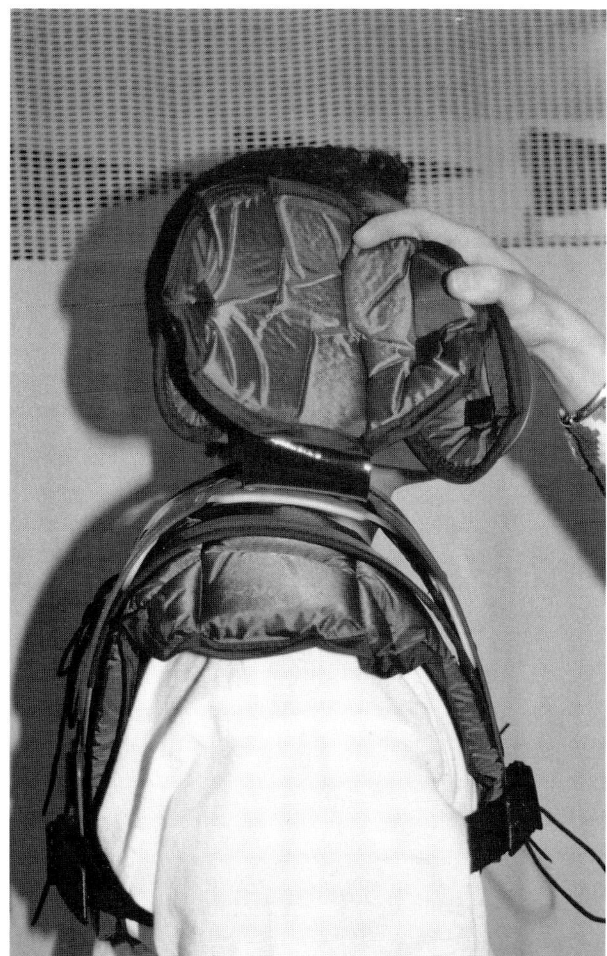

Figure 26-2. Cantilevered shoulder pad.

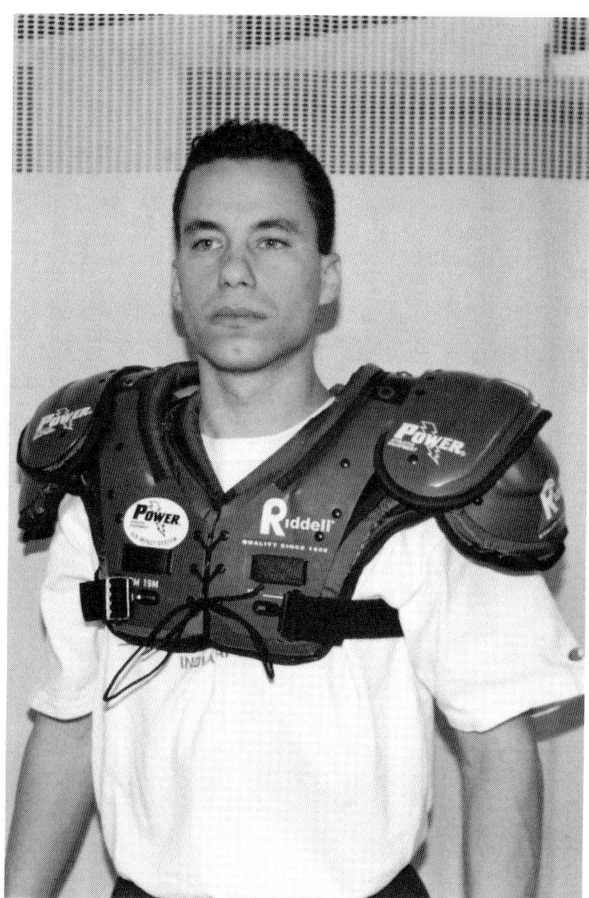

Figure 26-3. Cantilevered shoulder pad typically worn by football players and ice hockey players.

If a split clavicle shoulder pad is used, the channel for the acromioclavicular joint should be in proper position.

If an athlete has suffered a shoulder injury as the result of a direct blow while wearing shoulder pads, the pads should be re-evaluated for proper fit and sufficient padding before further play is permitted. On their own, athletes will sometimes choose equipment that is lightweight, minimally restrictive, and "looks good" rather than opting for the most effective and best-fitting device. Individual factors such as size, position, sport, strength, and physical development, as well as skill level, should be considered. Although using second-hand equipment is often unavoidable, older pads should be checked regularly for defects that might compromise the safety of the athlete.

Injury Trends

Selection and fit of pads can directly affect the players predisposition to injury. Pads that are too small will leave areas of the shoulder girdle exposed and can result in contusions to the deltoid, rotator cuff, and proximal humerus. Incomplete coverage of the anterior portion of the shoulder can result in posterior subluxation from a direct anterior blow. Conversely, anterior instability can result from a blow to the poorly protected posterior aspect of the shoulder. Injuries to the AC and sternoclavicular joints, as well as clavicle fracture, may occur if the pads are too large and shift with contact. Old or worn padding that has lost density can also contribute to injury.

Supplemental pads may be used to increase shock absorption or protect previously injured areas. These pads, often referred to as skeleton or shock pads, are typically made of vinyl foam and are worn beneath the shoulder pads (Fig. 26-4). Skeleton pads elevate the shoulder pads off the AC joint, sternoclavicular joint, and clavicle, which increases shock absorption.

Acromioclavicular Pads

Purpose

The purpose of the AC pad is to protect the AC joint by dispersing impact forces across the pad and away from the joint. AC pads can be used in both contact and noncontact sports. Depending on the rules of the sport, either rigid material or simple felt padding may be used.

Types

Three basic types of AC protection are available for use in athletics. Protection of the AC joint may involve simple taping using felt or foam for padding, forming a custom-made pad, or purchasing a prefabricated pad.

Taping

The purpose of AC joint taping is to provide support to the area by compressing the clavicle to the acromion. A felt donut pad can be used to protect the joint and distribute forces. Preparation for applying adhesive tape to the skin includes covering the nipple area on the affected side with bandaids or gauze. Excess chest hair should be removed.

Materials for shoulder taping include one roll of 3-in. elastic tape, scissors, adherent spray, AC pad, and bandaids or gauze pads.

Steps involved in applying AC protection include the following:

1. The athlete is instructed to look away from the affected shoulder to avoid eye irritation while spraying the area with adherent.
2. A piece of tape is placed partway around the torso from midline to midline to serve as an anchor.
3. The AC pad is positioned over the joint, with the donut hole directly over the acromion process.
4. The pad is secured in place with two or three anterior-to-posterior strips of elastic tape.

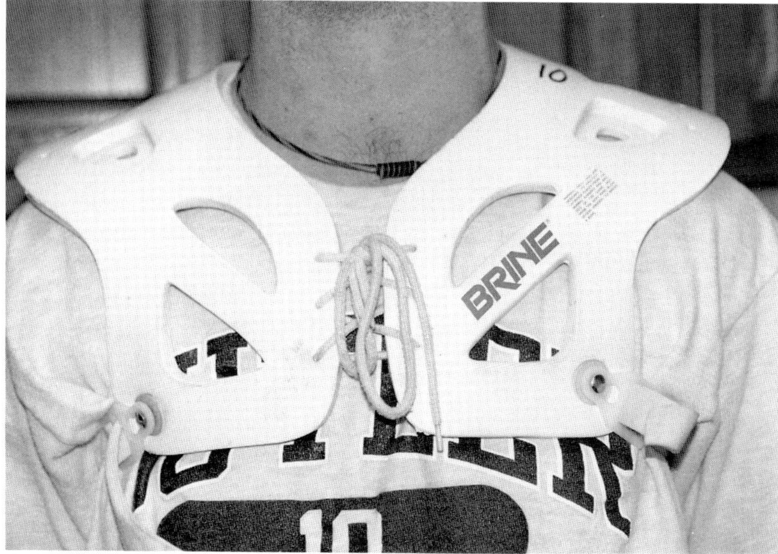

Figure 26-4. Supplemental pads are worn beneath shoulder pads to increase shock absorption.

5. The strips are secured with an additional anchor midway around the torso from midline to midline.

When applying AC protection to an athlete either with a custom-made pad, prefabricated device, or simple donut pad, the pocket must be positioned directly over the AC joint. If the AC pad will be attached directly to the shoulder pads, straps should be securely fastened to prevent the pad from slipping.

Simple protection in the form of a donut pad is also an option. These pads are typically cut from 0.5- to 0.75-in. felt or dense foam and are used for protection of athletes participating in sports such as wrestling, soccer, basketball, or other sports that prohibit hard plastic padding.

The custom-made pad is typically fabricated by an athletic trainer or physical therapist (Fig. 26-5). Materials needed for fabricating a custom-molded AC pad include thermoplastic material (i.e., Orthoplast, Ezeform, etc.), 0.75-in. adhesive-back foam padding, scissors, and hot water.

Steps in fabrication of this pad include the following:

1. Hot water is used to heat a piece of thermoplastic material large enough to cover the affected area. It should extend to the spine of the scapula posteriorly, over the clavicle anteriorly, and cover the area from the tip of the shoulder to the middle portion of the trapezius.
2. On removal of the material from the water, an object, such as a role of tape or adherent spray can top, is used to create a pocket in the middle of the material, and then it is applied to the athlete's shoulder. The pocket must be formed directly over the AC joint. When hot material is applied directly to the skin, it should be allowed to cool sufficiently to avoid burning. The material is firmly held to the shoulder until it becomes rigid. The material may be reheated and molded as necessary to obtain the best fit.
3. Donut-shaped 0.75-in. foam is adhered to the inside of the thermoplastic mold and around the area of the pocket.

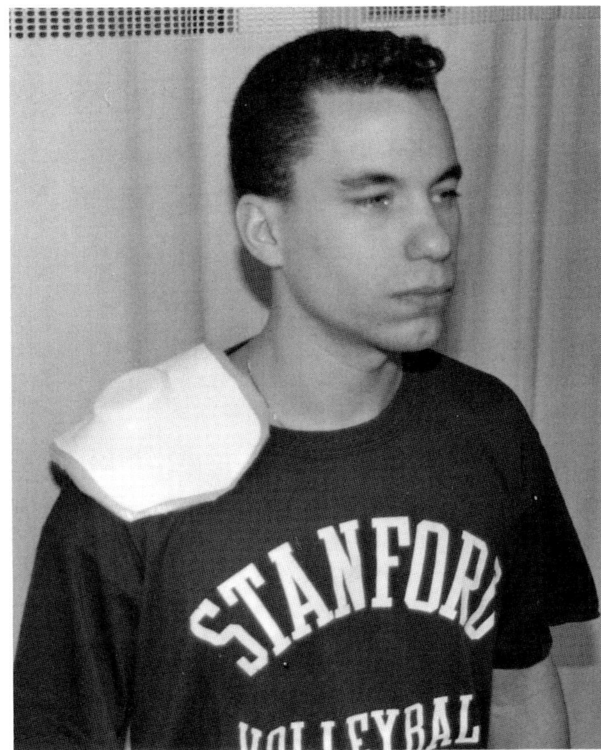

Figure 26-5. An example of a custom-made pad that is often fashioned by a trainer or therapist.

The completed AC pad can be held in place with adhesive stretch tape or an elastic wrap for competition. Taping the custom-molded pad in place involves the same steps as taping the simple AC donut pad in place. When worn under shoulder pads and properly fitted, the AC pad adds protection and does not interfere with shoulder motion.

A prefabricated AC pad can be purchased through a medical supply company. These pads are typically made from lightweight high-density polyethylene and must be molded in hot water or by using a heat gun. Placement of the pad is similar to the custom-made device.

Injury Trends

Football players are continuously at risk for shoulder injury as they use the upper body as a major source of contact. Injury to the AC joint is also commonly seen in wrestlers, who engage in repeated twisting and falling maneuvers.[2] Direct contact with the ground often results in contusions to the soft tissue of the upper arm; however, when the point of contact is the tip of the shoulder, injury to the acromion, AC joint, clavicle, and sternoclavicular joint may occur. Neurologic and muscular structures can also be injured as a result of direct blows beneath the outer shoulder pad.[5]

Glenohumeral Instability Taping and Bracing

Recurrent glenohumeral dislocation occurs frequently in athletes, especially those younger than 20 years of age. Instability of the glenohumeral joint is seen rather frequently in the scholastic and collegiate athlete. An 82 percent recurrence rate has been reported in athletes 20 years or younger, whereas the recurrence rate for nonathletes in the same age group was only 30 percent.[8] Other authors have reported up to a 95 percent recurrence of instability epidoses in teenagers.[4]

Immobilization and rehabilitation after the first-time dislocation remain controversial with respect to reducing the risk of recurrence with a more conservative treatment approach. Most high school and college athletes opt for a rather expedient return to competition, with a full understanding of the potential complications and risks of further problems. Attempting to prevent recurrent dislocation involves controlling motions that lead to instability, including abduction, extension, and external rotation.

Over the years, a variety of devices has been applied to the athlete's shoulder in an attempt to prevent further injury and allow participation. These devices have ranged from intricate strapping and taping techniques to combinations of neoprene, Velcro, and canvas.

The importance of administering a comprehensive rehabilitation program before returning an athlete to competition (after an incident of glenohumeral instability) cannot be overemphasized. Glenohumeral taping and bracing can be considered only after return of full and pain-free range of motion and strength. Once the rehabilitation goals have been met, the athlete should be counseled on competing with a restrictive shoulder device. If surgery is recommended, the possibility of completing the season in a brace and scheduling the procedure in the off-season can be discussed with the athlete and family.

Glenohumeral Taping

The purpose of glenohumeral taping and bracing is to decrease the likelihood of subluxation and dislocation by restricting upper extremity movement. It can be used in place of or in addition to glenohumeral bracing to help stabilize the shoulder joint. Preparation for this type of taping is similar to that of AC taping in that the athlete's nipple should be covered, chest hair removed, and adherent spray applied to the area. The shoulder may be taped for glenohumeral support using 3-in. elastic tape in the following steps:

1. An anchor strip is applied halfway around the torso and another strip anterior to posterior over the shoulder.
2. A third strip is applied from the anterior aspect of the shoulder, around the deltoid, to the posterior aspect of the shoulder. This strip may be wrapped under the noninvolved arm for additional support.
3. One or two more strips are applied in this fashion and an additional anchor strip is used to secure the taping (Fig. 26-6).

Taping and wrapping of the shoulder are not as common in sports as ankle or wrist taping but are often used to apply special padding or give added stability. There are differing opinions as to the value and effectiveness of shoulder taping. Shoulder stabilizing braces are a second option for controlling and limiting motion.

Glenohumeral Bracing

A variety of commercially produced shoulder braces are available on the market today. For the purposes of this chapter, we discuss three of the most widely accepted and currently prescribed braces for athletes.

The Duke Wyre vest (C.D. Denison Orthopaedic Appliance Corp., Baltimore, MD) (Fig. 26-7) was one of the original devices created for returning an athlete with glenohumeral instability to competition. The original shoulder harness was developed in the 1950s by the late Duke Wyre, former head athletic trainer at the University of Maryland, and the late Cedric Denison, former president and chief orthotist of C.D. Denison Corp.[6] The Duke Wyre vest is constructed of sturdy canvas with chrome eyelets sewn into reinforced leather. Nonstretch laces are used to secure the vest and limit motion. Sizing for the Duke Wyre vest

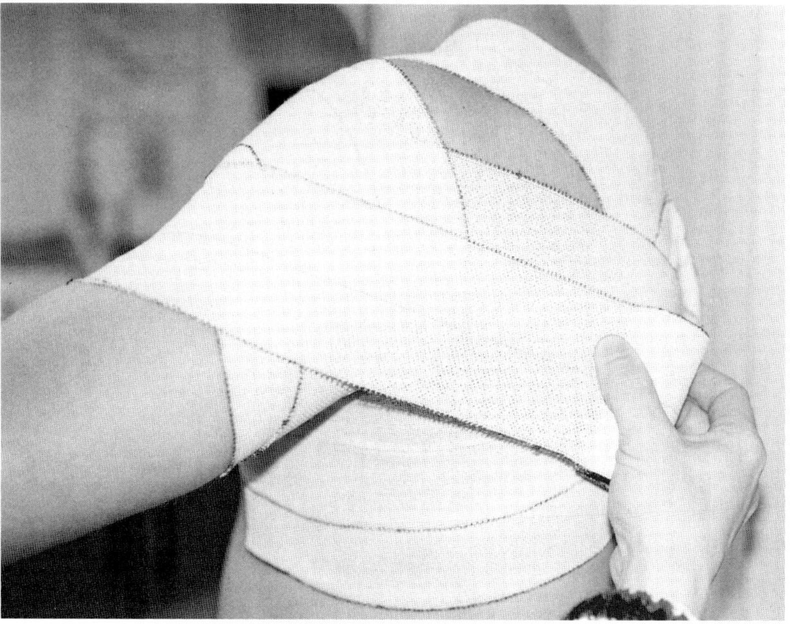

Figure 26-6. For the process of the glenohumeral taping, one or two strips of 3-in. elastic tape is applied from the anterior aspect of the shoulder, around the deltoid, to the posterior aspect of the shoulder. An anchor strip is used to secure the taping.

is based on chest and biceps circumference. Bilateral models are available, and sizes range to accommodate a chest circumference of 32 to 51 in. and biceps circumference of 14.5 to 17 in. The Duke Wyre shoulder vests cost approximately $100.00.

The Sawa shoulder orthosis (Brace International, Atlanta, GA) (Fig. 26-8) was developed in Canada in the mid-1980s by a chiropractor, Thomas Sawa. This device is composed of a blend of cotton/polyester and spandex and uses adjustable Velcro straps to limit motion. Success-

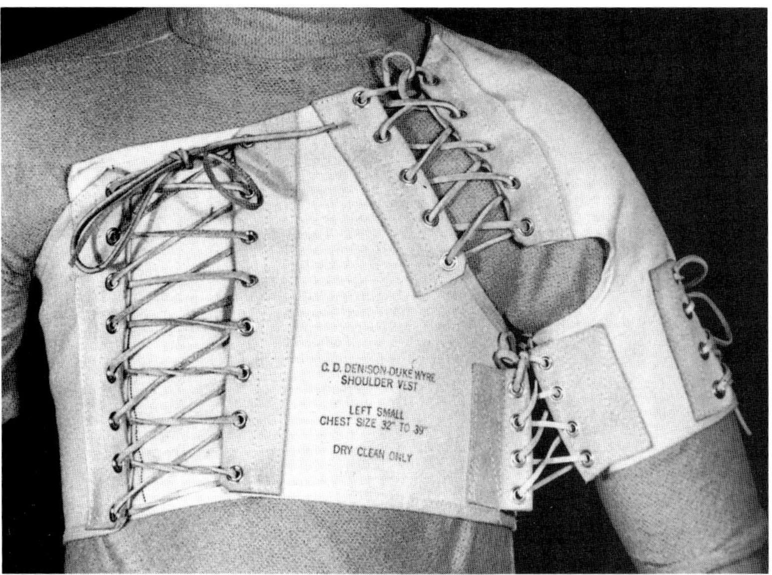

Figure 26-7. The Duke Wyre vest. One of the original devices created to enable the return of the athlete with glenohumeral instability to competition.

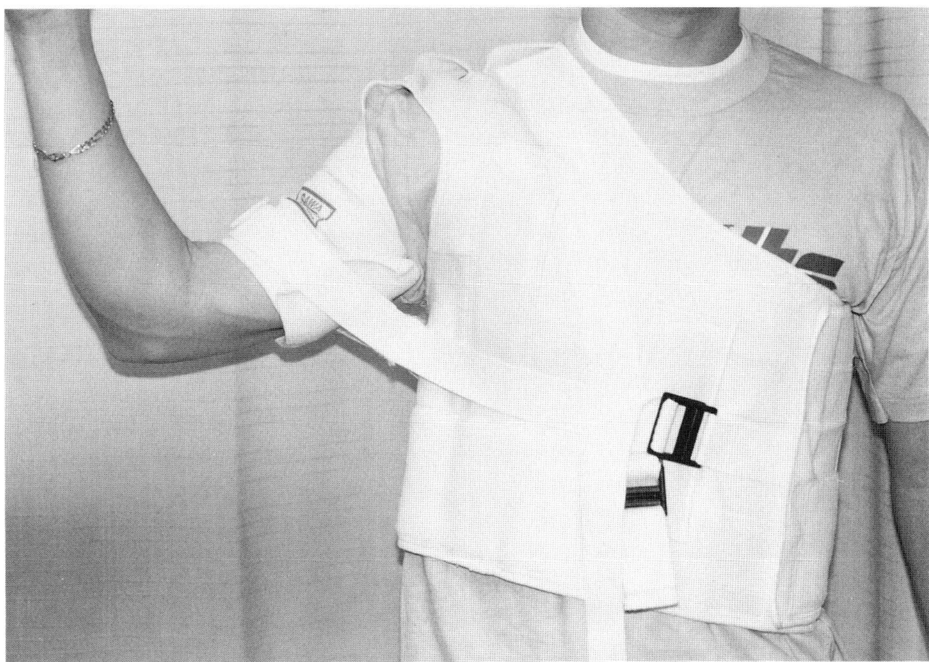

Figure 26-8. The Sawa shoulder orthosis, which limits shoulder motion and has enabled the return of amateur hockey players to the game.

ful return to sports after injury has been reported among amateur hockey players who wore the Sawa brace during therapy and competition.[7] Sizing of this brace is based on chest circumference. Bilateral devices are available, and sizes accommodate chest circumferences up to and including 48 in. The Sawa shoulder orthosis can be purchased for approximately $150.00.

The shoulder subluxation inhibitor (SSI) (Boston Brace International, Inc., Avon, MA) (Fig. 26-9) uses a polyethylene shell, pivot joints, and a posterior buttress to limit

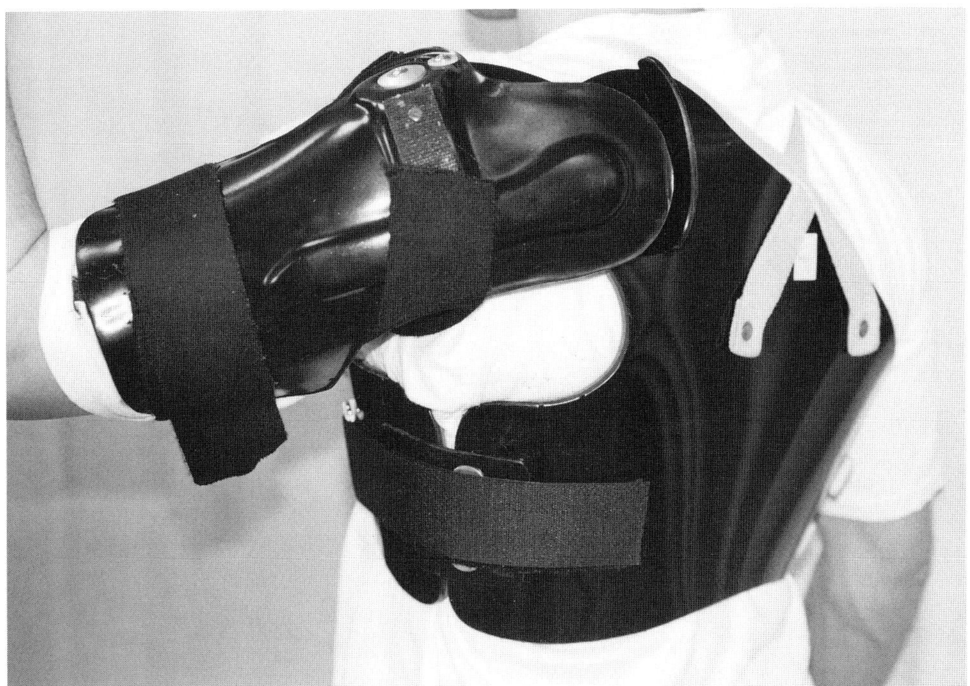

Figure 26-9. The shoulder subluxation inhibitor (SSI) limits horizontal extension.

horizontal extension. Determining size requires chest and biceps measurements, as well as height, weight, and sex, as specially molded braces are available for females. The SSI, which has its primary use in contact sports, is available in a bilateral model and accommodates chest sizes ranging from 29 to 49 in. The SSI, the most expensive of the three braces, can be purchased for approximately $300.00.

In bracing for glenohumeral instability, physician preference has been the primary method of selection. Opinions vary as to which brace is the most appropriate for returning athletes to sport. Each of the three shoulder braces discussed is used to allow injured athletes to participate in sports. Whether used prophylactically to prevent injury, after surgery, or before surgical intervention, the purpose of the brace is to prevent the shoulder from achieving motion that could lead to instability during participation. As previously discussed, these motions include abduction, extension, and external rotation for episodes of anterior instability.

Because no data could be obtained on the motion-limiting characteristics of the three braces, a clinical study was undertaken at our facility.[1] The purpose of this study was to determine the degree to which three braces maintain predetermined motion limitations after isokinetic exercise.

Ten male subjects with no prior history of glenohumeral joint instability performed isokinetic exercise in two planes of motion while wearing each of three types of shoulder braces, including the Sawa, Duke Wyre, and SSI. Range of motion was determined with a goniometer for each subject after brace fitting and isokinetic exercise. Measurements included the maximum range of active motion for forward flexion, abduction, and external rotation. Each subject performed 10 repetitions of forward flexion/extension and abduction/adduction at isokinetic speeds of 120 degrees per second and 180 degrees per second for each of the three braces. All subjects completed a subjective survey in which the braces were ranked according to comfort, ability to limit motion, and preference for sports participation.

From the study, we concluded that the most effective brace for use in (1) limiting motion leading to anterior instability and (2) providing maximum functional capabilities was the SSI. The SSI, while permitting overhead forward flexion, effectively maintained predetermined abduction limitations after exercise. The Sawa exhibited significant changes in both forward flexion and abduction after exercise. The Duke Wyre, like the SSI, did not exhibit significant change in abduction while allowing significant change in forward flexion. The difference, however, can be found in the degree of motion permitted (Table 26-1).

By design, the maximum abduction permitted in the Duke Wyre (determined at application by tightening the laces) directly affects the amount of forward flexion permitted. Both the Sawa and Duke Wyre use a "check reign" design that restricts arm movements away from the body by connecting the distal humerus to the lateral torso at the chest. This design, however, is not used in the SSI, which uses pivot joints in the shell to allow joint motion while providing adjustable hole settings to control maximum movement. Adjusting the brace to limit abduction does not directly affect its ability to limit forward flexion, as is the case with the Sawa and Duke Wyre. Anterior and posterior pivot joints control abduction, and a superior pivot joint (over the AC joint) controls forward flexion. A further benefit of the SSI is its ability to limit extension in a horizontal plane. A posterior buttress prevents this motion, which is known to compromise stability. When applying the SSI, the clinician can selectively limit or permit motion by determining placement of screws.

Subjects indicated that the Sawa was the most comfortable, followed by the SSI and the Duke Wyre. For subjective ability to limit motion, the Duke Wyre was indicated as the most limiting, followed by the SSI and the Sawa. The brace most preferred for sports participation (primarily football) was the SSI, followed by the Sawa and the Duke Wyre. Because this brace contains a plastic shell, it is most commonly used for participation in contact sports, primarily football.

Injury Trends

Although shoulder instability in athletics can be the result of a direct blow to the proximal humerus, indirect trauma is the most common cause of glenohumeral sublux-

Table 26-1. Mean Increase After Exercise

Brace	Flexion (degrees)	Abduction (degrees)	External Rotation (degrees)
Duke Wyre	13.60[a]	3.30	4.00
Sawa	12.30[b]	7.80[b]	3.00
SSI	14.30[a]	3.90	5.40

[a] Significant difference ($P < .01$).
[b] Significant difference ($P < .05$).

ation or dislocation.[9] Anterior dislocations, which occur more frequently than posterior dislocations, result from a combination of the forces of abduction, extension, and external rotation. Conversely, axial loading of the abducted, internally rotated arm produces posterior dislocation.[9]

CONCLUSIONS

Providing athletes with adequate shoulder protection during sports participation, especially contact sports, has continued to challenge physicians and athletic trainers, as well as equipment designers and manufacturers. Although some shoulder injuries may be unavoidable, muscular weakness can predispose athletes to risk of injury. As in other areas of medicine, the best protection against injury often involves prevention. In addition to providing properly fitted equipment, the incorporation of strength training and proper conditioning into practice sessions, along with stretching and an adequate warm-up, can contribute to injury prevention. The use of protective padding and taping secondary to injury is beneficial in allowing continued play and preventing further injury. The team physician should be familiar with the types of protective shoulder equipment available, as well as commonly used taping and wrapping techniques.

REFERENCES

1. DeCarlo MS, Malone KN, Gerig BH, Hunker MH: Analysis of shoulder instability bracing. Submitted
2. Hill JA: Epidemiologic perspective on shoulder injuries. p. 244. In Jobe FW (ed): Clinics in Sports Medicine. Vol 2. No 2. WB Sanders, Philadelphia, 1983
3. Hunter-Griffin LY (ed): Athletic Training and Sports Medicine. 2nd Ed. American Academy of Orthopaedic Surgeons, Park Ridge, IL, 1991
4. McLaughlin HL, McLellan DI: Recurrent anterior dislocation of the shoulder:II. A comparative study. J Trauma 7:191, 1967
5. Peterson TR: Sports injuries. p. 44. In Schneider RC, Kennedy JC, Plant ML (eds): Sports Injuries: Mechanisms, Prevention, and Treatment. Williams & Wilkins, Baltimore, MD, 1985
6. Reese RC, Burrus TP, Patten J: Shoulder equipment. p. 265. In Nicholas JA, Hershman EB, Posner MA (eds): The Upper Extremity in Sports Medicine. CV Mosby, St. Louis, 1990
7. Sawa TM: An alternate conservative management of shoulder dislocations and subluxations. Athl Train JNATA 27:4, 1992
8. Simonet WT, Cofield RH: Prognosis in anterior shoulder dislocation. Am J Sports Med 12:1, 1984
9. Wirth MA, Rockwood CA: Pathology and pathogenesis of major disorders of shoulder motion and stability. p. 290. In Matsen FA, Fu FH, Hawkins RJ (eds): The Shoulder: A Balance of Mobility and Stability. American Academy of Orthopaedic Surgeons, Rosemont, IL, 1992

CHAPTER TWENTY-SEVEN

Preventive Approach to the Athlete's Shoulder

David H. Janda

"Injury is probably the most underrecognized major public health problem facing the nation today, and the study of injury represents unparalleled opportunities for reducing morbidity and mortality and for realizing significant savings in both financial and human terms—all in return for a relatively moderate investment."[9]

The above statement, now 5 years old, continues to ring hollow in most medical research facilities in North America. All causes of injury have been estimated to kill more than 142,000 Americans each year and cause more than 62 million persons to require medical attention annually.[10] The U.S. Consumer Product Safety Commission has reported 5 million medically treated injuries associated with 15 of the most popular sports in a 1-year period.[13] Injuries are the greatest single killer of individuals from ages 1 to 44 years and cost the nation approximately $133.2 billion each year.[10] Thus, it is an understatement that injuries are an enormous public health problem that continue to usurp our limited health care financial resources.

In North America, a vast majority, if not all, of the training programs for sports medicine personnel including physicians focus on the treatment and rehabilitation of the injured individual. Little, if any, attention is given to teaching the skills required to evaluate a problem from a preventive approach, and the development of a preventive approach to a problem is consequently underemphasized or even nonexistent. Such is currently the case with sport medicine, a field in which prevention can take the form of modifications in training, preventive equipment, and elimination of unsafe practices.

Several published research studies emphasizing the preventive approach within the sports medicine field have yielded an enormous reduction in injury rates, as well as an enormous reduction in health care costs. Peterson's[12] 1970 analysis of injury rates in football led to the elimination of cross-body blocking and a substantial reduction in football injuries. The institution of passive preventive measures as recommended by the research of Pashby et al,[11] involving protective eye wear during racquet sports, has led to significant diminution in eye injuries and associated health care costs.

Similarly, in the United States more than 40 million individuals nationally participate in organized softball and baseball leagues, playing an estimated 23 million games a year in the United States. It has been estimated that softball and baseball injuries are two of the leading sports-related causes of emergency department visits in the United States. Previous studies conducted in Ann Arbor, Michigan, have elucidated that sliding is responsible for more than 70 percent of all recreational softball injuries. Also, break-away bases, which have been used in recreational softball leagues, have resulted in a 98 percent reduction of injuries and a 99 percent reduction in acute health care costs. An independent analysis by the Center for Disease Control in Atlanta, Georgia, has determined that the use of break-away bases has the potential of preventing 1.7 million injuries a year in the United States, with a savings of $2 billion a year nationally in health care costs. Also, in a recent study conducted within the NCAA and professional minor league baseball by the Institute for Preventa-

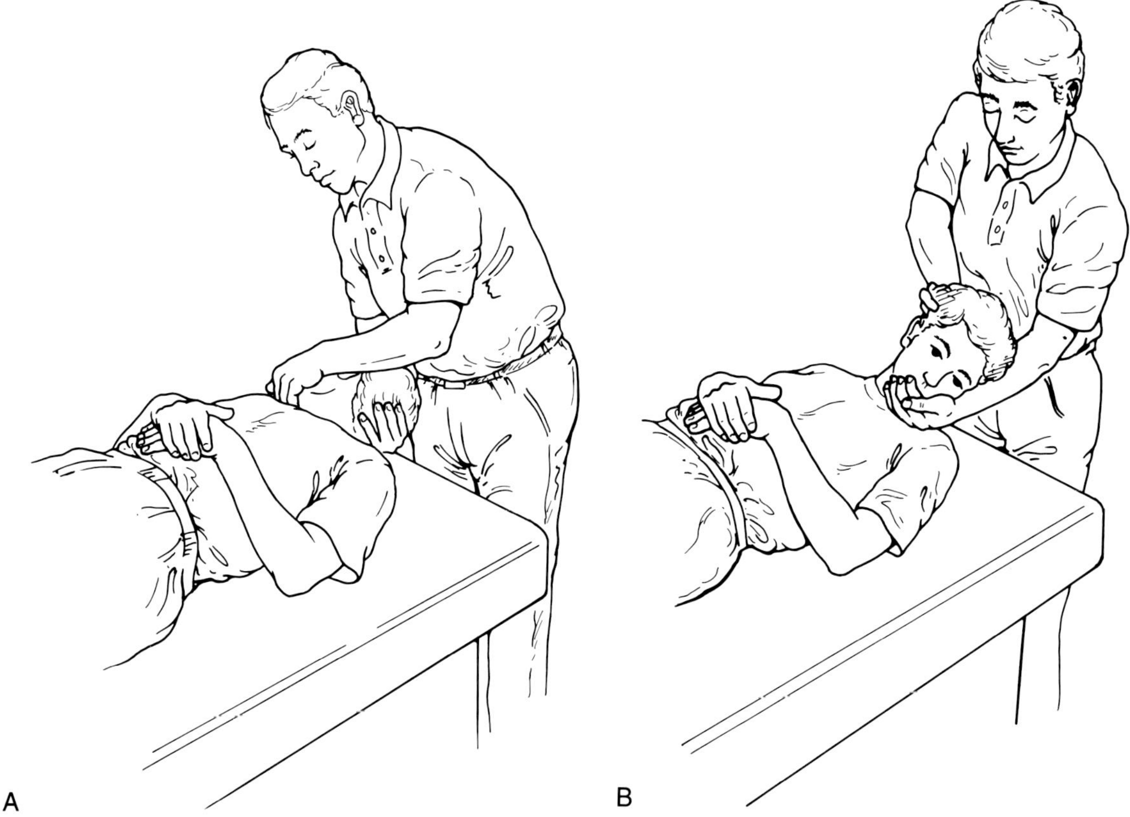

Figure 27-1. Neck exercise. Patients is in a supine position. Standing at patient's head, one hand is placed under chin (chin cupped in palm) and the other hand under occipital area. (**A**) In rhythm and with resistance, the patient should flex and rotate the neck until the chin reaches the center of the clavice. Then, in the reverse diagonal, the extension and rotation should be performed. This is repeated 10 times in each direction. (**B**) This and all proprioceptive neuromuscular facilitation exercises are isotonic and should be performed in rhythm and through the fullest range of motion. A diagonal pattern should always be used.

tive Sports Medicine, an 80 percent reduction ($P < .05$) was noted in this high-performance baseball population using break-away bases. This series of studies is a testimonial to the impact prevention-related research within the sports medicine community can have on a nationwide basis.[4]

On the one hand, research directed toward documenting the efficacy of preventive measures in sports seems to be logical, straightforward, and relatively simple. Unfortunately, this is not the case at present. Even with well-substantiated studies, the enforcement of protective rules and use of protective equipment continue to be shunned by the athletic community at large. Tradition has been one of the major obstructions to introducing new rules or equipment to prevent injuries. Implementing equipment changes such as break-away bases may offend the traditionalist and undermine traditional aspects of the sport. Also, other obstacles such as ignorance or lack of recognition of safety measures can delay or block instituting preventive measures.

Unfortunately, the general public can be misled by unethical and unsubstantiated prevention claims in product promotion. An example is the misleading use of medical research and testing by the Megg-Nets USA and Riley-Meggs Industries. A U.S. District Court judge has held these companies liable for unfair competition and false advertising for the unauthorized and improper use of research and test results in connection with their products—when, in fact, their products were *not* used in the testing or study. The medical community cannot stand by and allow the innocent public to be duped by unsubstantiated, false, and misleading advertising claims about safety.

Similar examples that can be brought to light focus on the chest and head impact fatality scenario that is occurring in youths between ages 5 and 14 years playing baseball in the United States. The Consumer Product Safety Commission has determined that baseball is the number one sport leading to fatalities in the United States. The two common scenarios for fatality include being struck either in the chest or in the head with a pitched or batted baseball.

Studies conducted by Janda and Viano at the Institute for Preventative Sports Medicine have, in fact, shown that manufacturers' safety claims are grossly exaggerated. The studies completed at the institute on the chest impact side of the equation reveal that softer baseballs and chest protectors for batters and pitchers, in fact, do not provide any protection, and some of these products actually enhance the impact when measuring force, momentum, energy transfer, and a measure of the risk of injury—viscous criterion. A similar study focusing on head impacts revealed that manufacturers' claims are grossly overexaggerated. This misinformation by several of the manufacturers imparts significant misinformation to the public and therefore leads to a public that is actually being exposed to further injury needlessly. Further, implementation of some protective equipment may be expensive and resisted by communities, schools, and organizations, because they must absorb the additional cost without benefiting directly from reduced insurance premiums.[5]

It is of paramount importance that citizens, organizations, and most important, physicians, researchers, and other health care professionals maintain persistent pressure on all organized sports groups, school leagues, city leagues, professional sports, and college sports to consider and promote improved equipment, safer techniques, and preventive measures. It is obvious that without this leadership by physicians and health care personnel, the necessary changes will not be instituted, and therefore, injury will continue to drain our already overburdened health care systems.

It has been well documented that throwing athletes, and, in particular, baseball pitchers at all levels of competition, face a substantial risk of injury.[3] It has also been reported that 50 percent of all professional baseball pitchers experience sufficient shoulder and elbow symptoms to keep them from pitching at various times in their careers.[2] Thurston has identified eight common causes of pitching injuries. They include fatigue such as the overuse syndrome, lack

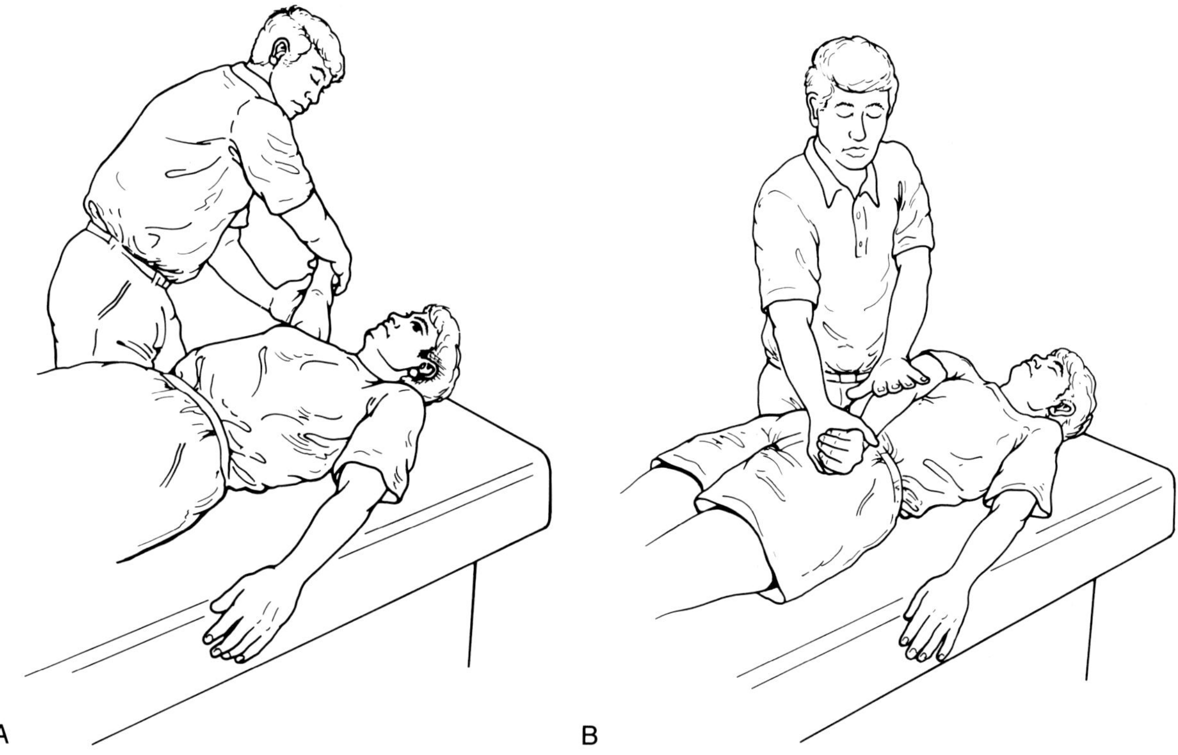

Figure 27-2. Left or right shoulder exercise. Patient is in a supine position. With the theropist standing at left or right side of patient. (**A**) The exercise should start on the right side. The arm should be entirely straight throughout the patterns, keeping the elbow stiff. The patient's hand is grasped with your right hand when you are standing on the right side. Your left hand should support the patients elbow. (**B**) You can start with either the upward or downward diagonal. As the patient moves the arm into extension internal rotation, the guideline should be anterior iliac crest. As the patient moves the arm up and out (flexion external rotation), the diagonal angle should be maintained in the oposite direction from the anterior iliac crest. It should be noted that the adduction can be added to the extension internal rotation pattern and that the abduction can be added to the flexion external rotation pattern. This exercise is repeated 10 times, with some resistance in both diagonal directions.

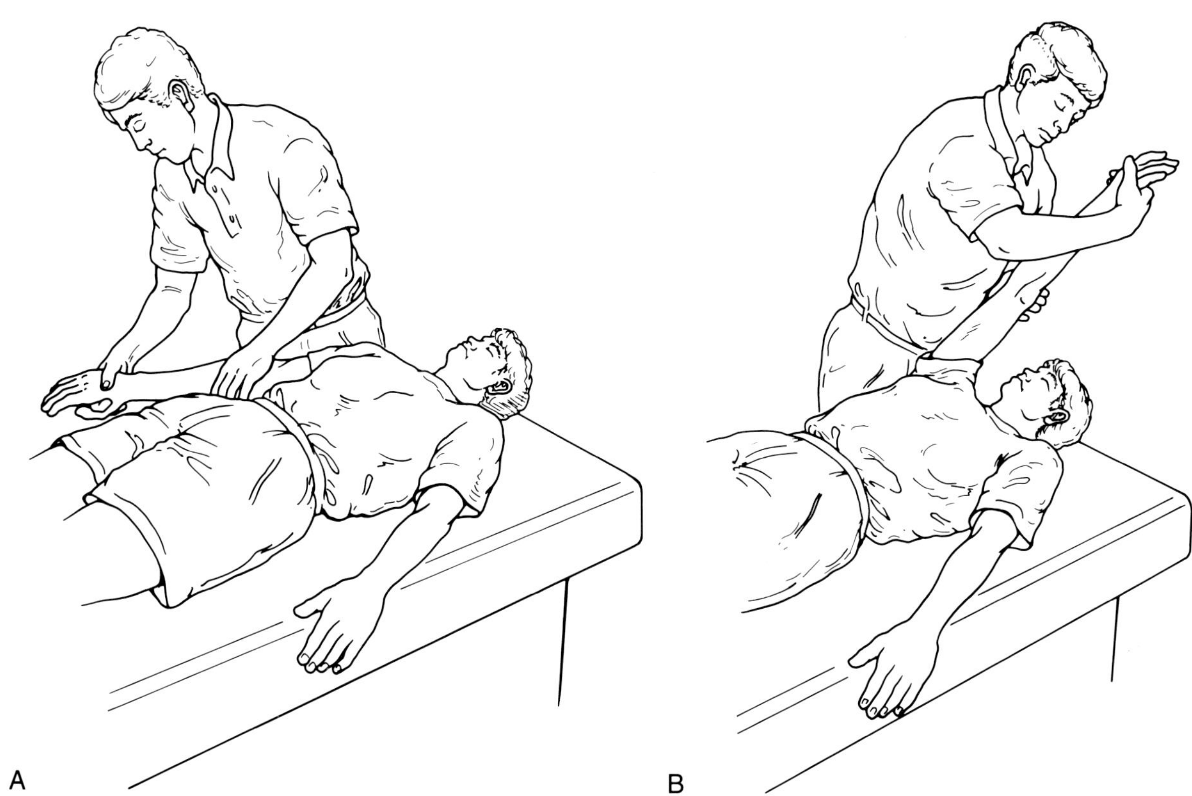

Figure 27-3. Left or right shoulder exercise. Patient is in a supine position. (**A**) Starting on the right side, you should keep the patient's elbow stiff. With your right hand, you grasp the patient's hand. With your left hand, you support the elbow. Our landmark will be the nose and its opposite diagonal. (**B**) Exercise is begun either up and in or down and out. When going up and in toward the nose (flexion external rotation adduction), you must remember to keep the elbow stiff. When going down and out (external abduction and internal rotation), you can follow the opposite diagonal from the nose. The pattern and rhythm should be kept. This exercise is repeated 10 times in each direction with some resistance. (It is important to always be careful not to administer too much resistance, only what each individual can handle through the fullest range.)

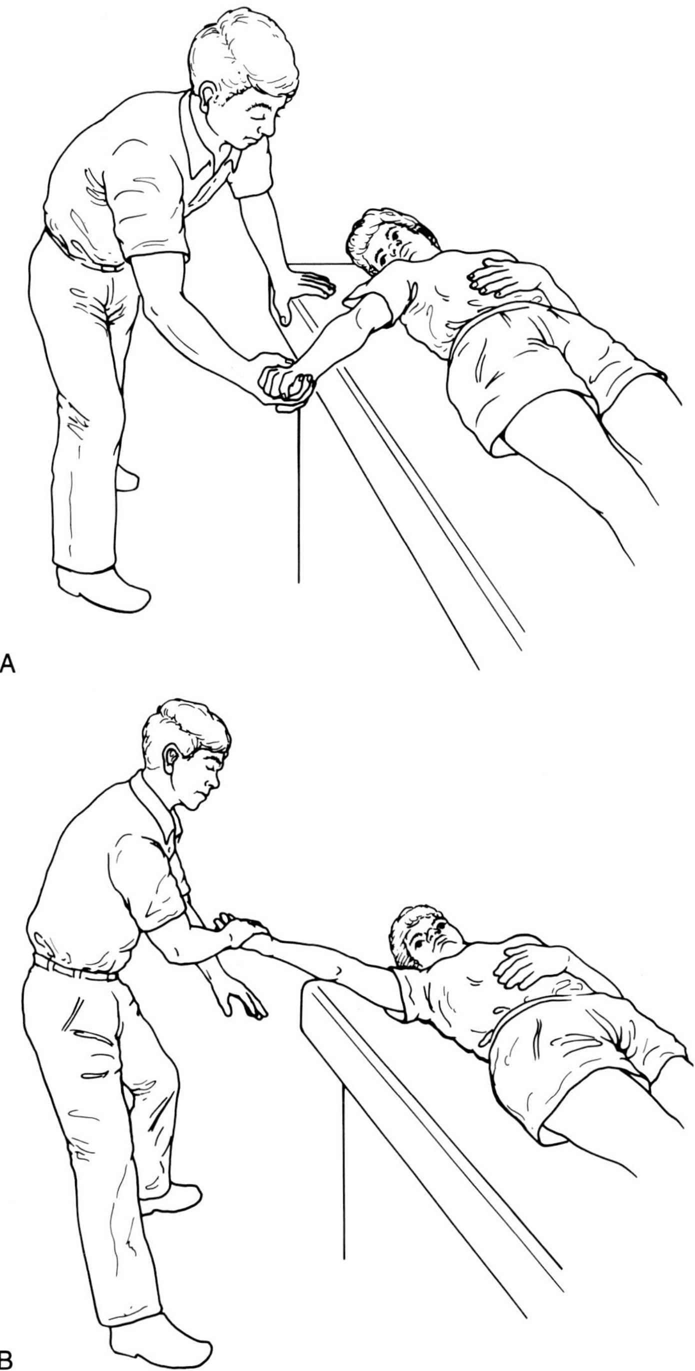

Figure 27-4. Shoulder joint and shoulder girdle exercise. Patient is in a supine position. (**A**) Starting on the right side, you should grasp the right hand of the patient with your right hand. You must support the elbow with your left hand. The elbow must be kept straight throughout this motion. The exercise is begun by placing the patient's arm along the side of the rib cage toward the posterior side. (**B**) You should follow the abduction external rotation, then adduction internal rotation toward the posterior side of the rib cage. As you take the arm away from the rib cage, the shoulder should be immediately rotated externally while abduction is also occurring. The upper extremity is taken through the fullest range of motion possible with some resistance. The motion is reversed going into adduction and immediately the shoulder adduction internal rotation toward the posterior side of the body is begun. You should follow the rhythm through the fullest range of motion with some resistance.

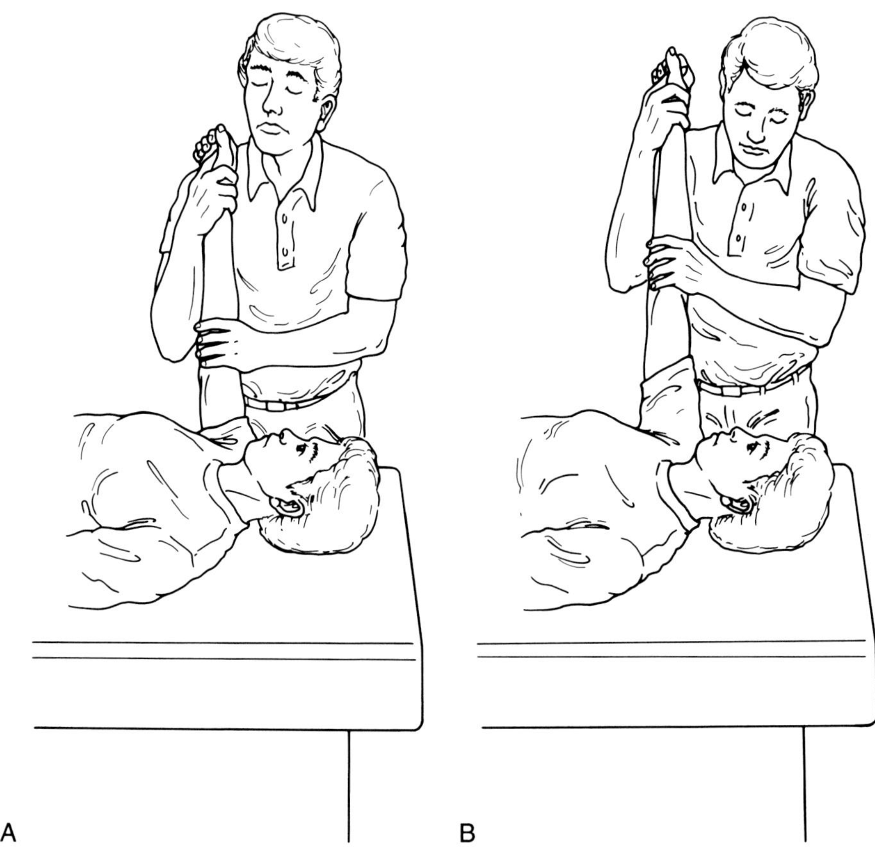

Figure 27-5. Should girdle and scapula stabilization exercise. Patient is in a supine position. (**A**) You stand on patient's side with arm pointed straight at ceiling and with the elbow kept stiff. (**B**) The arm is pushed straight up and down, again with the elbow kept stiff. You should apply resistance in both the up and down motion. The elbow must be kept stiff at all times. This exercise is repeated 10 times up and down.

of proper conditioning, lack of development of the pitching arm strength, lack of proper warm-up and stretching, lack of a recovery program or a recovery time between pitching rotations, attempting new techniques while throwing at full velocity, overstretching of the soft tissues about the shoulder joint, and improper throwing mechanics.[1]

It is imperative that orthopaedic surgeons turn the focus of their attention to the prevention of injury. This is of particular importance in the glenohumeral joint, where most injuries in the athletic and occupational populations are related to overuse. The countless hours of training and practicing are to be condemned if faulty technique or improper methods lead to damage to the musculoskeletal units about the glenohumeral joint. The underlying principle of prevention is applied common sense. A musculotendinous unit is only capable of resisting as much as it has been prepared to resist.

The basis of a preventive program designed for the glenohumeral joint is preparation. The preparation must invoke overall body conditioning, flexibility, and strengthening of the musculature about the glenohumeral joint and scapula.

Several rehabilitative exercise programs have been developed such as the program instituted by Jobe and Moynes,[6] which focuses on a stretching and strengthening program with free weights.

This chapter reintroduces the technique of proprioceptive neuromuscular facilitation (PNF). I have developed this approach into a preventive technique that is under clinical investigation at the institute for Preventative Sports Medicine.[3] PNF was developed at the Kabat-Kaiser Institute by Herman Kabat, MD. Techniques of PNF invoke placing a demand where a response is desired (Figs. 27-1 to 27-11).

These techniques may be defined as methods of promoting or hastening the response of the neuromuscular mechanism through stimulation of the proprioceptors. Emphasis is placed on the application of maximal resistance throughout the range of motion, using many combinations of motions in a pattern format. Motion is first performed in the strongest part of the range, with progression toward the weaker parts of the range of motion. Stretch is applied to groups of muscles, usually synergists, for greater proprioceptive stimulation. The technique of repeated contractions is used to gain range of motion as well as to improve endurance. The patterns used are spiral and diagonal in character and closely resemble the movements used in sports and in occupational activities.[7]

There are two diagonals of motion for the head and neck, the upper trunk, and the upper extremities. Each of the two diagonals is composed of two antagonistic patterns. Each of the spiral and diagonal patterns is a thee-component motion with respect to the glenohumeral joint. The three components include flexion or extension, abduction or adduction, and internal rotation. A pattern of motion permits the musculature to contract from a completely lengthened state to a completely shortened state when the pattern is performed through the full range of motion.[7]

The pattern of muscles contracting toward the shortened rate is termed the *agonistic pattern.* The pattern of muscles approaching the lengthened state in cooperation with those of the agonistic pattern is termed the *antagonistic pattern.*[8] Two types of muscle contraction are used in the PNF techniques. The first is an isotonic contraction, which is induced as the patient performs the particular pattern through a range of motion. The second is an isometric contraction, which is induced as the patient holds the upper extremity still without permitting a range of motion. The goal of this technique is a coordinated performance of patterns of facilitation through a full range of motion and with a balance of power between antagonistic patterns of both diagonals of motion.[7] In my current clinical investigation, I have implemented this technique as a purely preventive program in throwing athletes. The program that is currently being used focuses on the neck, upper trunk, and upper extremities. Initially, the patterns are implemented under the guidance of a trainer. Once the patterns are learned by the individual, a buddy system is used. The timing of these patterns is discussed later in this chapter.

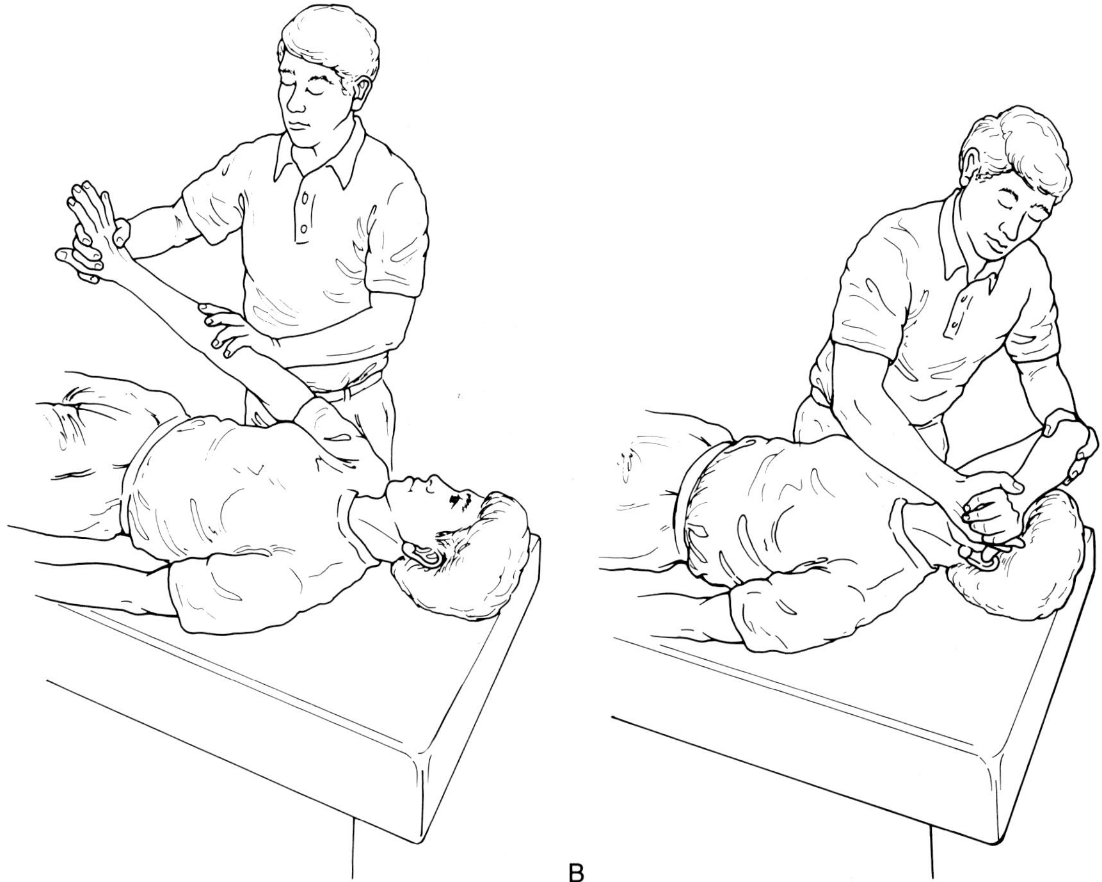

Figure 27-6. Combination shoulder and elbow exercise. Patient is in a supine position. (**A**) Standing at the patient's side, you start with the elbow bent to 90 degrees. If you are working the right arm, you grasp the patient's hand with your right hand and support the flexed elbow with your left hand. (**B**) This motion will include flexion of the shoulder and at the same time supination of the elbow and hand squeeze (finger flexion). When taking the arm up and over the head, the elbow is kept bent and the forearm supinate. When you start to return, you lead with the shoulder extension and elbow extension at the same time. The extension should be 45 degrees to the horizontal. Some resistance should be applied while maintaining the rhythm. This motion is repeated 10 times.

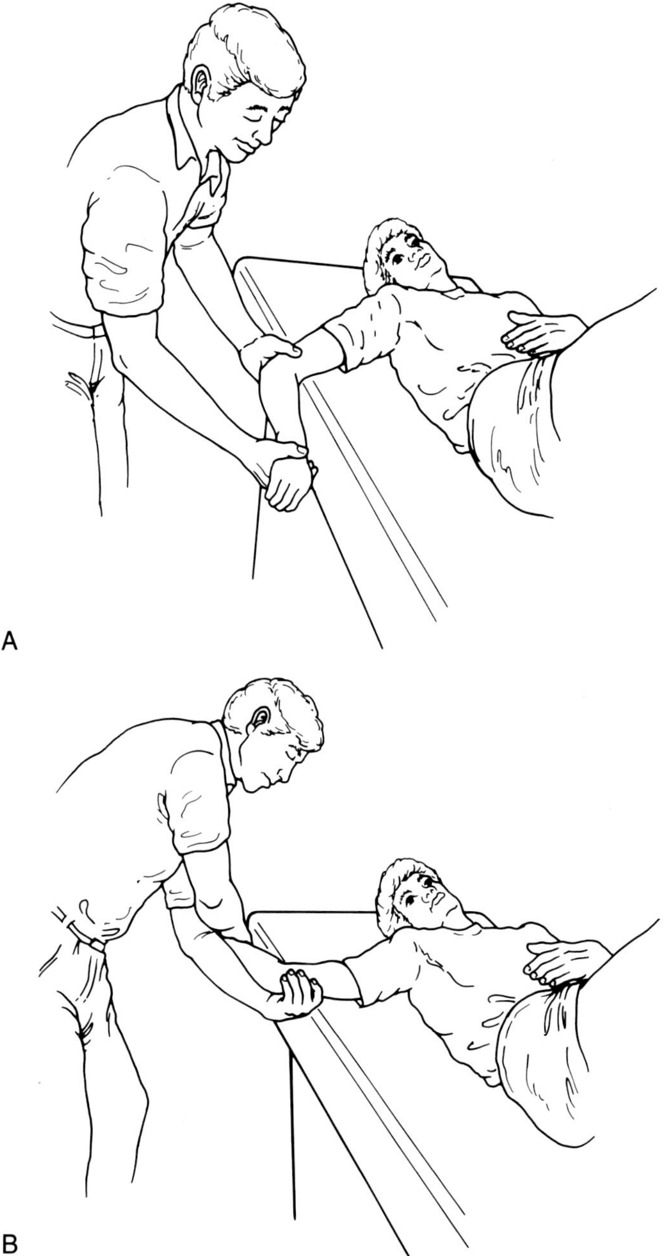

Figure 27-7. Shoulder exercise. Patient is in a supine position. (**A**) You stand at right side of patient. This motion will begin with the elbow bent at 90 degrees and with the shoulder abducted. This motion focuses on internal and external rotation through the fullest range possible, with resistance. (**B**) The right hand of the patient is grasped with your right hand and the elbow supported with your left hand. While applying these patterns, the shoulder should be kept in an abducted position. The elbow should not be allowed to slide downward from the abducted position. Tightness is indicated when the elbow wants to slide into a more adducted position. Motion should not be forced, and only the fullest range that the person can perform should be attempted.

PREVENTIVE PROPRIOCEPTIVE NEUROMUSCULAR FACILITATION PROGRAM

Implementation

For the program to be effective, a routine must also be used for throwing athletes. The routine that I have implemented is as follows:

Off-season
- Patterns every other day
- Lob tossing before patterns

During season
- Day 0: day of pitching game, ice on neck, shoulder, trunk
- Day 1: passive range of motion, patterns (light resistance), massage, lob toss
- Day 2: passive range of motion, patterns (more resistance), massage, lob toss
- Day 3: no patterns, throw as per pitching coach
- Day 4: pitch game

The program I have outlined is purely a preventive one for the upper extremities in the throwing athlete. I believe, however, that this program can be implemented in non-throwing athletes and in the occupational population involved in overhead activities. I have found this program to be easily used in an university setting. The keystone to this program is the participating individual. For optimal

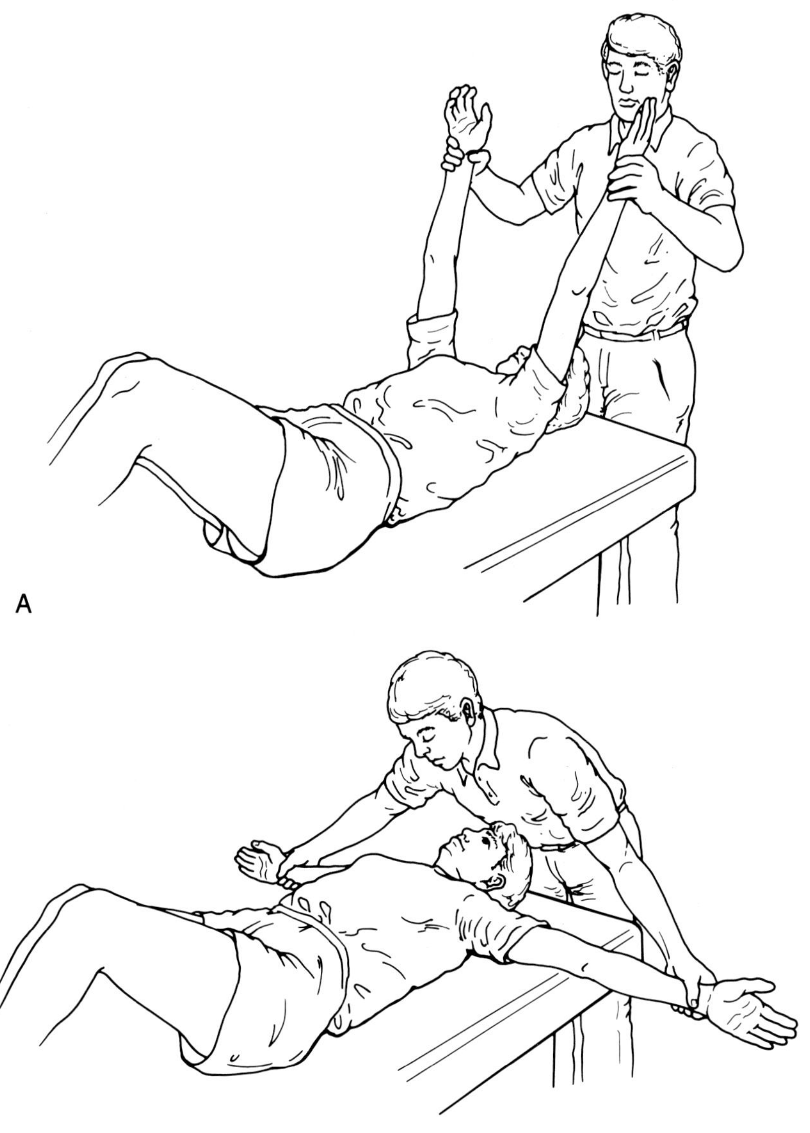

Figure 27-8. Shoulder girdle exercise. Patient is in a supine position. (**A**) You stand at the head of patient. The patient's arms should be straight and pointed toward ceiling. You grasp both hands. (**B**) The patient should horizontally abduct shoulders and then horizontally adduct shoulders. This is repeated 10 times with resistance.

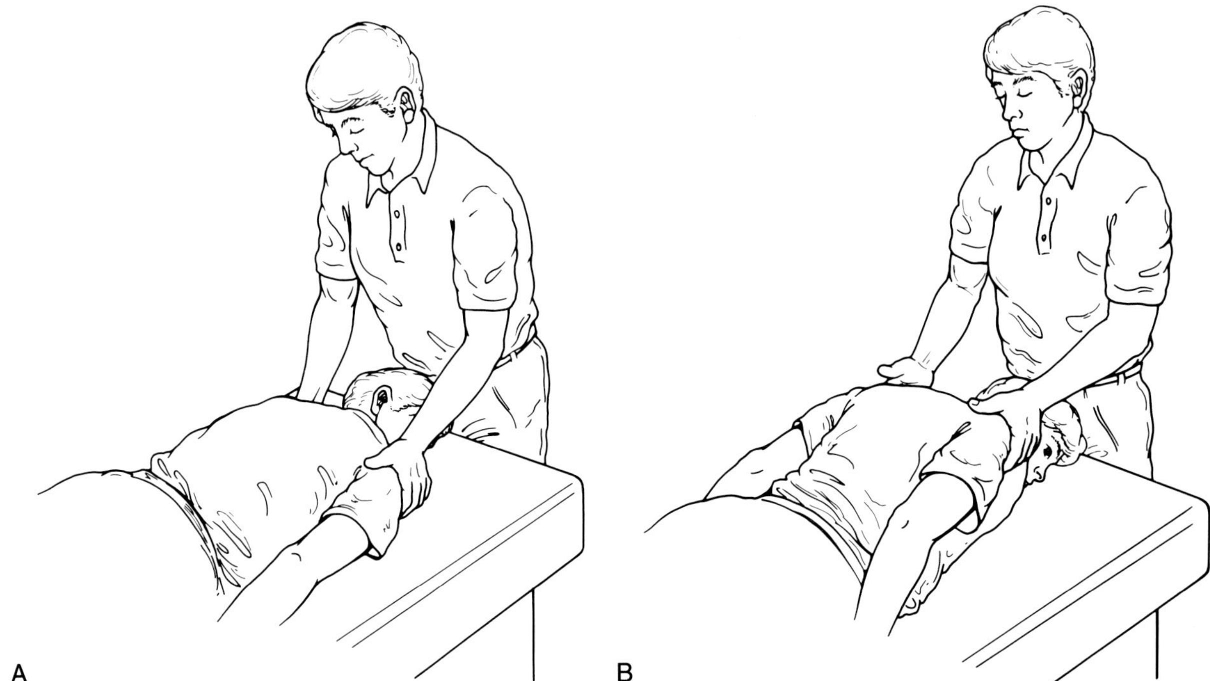

Figure 27-9. Scapular exercise. Patient is in a prone position. The head is turned onto the ear (not the cheek). (**A**) Arms should lay along the side of the body. (**B**) Only shoulders are worked up and down with some resistance. This exercise is repeated 10 times.

results, the program should be performed as outlined in this chapter.

With more people flocking into recreational and team sports for cardiovascular fitness, the likelihood that shoulder symptomatology will develop is high. It is therefore imperative that a preventive program be developed and used in both the athletic and occupational populations.

Testing Protocol Developed for Throwing Athletes

In addition to the preventive upper extremity program that I have implemented with the assistance of Warren G. Crouch, a testing protocol has also been developed with the assistance of Peter V. Loubert, Ph.D.[14] Both of these are under clinical investigation at the Institute for Preventative Sports Medicine. This testing protocol is designed for use as a repeatable performance measure for baseball pitchers or for throwing athletes participating in our sports injury prevention program. It is intended to provide objective performance data to accompany clinical and epidemiologic data. This information is believed to be necessary because it measures the performance effectiveness of the throwing athlete involved. This testing protocol has been designed to have both functional and controlled clinical components (i.e., to be easily carried out and, it is hoped, objective).

Six tests are performed. Four are performed on the Biodex (Shirley, NY) dynamometer, and two are functional activities involving throwing. Because pitching is the activity of interest, the two most important characteristics to measure that have a bearing on its effectiveness are speed and accuracy. These are described in tests 1 and 2, respectively. Of the Biodex tests, two are relatively common: internal/external rotation with the arm at the side and with the arm abducted to 90 degrees. These are described as tests 3 and 4, respectively. They provide a relatively good measure of strength of the rotator cuff musculature, one of the obvious potential limitations to a person performing high-intensity throwing tasks. The remaining two tests are for strength and endurance in the principal diagonal direction used for the throwing motion (i.e., moving from a flexed, abducted, and externally rotated position to an extended, adducted, and internally rotated position). The strength and endurance tests in the diagonal plane are described as tests 5 and 6, respectively.

Test 1—Maximum Throwing Velocity

Test 1 measures the maximum throwing velocity that a pitcher is capable of. It requires a testing site that is comparable with a normal pitching situation, specifically a pitcher's mound, a catcher, and a normal distance for the pitches. It is also requires a radar gun for measurement of pitch velocity.

Procedure

1. The participants should undertake a normal warm-up routine, including stretching, throwing lightly, and throwing at gradually increasing intensity, until they are warmed up. The throwing should include at least 20 pitches at near full effort.
2. Participants are then asked to throw five fast-ball pitches as hard and as fast as they can. It should be made clear that maximum velocity and not accuracy is important for this task. To be counted, a pitch need only come reasonably close to the home plate and be picked up on the radar.
3. After the maximum velocity throws, the participants should be instructed to cool down with about 5 minutes of light throwing.
4. The score for this task is the highest velocity of the five pitches.

Test 2–Throwing Accuracy

Test 2 measures the accuracy that the pitcher is capable of. It should be performed immediately after the participant completes the 5-minute cool-down from Test 1. The test requires a square target (18 in. to a side) placed on a

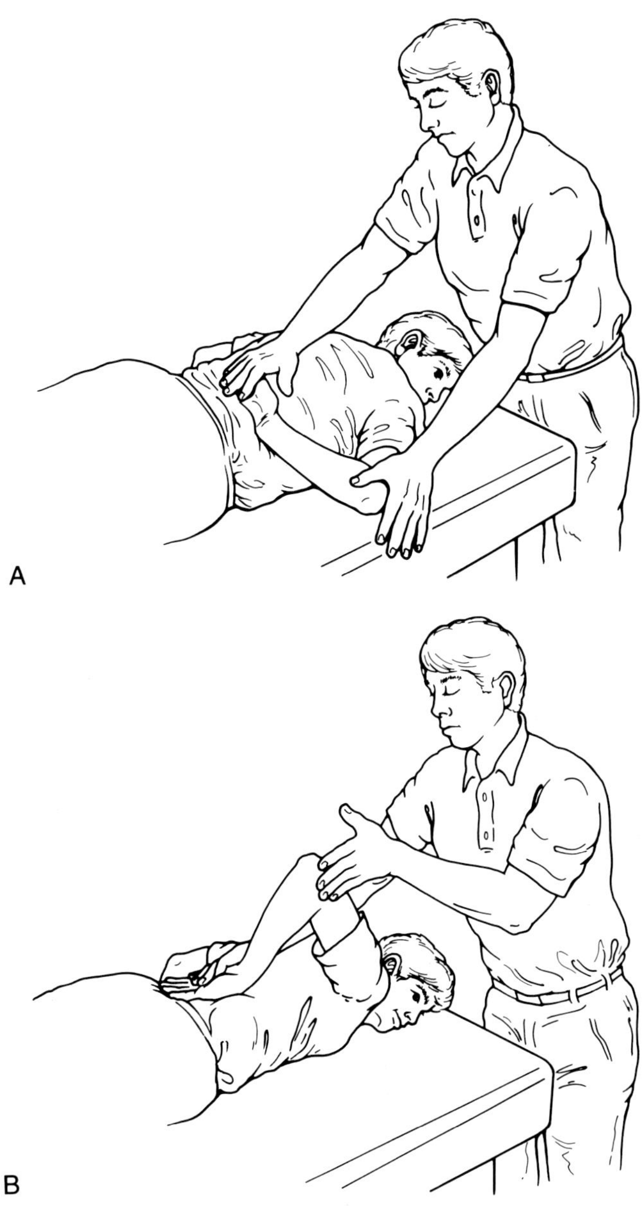

Figure 27-10. Shoulder girdle exercise. Patient is in a prone position. The head is turned onto the ear (not on cheek). (**A**) The shoulder is internally rotated until you can place the patient's hand onto the the lumbar area. (**B**) The hand that is on the lumbar area is held gently and carefully. With your other hand, you grasp the bent elbow. Again, the patient should carefully work the elbow up and down using some resistance. This exercise is repeated six to eight times.

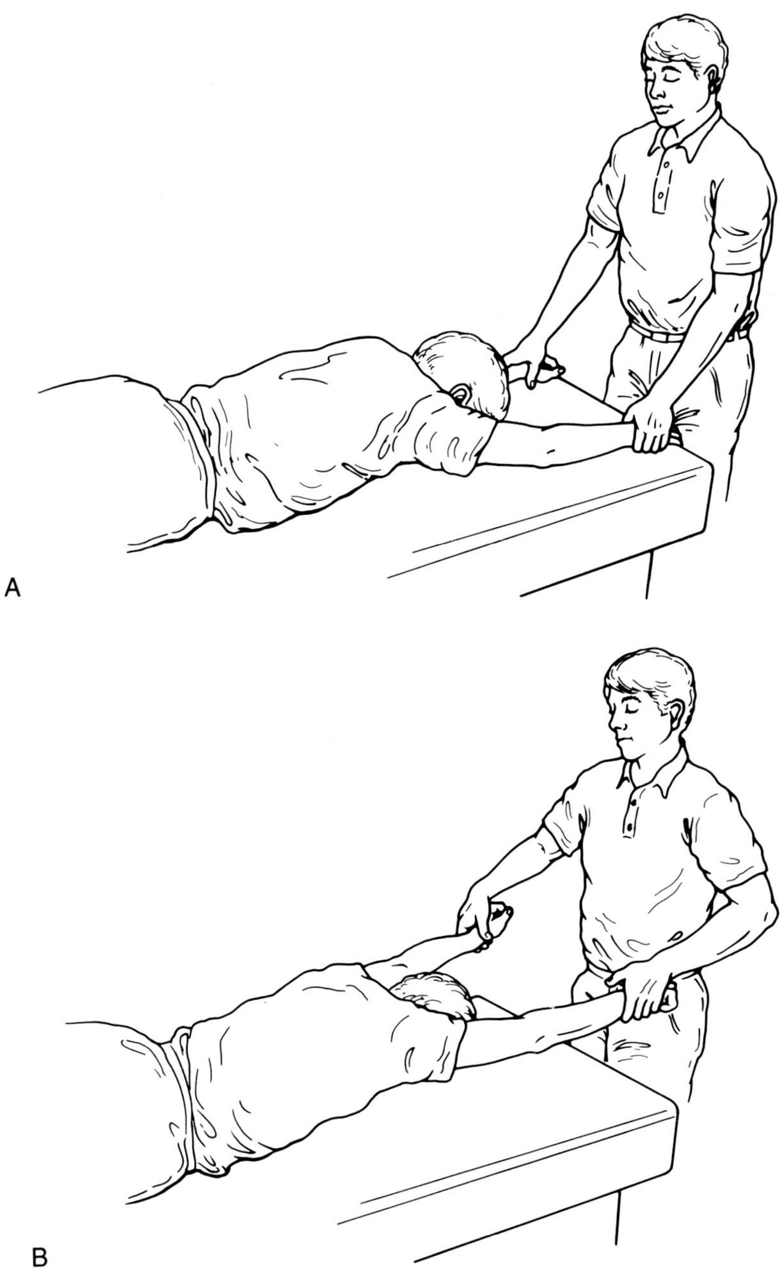

Figure 27-11. Shoulder girdle exercise. Patient is in a prone position with a pillow under the stomach. Elbows are straight with arms close to the ears. (**B**) You grasp each wrist with your hands. (**B**) The patient should lift the arms up and down using resistance in both directions. This exercise is repeated 10 times.

pitcher's screen 20 in. from the ground. The target should be placed the normal distance from the pitcher's mound to home plate.

Procedure

1. The participant is instructed to throw at 90 percent or more of maximum velocity and to attempt to hit the target. Each pitcher is asked to throw 20 "good" pitches.
2. Each throw is clocked with the radar gun and visually observed or videotaped to determine if it hits within the target area. Pitches are defined as "good" when they are at 90 percent or more of the maximum velocity, as determined in test 1. Each good pitch is recorded as "successful" or "unsuccessful" at hitting the target. The task is complete when the pitcher has thrown 20 good pitches (i.e., 20 pitches at 90 percent of maximum velocity).
3. The score for this task is the number of successful hits on the target of the 20 good pitches.

Tests 3 to 6

Tests 3 to 6 are performed in a single session after the session for tests 1 and 2. The second session should occur not less than 1 hour or greater than 5 days after the first session. Both the dominant and nondominant sides of the body should be tested for these four tasks.

Test 3—Shoulder Rotation From a Neutral Position

Test 3 is a standard Biodex test for internal and external rotation with the arm at the side.

Procedure

1. The subject should be in a standing position with the arm at the side. The axis of rotation of the dynamometer should be set at 180 degrees per second.
2. The subject is asked to perform 20 repetitions of internal and external rotation at 50 percent effort to warm-up.
3. The test consists of a set of five repetitions of external and internal rotation at maximum effort.
4. The scores for this task are the maximum torque and maximum work performed for each of the test directions.

Test 4—Shoulder Rotation From a Position of 90 Degrees of Abduction

Test 4 is a standard Biodex test for internal and externl rotation with the arm elevated 90 degrees from the side.

Procedure

1. The subject should be in a sitting position with the arm abducted 90 degrees. The axis of rotation of the dynamometer should be aligned with the long axis of the subject's humerus. The dynamometer speed should be set at 180 degrees per second.
2. The subject is asked to perform 10 repetitions of internal and external rotation at 50 percent effort to warm-up.
3. The test consists of a set of five repetitions of external and internal rotation at maximum effort.
4. The scores for this task are th maximum torque and maximum work performance for each of the test directions.

Test 5—Diagonal Strength

Test 5 is a strength test in a diagonal that is similar to the normal throwing plane and to one of the diagonals used in a strengthening exercise protocols. The set-up for this test and for test 6 requires the use of an alignment prop. The alignment prop should be a 2-ft-square piece of cardboard that can be laid on the floor in front of the subject being tested. It should have two bold lines that intersect at a 45 degree angle and that can serve as a visual guide to ensure consistency in setting up the subjects. The directions of the motion should be from a position of abduction, flexion, and external rotation (away from the body) to a position of adduction, extension, and internal rotation (across the body).

Procedure

1. The subject should be seated and aligned so that the midsagittal plane of the body intersects the plane of rotation of the dynamometer at a 45 degree angle. The dynamometer speed should be set at 180 degrees per second.
2. The subject is asked to perform 20 repetitions of the diagonal plane motion at 50 percent effort to warm-up. Demonstration and assistance by the tester may be necessary to familiarize the subject with the motion required for the task.
3. The test consists of a set of five repetitions of the diagonal plane motion (away from the body and across the body) at maximum effort.
4. The scores for this task are the maximum torque and maximum work performed for each of the test directions.

Test 6—Diagonal Endurance

Test 6 is an endurance task in the same diagonal plane as that for test 5.

Procedure

1. The set-up for this procedure is the same as that for test 5.
2. The test consists of a set of 20 repetitions of the diagonal plane motion (away from the body and across the body) at maximum effort.
3. The scores for this task are the percentages of maintenance of peak torque over the 20 repetitions for each direction.

SUMMARY

In summary, it is the responsibility of every health care provider within the field of sports medicine to make the practice of prevention the rule and not the exception. If we are truly serious about reducing morbidity, mortality, and the health care dollars spent on sports injuries, we, individually and collectively, must emphasize the development of preventive techniques that would lead to a significant reduction of injuries. Also, we must develop testing protocols that scientifically and thoroughly evaluate our efforts to truly monitor our effects. It has been my experience that the preventive PNF program outlined in this chapter, as well as the testing protocol outlined, accomplishes both goals.

REFERENCES

1. Fleisig GS, Dillman CJ, Andrews JR: Proper mechanics for baseball pitching. Clin J Sports Med 1:151–70, 1989

2. Janda DH: Prevention has everything to do with sports medicine. Clin J Sports Med 2:159–60, 1992
3. Janda DH, Loubert P: A preventative program focusing on the glenohumeral joint. Clin Sports Med 10:955–71, 1991
4. Janda DH, Maguire R, Mackesy D et al: Sliding injuries in college and professional baseball—a prospective study comparing standard and break-away bases. Clin J Sports Med 78–91, 1993
5. Janda DH, Viano DC, Andrzejak DV, Hensinger RN: An analysis of preventative methods of baseball induced chest impact injuries. Clin J Sports Med 2:172–9, 1992
6. Jobe FW, Moynes, DR: Delineation of diagnostic criteria and a rehabilitative program for rotator cuff injuries. Am J Sports Med 10:336–9, 1982
7. Kabat H: Proprioceptive facilitation in therapeutic exercises. pp. 327–43. In: Therapeutic Exercises. Waverly Press, Baltimore, MD, 1965
8. Knott M, Voss DE: Proprioceptive Neuromuscular Facilitation. Harper & Row, New York, 1968
9. National Academy of Sciences. p. 7 In: Injury Control. National Academy Press, Washington, DC, 1988
10. National Committee for Injury Prevention and Control: Injury prevention: meeting the challenge. Am J Prev Med, suppl.:1, 1989
11. Pashby TJ, Bishop PJ, Easterbrook WM: Eye injuries in Canadian racquet sports. Can Fam Physician 28:967–71, 1982
12. Peterson TR: The cross body block, the major cause of knee injuries. JAMA 211:211–4, 1970
13. Rutherford GE, Miles R: Overview of Sports Related Injuries. United Safety Consumer Product Safety Commission, Washington, DC, 1981
14. Thurston B: Throwing injuries. American Sports Medicine Institute, 1991
15. Tullos HS, King JW: Throwing mechanism in sports. Orthop Clin North Am 4:709–21, 1973
16. Viano DC, McCleary JD, Andrzejak DV, Janda DH: Analysis and comparison of head impacts using baseballs of various hardness in a hybrid III dummy. Clin J Sports Med 3:217–28, 1993

CHAPTER TWENTY-EIGHT

Throwing Sports

Frank W. Jobe
John T. Kao

The throwing athlete places extraordinary demands on the shoulder. Often, unnatural movements are performed to create extra velocity or an unusual movement on the ball being thrown. Because of the repetitive nature of throwing, the athlete pushes the shoulder to ''the limit,'' and often, the slightest aberration in form, whether caused by poor mechanics or fatigue, will result in injury. The rationale for this lies in the delicate balance between mobility and stability in the shoulder. To increase power, the athlete maximizes mobility to increase potential energy, which, in turn, will be eventually converted to the kinetic energy used to propel the ball. Unfortunately, this repetitive extreme motion stresses the inherent static stabilizers of the shoulder, which include the glenohumeral ligaments, the labrum, and the bony architecture. Initially, this stretching allows the athlete to perform better because of the increased motion, but eventually stretching of these stabilizers will result in shoulder instability and decreased performance. Thus, to avoid this, every throwing athlete's training must include the maintenance of this delicate balance between mobility and stability in the shoulder. This should be accomplished by tailoring an appropriate training program specifically designed for the shoulder, properly diagnosing any shoulder injury, treating a shoulder injury with appropriate exercises or surgical intervention, and having the injured athlete gradually return to sports in a monitored and controlled manner.

The athlete must be placed on an appropriate training program early in his or her career. The younger athlete must emphasize synchronous muscle motion and proper throwing biomechanics. Electromyographic (EMG) literature has demonstrated differences in muscle firing patterns between amateur athletes and professional throwing athletes as well as between the injured and normal athlete.[18,19,26] Therefore, along with muscle synchrony, proper throwing biomechanics should be strongly emphasized early during an athlete's development. Stretching, flexibility, and maintenance of strength are also important. The older athlete must concentrate more on maintenance of strength and flexibility to avoid attritional injuries such as rotator cuff tears or muscle strains. It is also important for the athlete of any age to maintain a general conditioning program to not allow an injury to another region of the body affect proper shoulder mechanics involved with throwing. This will further help to prevent injury and maximize the longevity of the athlete's career.

A coach, trainer, or therapist must play an integral role in learning to respect an athlete's limitations and restrain the athlete from ''going over the edge,'' which can lead to injury. Being cognizant of the early warning signs of fatigue such as an elbow dropping, excessive lumbar lordosis, scapular winging, or a loss of velocity while throwing will help to minimize injury. Parnianpour[39] demonstrated that, with muscle fatigue, muscle substitution occurs, which can lead to injury. Another key indicator in pitching is the number of innings pitched during a season. Wright and House[56] have suggested that pitchers pitching more than 170 innings per season during their early formative years in the minor and major leagues have a significantly shorter career, and the experience with professional pitchers at the Kerlan-Jobe Orthopaedic Clinic seems to correlate with this. Thus, it is the responsibility of the coaches and trainers to minimize overuse and recognize early pathology. Last, coaches and trainers must remember that stellar athletes are far and few between. Therefore, one must correlate training with potential because excessive training does not necessarily result in improved performance and can certainly result in cumulative injury, which may affect not only future athletic function but normal activities of daily living.

An understanding of the injury patterns, the typical presentation of the injured throwing athlete, the appropriate treatment options available, and the injuries specific to a sport or an athlete's age will help the orthopaedist play a vital role in minimizing shoulder injury and maximizing potential in the throwing athlete.

INJURY PATTERNS

Throwing injuries can usually be divided into two broad categories: macrotraumatic and microtraumatic injuries. The macrotraumatic injuries are usually catastrophic failures, and the athlete clearly remembers injuring the shoulder, whereas microtraumatic injuries are more commonly associated with overuse syndromes and have an insidious onset.

Macrotraumatic injuries to the shoulder include certain rotator cuff tears, shoulder dislocations, and fractures. Acute rotator cuff tears can often be pinpointed to a single pitch, and a ripping sensation is often perceived. Active shoulder motion is often limited, and a lidocaine injection into the bursa may help with relieving pain but will not improve shoulder function. Traumatic shoulder dislocations are also macrotraumatic injuries that usually require manual relocation by a trained specialist. In most young athletes, recurrent anterior instability is the rule, and future surgical intervention may be warranted. Fractures of the shoulder are a rare occurrence and usually involve either pathologic fractures, fractures from falls, or avulsion-type fractures. The usual tenants of fracture care apply concerning conservative or operative treatment. Because of the tremendous forces placed on the throwing shoulder, the athlete should not be allowed to return to throwing until the fracture has completely healed, and the athlete has undergone a supervised rehabilitation program.

Microtraumatic injuries of ''overuse'' syndromes include shoulder subluxation and shoulder impingement. Anterior shoulder subluxation is common in pitchers and is caused by the repetitive trauma on the anterior capsule during the throwing motion. Throwing biomechanics have been studied in great detail in professional-level pitchers, and the throwing motion can be broken down into six phases—windup, early cocking, late cocking, acceleration, deceleration, and follow-through.[6] During late cocking and acceleration, tremendous stress is applied to the anterior stabilizers of the shoulder because of the extreme shoulder external rotation with the arm at approximately 90 degrees of abduction. This repetitive stress during throwing leaves the anterior structures susceptible to microscopic injury and gradual stretching of these stabilizers. Rowe[43] reported that overhand athletes with this problem can present with a dead-arm syndrome, having symptoms of pain and weakness in the throwing extremity. These athletes can be broken down into two categories: (1) those who can sense that their shoulder is slipping out of the joint and (2) those who cannot. The classic presentation described in the literature includes an overhand athlete with a history of repetitive overuse or an acute injury with the shoulder in the abducted and externally rotated position who complains of pain and weakness with throwing, has a positive relocation test on examination, and is frustrated about his or her inability to perform.[5,25,27,45]

Posterior capsular tightness, another common finding in this population, only compounds the problems of anterior subluxation. With posterior tightness, the center of rotation of the humeral head will be forced anterior, placing further stress on the anterior static stabilizers and also leaving the patient susceptible to anterior impingement.[34] Therefore, the recommended conservative treatment regimen for anterior subluxation should include resistive exercises initially directed at rotator cuff strengthening combined with posterior capsular stretching, followed by a controlled program to return to throwing once the patient is asymptomatic. If the patient fails this program, surgical intervention must be considered.

HISTORY AND PHYSICAL EXAMINATION

The history and physical examination are critical in making the correct diagnosis in the throwing athlete. The dictum true in all medicine that one must ''first make the diagnosis'' is certainly true when addressing shoulder problems in the throwing athlete. A thorough history and physical examination are critical and will minimize the need for obtaining multiple imaging studies, which may cloud the diagnosis. These also will allow for proper treatment to begin in a timely fashion, thus minimizing the time loss from sports.

History

The history should determine the age, sport, handedness, activity level, location of pain, radiation of pain, trauma whether acute or repetitive, mechanism of injury, nature of onset, and any pertinent medical conditions of the athlete.

The age of the athlete is important because younger athletes (35 years or younger) often have shoulder problems associated with subtle instability whereas older athletes have attritional problems such as rotator cuff tears and muscle strains. There certainly can be exceptions to these rules, especially in the high-demand professional athlete, but often these generalizations allow one to quickly begin to narrow the diagnosis.

The involved sport is also important because of the injuries often associated with specific throwing sports such as baseball, football, and the javelin throw. Certainly, the diagnosis, treatment, and prognosis of the repetitive hard-throwing pitcher with an insidious onset of shoulder pain consistent with anterior subluxation will differ from the quarterback who was hit while throwing and complains of sharp and sudden shoulder pain along with gross deformity, consistent with a shoulder dislocation. Knowing the involved sport also will allow the physician to comprehend the demands that ultimately will be expected from the injured athlete's shoulder and will allow for an appropriate rehabilitation program to be instituted.

The handedness of the injured athlete is also important. Injury to the dominant throwing arm is certainly addressed differently from injury to the nondominant arm. An example of this, which has been well documented in the literature, is the baseball pitcher with anterior shoulder instability of the dominant arm treated unsuccessfully with standard reconstruction procedures, such as the Bankart procedure or Bristow procedure, because of the loss of external rotation, as compared with the athlete with anterior instability of the nondominant arm treated with a similar procedure with great success.[32]

The character, location, and nature of onset of shoulder pain are also vital information necessary in obtaining a diagnosis. The dull aching pain characteristic of a rotator cuff tear differs from the sharp pain often associated with crepitus, commonly seen in those patients with subacromial bursitis. The location of pain is also helpful in diagnosis such as when shoulder pain presents posteriorly during an apprehension-type maneuver, which may signify subtle instability, or when pain is noted down the upper arm, which may indicate a rotator cuff tear or a superior labral tear. The nature of onset also helps to differentiate the sudden macrotraumatic-type injuries from the insidious microtraumatic-type injuries.

Any radiation of the pain may indicate a cervical origin to the pain or a concomitant shoulder and neck injury, as has been described in the literature.[20] Although rare, cardiac, diaphragmatic, and pleural pathology have been noted to account for radiating shoulder pain.

Any history of prior trauma to the shoulder is useful in helping to diagnose a possible rotator cuff tear, a possible subluxation or dislocation event, a muscle tear, a neck strain, or a previous fracture. Also important is the severity of all previous injuries, which should be documented by noting the number of practices and games missed because of the injury and the treatment necessary to resolve the problem.

The pertinent medical history can also provide valuable information that can help in diagnosis as well as treatment. Examples of this include the athlete who has a history of ingesting anabolic steroids and who presents with shoulder pain caused by advanced degenerative arthritis of the shoulder joint or the diabetic patient who presents with shoulder stiffness and pain secondary to a recalcitrant adhesive capsulitis.

By performing a thorough history, one can classify an injury into either a macrotraumatic- or microtraumatic-type injury, as well as significantly narrow the list of differential diagnoses. The history also helps to indentify aggravating positions or activities, which may be avoided during rehabilitation, while helping to locate the region of pathology. This allows for an appropriately detailed physical examination, which enables one to arrive efficiently at the correct diagnosis. Thus, the importance of a good history cannot be overly emphasized.

Physical Examination

The physical examination should focus on the shoulder but must include an examination of the cervical spine, a neurovascular examination, and a cursory examination of the entire musculoskeletal system. The examination of the shoulder, specifically, should begin with the basic foundations of the physical examination, which include inspection to note any muscle atrophy, which may signify chronic muscle rupture or neurologic compromise, and palpation to identify the presence of acromioclavicular arthritis, subacromial bursitis, biceps tendinitis, or trigger points indicative of possible cervical involvement. Of lesser value are auscultation and percussion, although these modalities may help in locating the origin of any crepitus.

A comparison of the range of motion of the affected extremity as compared with the unaffected extremity in all planes of motion is also vital. The shoulder is a highly mobile joint with more than 16,000 possible positions differentiated by at least 1 degree, and therefore, a reproducible and structured system should be used to describe the range of motion.[40] Routinely documented motions include active and passive ranges of motion of both shoulders in forward flexion, abduction, external rotation with the arm abducted to 90 degrees, external rotation at the side, and internal rotation as measured by the spinal level the patient can reach posteriorly. The examiner must remember that increased external rotation and decreased internal rotation are normal in the dominant extremity of the throwing athlete.[23] While examining range of motion, it is also important to note any problems with synchronous scapulohumeral motion or winging of the scapula. Synchronous motion between glenohumeral and scapulothoracic articulation during abduction is also critical in the throwing athlete. Normal glenohumeral to scapulothoracic motion during the first 30 degrees of abduction is 4.3 : 1. During the remainder of abduction, this ratio decreases to 1.25 : 1.[41] Problems such as rotator cuff tears or adhesive capsulitis often exhibit increased scapulothoracic motion as compared with glenohumeral motion.

Strength testing should also be performed for the various muscle groups surrounding the shoulder, including the rotator cuff, scapular, deltoid, biceps, pectoralis major, and latissimus dorsi muscles. Pain on strength testing may indicate tendinitis, whereas profound weakness may represent a muscle tendon unit disruption or neurologic compromise. Special tests of benefit may include the supraspinatus test to diagnose supraspinatus rupture or tendinitis, the drop-arm test indicative of a rotator cuff tear, or the lift-off test indicative of subscapularis dysfunction. The lift-off test described by Gerber and Krushell[17] is performed with the dorsum of the hand of the affected extremity placed on the small of the back. The patient then attempts to lift the hand off his or her back. If the patient is unable to perform this maneuver and has normal range of motion, then subscapularis dysfunction is confirmed.

Shoulder impingement must be evaluated with thorough palpation of the acromioclavicular and periacromial regions. Pain from greater tuberosity impingement on the anterolateral acromion may be elicited with specific maneuvers described by Hawkins and Kennedy[21] and Neer and Welsh.[37]

Shoulder stability must also be assessed and is often the most difficult part of the examination to quantitate. The various components of instability are increased laxity, recreation of the symptoms, and pathology. A thorough physical examination will help to identify increased laxity as well as recreate the symptoms in a patient with instability. Pathology can then be confirmed through direct visualization arthroscopically.

The classic apprehension test with a positive examination being pain with a fear of dislocation is useful only in patients who have suffered a previous dislocation. More often, in patients with subluxation, this maneuver will elicit pain but no fear of dislocation. This pain is usually posterior in nature, and the relocation test can help to confirm a diagnosis of anterior instability.[27] This test involves pressure applied to the anterior upper arm while performing an apprehension maneuver (Fig. 28-1). If the patient notices relief of the pain through a similar range of motion, then the diagnosis of anterior instability is supported. If one suddenly removes the posteriorly directed force on the upper arm, the patient will again complain of a return of the shoulder pain. Other tests such as the sulcus sign, the posterior drawer test, and the push-pull test all help in determining instability in the inferior or posterior direction.

Another useful method to assess stability is to quantitate capsular tightness as described by Gerber and Granz[16] and Cofield and Irving.[9] By comparing the degree of external rotation required to obtain anterior capsular tightness of the involved shoulder as compared with the uninvolved shoulder, using an anterior drawer maneuver at 45 and 90 degress of abduction, one can determine if increased capsular laxity is present in the affected shoulder. When one uses this criterion, though, one must again remember that throwers may have a shift in the arc of rotation with increased external rotation and decreased internal rotation in the dominant extremity, and this shift in arc of motion also shifts the point at which anterior capsular tightness is noted.

The physical examination should also detail the tightness of the posterior capsule. It has been shown that a tight posterior capsule may increase the tendency for a shoulder to subluxate anterior. This "cam effect" has been well documented in the literature.[34] Posterior capsular tightness or laxity can be measured as described by Gerber and Granz[16] and Cofield and associates[9,10] in a similar manner as evaluating anterior capsular laxity or tightness. This is performed by quantitating the degree of translation during a posterior drawer maneuver at varying degrees of internal rotation and comparing the amount of internal rotation required to eliminate any significant posterior translation. Also important is a comparison of the degree of internal rotation in both the affected and normal shoulders.

Also, the physical examination should include an evaluation for generalized laxity.[4] These patients have an increased propensity for multidirectional instability and must be identified early to allow for appropriate conservative treatment. Last, a complete shoulder examination requires an evaluation of the cervical spine to rule out any radiating-type pain as well as a cursory examination of the entire musculoskeletal system to rule out any compounding problems that may secondarily be manifested as a throwing problem.

RADIOLOGY

Radiography may be useful in confirming the diagnosis. Plain radiographs are useful for identifying acromial spurs, degenerative changes, or bony avulsion injuries. Routinely obtained radiographs include an anteroposterior view with the arm internally rotated, an anteroposterior view with the arm externally rotated, an axillary view, and a scapular outlet view. An anteroposterior view with the arm internally rotated allows for identification of a Hill-Sachs lesion whereas an anteroposterior view in external rotation allows for an excellent view of the joint as well as the greater tuberosity. The axillary view is necessary to identify a bony Bankart lesion,[44] indicative of anterior instability, or a Bennett lesion,[2] indicative of posterior capsular traction, as well as any anterior or posterior subluxation or dislocation. A scapular outlet view allows for easy classification of acromial types as described by Bigliani et al,[3] which is helpful in identifying those patients prone to impingement.

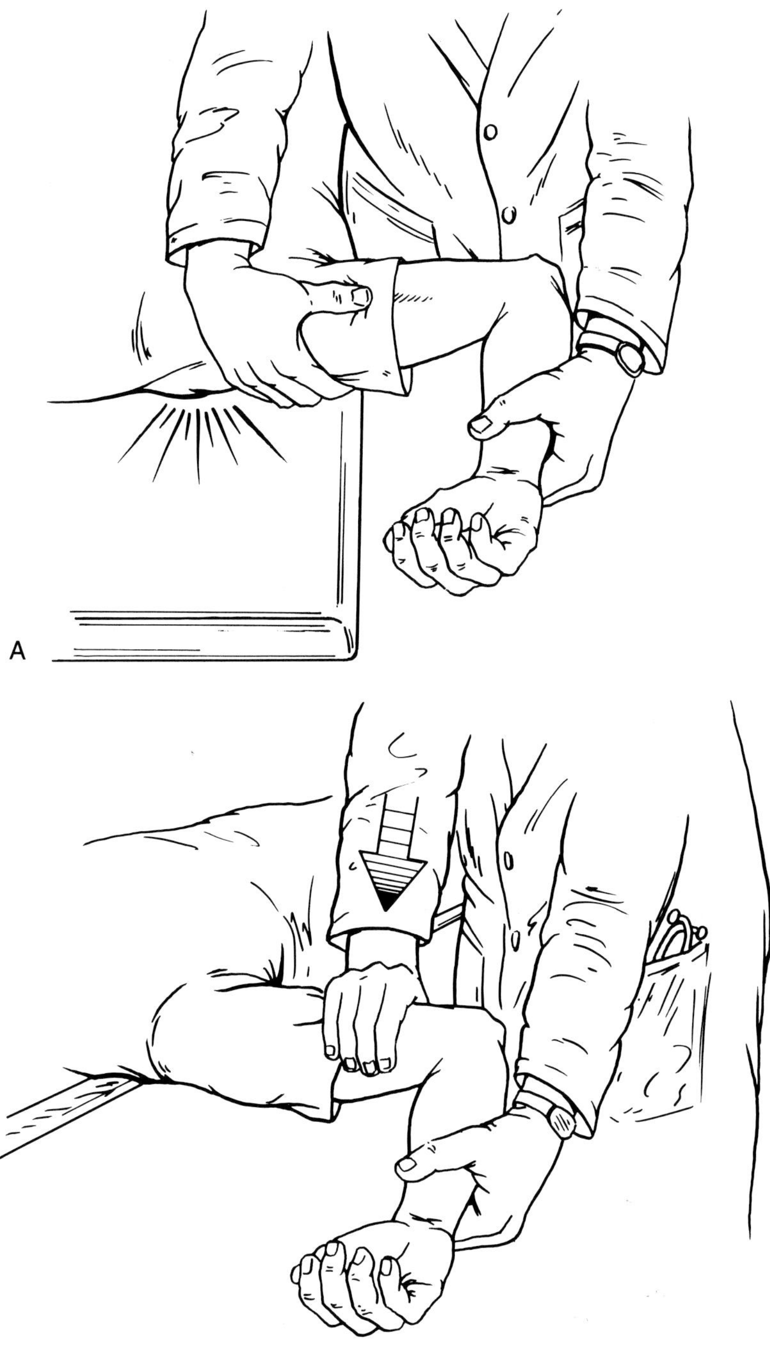

Figure 28-1. (**A**) The relocation test is initially performed as an apprehension test. This is usually uncomfortable for a patient with anterior subluxation. (**B**) A posterior force is then applied to the upper arm and humeral head while in the same position. Relief of the previous pain from the apprehension test is a sign of anterior subluxation.

Other radiographic examinations such as computer tomography (CT) scans, CT arthrograms, or magnetic resonance imaging (MRI) scans all may give added information to help confirm diagnoses but remain a poor substitute for a good history and physical examination. CT scans best allow one to visualize the bony anatomy as well as any intra-articular fractures. CT arthrograms are helpful in diagnosing labral lesions and instability with accuracy reported from 86 to 100%.[38,46] MRI scans provide excellent detail of the soft tissues surrounding the shoulder, allowing for diagnosis of rotator cuff tears, tendinitis, and impingement. It also may be used in diagnosing shoulder instability, but its accuracy appears to be inferior to CT arthrograms.[15,29] Presently, because of its noninvasive nature and an ability to demonstrate both bony and soft tissue pathology, MRI scans have gained great popularity, but it still has an unclear role in diagnosing subtle shoulder instability.

INSTABILITY VERSUS IMPINGEMENT

Most throwing athletes present with complaints of shoulder pain consistent with rotator cuff tendinitis and impingement syndrome. Rarely does one present with the classic "dead arm" syndrome. Early results treating these patients with subacromial decompression were sometimes successful at relieving the athlete's rest pain, but often, the athlete was unable to return to the previous level of competition.[48] Further investigation revealed that these patients younger than 40 years of age usually suffered from impingement secondary to instability unless an obvious spur or traumatic event was identified.[24]

Today, shoulder injuries involving instability or impingement in the throwing athlete are classified into four distinct groups. Group I is those patients exhibiting pure impingement signs and symptoms without any signs of instability. This group includes those patients with "classic" impingement as described by Neer.[36] Group II is patients with impingement signs and symptoms secondary to microtraumatic instability. This group would include the pitcher with anterior instability secondary to repetitive throwing. Group III is patients with impingement secondary to repetitive throwing. Group III is patients with impingement secondary to instability from generalized laxity. These patients would be those with Ehlers-Danlos types of laxity or those patients exhibiting classic signs of generalized laxity such as elbow and knee hyperextension, distal interphalangeal joint and metacarpal-phalangeal joint hyperextension in the hand, and a decreased thumb-to-forearm apposition distance.[4] Group IV includes patients who only exhibit signs and symptoms of instability. This group would include those patients with recurrent instability secondary to a traumatic dislocation or subluxation.

Treatment of patients within this classification should initially consist of a conservative exercise program, evaluation and modification of the athlete's mechanics, and an attempt to gradually return to throwing. Initially, rest, nonsteroidal anti-inflammatory medications, and various therapeutic modalities such as ice, heat therapy, ultrasound, phonophoresis, or electrical stimulation may be used to help decrease any tendinitis or inflammation. Next, a tailored exercise program is developed to help correct any muscular weaknesses or problems with synchronous motion. Stretching of the posterior capsule may also be necessary in those throwers with tight posterior structures. No stretching of the anterior structures is ever warranted. If this conservative treatment regimen is successful, then a throwing program may be implemented. If conservative treatment is unsuccessful, then surgical intervention may be necessary.

If group I patients fail a conservative treatment regimen after 3 to 6 months, a diagnostic arthroscopy may be performed to confirm the diagnosis of classic acromial impingement followed by an arthroscopic acromioplasty, resection of the coracoacromial ligament, and resection of the subacromial bursa. If a complete rotator cuff tear is noted at arthroscopy, an open repair should be performed. Also, if during arthroscopy, a clear subacromial space is noted along with signs of internal impingement, then group II secondary impingement with primary instability should be suspected.

If conservative treatment fails in group II patients, a diagnostic arthroscopy is performed to confirm the diagnosis followed by an anterior capsulolabral reconstruction (ACLR). These patients should then be started on a well-supervised rehabilitation program, with eventual return to throwing in 9 to 12 months.

If conservative treatment fails in group III patients, then a diagnostic arthroscopy is performed to confirm the diagnosis, followed by an ACLR. Postoperative rehabilitation in these patients should progress slowly, with absolutely no stretching or efforts to regain motion quickly because of the propensity of these patients to stretch out their repairs. No active attempt at regaining the extremes of motion should be made until after 6 months to 1 year.

Again, if conservative treatment fails in group IV patients, then a diagnostic arthroscopy is performed, followed by an ACLR. A structured rehabilitation program is then instituted with eventual return to sports.

One must appreciate that with continued microtrauma, any of the above groups may progress to a rotator cuff tear. Complete tears are noted most often in group I patients whereas group II to IV patients usually only show signs of partial undersurface tears. Complete tears in the throwing athlete are treated with open repair combined with an adequate acromioplasty. Undersurface partial tears are left alone or are minimally debrided. These partial tears are believed to be from an "internal" impingement of the undersurface of the rotator cuff on the posterosuperior glenoid rim and labrum. Also, shoulder pain in the throwing athlete caused by instability is believed to be from this internal impingement and not from the classic impingement as described by Neer,[36] which consists of rotator cuff and greater tuberosity trauma against the anterolateral corner of the acromion.[12,53] The existence of these "kissing lesions," recently documented in the literature, has been confirmed arthroscopically and in cadaveric models.[12,53] This accounts for the posterior shoulder pain often seen during an apprehension maneuver as well as the undersurface fraying of the rotator cuff noted on arthroscopy in these patients. During arthroscopy in these patients, the arm should be taken out of traction and placed into the late cocking position of throwing, the apprehension position, to evaluate any kissing lesions on the posterosuperior glenoid rim corresponding to undersurface fraying of the supraspinatus tendon (Plate 28-1 and Fig. 28-2). This internal impingement sign is another indication of anterior instability that helps to confirm the diagnosis of anterior instability and allows for initiation of a proper rehabilitation program followed by surgical intervention if conservative treatment fails.

REHABILITATION

Rehabilitation of the throwing athlete should be performed, taking into account the age of the athlete, the sport involved, and the future expectations of the athlete. Exercises should focus on shoulder stretching and synchronous muscle motion as well as on strengthening. Emphasis should be directed toward the shoulder positioning muscles (rotator cuff), the scapular muscles, and the power muscles (deltoids, latissimus dorsi, and pectoralis major). Sport-specific exercise must also be incorporated to allow for a successful return to the sport. Return to sports should be gradual, with a well-designed program starting with gentle tosses and advancing to an eventual return to the position that the patient plays. After successful reintegration into sports, a well-designed maintenance program must be continued to minimize reinjury.

Moseley et al[35] and Townsend et al[51] have identified a series of six exercises that help to strengthen all the muscles around the shoulder. These exercises include (1) scaption (shoulder elevation in the scapular plane) with the thumbs pointed down, (2) shoulder forward flexion, (3) horizontal abduction with the arms maintained in external rotation performed while in the prone position, (4) push-ups with a plus (a normal push-up adding maximum shoulder and scapular protraction with the elbows fully extended), (5) press-ups (a hand press elevating the buttocks off of a chair while in the seated position with the hands at the side), and (6) rowing (shoulder horizontal abduction with concurrent elbow flexion while in the prone position). These exercises are illustrated in Chapter 4.

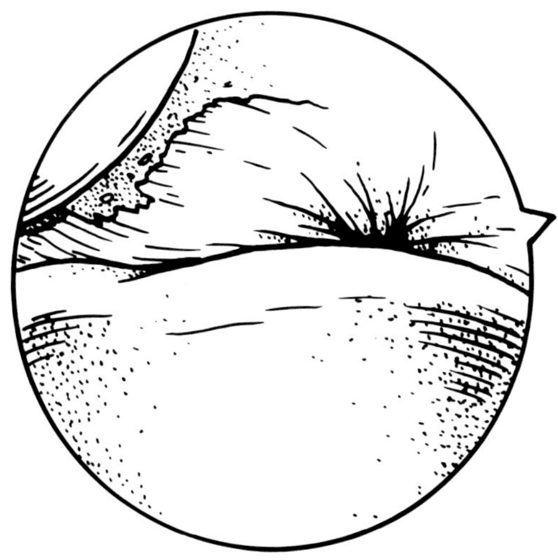

Figure 28-2. Diagram of the structures shown in Plate 2-1.

If isolated muscle weakness is diagnosed, then these exercises may be tailored toward the specific muscle injury. Specifically, the three heads of the trapezius were best exercised with scaption, horizontal abduction with the arms externally rotated, and rowing. The rhomboids and levator scapulae were best exercised with scaption, rowing, and horizontal abduction with the arms externally rotated. The serratus anterior was best exercised with scaption, flexion, and push-ups with a plus. The three heads of the deltoid were best exercised with scaption, flexion, horizontal abduction with the arms externally rotated, and rowing. The pectoralis major and latissimus dorsi were best exercised with a press-up. The supraspinatus and subscapularis were best exercised with scaption and flexion. The infraspinatus and teres minor were best exercised with flexion and horizontal abduction with the arms externally rotated. These six exercises, combined with appropriate stretching exercises, are important in maintaining adequate motor strength and flexibility.

Also important for the throwing athlete are sport-specific exercises. These exercises allow for appropriate rehabilitation and gradual return to sports in the injured athlete as well as provide the healthy athlete a therapy program necessary to maintain proper muscle synchrony and strength. An example of this program is a throwing program commonly used in throwing athletes.[28] In this program, the six core exercises previously described are emphasized, as well as other shoulder strengthening exercises such as shoulder shrugs, internal and external rotation with the patient in the lateral decubitus position, shoulder extension, and shoulder adduction with the patient supine. Also included are strengthening exercises of wrist, forearm, and elbow. Another key component is stretching exercises of the shoulder, elbow, and wrist. While performing these exercises, key elements that need to be addressed include a controlled effort by the athlete while performing the maneuver, synchronous movement in the entire upper extremity and torso, and maintenance of control and synchrony throughout a set of exercises. The amount of weight and number of repetitions should be tailored to the athlete to allow this to be accomplished.

The injured athlete must return to throwing using a well-supervised progressive throwing program. In baseball, a return to throwing should be instituted, starting with short lobs and progressing to lobs at longer distances. Throwing is performed three times a week, and all throwing is preceded with a proper warm-up and stretching program. Between throwing, the athlete must continue to work on the before-mentioned core exercises as well as sport-specific exercises. Once the player is able to make a throw from the outfield to home plate on a single bounce, he or she may begin throwing with gradually increasing velocity. The patient may then return to his or her sport position and continue advancing until the patient is performing at the prior level before surgery or injury. The throwing program should cover a period of approximately 2.5 to 3 months before the athlete is prepared to return to play.

This core of six exercises used to strengthen the shoulder muscles combined with sport-specific exercises to promote synchronous muscle firing patterns and flexibility will best prepare the athlete to return to his or her sport and avoid future injury.

SURGICAL PROCEDURES

Commonly performed surgical shoulder procedures for the throwing athlete include a diagnostic shoulder arthroscopy and an ACLR. Repairs of rotator cuff tears and subacromial decompression surgery, although not as common in the throwing athlete, are also performed if the appropriate pathology is noted. These injuries are usually secondary to attrition in the older athlete or from untreated shoulder subluxation with repetitive insults to the area. The selection of the proper procedure depends critically on the correct diagnosis.

Diagnostic Shoulder Arthroscopy

Diagnostic shoulder arthroscopy is routinely performed in throwing athletes undergoing any shoulder procedure. The diagnostic arthroscopy allows for identification of any intra-articular pathology, confirmation of a rotator cuff tear or instability, and identification of any other pathology such as a labral or articular lesion.

Shoulder arthroscopy is routinely performed in either the lateral decubitus position with the arm suspended with 10 lb of traction or in the semisitting position. A posterior portal is used approximately 1 cm medial and 3 cm distal to the posterolateral corner of the acromion. The scope is introduced into the joint, and a systematic examination is performed. In addition to the standard examination, it is important to note any difficulty in maintaining capsular distention, which is indicative of a rotator cuff tear; an easy "drive through" of the arthroscope from anterosuperior to anteroinferior, which supports a diagnosis of instability; a lack of anterior capsular tightening with external rotation of the arm; and an undersurface rotator cuff partial tear, which matches up with a kissing lesion on the posterior glenoid rim when the arm is in the late cocking position of throwing, indicative of internal impingement and instability. If any probing or resection is required, an anterior portal should be created. Rotator cuff repairs may be performed in this lateral decubitus position while those patients undergoing a shoulder reconstruction require repositioning. Also, very few arthroscopic shoulder reconstruction procedures are performed in the throwing athlete because of the difficulty, especially when the arm is distended with irrigation fluid, in assessing adequate tissue tension at repair to guarantee stability without loss of motion.

Anterior Capsulolabral Reconstruction

The ACLR was first devised to eliminate anterior shoulder instability while maintaining shoulder motion including external rotation, in particular. Today, this procedure is also used in traumatic anterior dislocators as well as in the multidirectional instability patient who has a primary anterior component.[14]

Briefly, the procedure preserves all muscle attachments and avoids medial-to-lateral shortening of the anterior capsule, allowing for maintenance of external rotation. After diagnostic arthroscopy, the procedure is performed through a saber-type incision developing the deltopectoral interval. The conjoined tendon is retracted medially, and the subscapularis tendon is split horizontally in line with its fibers at the junction of the upper two-thirds and lower third of the tendon. Anatomic dissection has revealed that this interval lies in the plane between the innervation of the upper and lower subscapular nerves.[30] The plane between the subscapularis and the anterior capsule is then developed, starting medially initially, which allows for easier identification of this interval. A horizontal capsulotomy is then made centered on the glenoid (Fig. 28-3). Tag sutures inserted on the upper and lower flaps should be placed at the level of the glenoid articular surface to identify the location of the capsulolabral attachment. The capsular flaps are then developed superiorly and inferiorly by subperiosteal dissection off the anterior glenoid neck. If multidirectional instability was the diagnosis, then inferior flap development should be performed to the 7-o'clock position. Suture anchors are then placed at the 3-o'clock, 4-o'clock, and 5-o'clock positions, and the flaps are imbricated in a pants-over-vest fashion. The capsular imbrication should still allow the arm to externally rotate to 90 degrees when the arm is at 90 degrees abduction. Care must be taken to

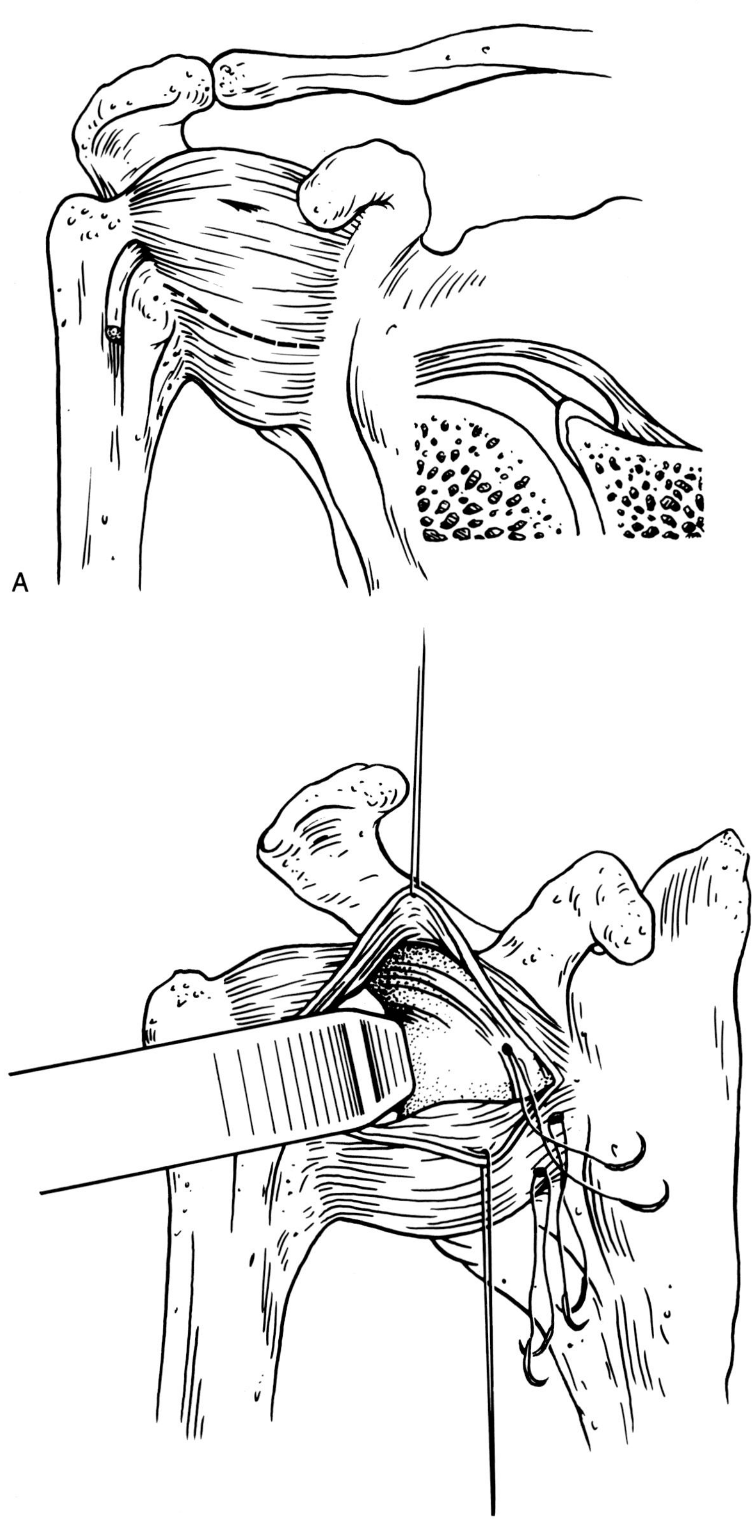

Figure 28-3. (**A**) Horizontal capsular incision used during the anterior capsulolabral reconstruction and (*inset*) redundant anterior capsule with an intact labrum commonly seen in the recurrent subluxator. (**B**) Inferior capsular flap shifted superiorly and "anchored" into position, eliminating the redundant capsule. After this, the superior flap is brought down to reinforce the repair.

avoid medialization of the capsule, which will cause a loss of external rotation. After imbrication, the horizontal capsulotomy is closed with a single absorbable suture followed by routine closure of the remaining layers. Pitchers and other high-level throwing athletes are placed in an abduction wedge or a custom orthotic that holds the arm in 45 degrees external rotation, 30 degrees horizontal adduction, and 90 degrees abduction for 3 weeks. Because no muscle origin or insertion was taken down, the patient is allowed immediate full passive and active range of motion except for full external rotation, which is limited to 90 degrees external rotation for 2 weeks. Full range of motion should be obtained by 2 months postoperatively. Once strength, motion, rhythm, muscle synchrony, and endurance are regained, the patient should be enrolled in a progressive throwing program starting at approximately 6 months postoperatively.

SPECIFIC SHOULDER PROBLEMS

The orthopaedist seeing the injured throwing athlete should be aware that other problems can be seen in this patient population other than instability, impingement, and rotator cuff tears. Some of these are described in further detail below.

Posterior Shoulder Problems

Primary posterior shoulder problems are much less common in the throwing athlete. They occur usually from microtrauma with repetitive stress on the posterior structures or from a traumatic dislocation. An example of microtrauma is the baseball pitcher with a Bennett[2] lesion that is thought to be from a microtraumatic traction injury to the posterior capsule. An example of a traumatic posterior dislocation is the baseball player or quarterback who falls on an outstretched hand. These patients usually complain of not only posterior shoulder pain but also rotator cuff and biceps tenderness. A detailed examination will help in properly diagnosing the subluxation of the shoulder posteriorly in the glenoid fossa. In muscular athletes, though, this can sometimes be difficult. In these situations, an examination under anesthesia with a diagnostic arthroscopy can aid in making the diagnosis. Arthroscopic findings usually reveal a redundant posterior capsule with the humeral head easily subluxatable posteriorly. Rarely is a true reverse Bankart lesion noted.

Patients with posterior instability are initially treated with a conservative therapy program. Emphasis is placed on strengthening of the external rotator cuff muscles, which include the teres minor and infraspinatus along with the posterior head of the deltoid. Concurrently, coaches and trainers must emphasize proper throwing mechanics, focusing on follow-through and lower body mechanics. Biofeedback has also been documented to be helpful in this patient population.[1] Conservative therapy is attempted for a minimum of 6 months and usually two-thirds of these patients eliminate their functional disability, although, often their posterior subluxation is still present on physical examination.

Treatment of those patients who fail conservative therapy is controversial because operative results have been disappointing.[22,50] If the patient understands the risks, though, and has failed a well-controlled and regimented therapy program, a posterior capsulorrhaphy may be performed. The procedure performed is similar to the ACLR and involves creating two posterior capsular flaps that are imbricated in a pants-over-vest fashion. These flaps are either anchored to an intact posterior labrum or to suture anchors placed in the posterior glenoid neck. Great care must be taken when developing the inferior flap because of the intimate relationship between the capsule and axillary nerve in this region. Postoperatively, the patient is placed in an abduction wedge, and isometric exercises are started immediately. Motion in the sagittal plane is avoided during the first 6 weeks. Thereafter, emphasis is placed on range of motion, strength, endurance, and muscle synchrony. Return to throwing is allowed at 9 to 12 months after surgery.

Another entity that has been noted in throwing athletes is posterior glenoid calcification or spurring. Bennett[2] first described this lesion, which is thought to be a traction-type injury. Although often asymptomatic, patients can complain of posterior deltoid pain and fatigue. Initial treatment consists of rest with gradual return to throwing. If this fails, spur resection through a posterior approach has had success in allowing the throwing athlete to return to sports.[31]

Acromioclavicular Problems

Acromioclavicular problems are rare in the throwing athlete. They are almost always caused not by throwing but by a fall directly on the shoulder or an outstretched hand. The diagnosis is usually easily made, and often rotator cuff tendinitis is also noticed. Treatment is almost always conservative unless severe displacement (grade IV to VI) is noted or an associated coracoid fracture is noted. Treatment consists of rest with a sling for several days to 1 week, followed by therapy emphasizing range of motion and strength. Tibone et al[49] noted no significant difference in shoulder strength between the injured and the uninjured shoulder after conservative treatment of a grade III dislocation. The throwing athlete can usually return to sports within 3 to 6 weeks.

Patients with late problems involving the acromioclavicular joint secondary to degenerative changes usually respond well to surgical intervention. Grade I and II dislocations do well after a distal clavicle resection. Slight weakness in the sagittal plane may be noted, but return to sports including pitching has been excellent after this procedure.[11] Patients with grade III dislocations are treated with a Weaver-Dunn procedure, with resection of the distal clavical along with reattachment of the coracoacromial ligament to the end of the clavicle.[54] Most patients undergoing these surgical procedures are able to return to sports within 4 to 6 months.

Neurologic Problems

The most common neurologic problems seen in throwing athletes are suprascapular nerve entrapment and quadrilateral space syndrome.

Suprascapular nerve entrapment can occur either at the scapular notch or at the scapular spine. Entrapment at the notch occurs secondary to hypertrophy of the transverse scapular ligament or from compression by a ganglion cyst. This is the most common location of suprascapular nerve entrapment in the general population, and excellent results are usually obtained from cyst removal, if necessary, and release of the transverse scapular ligament.[42] Athletes, though, usually develop this problem at the scapular spine distal to the notch, which spares the supraspinatus from denervation. The athlete often complains of vague shoulder pain, and misdiagnosis is common. Close examination will reveal infraspinatus atrophy and weakness with external rotation of the shoulder. Unfortunately, this lesion does not respond well to surgical intervention in the throwing athlete. Better results are usually obtained by maximizing the function of any residual infraspinatus because complete denervation is almost never seen. Because EMG literature demonstrates that only 30 to 40 percent of maximum infraspinatus activity is necessary during the pitching motion, this often will allow the athlete to continue to throw properly and return to the previous level of performance.[26]

The quadrilateral space syndrome was first described by Cahill and Palmer[8] and involves compression of the axillary nerve within the quadrilateral space posteriorly. Patients usually present with vague shoulder complaints, often in the area of the teres minor posteriorly and only when throwing or involved in physical activity requiring the arm to be positioned in the abducted and externally rotated position. The physical examination is usually normal, although some discomfort can be noted in the apprehension position. A misdiagnosis of instability is common. EMG studies are not of value because compression is activity-related. Diagnosis is made with the use of an arteriogram, which will reveal compression, only when the arm is abducted and externally rotated, of the posterior humeral circumflex artery that travels with the axillary nerve through the quadrilateral space. Treatment is usually successful with rest and cortisone injections in the region. If this fails, then a surgical release of the teres minor tendon has had favorable results in the athlete.[7]

Vascular Problems

Vascular problems in the throwing athlete usually involve the axillary artery. Occlusion of the artery when the arm is brought overhead has been documented in the normal athlete.[57] This occurs in the second portion of the axillary artery and is caused by compression from the pectoralis minor tendon. Tullos et al[52] have documented this phenomenon during pitching. With repeated hard throwing, sufficient trauma may lead to injury and eventual thrombosis of the axillary artery. The patient's complaints are usually vague, including pain, weakness, loss of endurance, and paresthesias, making diagnosis extremely difficult. Acute occlusion, though, may present with pallor, pulselessness, paresthesias, and extremity coolness, making the diagnosis obvious. The diagnosis is confirmed with an arteriogram, and treatment includes resection of the occluded segment with direct arterial reanastomosis or bypass graft.

Pediatric Problems

The pediatric throwing athlete is susceptible to injuries that are related to skeletal immaturity. One must appreciate the strength of the capsule and ligaments about the shoulder, which can approach five times the strength of the physeal plates. This is why physeal plate injuries are more common than sprains in the skeletally immature athlete.

Multiple epiphyses exist around the shoulder. The clavicle has a medial epiphysis that does not appear until 17 years of age and fuses between 18 and 24 years. The scapula contains seven or more epiphyses appearing between 1 and 18 years of age that fuse between 18 and 21 years. The proximal humerus contains three epiphyses that appear between 3 months and 5 years that fuse together by 6 years of age and fuse to the shaft between 18 and 21 years.

The most common areas of injury include the humeral physis and the distal clavicle. The humeral physis is usually injured from overuse. Dotter[13] described the classic presentation as a Little League pitcher or overhand athlete with a recent increase in throwing associated with aching shoulder pain. Physical examination may reveal local pain at the humeral physis, along with pain with resisted active internal rotation. Radiographs may be normal or show widening of the physis with lateral fragmentation. Late radiographs may show callus formation from periosteal stripping. Treatment consists of rest followed by gradual return to throwing after 1 to 2 months, with an emphasis on shoulder muscle strength and proper warm-up. No long-term problems have been associated with this problem.

Injury to the distal clavicle occurs from a fall on the shoulder or outstretched hand. Clinically, this injury presents similarly to an acromioclavicular separation, but clavicular fracture usually occurs in the immature athlete younger than the age of 13 years. Diagnosis is often obvious, and successful treatment is usually obtained with conservative treatment using a sling and emphasizing early range of motion.

Another serious injury seen in the pediatric and adolescent athlete is the traumatic shoulder dislocation. Recent literature has documented the poor long-term results associated with this injury, with a very high incidence of recurrence of up to 100 percent.[33,47] The patient and family must be warned of this and the possibility of a need for future shoulder reconstruction surgery. Although controversial, early stabilization of these patients may be warranted in certain situations. Wheeler et al[55] reported a reduction of the rate of recurrence from 92 to 22 percent after arthroscopic stabilization for acute dislocations in young athletes.

SUMMARY

The throwing athlete places incredible demands on the shoulder. A fine line is ''walked'' by every throwing athlete to balance shoulder mobility with stability. Skilled coaching and training emphasizing proper mechanics, avoidance of overuse, proper warm-up, and a maintenance program focusing on shoulder strength and mobility as well as general conditioning can help to maintain this balance throughout an athlete's career.

Shoulder injury involves disturbing this delicate balance between mobility and stability. Impingement and instability are the most common problems afflicting the throwing athlete when this delicate balance is disturbed, and the athlete may exhibit signs and symptoms of one or both of these entities. However, one must remember that several other specific shoulder problems also exist and that these entities are often misdiagnosed as recalcitrant tendinitis or impingement. Still, a careful history and physical examination will allow the astute clinician to diagnose properly both the common and the uncommon shoulder problem. If the correct diagnosis is made, treatment with rehabilitation and surgery, if necessary, can ensure the injured throwing athlete an excellent chance for recovery along with a successful return to sports.

REFERENCES

1. Beall SM, Dufenbach G, Allen A: Electromyographic biofeedback in the treatment of voluntary posterior instability of the shoulder. Am J Sports Med 15:175–8, 1987
2. Bennett GE: Elbow and shoulder lesions of baseball players. Am J Surg 98:484–8, 1959
3. Bigliani LU, Morrison D, April EW: The morphology of the acromion and its relationship to rotator cuff tears. Orthop Trans 10:228, 1986
4. Biro F, Gewanter HL, Baum J: The hypermobility syndrome. Pediatrics 72:701, 1983
5. Blazina ME, Satzman JS: Recurrent anterior subluxation of the shoulder in athletes—a distinct entity. J Bone Joint Surg [Am] 51:1037, 1969
6. Bradley JP, Perry J, Jobe FW: The biomechanics of the throwing shoulder. Perspect Orthop Surg 1:49–59, 1990
7. Brodsky JW, Tullos HS, Gartsman GM: Simplified posterior approach to the shoulder joint. J Bone Joint Surg [Am] 69:773–4, 1987
8. Cahill BR, Palmer RE: Quadrilateral space syndrome. J Hand Surg 8:65–9, 1983
9. Cofield RH, Irving JF: Evaluation and classification of shoulder instability. Clin Orthop 223:32, 1987
10. Cofield RH, Simonet WT: Symposium on sports medicine: part 2, the shoulder in sports. Mayo Clin Proc 59:157–64, 1984
11. Cook FF, Tibone JE: The Mumford procedure in athletes—an objective analysis of function. Am J Sports Med 16:97–100, 1988
12. Davidson PA, El Attrache NS, Jobe CM, Jobe FW: Rotator cuff injury associated with increased glenohumeral motion: a new site of impingement. J Shoulder Elbow Surg, in press
13. Dotter WE: Little Leaguer's shoulder: a fracture of the proximal humeral epiphyseal cartilage of the humerus due to baseball pitching. Guthrie Clin Bull 23:68, 1953
14. El Attrache NS, Jobe FW, Tibone JE: Anterior capsulolabral reconstruction in the treatment of traumatic glenohumeral instability. Paper presented at Specialty Day, Am Shoulder and Elbow Surg, San Francisco, 1993
15. Garneau RA, Renfrew DL, Moore TE: Glenoid labrum: evaluation with MR imaging. Radiology 179:519–22, 1991
16. Gerber C, Granz R: Clinical assessment of instability of the shoulder. J Bone Joint Surg [Br] 66:551, 1984
17. Gerber C, Krushell RJ: Isolated rupture of the tendon of the subscapularis muscle. J Bone Joint Surg [Br] 73:389, 1991
18. Glousman RE, Jobe, FW, Tibone, JE: Dynamic EMG analysis of the throwing shoulder with glenohumeral instability. J Bone Joint Surg [Am] 70:220–6, 1988
19. Gowan ID, Jobe FW, Tibone JE et al: A comparative EMG analysis of the shoulder during pitching: professional vs. amateur pitchers. Am J Sports Med 15:586–90, 1987
20. Hawkins RJ, Bilco T, Bonutti P: Cervical spine and shoulder pain. Clin Orthop 258:142–6, 1990
21. Hawkins RJ, Kennedy JC: Impingement syndrome in athletes. Am J Sports Med 8:151–8, 1980
22. Hawkins RJ, Koppert G, Johnston G: Recurrent posterior instability (subluxation) of the shoulder. J Bone Joint Surg [Am] 66:169–74, 1984
23. Jobe FJ, Bradley JP: The diagnosis and nonoperative treatment of shoulder injuries in athletes. Clin Sports Med 8:419–38, 1989
24. Jobe FW, Giangarra CE, Kvitne RS, Glousman RE: Anterior capsulolabral reconstruction of the shoulder in athletes in overhand sports. Am J Sports Med 19:428–34, 1991

25. Jobe FW, Jobe CM: Painful athletic injuries of the shoulder. Clin Orthop 173:117–24, 1983
26. Jobe FW, Moynes DR, Tibone JE, Perry J: An EMG analysis of the shoulder in pitching: a second report. Am J Sports Med 12:218–20, 1984
27. Jobe FW, Tibone JE, Jobe CM: The shoulder in sports. pp. 961–90. In Rockwood CA, Matsen FA (eds): The Shoulder. WB Saunders, Philadelphia, 1990
28. Jobe FW, Yocum LA, Schwab DR: Shoulder and Arm Exercises for Athletes. Champion Press, Inglewood, CA, 1986
29. Kieft GJ, Bloom JL, Rozing PM: MR imaging of recurrent anterior dislocation of the shoulder: comparison with CT arthrography. AJR 150:1083–7, 1988
30. King WD, Jobe FW, Levy SC: Anatomic and electromyographic studies of the subscapularis muscle. Paper presented at Specialty Day, Am Orthop Society Sports Med, New Orleans, 1994
31. Lombardo SJ, Jobe FW, Kerlan RK: Posterior shoulder lesions in throwing athletes. Am J Sports Med 5:106–10, 1977
32. Lombardo SJ, Kerlan RK, Jobe FW: The modified Bristow procedure for recurrent dislocation of the shoulder. J Bone Joint Surg [Am] 58:256–61, 1976
33. Marans HJ, Angel KR, Schemitch EH: The fate of traumatic dislocation of the shoulder in children. J Bone Joint Surg [Am] 74:1242–5, 1993
34. Matsen FA, Arntz CT: Subacromial impingement. pp. 623–46. In Rockwood CA, Matsen FA (eds): The Shoulder. WB Saunders, Philadelphia, 1990
35. Moseley JB, Jobe FW, Pink M et al: EMG analysis of the scapular muscles during a shoulder rehabilitation program. Am J Sports Med 20:128–34, 1992
36. Neer CS: Anterior acromioplasty for the chronic impingement syndrome in the shoulder. J Bone Joint Surg [Am] 54:41–50, 1972
37. Neer CS, Walsh RP: The shoulder in sports. Orthop Clin North Am 8:583–91, 1977
38. Nottage WM, Duge WD, Fields WA: Computed arthrotomography of the glenohumeral joint to evaluate anterior instability: correlation with arthroscopic findings. Arthroscopy 3:273–6, 1987
39. Parnianpour M: The effect of fatigue on the motor output and pattern of isodynamic trunk movement. Paper presented at the Annual Meeting of the International Society for the Study of the Lumbar Spine, Miami, FL 1988
40. Perry J: Normal upper extremity kinesiology. Phys Ther 58:265–78, 1978
41. Poppen NK, Walker PS: Normal and abnormal motion of the shoulder. J Bone Joint Surg [Am] 58:195, 1976
42. Post M, Grinblat E: Suprascapular nerve entrapment: diagnosis and results of treatment. J Shoulder Elbow Surg 2:190–7, 1993
43. Rowe CR: Recurrent transient anterior subluxation of the shoulder: the dead arm syndrome. Clin Orthop 223:11–19, 1987
44. Rowe CR, Patel D, Southmayd WW: The Bankart procedure: a long-term end-result study. J Bone Joint Surg [Am] 60:1–16, 1978
45. Rowe CR, Zarins B: Recurrent transient subluxation of the shoulder. J Bone Joint Surg [Am] 63:863, 1981
46. Shuman WP, Kilcoyne RF, Matsen FA: Double-contrast computed tomography of the glenoid labrum. AJR 141:581–4, 1983
47. Tibone JE: Shoulder problems of adolescents: how they differ from those of adults. Clin Sports Med 2:423–7, 1983
48. Tibone JE, Jobe FW, Kerlan RK: Shoulder impingement syndrome in athletes treated by anterior acromioplasty. Clin Orthop 188:134–40, 1985
49. Tibone JE, Sellers R, Tonino P: Strength testing of third degree AC separations. Am J Sports Med 20:328–31, 1992
50. Tibone JE, Ting A: Capsulorrhaphy with a staple for recurrent posterior subluxation of the shoulder. J Bone Joint Surg [Am] 72:999–1002, 1990
51. Townsend H, Jobe FW, Pink M, Perry J: Electromyographic analysis of the glenohumeral muscles during a baseball rehabilitation program. Am J Sports Med 19:264–72, 1991
52. Tullos HS, Erwin WD, Woods WG: Unusual lesions of the pitching arm. Clin Orthop 88:169, 1972
53. Walch G, Liotard JP, Boileau P: Postero-superior impingement in the throwing athlete. Paper presented at the 5th International Conference on Surgery of the Shoulder, Paris, 1992
54. Weaver JK, Dunn HK: Treatment of acromioclavicular injuries, especially complete acromioclavicular separation. J Bone Joint Surg [Am] 54:1187–97, 1972
55. Wheeler JH, Ryan JB, Arciero RA: Arthroscopic versus nonoperative treatment of acute shoulder dislocation in young athletes, Arthroscopy 5:213–7, 1989
56. Wright CR, House T: The Diamond Appraised. Simon & Shuster, New York, 1989
57. Wright IS: The neurovascular syndrome produced by hyperabduction of the arm. Am Heart J 29:1, 1945

CHAPTER TWENTY-NINE

Tennis Injuries

Larry D. Field
David W. Altchek

The current popularity of tennis not only at the professional level but as a recreational sport for people all ages has led to an increased number of injuries of all types. Shoulder injuries are very common and are most often related to overuse. Several factors contribute to overuse injury including poor mechanics, improper equipment, increased age, and poor conditioning of the players. Another contributing factor is the perception of the game itself, which has undergone a transition over the past two decades from one in which technique is emphasized to the game today, which is often characterized by the power, speed, and endurance of the athletes.

EPIDEMIOLOGY

Tennis players range from the very young to the very old and represent one of the most diverse groups of athletes of any sport. More than 14 million people play tennis every year[18] on approximately 140,000 tennis courts.[21] Although lateral epicondylitis is common, with more than half of all tennis players developing symptoms at one time or another,[21] shoulder complaints are very common as well.[17,34] Priest and Nagel[27] found, in a review of some of the world's best tennis players, that more than 50 percent had experienced shoulder symptoms at some time during their careers. Kibler et al[17] reported that among 97 junior tennis players, shoulder injuries occurred more commonly than other injuries.

TENNIS KINEMATICS

Tennis players are prone to shoulder injuries because of the high demands placed on the shoulder as a result of repetitive strokes. The serve and overhead smash are especially demanding and are the strokes that most commonly produce shoulder symptoms.[27] The tennis racquet also contributes to force generation about the shoulder through the effect of an increased lever arm during the stroke.

Several articles have described the tennis stroke and divided it into components in an effort to better understand the complex coordination and sequence of muscle activity required.[9,22,25,29] The tennis serve and forehand and backhand strokes have been studied using dynamic electromyography and synchronized high-speed photography.

The tennis serve is divided into four stages similar to the stages of baseball pitching.[13,14] Stage I (Fig. 29-1A) represents the windup and ends at the time of ball release. It is characterized by shoulder abduction, extension, and external rotation. Stage II of the serve (Fig. 29-1B) begins at ball release and continues until both shoulder are level and the arm is in maximal external rotation. Muscle activity during this cocking phase is similar to that for stage I. Serratus anterior function has been shown to be important during this phase in stabilizing the scapula against the thoracic wall.[29] Stage III of the serve (Fig. 29-1C) involves acceleration of the arm in coordination with forceful internal rotation and adduction of the shoulder and continues until impact of the racquet with the ball. Again, serratus anterior function is maximal during this stage. Stage IV

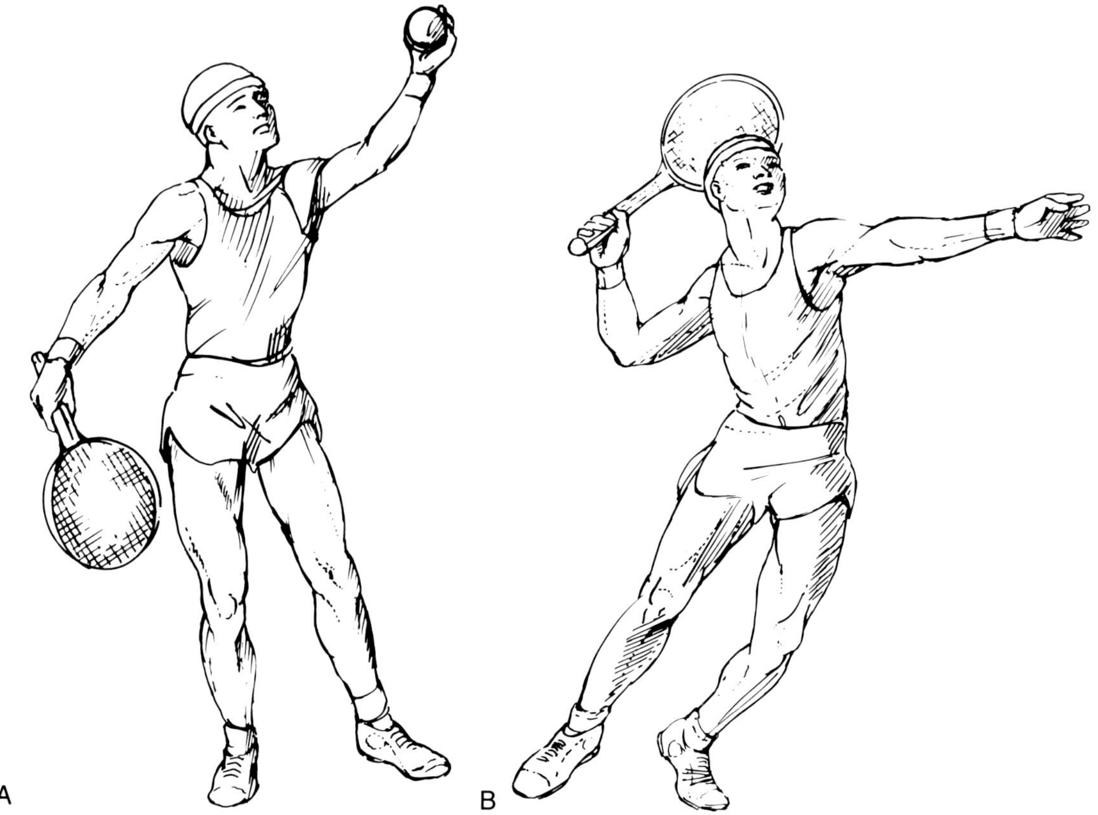

Figure 29-1. The four stages of the tennis serve. (**A**) Windup begins the serve and (**B**) the cocking follows. (*Figure continues.*)

(Fig. 29-ID) completes the service motion and is referred to as follow-through. The arm crosses the body during this phase as the shoulder adductors and internal rotators continue to show activity. A deceleration force is also prominent during this phase.

The forehand and backhand strokes can be divided into three stages.[29] Stage I of the forehand stroke (Fig. 29-2A) begins with racquet preparation as the shoulder rotates. Shoulder abduction and external rotation are prominently seen during this stage. Stage II (Fig. 29-2B) involves acceleration of the arm to the point of ball impact and is characterized by internal rotation and adduction of the shoulder, with high levels of muscle activity present in the biceps brachii, subscapularis, pectoralis major, and serratus anterior.[29] Stage III (Fig. 29-2C) continues after ball strike as follow-through and is characterized by decreased muscle activity.

Stage I of the backhand stroke begins with racquet preparation (Fig. 29-3A) just as for the forehand stroke. In stage II (Fig. 29-3B), acceleration of the arm in coordination with abduction and external rotation occurs at the shoulder. The middle deltoid, supraspinatus, and infraspinatus muscles show high activity levels during this stage.[29] Stage III of the backhand stroke (Fig. 29-3C) begins at ball strike with deceleration and produces reduced muscular activity similar to the follow-through stage of the forehand stroke.

Proper tennis stroke technique requires proper coupling of trunk rotation with arm acceleration. Correct coupling of rotation between the arm and trunk helps to reduce the demands on the shoulder by effectively adding the body weight to the power of the stroke at ball contact. Just as a pitcher's ball velocity is significantly increased by using the legs and body to step toward the batter, a tennis player's stroke power is improved by coordinated rotation of the trunk at ball contact (Fig. 29-4A). Premature trunk rotation greatly reduces its relative contribution to racquet velocity. The player must compensate by increasing the demands on the arm and shoulder to maintain stroke power (Fig. 29-4B). This uncoupled motion of the trunk is otherwise referred to as "opening up too early" and can increase the extension required of the shoulder during the acceleration stage of the stroke. Repetitive overloading, along with increased extension of the shoulder, can lead to overuse-related symptoms.

Another important factor regarding proper technique concerns the point at which contact of the ball with the racquet is made. Ball contact should remain anterior to the sagittal plane of the body. Striking the ball anterior to this

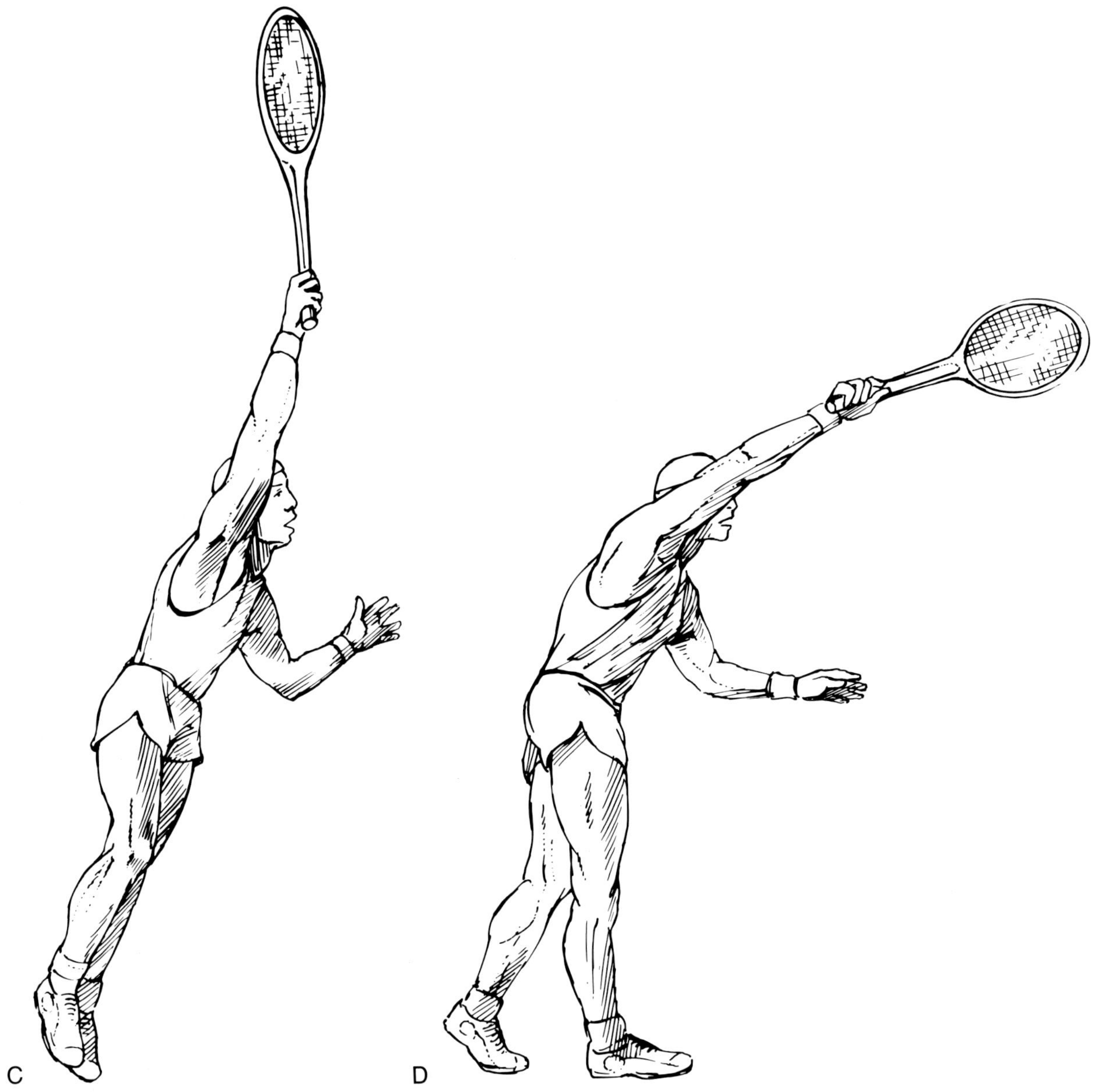

Figure 29-1 (*Continued*). (**C**) The acceleration stage proceeds until ball strike, and (**D**) follow-through completes the service stroke.

plane, otherwise known as striking the ball "out in front," allows for maximum energy transfer to the ball because racquet velocity continues to increase throughout the stroke and peaks at this anterior position. Also, maintaining the point of ball contact anteriorly indirectly aids stroke power by accommodating a stroke that incorporates forward movement of the body toward the ball. Stepping in the direction of the ball increases the transfer of energy to the ball and can reduce the demands on the shoulder. By contrast, when ball contact occurs behind the body, the time allowed for the arm to attain adequate stroke velocity is reduced. This increased acceleration rate on the arm along with the negative effect that this ball contact point has toward accommodating forward thrust of the body can contribute to overuse symptoms.

ROTATOR CUFF INJURY

Rotator cuff injury is the most common cause of shoulder pain in tennis players,[20,27] and the spectrum covers the entire range from the mild dysfunction associated with rotator

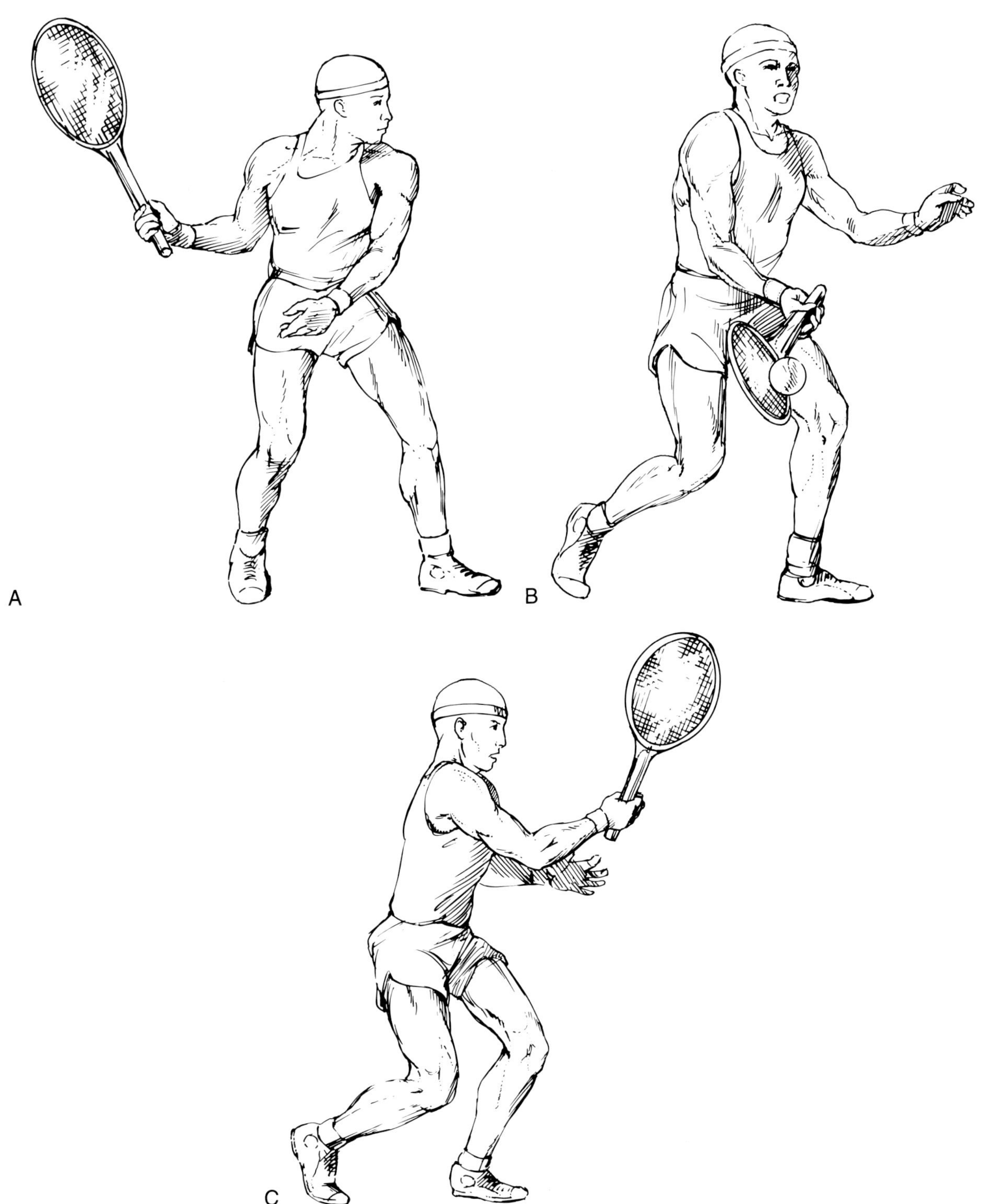

Figure 29-2. Stages of the forehand stroke. (**A**) Racquet preparation is followed by (**B**) the acceleration stage. (**C**) The stroke is completed with follow-through.

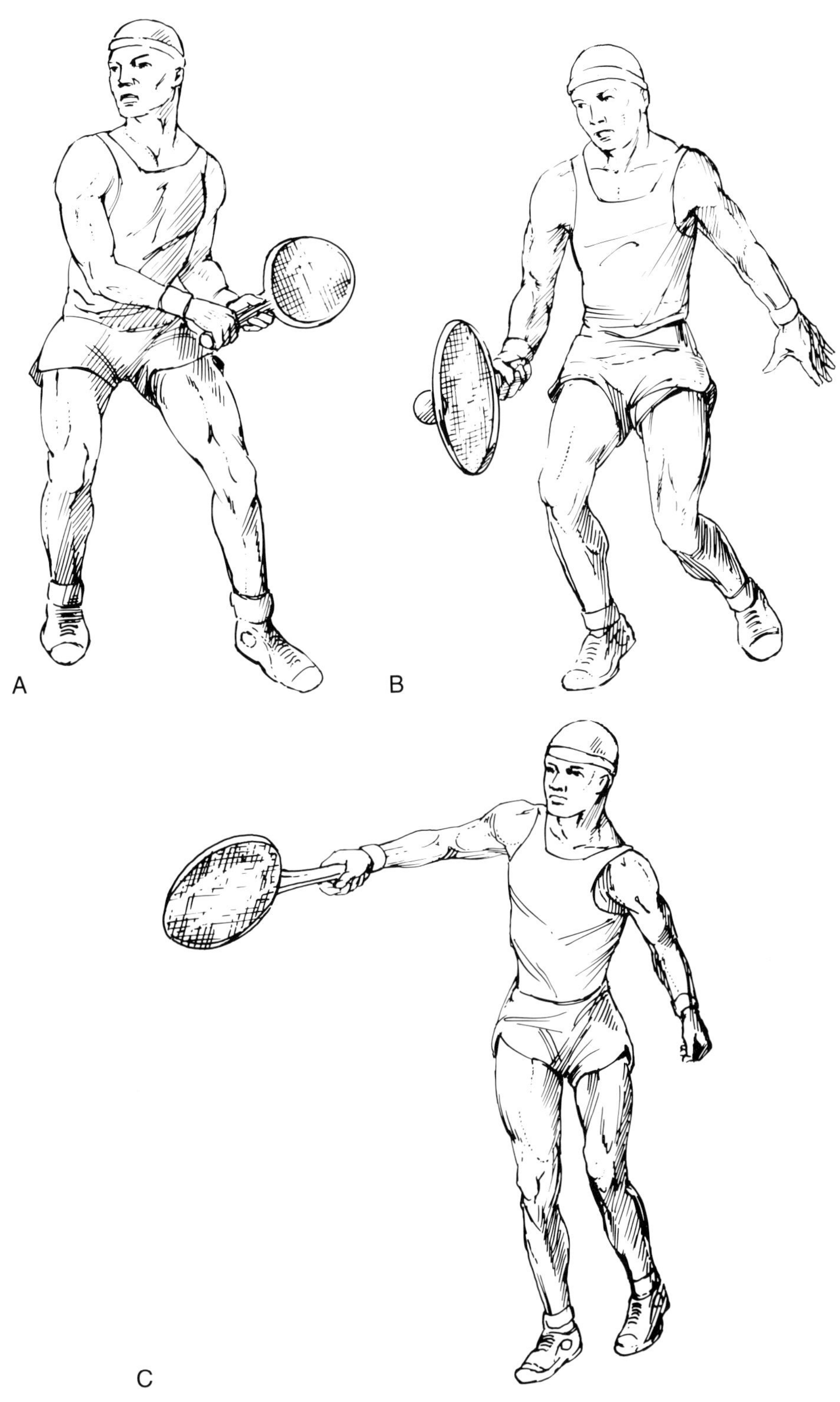

Figure 29-3. Stages of the backhand stroke. (**A**) Racquet preparation is followed by (**B**) the acceleration stage. (**C**) The stroke is completed with follow-through.

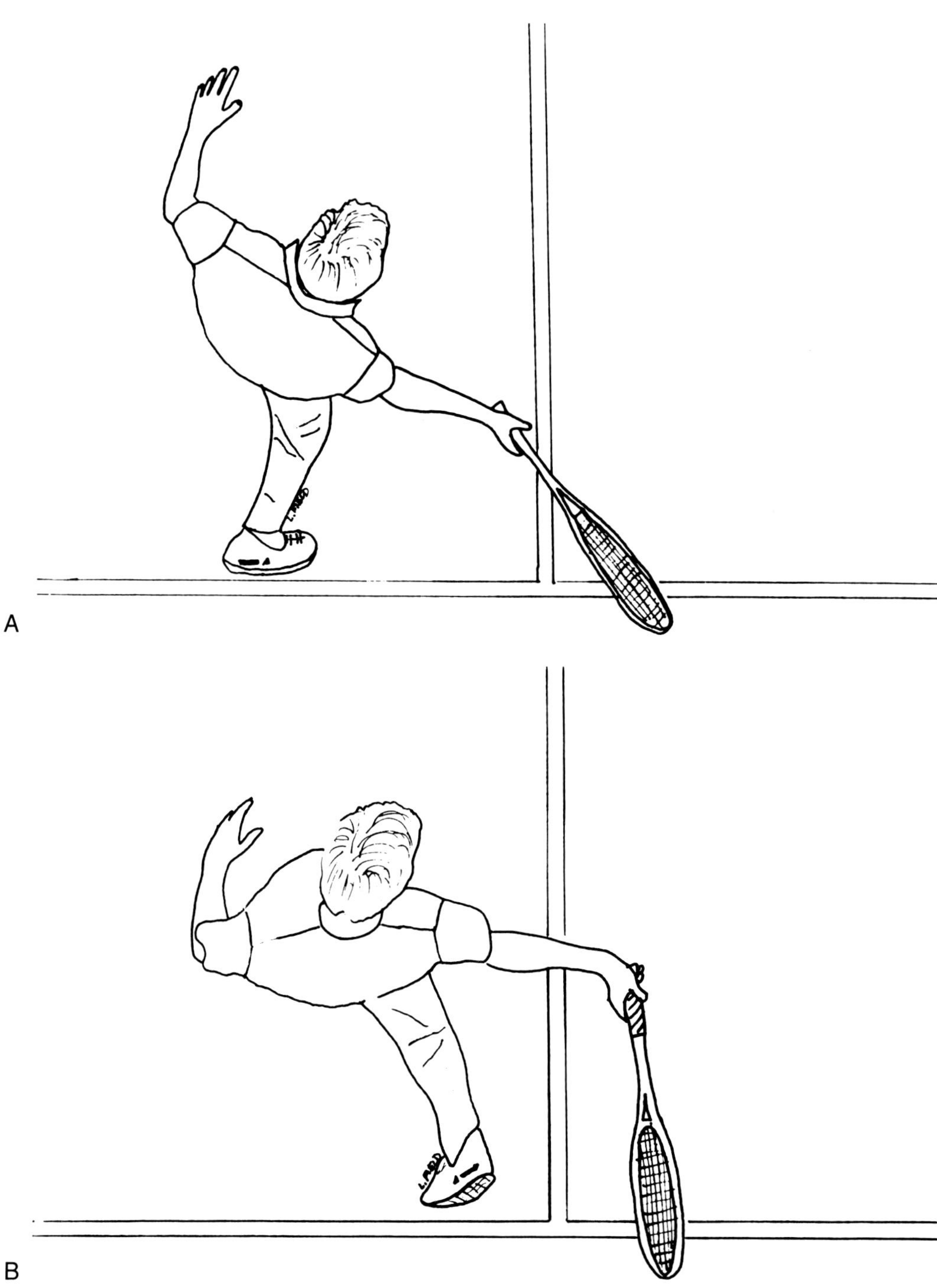

Figure 29-4. Proper and improper techniques for the tennis forehand stroke as seen from above the player. (**A**) Properly coordinated motion of the trunk with the arm maximizes energy transfer to the ball. (**B**) Improper technique or "opening up too early" characterized by premature trunk rotation results in loss of power at ball strike and contributes to injury by increasing demands on the shoulder.

cuff overload to the significant disability associated with large full-thickness tears of the rotator cuff. The supraspinatus muscle is subject to intrinsic overload throughout the various stages of the tennis stroke. This repetitive overloading can generate a microtraumatic injury pattern within the tendon that in the early stages responds through attempts at repair. Repeated injury to the tendon, however, can lead to changes within its substance through degeneration or the production of pathologic reparative tissue.

The rotator cuff acts as a dynamic stabilizer of the shoulder by acting to compress the glenohumeral joint and depress the humeral head. Injury to the rotator cuff in a young adult tennis player usually occurs as a result of the tensile overload generated by repetitive strokes and weakens the cuff's effect on stability and humeral head depression. The microtraumatic tearing of the muscle and tendon unit directly reduces the strength of the rotator cuff but also detrimentally affects rotator cuff function indirectly through inhibition secondary to pain. This inhibition leads to progressive weakening as the player avoids the positions or motions that cause discomfort. As the effectiveness of the rotator cuff musculature on humeral head depression is reduced, the upward pull of the deltoid on the humerus begins to dominate. The relative overpull of the deltoid leads to a reduction in the space available under the coracoacromial arch. This muscle imbalance secondarily causes direct injury of the tendinous portion of the supraspinatus as it moves into close proximity with the coracoacrominal arch.[30] Also, because the contribution of the injured rotator cuff is diminished, its important function as a dynamic stabilizer in reducing humeral head translation is decreased. Paletta et al[24] have recently shown in a radiographic study that abnormal superior humeral head translation does occur in patients with instability symptoms. This destabilizing effect can exacerbate impingement symptoms or can contribute to functional instability. These authors think that initial rotator cuff injury followed by secondary rotator cuff dysfunction is the sequence responsible for impingement-related symptoms in young adult tennis players.

A thorough history and physical examination of the tennis player's shoulder are the keys to proper diagnosis and treatment. A careful examination of the cervical spine along with a neurovascular assessment are important toward ruling out alternative sources for upper extremity symptoms. Also, active and passive range of motion in forward flexion and internal and external rotation should be measured. A positive impingement sign is produced when passive forward flexion in the terminal 10 to 15 degrees causes pain and is valuable evidence of rotator cuff injury in tennis players as in other overhead athletes. Strength testing is also important in evaluating rotator cuff function and should be recorded. Tests for shoulder stability are best performed with the tennis player supine and the arm in 90 degrees of abduction and neutral rotation. Increased anterior, posterior, or inferior translation as compared with the opposite extremity, especially when associated with a positive apprehension test, is suggestive of clinical instability and has significant implications on treatment. The anterior apprehension test, performed with the arm abducted and externally rotated, closely approximates the position of the tennis serve and is an important test to include in physical examination.

Impingement of the supraspinatus tendon under the coracoacromial arch can be exacerbated by the tennis serve as the shoulder is forcefully internally rotated from an abducted, elevated, and externally rotated position, especially when rotator cuff fatigue or dysfunction is present. Muscle weakness resulting from fatigue reduces the depressor and stabilizing effect of the rotator cuff on the humeral head and can contribute to symptoms. Another factor that may have a negative influence on rotator cuff health is a deformity sometimes seen in highly skilled tennis players and is described as tennis shoulder.[26,27] It is characterized by a depression of the exercised shoulder most likely due to stretching of the elevating muscles and hypertrophy of the extremity. This shoulder depression results in downward rotation of the scapula and relative abduction of the humerus, which may diminish the space available for the supraspinatus and predispose players to rotator cuff injury or exacerbate symptoms already present.

Rotator cuff injury can be further subdivided into one of three stages, and proper management for tennis players varies according to each stage. Tennis players younger than 25 years of age generally present with stage I injury, characterized by edema, and hemorrhage of the rotator cuff and surrounding tissues.[23] These younger players are best treated initially using modalities to reduce the acute pain component along with temporary activity modifications. Once a painless and full range of motion is restored, an aggressive, well-monitored rehabilitation program is instituted to strengthen the rotator cuff musculature and regain balance about the shoulder. A well-monitored exercise program ensures compliance and helps maximize effort that, in most cases, results in resolution of symptoms. Subacromial corticosteroid injections are usually not necessary, and surgical intervention in these players is rarely indicated. In our experience, these changes are reversible. Stage II injury is generally seen in adults older than 25 years of age, whereby subacromial scarring and fibrosis resulting from chronic injury with repeated attempts at repair are present. Partial-thickness undersurface rotator cuff tears are not uncommon during this stage. An exercise and rehabilitation program for these players, although usually effective in helping to alleviate symptoms, does not always provide significant long-lasting improvement as reliably as in younger adults in whom no permanent subacromial soft tissue and bony changes are present. These patients with stage II injury occasionally require surgical intervention to provide long-lasting relief. Magnetic resonance imaging (MRI) can be valuable as a staging tool in some patients with stage II injury and should be considered. Stage III rotator cuff injury is characterized by frank tearing of the rotator cuff and is often associated with significant bony spurring of the acromion, particularly in older players.

The exercise program for subacromial rotator cuff injury in tennis players generally follows standard guidelines for rehabilitation.[28] Certain aspects of the rehabilitative effort deserve emphasis, however, due to the specifics of the tennis stroke and as a consequence of the changes in strength and flexibility of the upper extremity that result. Tennis players can lose flexibility in internal rotation,[5] and emphasis on regaining this flexibility can be valuable in maximizing recovery. Loss of internal rotation is due to a contracture of the posterior capsule. Asymmetric tightness of the posterior capsule causes increased anterior and superior humeral translation on the glenoid.[12] The abnormal mechanics that result contribute to symptoms and may predispose a subacromial impingement. Once range of motion exercises can be performed without pain, rehabilitation can be graduated to a Theraband program, and use of the Therabands to simulate the various tennis strokes including the serve, forehand, and backhand can help isolate and strengthen the shoulder musculature necessary to prevent recurrence. Tennis players often have disproportionately strong internal rotators,[4] and an exercise program that emphasizes external rotator strengthening can help recover rotator cuff balance and aid in reducing the incidence of reinjury. Kennedy et al[16] have recently shown that the external rotators of the dominant extremity in competitve tennis players are able to generate statisically higher torque values and work output than the nondominant extremity. This study also highlights the important function of the external rotators in decelerating the arm in follow-through, suggesting tht rehabilitation of the external rotators focuses on their eccentric function. Finally, emphasis must be placed on the trunk and pelvic musculature. These muscles are necessary for the development of a powerful tennis stroke and are particularly important when the player is recovering from shoulder injury.

Persistent symptoms and shoulder dysfunction that are not alleviated by a comprehensive strengthening and flexibility program are indications for surgical intervention. MRI can be of value as a staging study in selected patients for whom the degree of rotator cuff injury is difficult to clarify. If surgical intervention is carried out, shoulder arthroscopy can play a valuable role in precisely defining the injury pattern to the rotator cuff. Small partial-thickness tears of the undersurface of the rotaor cuff identified at arthroscopy are debrided in an attempt to stimulate a healing response. Partial-thickness tears of greater than 50 percent of the thickness of the tendon as determined by visualization and probing of both the undersurface and bursal sides of the tendon are repaired in active tennis players. This is accomplished by localizing the skin incision site over the lateral deltoid with a spinal needle. The spinal needle is then used as a conduit to place a suture through the partial tear. The suture is then followed to the location of the partial tear through a mini-open deltoid-splitting incision. The supraspinatus tendon is then incised in line with its fibers through the partial-thickness tear and the edges imbricated and reduced into a prepared tuberosity bed using a suture anchor. In the absence of a partial tear but when subacromial inflammation or spurring is present, an arthroscopic acromioplasty is performed.

Full-thickness rotator cuff tears are a common occurence in older tennis players as a result of chronic repetitive injury to the rotator cuff tendons and musculature. Of interest, however, is the fact that few overhead athletes continue to regularly participate in their respective sports as they age beyond young adulthood. Tennis players, however continue to play often at high skill levels into middle and advanced age. This creates a unique situation in which an older tennis player may place unusually high demands on the shoulder. A tennis player's desire to return to the presymptomatic level of play is often an indication for a more aggressive management plan for these patients. Bigliani et al[13] found that 19 of 23 tennis players were able to return to their presymptomatic level of play after repair of a full-thickness rotator cuff tear. These patients averaged 58 years of age, and all patients except for one were able to return to playing tennis at some level. Although repair of a torn rotator cuff tendon in overhead athletes does not guarantee return to a presymptomatic level of play,[32] symptoms attributable to a torn rotator cuff often preclude these players from participation in tennis at any level, and operative repair can be of significant benefit. Conversely, many older tennis players with massive rotator cuff tears participate regularly. Management of players with irreparable rotator cuff tears should consist of an exercise program emphasizing scapular and rotator cuff strengthening and specific therapeutic modalities as symptoms dictate. Occasionally, arthrospcopic soft tissue debridement may be helpful in players who do not respond to these interventions. Acromioplasty, however, is not usually performed in players with massive tears and associated superior humeral head migration.

INSTABILITY

Shoulder instability occurs in the tennis player but less commonly than in the throwing athlete. Instability is important but sometimes difficult to distinguish from rotator cuff injury because their symptoms are often very similar. The tennis player with subtle instability will often relate only symptoms of anterior shoulder pain. Also, rotator cuff injury can occur in combination with underlying shoulder instability. The tennis serve, which is the stroke most commonly reported as problematic by tennis players,[27] places the arm in abduction, extension, and external rotation. This is also the classic position of apprehension for patients with anterior instability, making these two diagnoses sometimes difficult but important to distinguish. Manual shoulder testing is instrumental in diagnosing instability and in structuring an appropriate treatment plan.

Shoulder instability can produce symptoms due to anterior subluxation, posterior subluxation, or multidirectional instability. Symptoms due to anterior subluxation in the tennis player are most often reproduced by overhead strokes and may consist of pain alone, popping, or a sense that the arm "goes dead" or "goes out." This symptomatic anterior subluxation most often results from the high levels of repetitive intrinsic forces generated during each tennis stroke in players who possess increased capsular laxity.

An exercise program emphasizing recovery of a full range of motion followed by scapular and rotator cuff musculature strengthening is often effective in reducing or eliminating instability symptoms, but arthroscopic or open stabilization procedures may be required. If an arthroscopic stabilization is being considered, significant inferior laxity must be ruled out. Excessive inferior translation indicates that an element of multidirectional instability is present and is probably best treated with an open capsular shift procedure.

Posterior dislocation in the tennis player is very unusual, but symptoms related to posterior subluxation do occur. These symptoms are primarily related to pain alone rather than instability and usually occur late in the tennis stroke as the humeral head internally rotates, which stresses the posterior capsular structures and labrum. Initial treatment for posterior instability should include a flexibility and strengthening program. If this exercise regimen fails to improve symptoms, then surgical stabilization should be considered. Preoperatively, an evaluation of glenoid version using a computed tomography scan is recommended, along with an assessment of the player's generalized ligamentous laxity. A stabilization procedure using an open technique is generally performed so that the infraspinatus tendon, transected obliquely during the surgical approach, can be used to reinforce the thin posterior capsule at the time of closure. In those patients without generalized laxity, a capsular repair is performed in a manner similar to the anterior Bankart procedure. If excessive inferior subluxation is identified, a capsular shift procedure is performed to reduce the volume of the inferior axillary recess.

Labral lesions can also contribute to symptoms of instability. Bankart lesions in association with corresponding capsular injury can allow for recurrent anterior subluxation and produce true instability symptoms. Isolated anterior and posterior labral tears, however, more commonly produce pain and clicking but are also often associated with a less dramatic yet significant sense of functional stability. Surgical treatment of these isolated labral tears can usually be accomplished with the arthroscope, but management can be problematic. These tears may be representative of significant underlying instability, and this must be ruled out. Also, simple debridement of isolated labral tears may not yield good long-term results,[2] and an effort to stabilize the labrum may be more desirable. Superior labrum anterior and posterior (SLAP) lesions[31] can cause pain and disability, especially when associated with detachment of the labral-biceps tendon complex from the superior glenoid (type II and type IV SLAP lesions). Detachment of the biceps tendon reduces its contribution toward glenohumeral stability and can produce symptoms suggestive of a functional or microinstability. Although debridement of loose or torn superior labral tissue may improve symptoms, we think that glenoid abrasion and superior labrum stabilization is preferrable because it allows for reduction and subsequent healing of the biceps tendon onto its insertion at the supraglenoid tubercle.[8]

EQUIPMENT VARIABLES

The use of proper tennis equipment is important not only in maximizing the speed of recovery after a shoulder injury but also in helping to prevent injuries. Variables such as racquet type, racquet size and shape, string type and tensioning, and tennis balls all play a part in reducing such injuries. Tennis racquets are currently designed most often in a Y-shaped throat configuration in association with a medium-to-large head size. This Y throat design reduces air resistance during the stroke[19] (Fig. 29-5). Other racquet considerations include a relatively heavy or light racquet head. Heavy racquet heads increase the torque about the shoulder joint by shifting the effective moment arm away from the shoulder and are not recommended for players recovering from a shoulder injury. String tension is also important, and Lehman[19] recommends decreasing string tension by 3 to 5 lb below the tension typical for a particular injured athlete because as string tension is reduced, less stress is transferred to the arm. Natural gut strings are also recommended over nylon or synthetic strings at least for the competitive tennis player to help prevent or speed the resolution of overuse injuries to the shoulder. Finally, new tennis balls should be used during the recovery phase because greater racquet speed is required to achieve comparable ball speed when "dead" balls are used.[19] Thus, older balls can increase the demands on a shoulder recovering from injury.

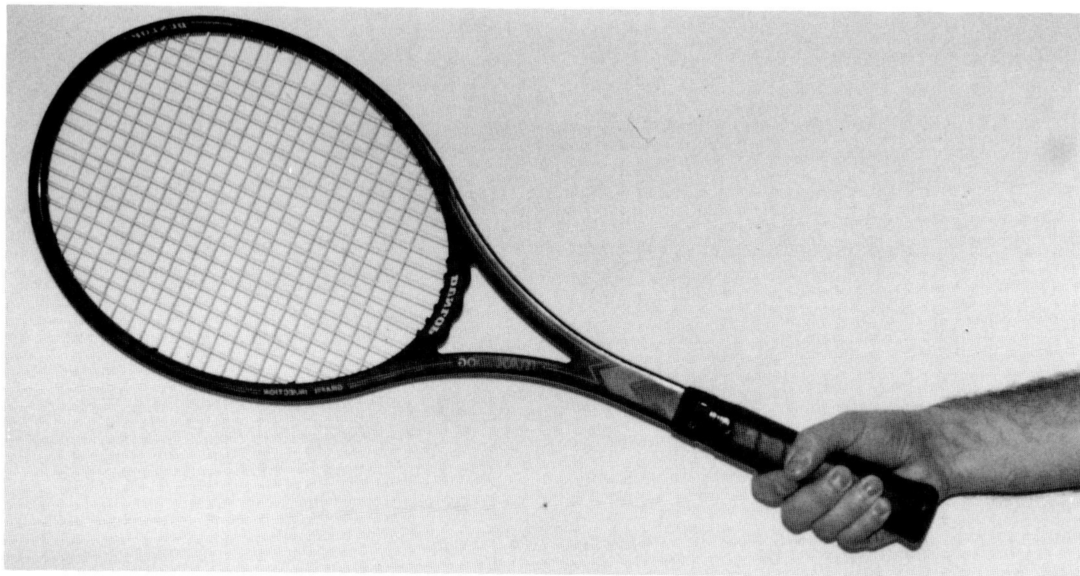

Figure 29-5. A modern tennis racquet with a Y-shaped throat design.

ELDERLY AND ADOLESCENT TENNIS PLAYERS

Individuals of all ages from the very young to the very elderly participate in tennis, and this age variability is greater than in most other sports. Shoulder symptomatology, relatively common among middle-aged and elderly persons, can present itself or be exacerbated by the demands of tennis.

Tennis is a popular sport among children and teenagers, with approximately 500,000 participating regularly each year.[10] Shoulder complaints are common, and treatment plans must often be individualized to this population of players as etiologly of their complaints sometimes differs from that of adults. In a study of 270 competitive junior tennis players, 24 percent reported either a current or prior history of shoulder pain. These shoulder symptoms in adolescents are most often due to rotator cuff overload with or without glenohumeral subluxation,[20] but other etiologies can act as a source of symptoms. Shoulder injuries exclusive to children and adolescents are related to the proximal humeral physis and apophyses. During ossification, these apophyses are susceptible to repetitive stress from overuse and can result in localized pain. Injuries to the proximal humeral physis have been described in baseball throwers[1,7,15,33] and recently in an adolescent tennis player.[6] Symptoms consist of tenderness localized to the area adjacent to the proximal humeral growth plate and to pain during and after the serve. The diagnosis is confirmed by radiologic evidence of widening of the lateral aspect of the proximal humeral physis with demineralization and fragmentation of the lateral aspect of the adjacent metaphysis. The mainstay of treatment is rest until symptoms resolve.

Repetitive stress injuries to the rotator cuff humeral insertions onto the greater and lesser tuberosities of skeletally immature athletes can result in what has been described as "Osgood-Schlatter disease of the shoulder."[10] The child typically presents with impingement symptoms in association with localized rotator cuff insertion site tenderness and radiographic abnormalities as a result of the abnormal ossifications.[10]

Impingement symptoms in adolescents most often result from repetitive strokes and overhead serves, just as in adults. Treatment, however, may differ in some respects in these patients. Most components of the rehabilitation program, including restriction from certain activities and exercise protocols, mirror that for adults, but we do not use steroid injections in children and adolescents and rarely use nonsteroidal anti-inflammatory medications. Also, because junior tennis players have been shown to sometimes have significantly decreased internal rotation,[5] we think that the rehabilitation program should also emphasize improving this component of shoulder motion. Increasing internal rotation toward normal will hopefully aid in improving rotator cuff balance and thus promote recovery and reduce the incidence of reinjury.

As is true of this older population in general, elderly tennis players more commonly develop symptoms related to rotator cuff injury. Underlying degenerative disease of the glenohumeral or acromioclavicular joints can also cause symptoms primarily or can predispose to impingement symptoms. Management of impingement symptoms in-

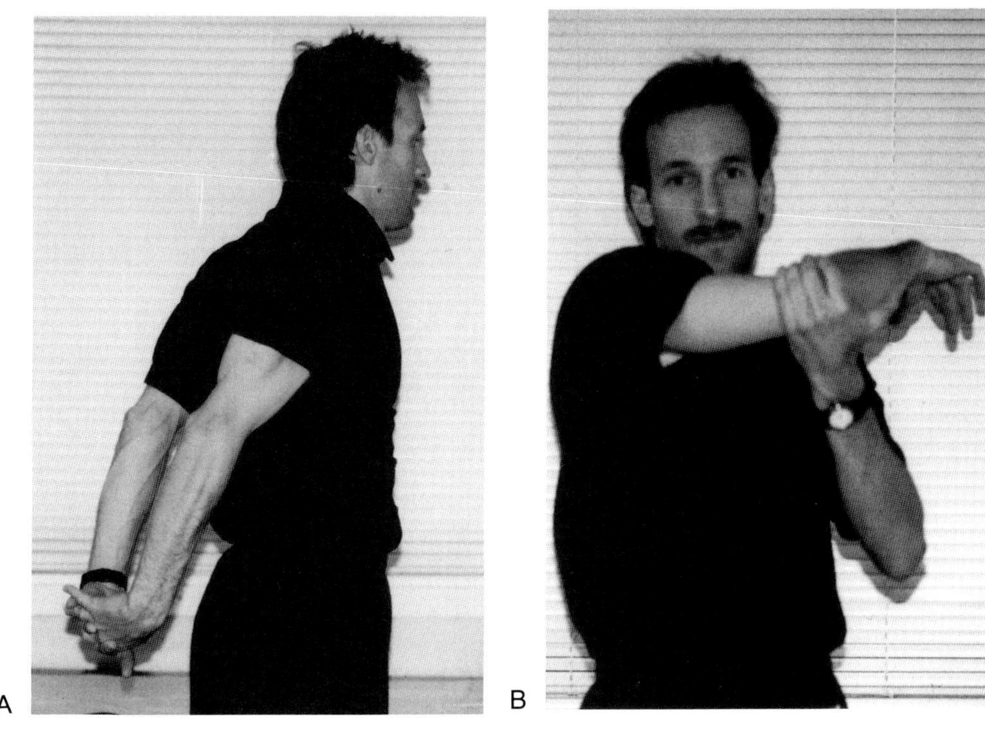

A B

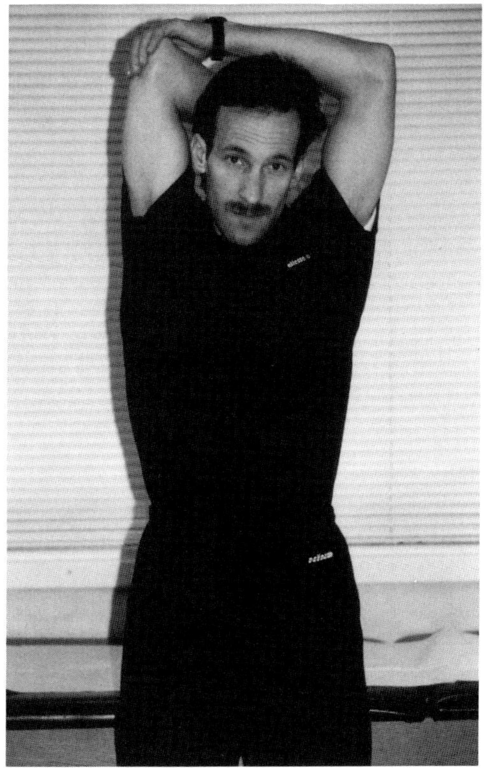

C

Figure 29-6. (**A**) Shoulder stretching consists of stretching of the anterior shoulder structures by progressively raising and hyperextending both arms. (**B**) Posterior shoulder stretching is effectively accomplished by adducting the shoulder in the horizontal plane and by using the opposite arm to increase and maintain the stretch. (**C**) Bringing the arm directly over the head serves to stretch the shoulder in the coronal plane.

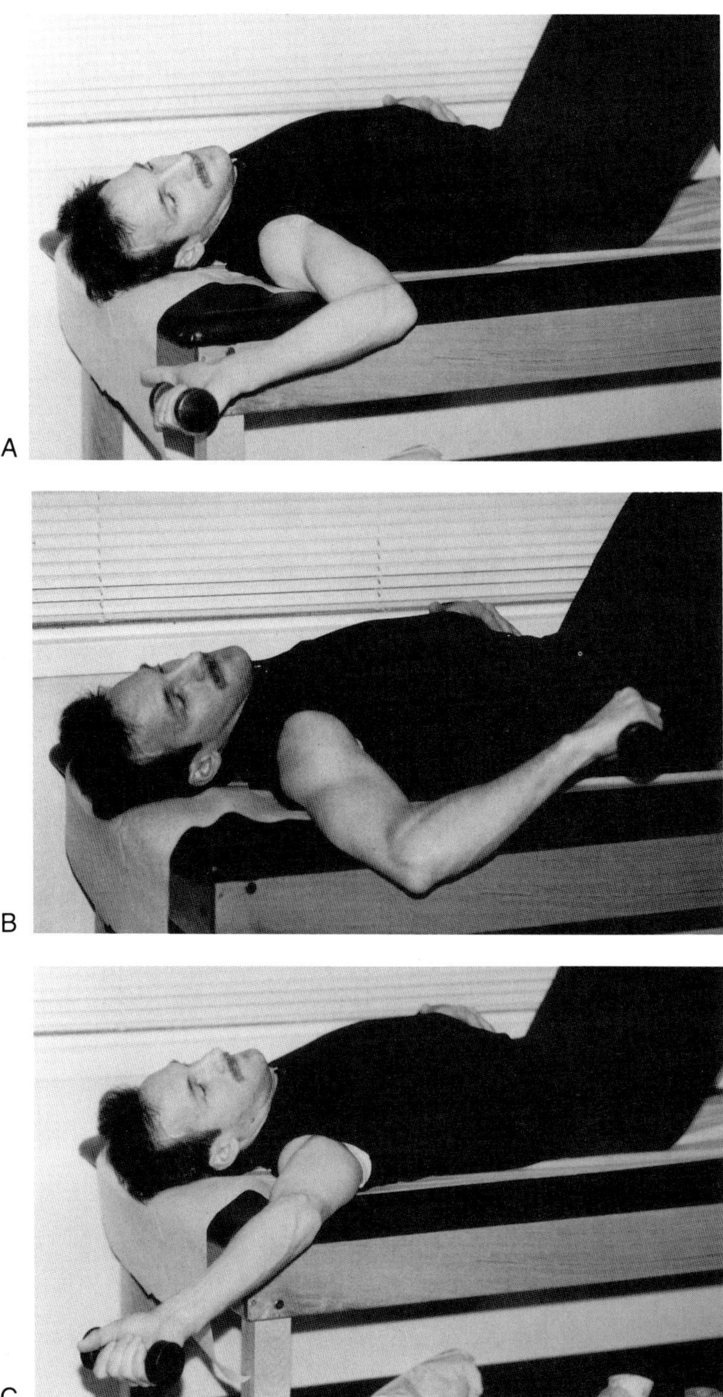

Figure 29-7. Stretching of the shoulder internal and external rotators is most easily accomplished supine. (**A**) The internal rotators are stretched with the arm over the table side and at 90 degrees of abduction. (**B**) The external rotators are likewise stretched. (**C**) The anterior capsule can be effectively stretched by extending the elbow and forward flexing the shoulder as shown.

volves pursuing standard rehabilitative protocols.[28] However, the increased functional demands of many of these patients often dictate a more aggressive approach to management. For middle-aged to elderly tennis players with impingement-related symptoms, we recommend a 6-week to 3-month period of rehabilitation, with the addition of a shoulder MRI or arthrogram for those patients who do not respond to this exercise regimen or in whom a rotator cuff tear is suspected. Also, for those players who do report a specific injury to the shoulder and in whom an MRI or arthrogram shows a rotator cuff tear, consideration should be given to early repair.

Elderly tennis players, although only rarely symptomatic from problems attributable to shoulder instability, are far more likely to experience symptoms related to degenerative arthritis in the shoulder or acromioclavicular joint than are young adults. Treatment of symptoms due to these degenerative changes, such as stiffness and pain, is primarily accomplished through range of motion and strengthening exercises. Nonsteroidal anti-inflammatory medications are generally reserved for patients with more significant disease or for patients who fail to respond to exercises alone.

PREVENTION

Shoulder girdle flexibility, strength, and balance along with proper mechanics including coupled rotation and early ball contact are the keys to prevention of shoulder injuries in tennis. The repetitive intrinsic loads placed on the rotator cuff musculature and scapular stabilizers place high demands on the shoulder joint, and failure to incorporate a comprehensive conditioning program into a training schedule or use of poor technique will significantly increase a player's risk of injury.

Flexibility of the shoulder should be maintained. Chandler et al[5] has shown that junior elite tennis players are significantly tighter in dominant shoulder internal rotation. An exercise regimen designed to improve internal rotation flexibility should be used to reduce this imbalance, or loss of shoulder motion can result. Restrictions in motion could then predispose the player to injury. A flexibility program, although focusing on the internal rotators of the shoulder, should also incorporate the other muscles about the shoulder. Proper stretching exercises for the shoulder as detailed by Hageman and Lehman[11] include overhead and horizontal upper extremity stretches using the opposite arm to increase and maintain the degree of stretch (Fig. 29-6). Shoulder internal and external rotator stretching (Fig. 29-7) is best performed supine and can include the use of small weights or the tennis racquet itself. Theraband devices can be used to simulate the various tennis strokes, and the Theraband can even be applied to the racquet to more closely reproduce the tennis stroke.[11]

Shoulder strength and muscular balance about the shoulder are also important components in preventing tennis injuries. Repetitive strokes can lead to muscle fatigue and weakness, which can increase the risk of injury. Also, unlike a baseball pitcher who can control the number of overhead pitches thrown, the tennis player is committed to serving throughout a tennis match. Chandler et al[4] showed that the shoulder external rotators, responsible for decelerating the arm after the tennis serve, are disproportionately weaker relative to the strong internal rotators. This relative muscle imbalance can predispose to injury. Therefore, emphasis should be placed on external rotator strengthening to maintain shoulder girdle balance, with the eccentric component of external rotator function especially important to rehabilitate in the tennis player.[16] Also, Ryu et al[29] has illustrated in an electromyographic study the high activity levels of the serratus anterior muscle during the tennis serve and forehand and backhand strokes. As a result of this study and our own experience, we emphasize strengthening of the scapular stabilizers in our conditioning protocol for tennis players.

Although maintaining good shoulder flexibility, strength, and balance are most important in preventing shoulder injuries in tennis, other factors play a role. Even the best conditioned tennis player must set realistic limits on duration and level of play. Excessive tournament play as well as participation against a partner of greatly superior ability can predispose the player to injury. Proper technique is also important in preventing injuries because poor technique can result in overloading one or more of the tendinous components of the shoulder girdle. Finally, use of proper equipment can reduce load transfer to the shoulder and decrease the risk of injury.

REFERENCES

1. Adams JE: Little League shoulder: osteochondrosis of the proximal humeral epiphyses in boy baseball pitchers. California Med 105:22, 1966
2. Altchek DW, Warren RF, Wickiewicz TL, Ortiz G: Arthroscopic labral debridement. A three-year follow-up study. Am J Sports Med 20:702, 1992
3. Bigliani LU, Kimmel J, McCann PD, Wolfe I: Repair of rotator cuff tears in tennis players. Am J Sports Med 20:112, 1992
4. Chandler TJ, Kibler B, Stracener EC et al: Shoulder strength, power, and endurance in college tennis players. Am J Sports Med 20:455, 1992
5. Chandler TJ, Kibler WB, Uhl TL et al: Flexibility comparisons of junior elite tennis players to other athletes. Am J Sports Med 18:134, 1990

6. Deutsch A, Potter HG, Veltri DM et al: MRI findings of Little League shoulder syndrome in an adolescent tennis players: a case report. Submitted
7. Dotter WE: Little Leaguer's shoulder: a fracture of proximal epiphyseal cartilage of the humerus due to baseball pitching. Guthrie Clin Bull 23:68, 1953
8. Field LD, Savoie FH: Arthroscopic suture repair of superior labral detachment lesions of the shoulder. Am J Sports Med 21:783, 1993
9. Glousman R: Electromyographic analysis and its role in the athletic shoulder. Clin Orthop 288:27, 1993
10. Gregg JR, Torg E: Upper extremity injuries in adolescent tennis players. Clin Sports Med 7:371, 1988
11. Hageman CE, Lehman RC: Stretching, strengthening, and conditioning for the competitive tennis player. Clin Sports Med 7:211, 1988
12. Harryman DR, Sidles JA, Clark JM et al: Translation of the humeral head on the glenoid with passive glenohumeral motion. J Bone Joint Surg [Am] 72:1334, 1990
13. Jobe FW, Moynes DR, Tibone JE, Perry J: An EMG analysis of the shoulder in pitching. A second report. Am J Sports Med 12:218, 1984
14. Jobe FW, Tibone JE, Perry J, Moynes D: An EMG analysis of the shoulder in throwing and pitching. A preliminary report. Am J Sports Med 11:3, 1983
15. Kalhill BR, Tullos HS, Fain RH: Little league shoulder: lesions of the proximal humeral epiphyseal plate. Am J Sports Med 2:150, 1974
16. Kennedy K, Altchek DW, Glick IV: Concentric and eccentric isokinetic rotator cuff ratios in skilled tennis players. Isokinetics Exerc Sc 3:155, 1993
17. Kibler WB, McQueen C, Uhl T: Fitness evaluations and fitness findings in competitive junior tennis players. Clin Sports Med 7:403, 1988
18. Koplan JP, Siscovick DS, Goldbaum GM: The risks of exercise: a public health view of injuries and hazards. Public Health Rep 100:189, 1985
19. Lehman RC: Surface and equipment variables in tennis injuries. Clin Sports Med 7:229, 1988
20. Lehman RC: Shoulder pain in the competitive tennis player. Clin Sports Med 7:309, 1988
21. Maylack FH: Epidemiology of tennis, squash, and racquetball injuries. Clin Sports Med 7:233, 1988
22. Moynes DR, Perry J, Antonelli DJ, Jobe FW: Electromyography and motion analysis of the upper extremity in sports. Phys Ther 66:1905, 1986
23. Neer CS: Impingement lesions. Clin Orthop 173:70, 1983
24. Paletta GA, Warner JP, Warren RF, Altchek DW: Biplanar x-ray evaluation of patients with rotator cuff tears or anterior instability. Paper presented at the American Academy of Orthopaedic Surgeons Annual Meeting, Washington, DC, 1992
25. Perry J: Anatomy and biomechanics of the shoulder in throwing, swimming, gymnastics, and tennis. Clin Sports Med 2:247, 1983
26. Priest JD: The shoulder of the tennis player. Clin Sports Med 7:387, 1988
27. Priest JD, Nagel DA: Tennis shoulder. Clin Sports Med 4:28, 1976
28. Rockwood CA, Matsen FA (eds): The Shoulder. Vol. 2. WB Saunders, Philadelphia, 1990
29. Ryu RK, McCormick J, Jobe FW et al: An electromyographic analysis of shoulder function in tennis players. Am J Sports Med 16:481, 1988
30. Schwartz E, Warren RF, Otis JC et al: Superior migration of the humeral head in rotator cuff dysfunction. Orthop Trans 12:497, 1988
31. Snyder SJ, Karzel RP, Del Pizzo W et al: SLAP lesions of the shoulder. Arthroscopy 6:274, 1990
32. Tibone JE, Elrod B, Jobe FW et al: Surgical treatment of tears of the rotator cuff in athletes. J Bone Joint Surg [Am] 68:887, 1986
33. Torg JS, Pollack H, Sweterlitsch P: Ther effect of competitive pitching in the shoulders and elbows of preadolescent baseball players. Pediatrics 49:267, 1972
34. Winge S, Jorgensen U, Nielsen AL: Epidemiology of injuries in Danish championship tennis. Int J Sports Med 10:368, 1989

CHAPTER THIRTY

Swimming

Peter J. Fowler

Shoulder pain is a problem in a significant number of competitive swimmers and is, in fact, the most common orthopaedic complaint. Reports have cited incidences that range from 47 to 73 percent.[7,9,11,12] Several factors (Table 30-1) are implicated in what is typically known as *swimmer's shoulder,* the term introduced to the clinical literature by Kennedy and Hawkins in 1974.[6] This referred to what was thought to be a tendinitis of the rotator cuff, usually the supraspinatus or biceps tendon.[6] Inflammation has not been noted histologically or under direct vision, however, and the term *tendinopathy* is a more appropriate description of this disorder.

The demands of competitive swimming are excessive in terms of repetition and force. These stress the shoulder muscles and their tendons far beyond their design and normal use and make the swimmer vulnerable to shoulder injury. It is important that prevention of injury be given a central role in training programs as swimmers and coaches work together to optimize performance.

The four competitive swimming strokes are freestyle (front crawl), backstroke, butterfly, and breaststroke. In the freestyle, backstroke, and butterfly, the arms provide 75 percent of propulsion. In the breaststroke, the arms and legs contribute equally. Each stroke consists of four phases: the reach, the catch, the pull, and the recovery. During the catch position in all strokes but the breaststroke, the shoulder begins to extend, abduct, and medially rotate. This is where maximum impingment can occur, and most swimmers describe the occurrence of their pain as just after the catch.

INTENSITY OF TRAINING PROGRAMS

Training programs for competitive swimming have become increasingly rigorous. Typically, the national caliber swimmer practices in the water in sessions lasting 2 hours twice daily for a minimum of 5 days a week. Also, dry land training is performed to increase strength and endurance. Opinions regarding ideal training distances vary among coaches, but ranges average from 4,000 to 8,000 m each practice. The time in the pool is used to not only improve conditioning but to work on starts, strokes, and turns. These schedules, which can contribute to fatigue, can be a major factor in the development of swimmer's shoulder.[11]

OVERWORK

The shoulder is the most mobile and least stable joint, and as such it is most vulnerable to injury in the overhead position. The continuous, repeated demands of competitive swimming may require the rotator cuff muscles to work excessively hard to stabilize and contain the humeral head. This workload can lead to fatigue of the muscles and to the onset of a chronic tendinopathy condition. With rotator cuff fatigue, superior migration of the humeral head, which can increase subacromial loading, can occur. This, in turn, may be a factor precipitating the onset of a tendinopathy. As well, the mechanics of the entire shoulder complex may be altered if there is scapular muscle fatigue.

Table 30-1. Factors Implicated in Swimmer's Shoulder

Intensity of training programs
Overwork
Impingement—subacromial loading
Stroke mechanics
Shoulder joint laxity
Shoulder instability
Acromial shape
Hypovascularity

IMPINGEMENT—SUBACROMIAL LOADING

The coracoacromial arch is formed by the coracoid process, the rigid coracoacromial ligament, and the anterior acromion. The supraspinatus and biceps tendons insert on or across the humerus directly below the coracoacromial arch. This anatomic arrangement makes them particulary susceptible to impingement. In the catch phase of all swimming strokes, the arm is in abduction, forward flexion, and internal rotation and the humeral head moves under the arch, where the tendons may be repeatedly impinged. If the mechanics of the scapula have been altered, the tendons may be impinged against the arch, causing a mechanical irritation and tendinopathy that can further compromise the available space here. Untreated, this can progress to involve the subacromial bursa and acromioclavicular ligament.

STROKE MECHANICS

At entry and the first half of the pull, the shoulder is in forward flexion, abduction, and internal rotation. The humeral head is forced under the anterior acromion and coracoacromial ligament. Impingement of the supraspinatus and biceps tendons may occur, especially when the cuff is fatigued.

Lateral impingement may be related to the recovery phase of the freestyle and butterfly. Here, the shoulder is in abduction and internal rotation, and the humeral head comes up against the lateral border of the acromion. This is particularly true when the shoulder leads the rest of the arm. When the humeral head leads the arm through recovery, there is less potential for lateral impingement.

At the end of the pull phase, the shoulder is in adduction and internal rotation, a position that corresponds to the "wringing out" mechanism described later in this chapter.

An analysis of the freestyle arm position at the time swimmers experienced pain suggested a correlation with the biomechanical factors implicated in tendinopathy.[12] Almost one-half of the swimmers with shoulder pain said it occurred during entry or the first half of the pull phase; 14 percent reported pain during the second half of the pull phase; and 23 percent had pain during the recovery. The remaining 17.8 percent had pain during the entire pull or the recovery phase. Some of these swimmers experienced pain throughout the entire stroke.

SHOULDER JOINT LAXITY

In the athlete with loose or lax shoulders, the muscles of the rotator cuff may already be working hard just to contain the humeral head. The added rigor of training makes further demands on these fatigued or fatiguing muscles. Fowler and Webster[4] evaluated 188 competitive swimmers and compared them with a control group of 50 recreational athletes. The investigators found that 50 percent of the swimmers had a history of shoulder pain. As well, 55 percent of the swimmers and 52 percent of the control group had some degree of posterior laxity in one or both shoulders. These results suggested that swimming does not predispose an athlete to increased posterior laxity. Twenty-five percent of the swimmers had a history of tendinopathy and increased posterior laxity. The tendinopathy was always present in the lax shoulder, suggesting an association between tendinopathy and increased laxity.

At manual testing on these same swimmers, 40 had external rotator weakness in one or both shoulders. Thirty-three had both weakness and a history of tendinopathy in the same shoulder. Based on these findings, a second study was conducted to measure rotation strength about the shoulder. The Cybex II dynamometer (Lumex Inc., Ronkonkoma, NY) measured internal and external rotation strength in neutral, 90 degrees abduction, and 90 degrees flexion in 119 swimmers and 51 controls (participants in activities not requiring arm rotation strength primarily). There was a significant difference in the torque ratio between the two groups in abduction and neutral[3] (Table 30-2). This imbalance was attributed to the swimmer's greater strength in internal rotation, a result of the emphasis placed on strengthening the internal rotators and extensors to improve speed and endurance.

SHOULDER INSTABILITY

Pain as a result of shoulder instability alone is seldom seen in competitive swimmers. Anterior instability is often secondary to a traumatic incident in another sport. Compared with the throwing mechanism, the arm is seldom in the provocative position during any swimming stroke.

In contrast to anterior instability, swimmers with frank posterior instability may have pain from being dislocated

Table 30-2. Rotation Strength Ratio about the Shoulder: Comparison of Competitive Swimmers and a Control Group of Athletes[a]

Position	Swimmers	Controls
Neutral	53.7 (SD = 17)	65 (SD = 15)
90 degrees abduction	62.1 (SD = 14)	78.2 (SD = 17)
90 degrees flexion	Right 46 (SD = 18.4) Left 42 (SD = 19.7)	52 (SD = 17)

[a] External rotation/internal rotation × 100 = rotation ratio.

in the swimming stroke cycle. The ''at-risk'' position of forward flexion and internal rotation is a component of all strokes. Those with multidirectional instability, congenital or acquired, are susceptible to this. It is important to differentiate between pain from instability alone and painful tendinopathy with concomitant increased laxity.

HYPOVASCULARITY

Rathbun and Macnab[10] have demonstrated that the blood supply to the supraspinatus and biceps tendons is affected by arm position. In adduction and neutral rotation, there is an area of avascularity close to the musculotendinous junction where the tendons are stretched tightly over the humeral head. In abduction, circulation is restored as the vessels fill. This repeated avascularity, known as the ''wringing out'' mechanism, occurs in the area of the tendon most vulnerable to loading. Repeated interruption of the vascular supply may contribute to early degenerative changes and increase the potential for rotator cuff damage.

ACROMIAL SHAPE

In a cadaveric study, Bigliani and associates[1] identifed three acromial shapes: type I, flat: type II, curved; and type III, hooked. There were classified according to shape, angle of anterior slope, and the presence of spurs. A disproportionate number (70 percent) of rotator cuff tears were identified in those specimens with type III acromions. These findings suggested that the presence of an anatomic factor leading to a refractory tendinopathy. A competitive swimmer with a type III acromion may be predisposed to impingement because the dimensions of the acromial arch are decreased to begin with. A tendinopathy may more easily develop and be more resistant to treatment.

PHYSICAL EXAMINATION

The physical examination includes inspection, palpation, assessment of range of motion with associated pain, crepitus, stability, and motor strength.

Clinical Tests

1. *Palpation of supraspinatus tendon:* tenderness elicited by palpation of the supraspinatus tendon medial to its insertion on the greater tuberosity suggests a tendinopathy. If the long head of biceps is involved, there will be tenderness over the bicipital groove as well.
2. *Painful arc syndrome:* there is pain with active abduction, which is most pronounced between 60 and 100 degrees. The pain may be intensified when the examiner provides resistance.
3. *Resisted forward elevation:* the examiner applies pressure to the fully forward elevated arm. This drives the head of the humerus against the anteroinferior border of the acromion. Pain may be reproduced if already injured tendons are impinged against the anterior acromion.
4. *Forced internal rotation at 90 degrees forward flexion:* as the examiner internally rotates the arm that is 90 degrees forward flexed, the tendons are impinged between the humeral head and the coracoacromial arch (anterior acromion and coracoacromial ligament), reproducing pain (Fig. 30-1).
5. *External rotation weakness:* with the arms in external rotation and adduction and the elbows flexed to 90 degrees, the patient resists internal rotation force applied by the examiner. Gross weakness will be readily apparent. Pain may accompany this test.
6. *Apprehension test (anterior instability):* generalized laxity in the swimmer is assessed particularly as it relates to the shoulder. Increased laxity or frank instability should be documented as it contributes to the progression of tendinopathy or as the total cause of the pain. For anterior instability to be assessed, the patient lies supine and the examiner abducts the arm to 90 degrees and externally rotates the humerus. A positive sign is obtained when the patient exhibits a feeling of anxiety,

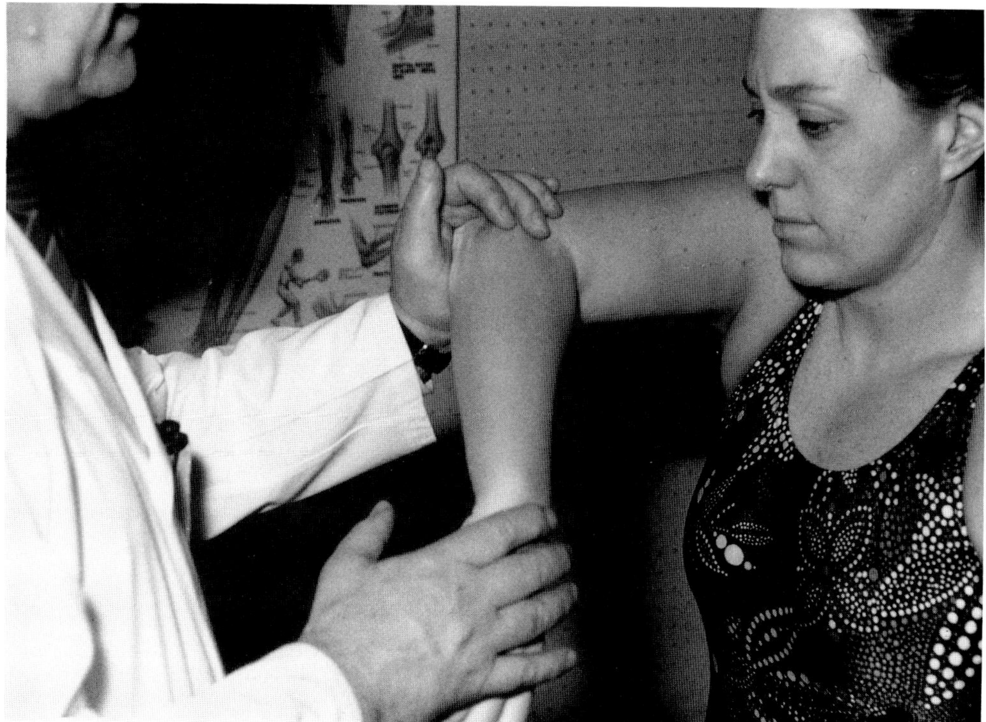

Figure 30-1. In this test, the tendons are impinged under the coracoacromial arch. Care must be taken, as very little pressure will elicit a painful response.

often with pain, and will not allow further external rotation. The anxiety is alleviated when the examiner applies posterior pressure on the upper arm, which contains humeral head.

7. *Load-and-shift tests—assessment of posterior translation:* with the patient sitting, the examiner stabilizes the shoulder girdle with one hand and with the opposite hand applies posterior pressure to the humeral head and assesses the amount of movement. This may be more easily performed with the patient supine with the examiner holding the arm in 90 degrees of abduction and applying posterior pressure to the upper humerus. Movement of the humeral head 50 percent of the glenoid is considered normal. Motion greater than this, although not necessarily abnormal, can influence the mechanics of the shoulder by creating an increased workload for the rotator cuff. Applying an axial load to the humeral head may reproduce symptoms of clinical instability (load-and-shift test).

Clinical Picture

Blazina's classification of jumper's knee, which associates pain with level of activity, is useful in assessing the clinical severity of shoulder tendinopathy.[2] In grade I, there is pain with activity; grade II, pain (not disabling) during and after activity; and grade III, pain (disabling) during and after activity. In a fourth category, there is pain with activities of daily living, even after cessation of sport.

The progression of tendinopathy is insidious. Pain becomes generalized about the shoulder and is often present at night or at rest. The athlete tends to avoid painful positions and develops subtle changes in stroke mechanics to minimize pain. In other activities as well, the athlete will modify all positions that aggravate the symptoms.

PREVENTION

A training program that focuses on prevention of overuse syndromes about the shoulder, as well as on improving speed and conditioning, will ultimately be more successful. Principles for prevention (Table 30-3) should be included in the training program from the outset of a swimmer's career. The importance of an informed coach cannot be overstated. Ongoing stroke analysis, advice concerning stroke errors, careful planning of practice sessions, and regular monitoring of performance to prevent rotator cuff fatigue are among the responsibilities of the coaching staff.

Training

Overwork is a primary cause of tendinopathy and is often the result of an increased intensity or distances of training sets. Rigorous training sessions or "extra hard" practices at the beginning of a training program before the athlete is ready can trigger the onset of a rotator cuff tendinopathy. Demands on swimmers should be increased gradually as the schedule progresses. Work-outs should be

Table 30-3. Prevention of Shoulder Tendinopathy in the Swimmer

Training regime
Proper warm-up and warm-down (every practice)
Gradually increase distance
Gradually increase intensity
Most rigorous sets at beginning of work-out
Strengthening (no pain involved)
Proper warm-up and warm-down (every practice) with dry-land training
Include external rotators in dry-land program
External rotator strengthening more than three times per week
Strengthening exercises for muscles surrounding scapula
Stretching (no pain involved)
Daily
Less than 15 years of age, single stretching
More than 15 years of age, pairs stretching
Passive or proprioceptive neuromuscular facilitated stretching
No ballistic stretches
Stroke mechanics
Pay particular attention to proper stroke mechanics when shoulder is fatigued
Use proper body roll

designed so that the difficult portion is completed early in the practice when the athlete is not severely fatigued. The session can then continue with emphasis on stroke drills and with alternating strokes with leg work or with start-and-turn techniques. In this way, the structures at risk will be provided with relative rest. Proper instruction will enable the swimmer to guard against the damaging effects of fatigue and to minimize the potential for injury by using increased awareness and good stroke mechanics.

Strengthening

Imbalance in muscle strength about the shoulder results from swimmers emphasizing, both during pool and dry-land training, muscle groups that improve propulsion and neglecting those that stabilize the shoulder. This contributes to overwork for the cuff muscles. A balanced exercise program to include external rotation strengthening may reduce the incidence of tendinopathy, particularly that associated with glenohumeral laxity. It is also important to condition the scapular muscles. When doing weight training, painful subacromial loading positions should be avoided. Paddles, which swimmers use to increase resistance, must be used with caution as the increased leverage can overload the rotator cuff muscles.

Stretching

Stretching should be performed regularly as part of the daily training warm-up. Three times weekly is not sufficient. Griep[5] studied the relationship between shoulder flexibility and the incidence of tendinopathy in swimmers. He found that regardless of sex and the stroke most frequently used, those swimmers with restricted flexibility were more likely to develop a tendinopathy than those who maintained and improved flexibility with a stretching program. Stretching can be performed individually or in pairs (Figs. 30-2 and 30-3). Pairs stretching should be both taught and performed carefully and should be restricted to swimmers older than the age of 15 years. It is important for coaches to stress that overstretching and forcing the shoulder to an excessive range of motion can increase the irritation to the rotator cuff tendons.

The stretching techniques used by pairs can be either passive or proprioceptive neuromuscular facilitated (PNF). In passive stretching, the partner slowly and gently moves the swimmer to the pain-free limit and then holds the position. In PNF stretching, the swimmer to be stretched moves to the limit of range. The partner maintains the position while the swimmer contracts against the partner's resistance.

Stroke Mechanics

Poor stroke mechanics cannot only slow a swimmer down but can also be a major contributor to shoulder pain. The coach should examine the execution of strokes that cause pain and help the swimmer to modify them. Analysis of changing stroke technique during fatigue is essential. Insufficient body roll in freestyle or backstroke can contribute to lateral shoulder impingement. A high elbow position during recovery must be achieved with body roll rather than muscle activity. Forcing the elbow into a higher position without body roll may induce subacromial humeral head impingement.

In the catch phase of all strokes, the swimmer is preparing for maximal propulsion. Overreach with excessive in-

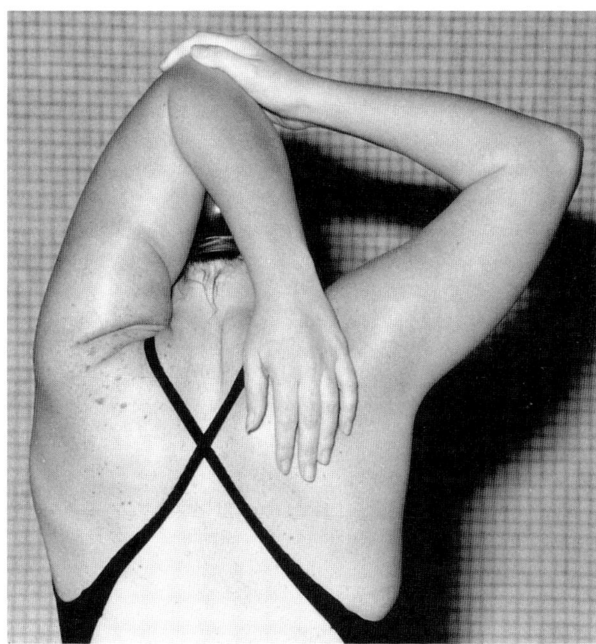

Figure 30-2. Stretching alone can accommodate all muscle groups.

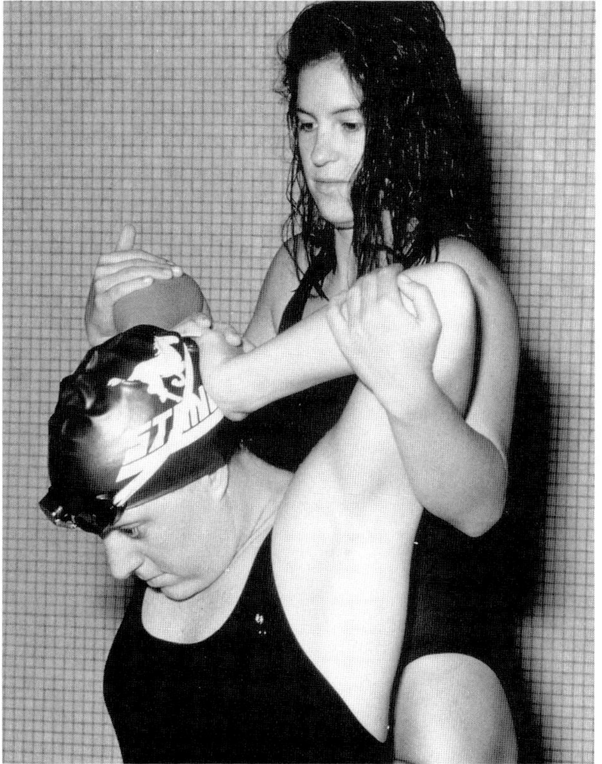

Figure 30-3. Pairs stretching can be performed by older swimmers. Knowledge of proper technique and dangers of overstretching is important.

ternal rotation at the end of the stroke may cause undue subacromial loading and may require excessive activity for the cuff muscles to contain the humeral head. As well, too much internal rotation at the end of the stroke may intensify the "wringing out" mechanism.

TREATMENT

A grade I tendinopathy responds well to conservative management (Table 30-4). The swimmer is instructed to increase time spent in both prepractice stretching and in-the-pool warm-up. Proper stretching can restore full range of motion, increase blood flow, and reduce potential for further impingement injury. The in-the-pool warm-up should be prolonged, at a very slow pace and in pain-free strokes. Kicking drills can be emphasized, and training sessions should conclude with a swimming warm-down period.

Icing the shoulder after each practice, with ice cups or ice bags for no more than 15 minutes, will reduce pain. External rotator weakness should be corrected with exercises that begin in adduction and progress to varying degrees of abduction (Fig. 30-4). This will improve the control of the glenohumeral joint, which will result in more efficient muscle work and a better performance potential. It is important that the swim practice be as pain-free as possible. If the swimmer has pain only when the work load is too heavy, it should be reduced for a time and then gradually increased. Any stroke causing symptoms should be temporarily discontinued and gradually reintroduced, with any faults corrected, once the symptoms have subsided.

A grade II tendinopathy requires relative rest, physiotherapy, and in some instances, medication. Relative rest does not suggest that there be total abstinence from the sport but rather that the athlete use strokes that do not elicit pain. Again, leg work can be emphasized. Kick boards should not be used because they place the shoulder in the pain-provoking position. For aerobic training, running and cycling can supplement the swim work-outs. Along with these measures, a short course of anti-inflammatory medication will often help provide symptomatic relief.

At this stage, physiotherapy is indicated. The therapist will assess the athlete's shoulder to determine intensity and duration of pain, loss of shoulder motion, and any loss of strength in the arm or shoulder girdle muscles. These findings will determine choice of treatment, which may include modalities such as ultrasound, interferential therapy, or transcutaneous electrical nerve stimulation. Loss of shoulder motion is treated with passive mobilization techniques and range of motion exercises. Biofeedback techniques allow the swimmer to train specific muscles. A strengthening program is planned to correct any imbalance in muscle strength or significant weakness in any muscle

Table 30-4. Treatment of Tendinopathy

Grade I
Increase prepractice strengthening and warm-up times
Emphasize pain-free strokes
Emphasize warm-down after training
Use icing techniques to reduce pain and inflammation
Correct weakness in external rotators
Grade II
Relative rest (i.e., emphasize leg work and pain-free strokes)
Anti-inflammatory medication
Physiotherapy modalities (e.g., ultrasound, transcutaneous electrical nerve stimulation
Strengthening program (free weights, rubber tubing, etc.)
Mobilization techniques
Consider steroid injection if no response to above
Grades III and IV
Conservative treatment may not relieve symptoms
Options include change in activity, surgery
Surgical treatment may include subacromial decompression, resection affected tendon ± adjacent subacromial bursa
Counseling, teaching, careful evaluation of options and related implications important

group. The exercises will be isometric, isotonic, or where possible, isokinetic, depending on the nature and presentation of the pain, joint range of motion, and weakness. Effective treatment programs can be developed using free weights or surgical tubing. Exercises should not reproduce pain. If pain is felt at certain positions, the exercise should be performed around these. Exercises that are painful throughout range should be discontinued or decreased in repetition or resistance to a pain-free level.

A successful treatment program will enable the swimmer to return gradually to a full training schedule. Therapy should continue until the preinjury level of activity is attained.

A corticosteroid injection into the subacromial space should be considered only if there is no response to treatment and if impingement-aggravated tests continue to elicit pain. These should not be used routinely.

In some cases, none of these measures is successful and

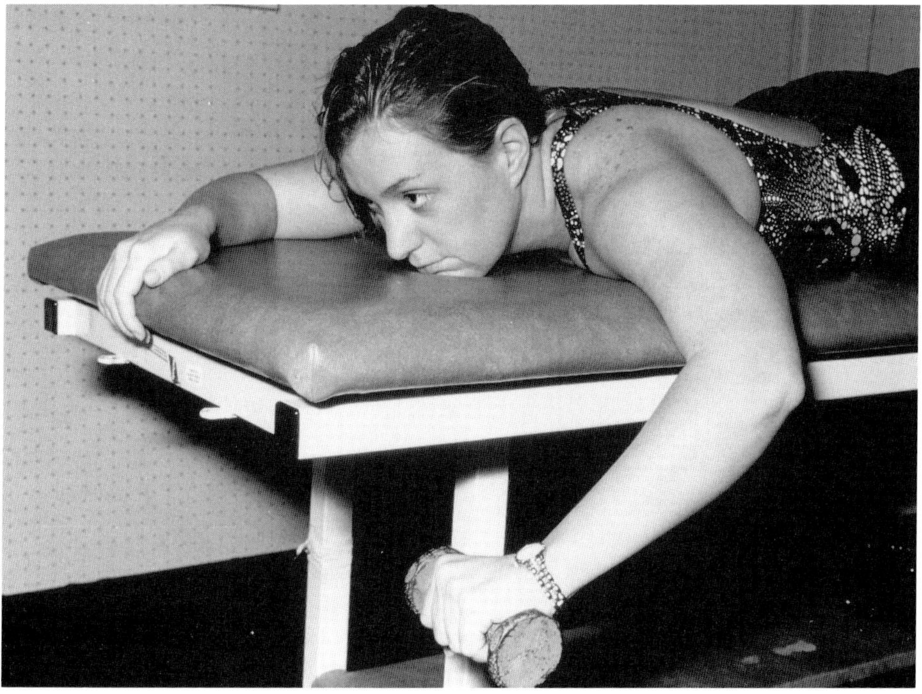

Figure 30-4. Free weights are used to strengthen external rotators in 90 degrees of abduction.

the tendinopathy progresses to grade III or beyond. In this instance, options available to the swimmer include a change of sport or surgery. Unless a high-caliber career at the national or international level is possible, most young swimmers correctly select the former option. In most cases, this is a decision to be encouraged. Surgical options include resection of the diseased segment of tendon along with adjacent subacromial bursal tissue if involved or decompression of the same area.

Before surgery is selected as an option, the clinician should make clear to the athlete that the postoperative recovery period requires a firm personal commitment. During this time, rehabilitation will include a progressive exercise program designed to restore range of motion and balanced muscle strength. The athlete must understand that the level of cooperation and compliance with the program will directly affect the outcome of the surgery. Return to the pool should begin with slow swimming, and progress to interval training and guided stroke modification. An overlapping period between formal rehabilitation and return to the sport is important. The significance of the coach to an athlete's successful return cannot be overemphasized.

A grade IV clinical presentation, pain with all activity, is most often seen in the mature athlete and may indicate a rotator cuff tear. Conservative measures may be insufficient to effect relief of symptoms. Although the diagnosis may be made clinically, imaging techniques such as arthrography, ultrasonography, and magnetic resonance imaging can provide confirmation. Arthroscopy of the shoulder joint and the subacromial space can help identify such lesions as partial-thickness tears and thickened subacromial bursae. Although not a frequent cause of pain, particularly in the younger swimmer, quadrant labral tears, anterior or superior, can cause pain and may be successfully treated with arthroscopic excision.[8]

In younger athletes, bursectomy alone followed by appropriate rehabilitation can provide relief. A more radical decompression to include resection of the anteroinferior acromion and a portion of the coracoacromial ligament is usually recommended. A torn rotator cuff is repaired to provide symptomatic relief and prevent progressive tearing. This may be noted in the older swimmer competing at the master's level. Return to the preinjury level of participation is unlikely, and this should be underscored preoperatively.

Formal physiotherapy plays a significant role postoperatively because range of motion is often lost and muscle strength, endurance, and power deteriorate. Typically, the abductors and external rotators are the weakest, but the rehabilitation program must ensure that all the muscle groups about the shoulder girdle are exercised.

SHOULDER INSTABILITY

Anterior Instability

Anterior instability is not often the cause of pain in competitive swimmers but is usually secondary to a traumatic incident in another sport. Primary conservative treatment is stroke modification and balanced strengthening exercises. If symptoms do not subside, examination under anaesthesia or arthroscopy will confirm an intra-articular lesion such as the Bankart or Hill-Sachs. An anterior stabilizing procedure can provide relief, and the athlete may return to preinjury levels if former strength and motion are regained.

Multidirectional Instability

Persistence with a nonoperative program is suggested for prolonged periods of multidirectional instability. In most cases, stroke modification, correction of strengthening deficits, and adjustment of training programs to minimize the magnitude and incidence of abnormal motion can be used successfully. Surgical intervention such as an inferior capsular shift, a "reefing procedure" to the posterior cuff and capsule, or a glenoid osteotomy should be considered only when all nonoperative treatments have been exhausted. The goal of these procedures is to provide symptomatic relief for activities of daily living. Although sports (swimming included) at a recreational level may be possible, a return to swimming at a highly competitive level occurs only occasionally.

REFERENCES

1. Bigliani NU, Morrison DS, April EW: The morphology of the acromion and its relationship to rotator cuff tears. Orthop Trans 10:216, 1986
2. Blazina ME: Jumper's knee. Orthop Clin North Am 4:65, 1980
3. Fowler PJ: Shoulder injuries in the mature athlete. pp. 225–38. In Grana WA (ed): Advances in Sports Medicine and Fitness. Year Book Medical Publishers, Chicago, 1988
4. Fowler PJ, Webster MS: Shoulder pain in highly competitive swimmers. Orthop Trans 7:170, 1983
5. Griep JF: Swimmers shoulder: the influence of flexibility and weight training. Orthop Trans 10:216, 1986
6. Kennedy JC, Hawkins RJ: Swimmer's shoulder. Phys Sports Med 2:35, 1974

7. Lo YPC, Hsu YCS, Chan KM: Epidemiology of shoulder impingement in upper arm sports events. B J Sports Med 24:173–7, 1990
8. McMaster WC: Anterior glenoid labrum damage: a painful lesion in swimmers. Am J Sports Med 14:383, 1986
9. McMaster WC, Troup J: A survey of interfering shoulder pain in United States competitive swimmers. Am J Sports Med 21:67, 1993
10. Rathbun JB, Macnab I: The microvascular pattern of the rotator cuff. J Bone Joint Surg [Am] 54:540–53, 1979
11. Stocker D, Pink M, Jobe FW: Comparison of shoulder injury in collegiate and master's level swimmers. Clin J Sport Med 5:4–8, 1995
12. Webster MS, Bishop P, Fowler PJ: Swimmer's shoulder. Undergraduate thesis. University of Waterloo, Waterloo, Ontario, 1981

CHAPTER THIRTY-ONE

Golf

William J. Mallon

Shoulder injuries constitute a major source of injuries to active golfers. Several factors cause the shoulder to be frequently injured in golfers, including the necessity for professionals and competitive amateurs to practice many hours per day, which can lead to a cumulative trauma disorder. The biomechanics of the golf swing also put the shoulder, particularly the left shoulder (in right-handed players), at risk for shoulder injuries.

Pink et al[17] and McCarroll et al[12,13] studied the incidence of injuries to both amateur and professional golfers in two separate studies. Among amateur golfers, they showed that the shoulder was the fourth most commonly injured area, with 12 percent of all injuries, following the lower back, the elbow, and the wrist.[13] But among professional golfers, the shoulder trailed only the lower back and wrist as a source of injuries.[12] Jobe et al[6] found that 21 percent of patients presenting with golf injuries had shoulder problems.

In particular, McCarroll and Gioe[12] showed that injuries to the left shoulder are particularly common (7 percent), with the right shoulder being less frequently injured (3 percent). Jobe's group noted that all the right-handed golfers seen at their office for shoulder problems had involvement of the left shoulder[17] Jobe et al[7] also noted that there is no difference between the incidence of shoulder injuries on the men's and women's professional golf tours.

BIOMECHANICS OF THE GOLF SWING

No good medical study has ever looked at the exact biomechanics of the motion of the shoulder during a golf swing. Jobe et al[6] have studied the function of the rotator cuff during the golf swing. However, without a precise explanation of the motions made by the shoulder girdle during the golf swing, this study is difficult to interpret and apply to golfing situations.

The golf swing is unusual among sports in that it is a bilateral motion, with each arm performing very different actions because of their attachment to the golf club. In actuality, each arm performs essentially the same motions during a golf swing, but they are not performed concurrently. The left arm backswing action is mirrored by the right arm during the follow-through, and vice versa.

We deal here with a right-handed golfer, which constitutes most players. A basic understanding of the motions of the arms, primarily the left arm, has been elucidated by the seminal work by Cochran and Stobbs.[4] They broke the model backswing into five segments (Figs. 31-1 to 31-5). Not all segments involve motion of the shoulders.

Movement 1 is defined as the turning of the shoulders around the spine as an axis (Fig. 31-1).[4] Termed a *shoulder turn* by golf professionals, the motion is in reality a trunk rotation performed by the spine and the muscles of the lower back and has nothing at all to do with the shoulders. Movement 2 is defined as raising the left arm "vertically from the shoulder"[4] (Fig. 31-2). This motion is actually forward flexion of the left shoulder. Movement 3 consists of "cocking" (radial deviation) of the left wrist and does not affect the shoulders (Fig. 31-3). Movement 4 (Fig. 31-4) consists of swinging the left arm across the chest, such that the left hand and elbow are brought nearer to the right shoulder.[4] This can be defined as cross-body adduction or, more properly to the kinesiologists, horizontal adduction. Finally, movement 5 (Fig. 31-5) consists of the "roll of the left forearm putting the clubhead into plane."[4] This motion probably does affect the left shoulder to some degree. Although it consists primarily of forearm rotation, specifically the left forearm is pronated a certain amount,

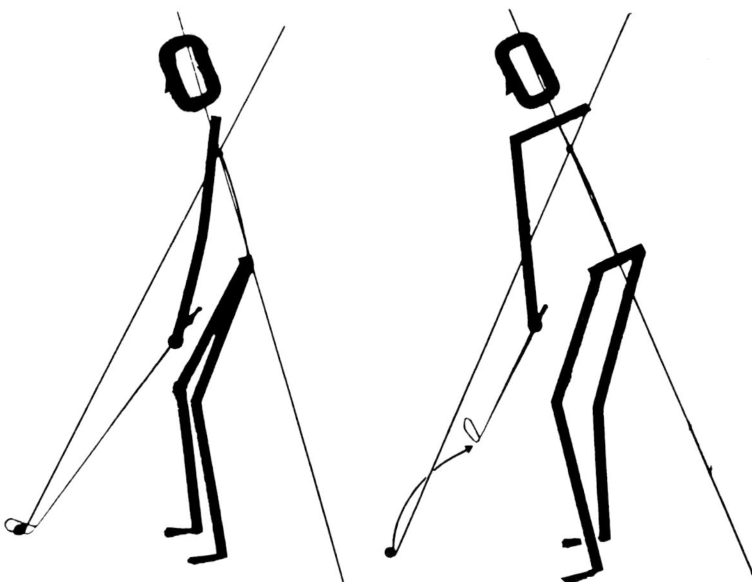

Figure 31-1. Movement 1 is defined by Cochran and Stobbs[4] as the turning of the shoulders around the spine as an axis. (From Cochran and Stobbs,[4] with permission.)

some of this motion is likely performed by the humerus and consists of internal rotation at the glenohumeral joint.

In an efficient golf swing, these five motions are performed smoothly and synchronously rather than as isolated movements. A good description of the motion of the left arm during the backswing is as follows: the golfer bends slightly from the waist, allowing the left arm to hang freely. It then begins in the address position at close to neutral abduction/adduction but is probably forward flexed about 20 degrees. During the golf swing, the above movements 2, 4, and 5 are performed concomitantly. This causes the left shoulder to forward flex to 90 degrees or greater, to

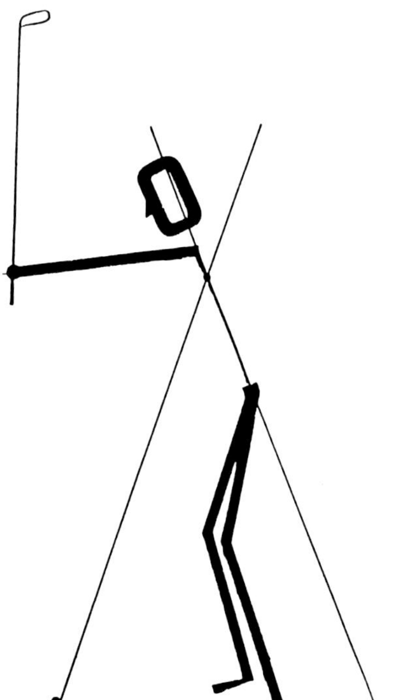

Figure 31-2. Movement 2 is defined by Cochran and Stobbs[4] as raising the left arm "vertically from the shoulder." (From Cochran and Stobbs,[4] with permission.)

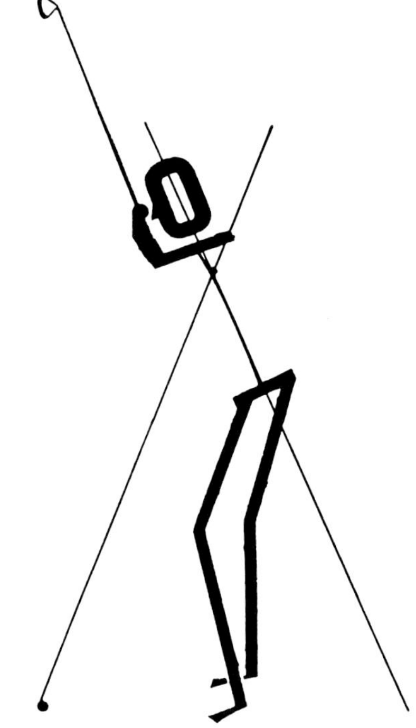

Figure 31-3. Movement 3 consists of "cocking" (radial deviation) of the left wrist and does not affect the shoulders. (From Cochran and Stobbs,[4] with permission.)

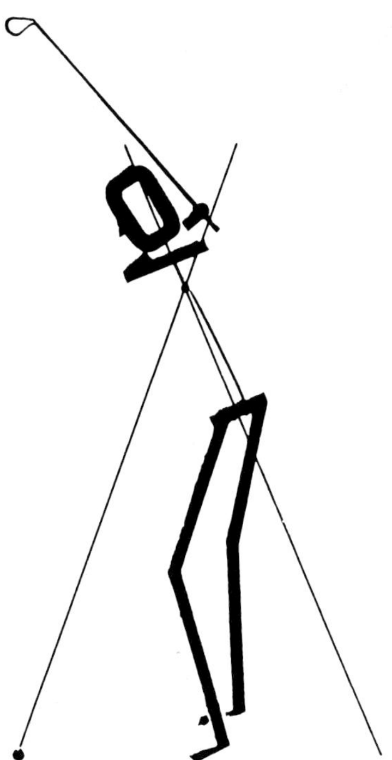

Figure 31-4. Movement 4 consists of swinging the left arm across the chest such that the left hand and elbow are brought nearer to the right shoulder. (From Cochran and Stobbs,[4] with permission.)

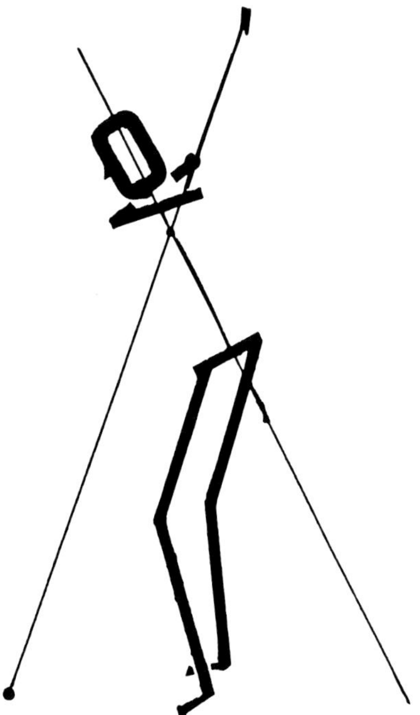

Figure 31-5. Movement 5 consists of the "roll of the left forearm putting the clubhead into plane." (From Cochran and Stobbs,[4] with permission.)

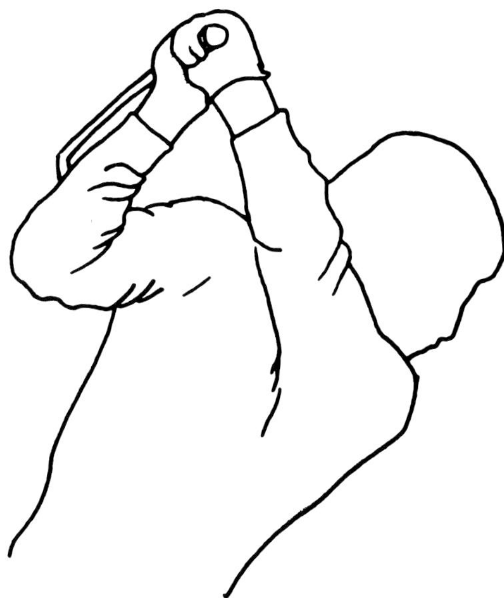

Figure 31-6. A drawing based on a photograph taken from behind a modern professional at the top of the backswing, demonstrating the amount of elevation (well above the shoulder plane or 90 degrees of elevation) and cross-body adduction of the left arm.

horizontally adduct (cross-body adduct) as much as 60 degrees relative to a sagittal plane intersecting the left glenohumeral joint, and to internally rotate slightly (Figs. 31-6 to 31-9).

The right arm is connected to the golf club by the grip while the left arm performs the above motions. But the

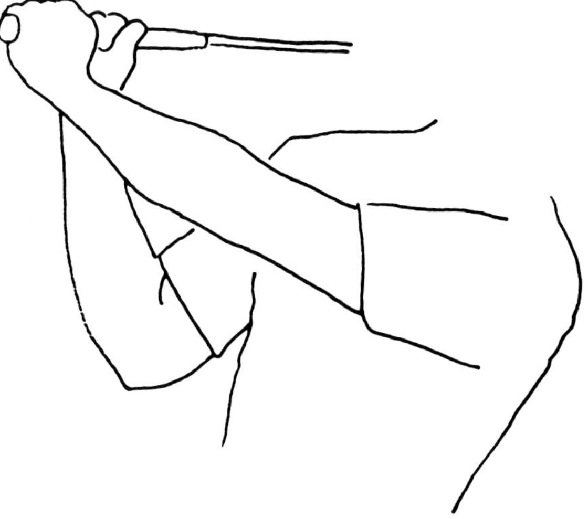

Figure 31-7. A drawing based on a photograph taken from behind a modern professional at the top of the backswing, demonstrating nicely the cross-body adduction of the left arm and also showing the minimal motion that has occurred at the right shoulder during a backswing.

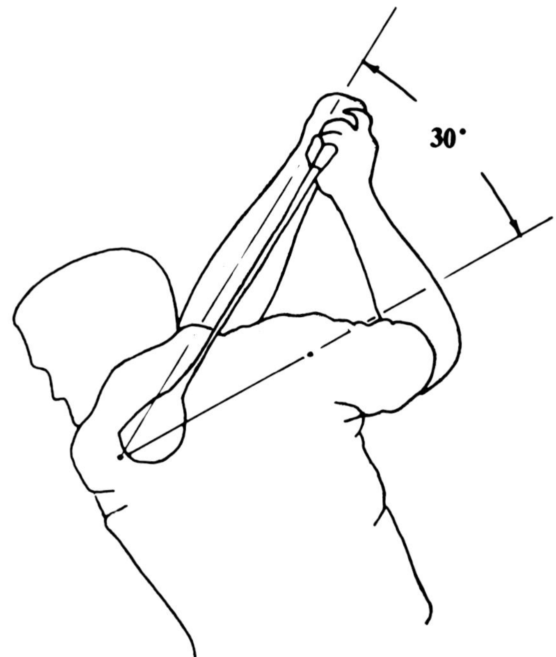

Figure 31-8. A drawing based on a photograph taken from in front of a modern professional at the top of the backswing, demonstrating the amount of elevation (30 degrees above the shoulder plane or 120 degrees of elevation) and cross-body adduction of the left arm.

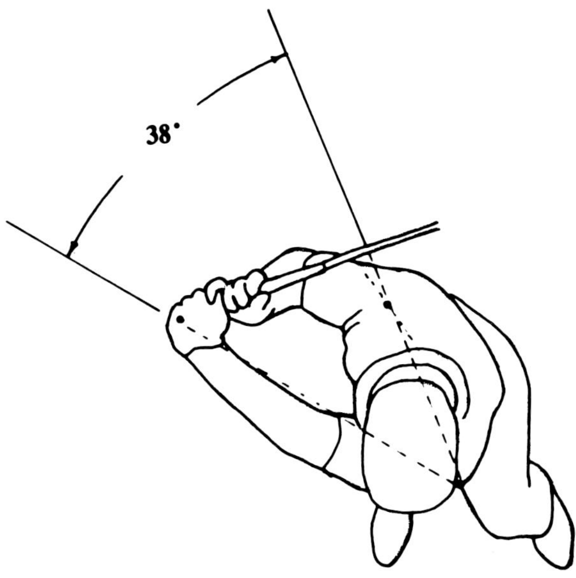

Figure 31-9. A drawing based on a photograph taken from overhead of a modern professional at the top of the backswing, demonstrating the cross-body adduction of the left arm (52 degrees, brings the arm within 38 degrees of the plane of the shoulders).

right shoulder performs very dissimilar motions during the backswing. In fact, the right shoulder does not move much at all during a normal backswing. It is abducted slightly and externally rotated as much as 90 degrees but not approaching the apprehension position of anterior instability (Figs. 31-6 and 31-8). The degree of abduction of the right arm is variable, but even in players with a "flying right elbow," it is probably not abducted more than 60 degrees.

During the forward swing to impact and through to follow-through, the right and left shoulders basically reverse their positions. At the end of follow-through, if carried out fully, the right shoulder will assume a position similar to that of the left shoulder at the top of the back swing—forward flexed (but less so) and horizontally adducted across the chest. The left shoulder at the end of a follow-through is abducted slightly and externally rotated as is the right shoulder at the end of a backswing.

It is important to remember that between the top of a backswing and the end of follow-through, the golfer must hit the ball. Thus, between these two extremes, the golf club and the shoulders are swung through the impact position. Impact position of the shoulders essentially duplicates their position at address, although only transiently and at very high speed (clubhead speed among professionals with a driver can exceed 200 km/h).

In three separate studies, Jobe et al[6,7] and Pink et al[17] looked at electromyography of the shoulder and rotator cuff function in professional golfers. They found that the deltoid was remarkably quiescent during the golf swing. They also found that in right-handed golfers, the total firing patterns were similar for the left and right shoulders. The subscapularis was the rotator cuff muscle with the most activity. They concluded that golfers should preferentially strengthen the rotator cuff bilaterally as well as the latissimus dorsi and the pectoralis major.[5,6]

Jobe et al[6] note that golf does not require extreme range of motion requirements. They state that elevation is less than 90 degrees, but photos of top professionals (Figs. 31-6 and 31-8) contradict this statement, as elevation in both cases approaches 130 degrees, in adduction to the position of maximal cross-body adduction.[6] As described above and elsewhere, the left shoulder especially is moved through a wide, rather unusual range of motion at very high speed.[11]

CLINICAL IMPLICATIONS

Shoulder problems in golfers can be from various sources, as in nongolfers. An important differentiating feature is to ask the golfer at what stage of the golf swing the pain or instability is felt. This may give some clues as to the etiology of the problem. Even better is to ask the golfer to demonstrate the swing and attempt to isolate the exact timing and movement that causes the pain.

Injuries to the left shoulder are more common (7 percent) than to the right shoulder (3 percent).[12] In my own practice, this incidence has been closer to 10 : 1 than 2 : 1,[10] similar to the study of Pink et al,[17] in which 100 percent of professional golfers they saw with shoulder problems had them affect the left shoulder. Examining the motions of the normal backswing helps explain this. At the top of the backswing, the left arm in a right-handed golfer is in a fairly awkward position of forward flexion, internal rotation, and cross-body adduction.

The position of forward flexion and internal rotation may predispose to impingement-type problems, as in this position, the greater tuberosity is driven under the acromion. At the end of the backswing, the position of cross-body adduction is a provocative position for both problems in the acromioclavicular joint and for posterior subluxation of the glenohumeral joint. These seem to be the most common problems in golfers who have pain during the backswing. Forces at the acromioclavicular joint in cross-body adduction have been shown to be high,[1] which may contribute to the high incidence of problems in this joint among golfers.[10]

Pain during the forward swing and follow-through is less common but also may be of several causes. Pain early in the forward swing is an unusual occurrence that I have seen only twice in my practice. In both cases, the patients had posterior instability of the shoulder that did not manifest until a palpable "clunk" of reduction occurred during the beginning of the forward swing. This could be heard but could also be felt by a hand placed on the posterior shoulder while the swing was demonstrated. At the beginning of the forward swing, the left arm is swung downward so that it no longer is in as much cross-body adduction, and in addition, the arm, and likely the humerus, externally rotates slightly. These two maneuveurs seem to have caused a rather violent reduction of the position of posterior subluxation. Neither patient had symptoms of instability during the backswing.

Pain in the left shoulder near the end of the follow-through may occur from symptoms of anterior instability. In this position, the left arm is abducted slightly and is in about as much external rotation as ever occurs in the left arm during the golf swing.

Although the golf swing symptoms may lead one to a tentative diagnosis, the symptoms and signs demonstrated during a golf swing should be confirmed by a careful clinical examination. The examiner should check for evidence of impingement, anterior instability, posterior instability, multidirectional instability, and symptoms referable to the acromioclavicular joint. In the older patient, a rotator cuff tear may be present. O'Driscoll[15] has emphasized that impingement testing may mimic a test for posterior instability and has recommended a provocative lidocaine injection test to differentiate the two.

Radiologic imaging of the shoulder will also help with the diagnosis. A supraspinatus outlet view of the shoulder may show evidence of a hooked acromion,[2,14] but by itself, this is not important unless it is associated with signs and symptoms of impingement or rotator cuff derangement. An anteroposterior radiograph of the shoulder aimed cephalad approximately 15 degrees will isolate the acromioclavicular joint well and demonstrate any possible osteoarthritis of that joint or osteolysis of the distal clavicle.[3] True anteroposterior and axillary lateral views are usually also obtained. However, very few avid golfers have abnormalities on these views, as osteoarthritis, large Hill-Sachs defects, or gross instability visible on an axillary lateral will usually preclude golf from being played effectively.

Should the diagnosis still be in doubt after a history, examination of the shoulder during a golf swing, and a routine physical and with standard radiographs, a magnetic resonance imaging (MRI), arthrogram, or ultrasound of the shoulder may be obtained to look for other pathology. Specifically, these may demonstrate a rotator cuff tear, and the MRI can show evidence of labral tears, which may be manifestations of subtle shoulder instability.

PREVENTION AND TREATMENT

Methods to decrease injury risk in golf have previously been discussed.[11] Proper warm-up was emphasized, especially by spending some time on the practice tee, beginning with short shots and working up to full swings with a drive before playing. It is recommended that golfers perform both flexibility and strength conditioning to also decrease the risk of injury, especially in the winter months. The study of Jobe et al[6] noted that the emphasis of strengthening should be on the rotator cuff muscles, the latissimus dorsi, and the pectoralis major.

Jobe and Moynes[5] have shown that professional golfers use a lower percentage of their muscular strength than do amateur golfers. This is likely related to the greater efficiency of the professional swing and may help to protect against injuries. To help avoid shoulder injuries, amateur golfers should spend time with a professional to help develop optimal swing techniques.[11]

Treatment of golfers with established shoulder problems is similar to treatment of shoulder problems in nonathletes or nongolfing athletes. For problems of pure rotator cuff tendinitis or impingement, it usually begins with active rest of the involved shoulder, emphasizing avoidance of provocative positions while rehabilitating the rotator cuff in nonprovocative positions. Also, use of nonsteroidal medication and thermal modalities of ice and heat may also help during the recovery period. Diagnostic and therapeutic use of cortisone injections is advocated by some, although the use is controversial because of the possibility of causing weakening of the collagen tissue and possible rotator cuff rupture. Finally, in recalcitrant cases, surgery may be recommended.

Treatment of instability usually also begins with rehabilitation of the muscles about the shoulder, preferentially strengthening the muscles on the side of the instability. During the painful acute injury phase of this problem, nonsteroidal anti-inflammatories may help recovery, but cortisone injections have absolutely no use in these problems. Again, surgery is available in cases that do not respond to conservative therapy.

Treatment of problems about the acromioclavicular joint tend to have an arthritic component, and rehabilitation may be less successful. Here, cortisone can be very helpful, as can resection of the distal clavicle. Golfers who have had resection of the distal clavicle are usually able to resume their former level of play.[10]

In addition to standard treatments of golfers with shoulder problems, modification in playing techniques can be attempted to decrease symptoms. In high-class golfers, any modification of the swing will often cause a decrease in playing ability, and the player should be warned that this may occur.

All golfers with shoulder problems—whether arthritic, inflammatory, or instability—should benefit from shortening the backswing. Most shoulder pain seems to occur during the backswing, and by shortening this, the arc of motion of the left shoulder will likely be less. Also, Palmer[16] has commented that shortening the backswing rarely causes a decrease in length and will likely increase accuracy. A mathematical analysis of the golf swing supports this fact, noting that the backswing may be decreased in length substantially with a minimal decrease in clubhead speed.[8]

Bending over more from the waist at address may also help golfers with shoulder problems, although at first this may seem contradictory. However, this will encourage a steeper, more upright "shoulder turn" as trunk rotation occurs at 90 degrees to the angle of the spine. The increased steepness of the shoulder plane allows the golfer to elevate the left arm less and still achieve a reasonably upright swing plane. The decreased elevation may take stress off the left shoulder on the backswing.

Finally, golfers with posterior instability or acromioclavicular problems during the backswing may benefit by attempting to swing with the left arm farther from the body during the backswing. This will decrease cross-body adduction and decrease the tendency to posteriorly subluxate or to cause stress across the acromioclavicular joint. However, this position is not recommended at all by current golf-teaching theory.

Many older golfers will develop a rotator cuff tear, although this may be more related to the degenerative process than to any effect of the golf swing on the rotator cuff. As many older patients wish to play golf in their retirement years, they frequently ask about the possibility of return to golf with a rotator cuff tear or after rotator cuff repair.

The rhythm of glenohumeral elevation has been a critical test in this regard. Patients unable to elevate their left arm to shoulder height in a smooth, synchronous glenohumeral rhythm have not been able to return to golf, even when the shoulder may become pain-free for other activities. The same caveat has seemed to be true after rotator cuff surgery and can be used to guide any rehabilitation program.

Rehabilitation after rotator cuff surgery should be highly individualized, based on the size of the tear, the mobility and quality of the tissues, the stability of the repair, and the patient's age and ability to follow the postoperative regime. Small tears with a stable repair can be treated similarly to those patients who have had an acromioplasty with no repair. In these patients, one can expect a return to chipping and pitching by 6 weeks after the surgery and to full shots and playing within 3 months after the surgery.

At the other extreme is the patient with a large or massive tear that requires aggressive mobilization of tissue to close the defect. These patients may not play golf again. If they do, the glenohumeral rhythm should be used as a guide for allowing resumption of golf. However, it is likely that only short putting will be possible for the first 6 weeks after surgery. Even with a good result, the patient will not be able to hit full shots for at least 6 months, and more likely 1 year, after the rotator cuff repair.

SUMMARY

The shoulder is a common source of problems in golfers. The left shoulder in right-handed players seems to be particularly vulnerable. This is likely due to the biomechanics of the golf swing, which place the left shoulder into an unusual position of forward flexion, internal rotation, and cross-body adduction at the top of the backswing.

The causes of shoulder problems in golfers include rotator cuff tendinitis, acromioclavicular disorders (arthritis, distal clavicular osteolysis), and instability of the shoulder, primarily posterior. In addition to standard methods of treating and preventing these problems, possible adaptations of the golf swing can be used to relieve stress on the affected structures during the swing.

REFERENCES

1. Bell RH, Acus R, Noe D, Askew M: A study of acromioclavicular joint forces. J Shoulder Elbow Surg, suppl. 1–2, 2:S24, 1993
2. Bigliani LU, Morrison DS, April EW: Morphology of the

acromion and its relationship to rotator cuff tears. Orthop Trans 10:216, 1986
3. Cahill BR: Osteolysis of the distal part of the clavicle in male athletes. J Bone Joint Surg [Am] 64:1053–8, 1982
4. Cochran A, Stobbs J: The Search for the Perfect Swing. JB Lippincott, Philadelphia, 1968
5. Jobe FW, Moynes DR: 30 Exercises for Better Golf. Champion Press, Inglewood, CA, 1986
6. Jobe FW, Moynes DR, Antonelli DJ: Rotator cuff function during a golf swing. Am J Sports Med 14:388–92, 1986
7. Jobe FW, Perry J, Pink M: Electromyographic shoulder activity in men and women professional golfers. Am J Sports Med 17:782–7, 1989
8. Jorgensen T: On the dynamics of the swing of a golf club. Am J Physics 38:644–51, 1970
9. Mallon WJ: Epidemiology of golf injuries. In McCarroll JR, Stover CS, Mallon WJ (eds): Feeling Up to Par: Medicine from Tee to Green. FA Davis, Philadelphia, 1994
10. Mallon WJ, Colosimo AJ: The acromio-clavicular joint as a source of shoulder pain in professional and low-handicap golfers. J Southern Orthop Assoc, in press
11. Mallon WJ, Hawkins RJ: Prevention of shoulder injuries in athletics. In Renström P (ed): Prevention of Injuries in Sports. International Olympic Committee, Lausanne, 1994
12. McCarroll JR, Gioe TJ: Professional golfers and the price they pay. Phys Sports Med 10:54–70, 1982
13. McCarroll JR, Rettig AC, Shelbourne KD: Injuries in the amateur golfer. Phys Sports Med 18:122–6, 1990
14. Morrison DS, Bigliani LU: Roentgenographic analysis of acromial morphology and its relationship to rotator cuff tears. Orthop Trans 11:439, 1987
15. O'Driscoll SW: A reliable and simple test for posterior instability of the shoulder. Orthop Trans 15:762–3, 1991
16. Palmer AD: My Game and Yours. Simon & Schuster, New York, 1963
17. Pink M, Jobe FW, Perry J: Electromyographic analysis of the shoulder during the golf swing. Am J Sports Med 18:137–40, 1990

CHAPTER THIRTY-TWO

Volleyball

Douglas A. Foulk
Gary W. Misamore

Since the invention of volleyball in 1895, participation at both the recreational and competitive level has increased significantly. The International Volleyball Federation represents approximately 150 million players. Although studies regarding injuries have been few, surveys demonstrate that less than 10 percent involve the shoulder and nearly 90 percent involve the lower extremity.[4,7]

Because volleyball requires the rapid and repetitive use of the upper extremity, both acute and overuse-type injuries occur, with the latter being more common and underreported. Schafle et al,[7] in a prospective study of injuries in the 1987 National Amateur Volleyball Tournament, found that shoulder injuries accounted for 8.4 percent of the total reported injuries, with greater than 90 percent being overuse. Gerberich et al[4] found similar results, with no significant gender differences.

Although most injuries sustained while playing volleyball are not unique to the sport, the sport itself differs in some regards from other overhead activities. The game is usually played on a hard surface and involves not only diving and rolling but also hitting a ball while at maximum vertical leap. Muscles of the trunk and shoulder are used to accelerate, decelerate, and rotate the extremity during the acts of serving and spiking. Schafle et al[7] found that the middle and strong side hitter had the highest overall injury rates. Middle hitters require more spin on their hits to pass defending blockers, thus requiring rotation of the extremity at high speeds. Schafle et al,[7] as well, demonstrated that hitting and blocking were the most common mechanisms of injury.

EVALUATION

As with any other shoulder problem, evaluation of the volleyball player's shoulder begins with a thorough history. Questioning should focus on the events surrounding the onset of the problem. Date of onset, player position, number of years played, level of competition, and change in level of competition should be elicited. At the collegiate level, freshmen and sophomores are more likely to be injured than upperclassmen. This is most likely attributed to longer points and matches as well as an increase in the speed of the game and the necessity for the player to develop techniques in college that were not needed at the high school level. These injuries can be grade I, II, or III sprains, the treatment of which has been well described in Chapter 17. Somewhat unique to the sport of volleyball is suprascapular neuropathy. Although we have not seen this entity in the volleyball teams we have cared for, its description and suspected etiology are discussed.

From our experience, it would appear that most volleyball players at some point in their career develop a sore shoulder. Many of these athletes are never evaluated because the severity and duration of symptoms are not great enough for them to bring it to the attention of anyone other than their coach or trainer. Games are infrequently missed at the collegiate level because of a sore shoulder, but icing before and after practice and competition is common place because of minor symptoms. Soreness in the shoulder most

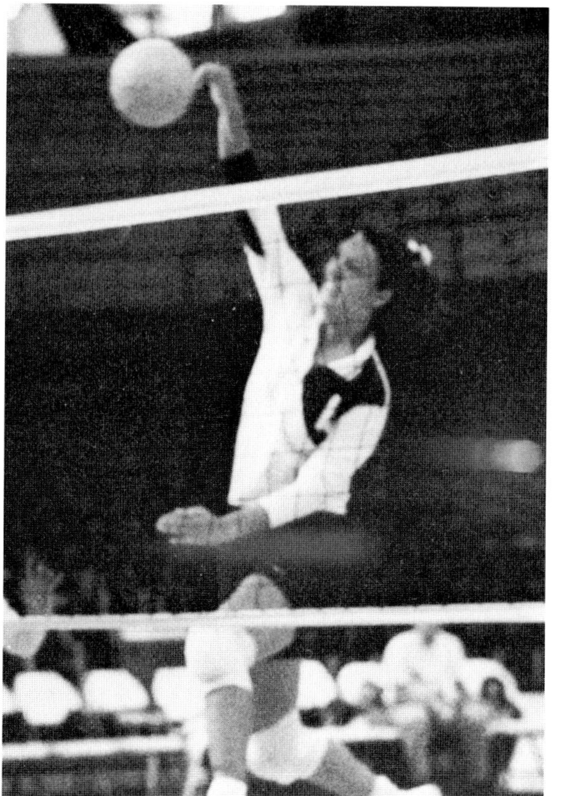

A

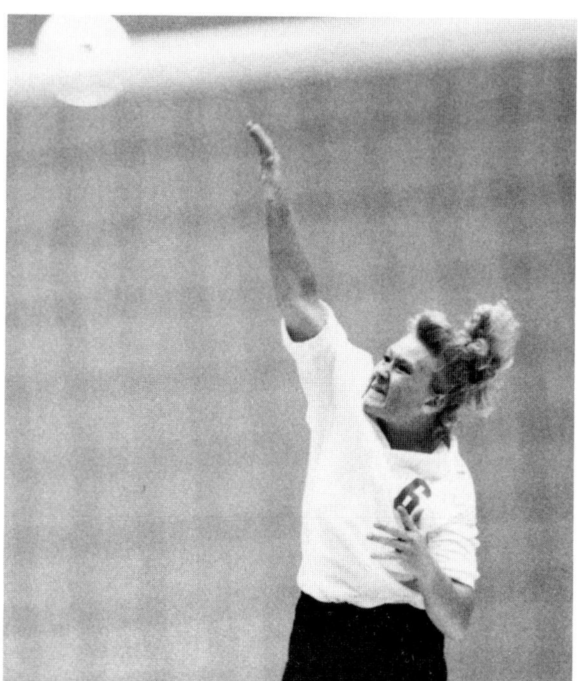

B

Figure 32-1. (**A & B**) Hitting with the elbow extended and contact with the ball occurring just anterior to the plane of the body.

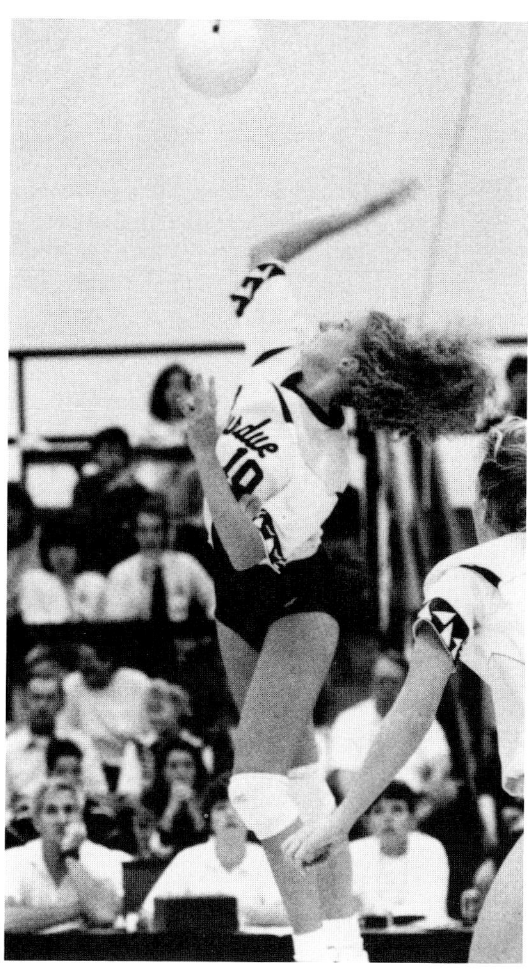

Figure 32-2. This player is hitting with the bent arm technique. This puts greater strain on the rotator cuff.

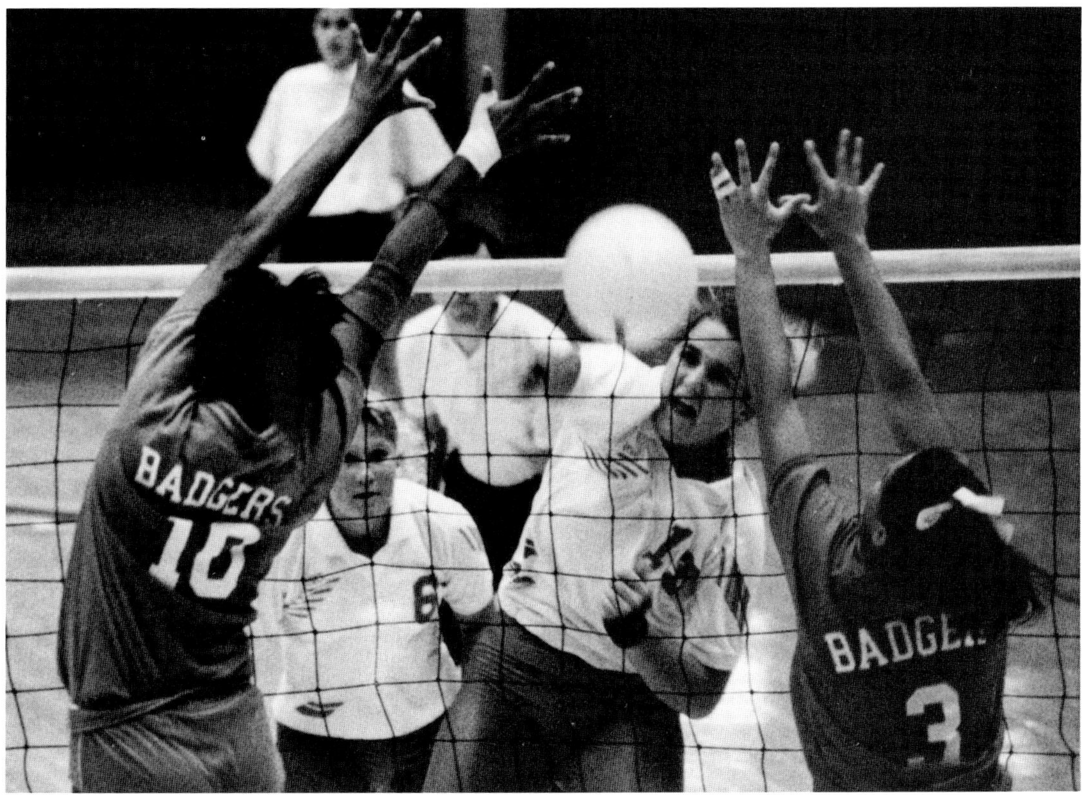

Figure 32-3. The follow-through phase of hitting stresses the posterior capsule similar to other overhead athletes.

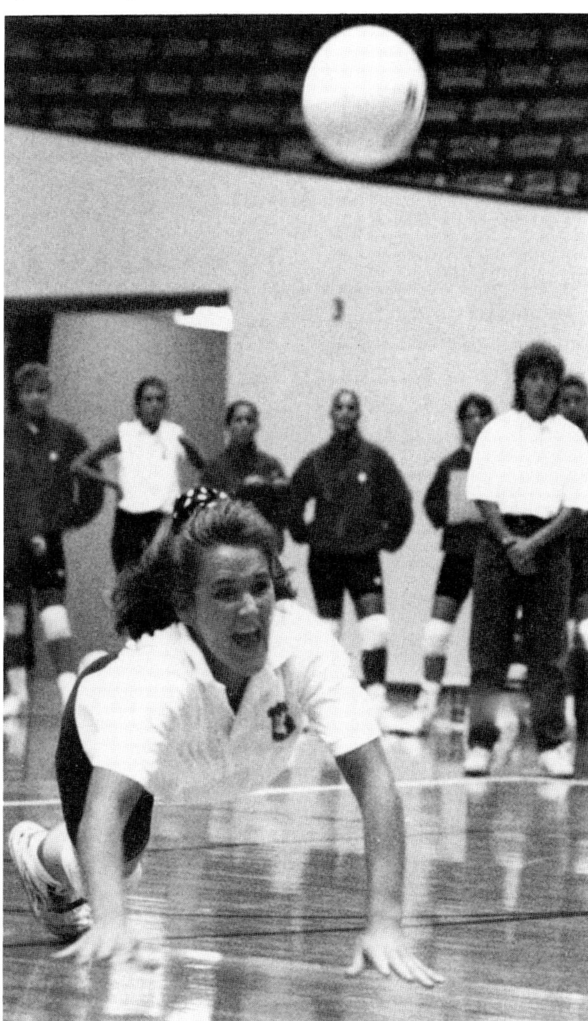

Figure 32-4. Landing on the outstretched hand can injure the anterior or posterior capsule, depending on the degree of adduction or abduction present. This player's arm is adducted, which could result in posterior capsule injury as her hand makes contact with the floor.

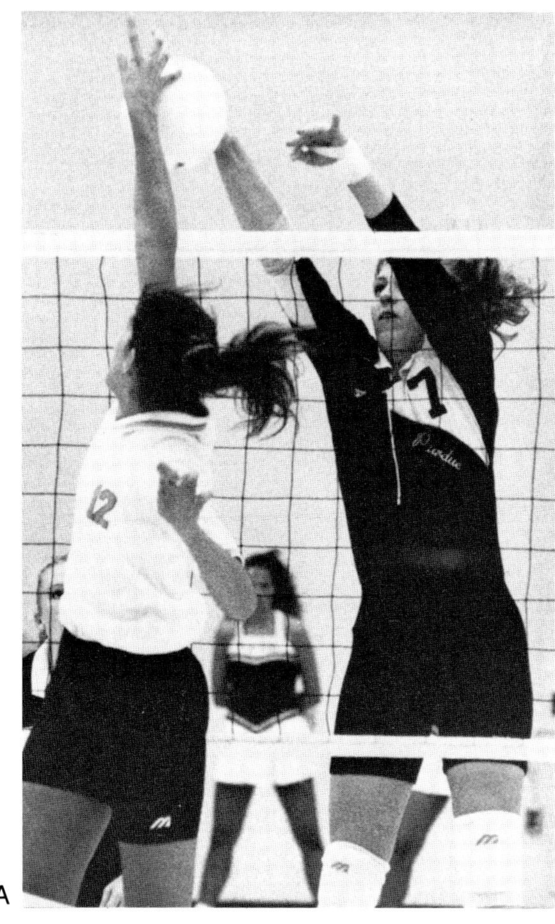

A

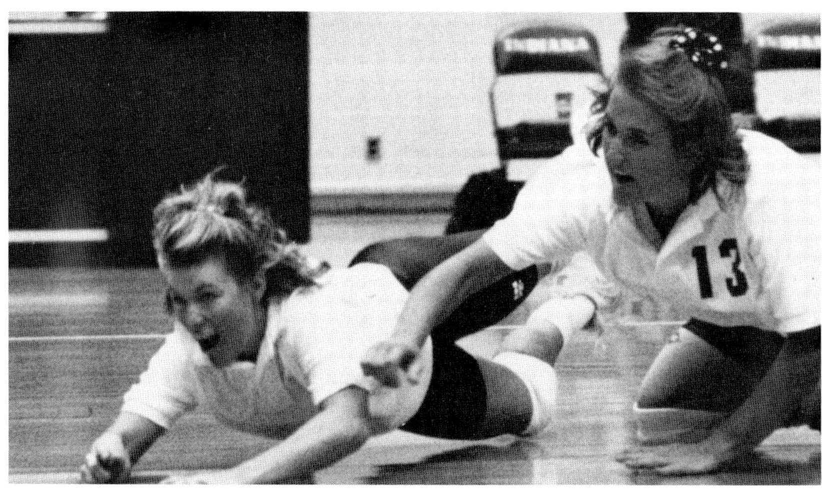

B

Figure 32-5. (**A–C**) A blocked hit at the net can result in the arm being forced into an abducted externally rotated position. This can also occur from falling on an outstretched arm. Both mechanisms can injure the anterior shoulder capsular structures. (*Figure continues.*)

frequently occurs 4 to 6 weeks after competition has begun. Players who are hitting at least 50 to 70 times per game are most likely to develop soreness. Although little has been written concerning hitting technique, players who strike the ball with the elbow extended, arm close to ear, with contact occurring just anterior to the plane of the body, seem to develop shoulder pain less frequently (Fig. 32-1). Muscles of the back and trunk are used to generate power with this technique. This is in contrast to the "bent arm" technique, which places greater strain on the rotator

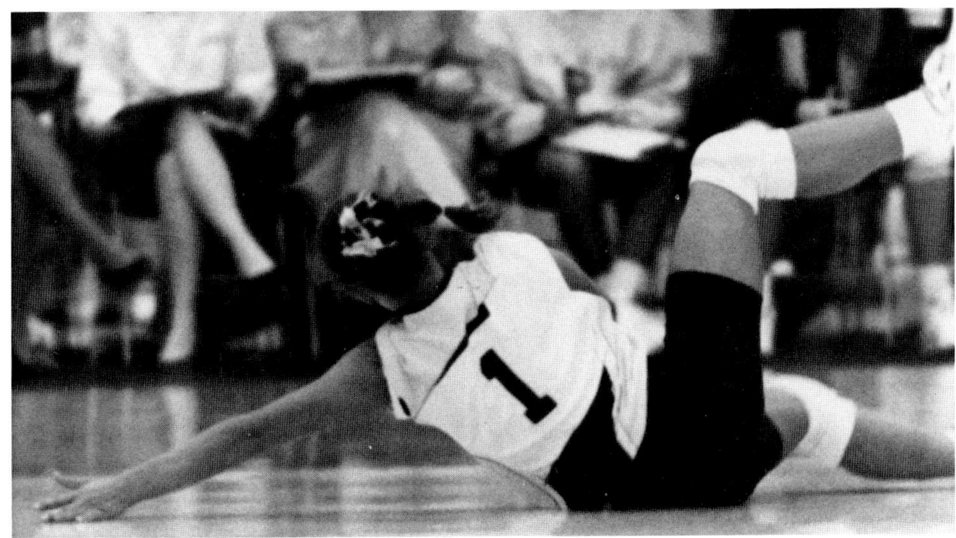

Figure 32-5 *(Continued).*

cuff, because the muscles of the shoulder are used more for generation of force with this technique (Fig. 32-2).

ROTATOR CUFF TENDONITIS

Tendinitis and tendonosis of the rotator cuff can occur with or without underlying impingement. As with other overhead athletes, careful evaluation is necessary to rule out an associated instability pattern. Regardless of the etiology, the tendonitis may become severe enough that practice modification or cessation may be necessary in the initial stages of treatment. This period of rest combined with nonsteroidal anti-inflammatory agents is the method we have found to be the most effective. This is then followed by a specific rehabilitation protocol as described in Chapter 24.

We have on occasion seen volleyball players with impingement not associated with instability who have failed to improve with conservative management. In none of these athletes have we found acromial pathology such as spurs or "hooked" morphology (type III). We have rarely found it necessary to perform acromioplasty in these athletes, but when it has been performed, it has been quite successful. The volleyball players whom we have treated with arthroscopic acromioplasty for isolated impingement have all returned to full competition without further symptoms. Finally, questions regarding technique or change in technique, practice habits, off-season preparation, and a history of a previous shoulder problem and its treatment are important.

Examination of the shoulder, covered in Chapter 2, does not need to be modified when examining a volleyball player. It is useful, however, to observe the player at practice or competition and to discuss the player's technique and practice habits with the coach. Minor changes in serving and spiking technique may be the cause of the player's problem. After a thorough history and physical examination, plain radiographs of the shoulder should be obtained. If at this point further information is needed to direct treatment, studies including magnetic resonance imaging, arthrography, and electromyography (EMG)/nerve conduction velocities may be ordered in certain circumstances.

DISORDERS

In our experience, rotator cuff tendonitis with or without impingement, along with shoulder instability, is the most common problem we have encountered. Although covered in previous chapters, we present our approach to these problems and point out the mechanisms in volleyball causing them. Injuries involving the acromioclavicular joint can occur as a result of landing on the point of the shoulder after a dig for the ball.

INSTABILITY

Although both anterior and posterior shoulder instability occur in volleyball players, in our experience, posterior instability has been more common. Many of the volleyball players with symptomatic posterior instability whom we have seen have some degree of multidirectional instability. Often, only the posterior component is symptomatic. Repetitive stressing of the posterior capsule can occur in volleyball players much the same way as it does in other throwing athletes. During the follow-through phase of hit-

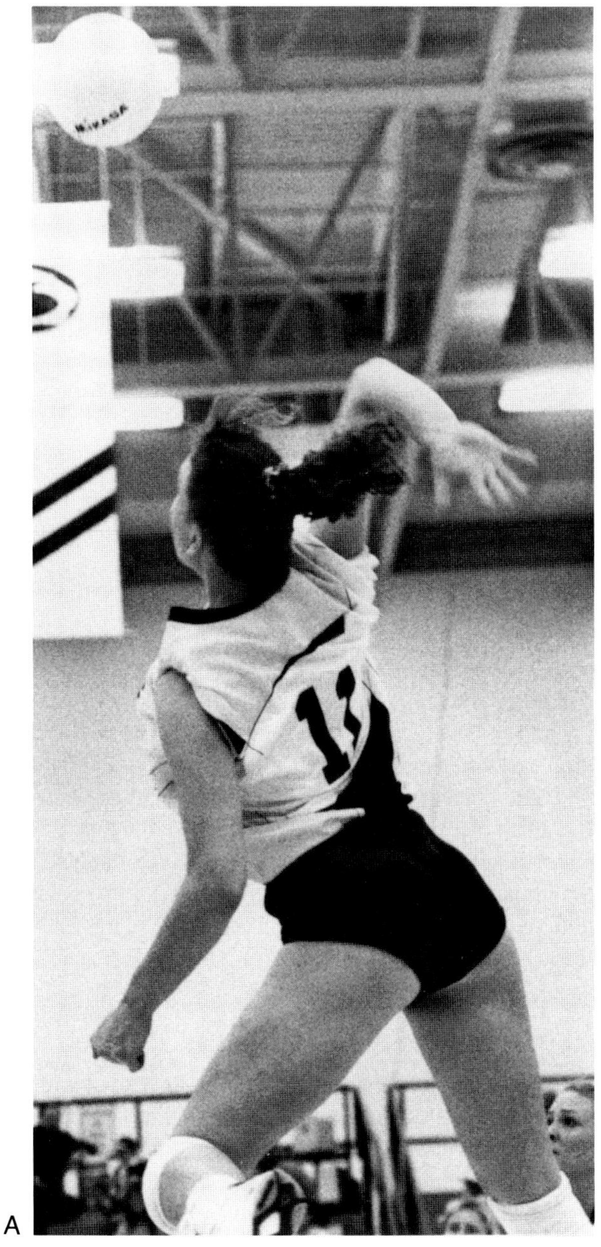

A

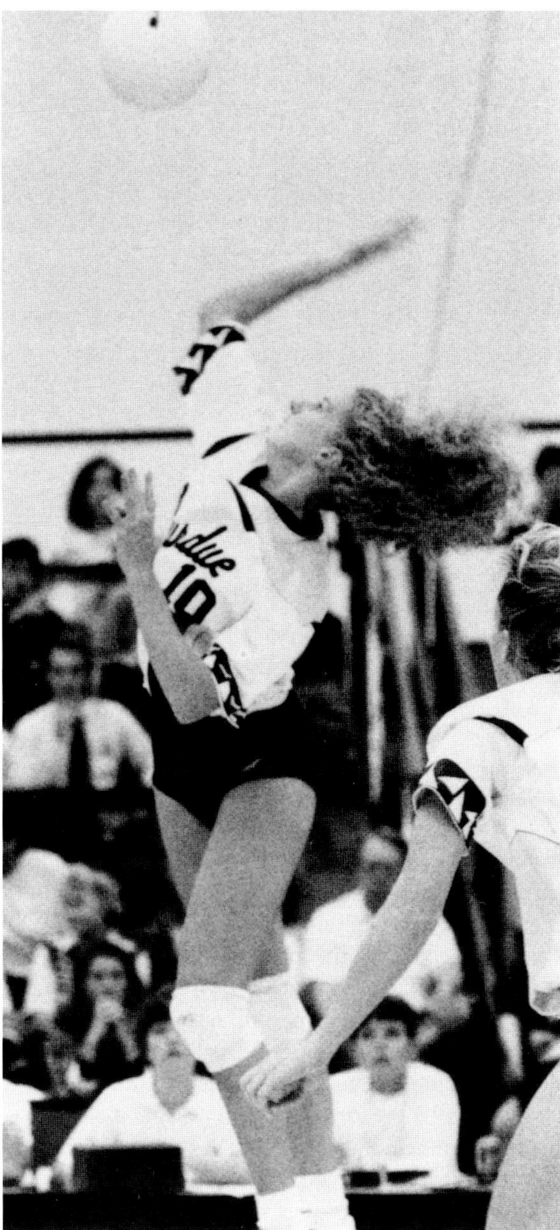

B

Figure 32-6. (A & B) Repetitive abduction and hyperrotation can result in anterior shoulder laxity secondary to capsular stressing.

ting, the posterior capsule is stressed (Fig. 32-3). Over time, this can lead to laxity and the development of symptoms secondary to subluxation. Also, posterior instability could occur secondary to trauma when falling onto the hard court surface landing on an outstretched flexed arm or directly on the front of the shoulder (Fig. 32-4). However, this type of traumatic posterior instability is less common than that associated with repetitive microtrauma from overuse.

The treatment of posterior instability has been covered in Chapter 15. Conservative management with emphasis on strengthening the external rotators of shoulder is always the first step. Unfortunately, some players will not improve to the point that play can resume at their preinjury level. At this point, surgical intervention may be indicated, depending on athlete's desire to continue play. Although posterior capsulorrhaphy is the preferred treatment for this problem, we have on occasion simply performed arthroscopic debridement of the labral damage in an effort to effect a quick return to competition. In our experience, a small percentage of athletes (approximately one in three) is improved enough with that minor surgery that they can successfully return to competition. Usually their symptoms are not completely resolved but instead simply improved significantly.

Anterior laxity can occur as the result of an acute event such as a fall with the shoulder hyperabducted or from blocking at the net (Fig. 32-5). Repetitive stressing of the anterior capsule in the cocking phase of hitting can also result in anterior laxity (Fig. 32-6). Frequently, the player's first examination is not specific enough to make the diagnosis. Repeat evaluation, particularly when the pain and guarding have subsided, may allow one to detect subtle instability.

Treating anterior shoulder instability in the volleyball player is not different from other overhead athletes. Instability that is the result of repetitive stress may respond to the point that play can resume at their preinjury level. At this point, surgical intervention may be indicated, depending on athlete's desire to continue play. Although posterior capsulorrhaphy is the preferred treatment for this problem, we have on occasion simply performed arthroscopic debridement of the labral damage in an effort to treating anterior instability. If surgery is needed, then we prefer an anterior capsular repair.

SUPRASCAPULAR NEUROPATHY

Ferretti et al[3] studied 96 top-level volleyball players and found that 12 had asymptomatic isolated paralysis of the infraspinatus muscle on the dominant side. Although no athlete had any history of injury, pain, or loss of function, all had obvious infraspinatus atrophy and four-fifths strength with resisted manual testing of external rotation. Three players underwent additional testing including EMG and isokinetic strength evaluation. All demonstrated spontaneous potentials in the infraspinatus consistent with denervation and a 15 to 30 percent decrease in external rotation power.[2]

Hama et al[6] reported that 3 of 26 volleyball players with infraspinatus weakness complained that they could not rotate the shoulder enough externally during cocking and could not strike the ball as forcefully as they previously could. They described an infraspinatus test to detect early weakness. Inability to externally rotate the shoulder against at least 3 kg (holding a dumbbell) while lying in the lateral position with the elbow flexed to 90 degrees in neutral rotation is indicative of infraspinatus weakness.

Drez[2] described compression of the common trunk of the suprascapular nerve at the suprascapular notch. Ferretti et al[3] pointed out that in approximately 30 percent of the population, the nerve makes an acute angle around the base of the scapular spine. When the arm is abducted and externally rotated (cocking stage of the serve), the terminal branches of the nerve are shifted medially, tensing the nerve against the spine of the scapula. Also, at the conclusion of the serve, the infraspinatus must eccentrically contract to brake the movement of the scapula, again stretching the nerve. Whether this is the mechanism of injury or the spinoglenoid ligament (present in 50 percent of the population) causes compression is not clear at this point.

EMG studies performed to evaluate pitching suggest that in throwing the infraspinatus is required to perform at only 30 to 40 percent of its maximal strength.[4] Extrapolating this data and recognizing that asymptomatic athletes are unlikely to change practice and competitive routines, it is probably more important to be aware that this can be a cause of player complaints in relation to serving and spiking, and treatment may not be necessary.

INJURY PREVENTION

It seems that upper extremity conditioning has not been a priority for most high school and collegiate volleyball teams that we have evaluated. It would seem that more athletic trainer involvement during off-season and preseason conditioning and education of coaches to the importance of shoulder and trunk condition would be beneficial to these athletes. A conditioning program, as described in Chapter 25, should be encouraged for these athletes.

A specific rotator cuff strengthening program is recommended in addition to other upper body programs.[1] Many volleyball players have never specifically strengthened their rotator cuff muscles and thus will have to start this program slowly, using light, if any, weights and emphasizing repetition. Stretching should be carried out before and after each session. Bands or light dumbbells can be used to perform internal and external rotation, either standing or lying. Along with concentric strengthening, eccentric strengthening is critical as the rotator cuff functions to a significant degree as a decelerator of the upper extremity during hitting and serving. Most important is that players need the time either before or after practice to be able to complete the exercises, particularly during the season. If shoulder pain develops, it is important to pay attention to the complaint so that modifications in the practice schedule can be made, including avoidance of hitting and serving with an emphasis on passing and digging skills until the soreness resolves.

REFERENCES

1. Breslin G: Integrating rotator cuff exercises into a volleyball training program. Performance Conditioning for Volleyball 1:7–8, 1993
2. Drez D: Suprascapular neuropathy in the differential diagnosis of rotator cuff injuries. Am J Sports Med 4:43–45, 1976
3. Ferretti A, Guglielmo C. Giovanni R: Suprascapular neuropathy in volleyball players. J Bone Joint Surg [Am] 69: 260–3, 1987

4. Gerberich S, Luhmann S, Finke C et al: Analysis of severe injuries associated with volleyball activities. Physician Sportsmed 15:75–79, 1987
5. Gowan I, Jobe F, Tibone J: A comparative EMG analysis of the shoulder during pitching. Am J Sports Med 15:586–90, 1988
6. Hama H, Morinaga T, Suzuki K et al: The infraspinatus test: an early diagnostic sign of muscle weakness during external rotation of the shoulder in athletes. J Shoulder Elbow Surg 2:257–9, 1993
7. Schafle M, Requa R, Patton W, Garrick J: Injuries in the 1987 National Volleyball Tournament. Am J Sports Med 18:624–31, 1990

CHAPTER THIRTY-THREE

Weight Lifting

Mark S. Schickendantz

The term *weight lifting* encompasses a spectrum of various athletic activities that involve the use of muscular strength and power to move weights or other forms of resistance. These activities include Olympic weight lifting, power lifting, body building, and recreational weight training or conditioning. Olympic lifting and power lifting involve the performance of one maximal repetition of a few select lifts. The Olympic weight lifter combines incredible strength, speed, and flexibility to perform two basic lifts, the snatch and the clean-and-jerk. Power lifting involves the performance of three lifts, the supine bench press, squat, and dead lift. Both Olympic and power weight lifters train with heavy weights and relatively low repetitions and limit the number of exercises to a few basic movements (e.g., bench press, squat, dead lift). The primary goal of training in these athletes is to increase muscular strength and power.

Body builders, however, train to increase muscular size, definition, and quality, with strength and power being less important. As such, these athletes train typically with moderate amounts of weight, lifting for many repetitions, and often will perform several if not many different exercises for a given body part during a work-out.

Weight training or conditioning is the use of resistance exercises to enhance performance in the athlete's primary sport. Once associated only with the "power" sports such as football, many recreational and almost all high school, collegiate, and professional sports programs and teams now include weight training as a part of their conditioning programs. Most of these weight training programs are sports-specific and, as such, involve a limited number of exercises. Athletes involved in the power sports tend to train with heavier weights for fewer repetitions, whereas endurance and agility athletes (e.g., swimmers and runners) train with lighter weights for more repetitions.

Also, many individuals now use weight training as a form of general conditioning or exercise. These recreational weight lifters typically perform a variety of different exercises using relatively light-to-moderate amounts of weight for a moderate-to-high number of repetitions.

Weight lifting has been shown to be a relatively safe recreational activity. Requa et al[49] determined that weight lifting had low-to-medium rates of injury, comparable with those associated with cardiovascular fitness activities such as aerobic dance and step climbing. Of those study participants reporting injuries, the shoulder was the second most commonly injured area. No difference was noted between the use of free weights and machine exercises. Brady et al[7] reported no shoulder injuries in a group of 89 high school athletes seen for weight lifting-related injuries over a 4-year period. Most reported weight lifting injuries are due to improper technique or attempting to lift too much weight.

Weight lifters who train and compete with very heavy weights are prone to more severe injuries of the shoulder than those athletes who train with relatively less weight. Kulund et al[25] found a relatively high rate of shoulder injuries in a group of 80 competitive-style weight lifters. Twenty-six athletes reported significant injuries to their shoulders, most occurring during the clean-and-jerk lift. These authors point out that improper technique and poor flexibility predispose to injury, especially if the athlete must "rotate out" of a lift he or she cannot handle (Fig. 33-1). To do this, the athlete must allow the shoulders to rotate into a position of extreme horizontal abduction and external rotation, allowing the athlete to get out from beneath the weight. This movement places a tremendous amount of strain on the anterior aspect of the shoulder and, if performed improperly, could result in significant injury.

Weight training in preadolescence and adolescence has been shown to be relatively safe when carried out with

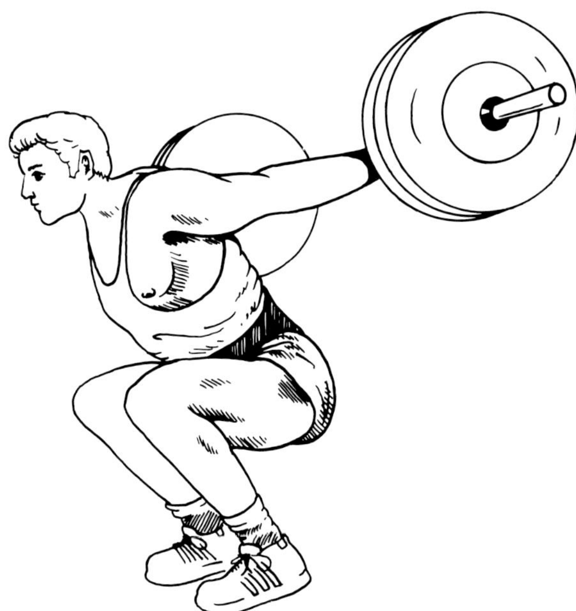

Figure 33-1. Rotating out of a failed lift. (Adapted from Kulund et al,[25] with permission.)

proper technique, guidance, and supervision.[28,48] Most injuries reported in this age group occur in unsupervised settings. Rians et al[50] reported only one shoulder strain in a group of 19 young men (mean age, 8.3 years) who trained three times per week for 14 weeks on hydraulic resistance equipment in a controlled setting. No other injuries were reported.

BIOMECHANICAL CONSIDERATIONS

In an effort to identify risk factors associated with injury while performing the bench press, Madsen and McLaughlin[33] filmed 17 novice recreational lifters and reviewed film of 19 expert lifters performing this exercise. Analysis of the digitized data collected revealed that the bar path used by the expert groups was closer to the shoulder than that used by the recreational group. As such, the relative moments produced about the shoulder in the expert group were smaller than those produced by the recreational lifter exerting a similar amount of force. Also, the experts generated a much more uniform force during the lift, exhibiting less variation between maximal and minimal force generated throughout the movement. Also, expert lifters lowered the bar more slowly to the chest than did their novice counterparts, resulting in a relatively smaller amount of force being required to bring the bar to rest on the chest. Thus, it appears as though the expert lifter is much more mechanically efficient than the novice. This may help explain why well-trained and supervised weight lifters have a relatively lower rate of injuries to their shoulders than the unsupervised novice.

The inferior glenohumeral ligament complex (IGHLC) has been shown to be the primary static restraint to both anterior and posterior subluxation of the abducted shoulder.[54,60] O'Brien and colleagues[42] further defined the anatomy and histology of the IGHLC and determined that with progressively increasing external rotation of the abducted shoulder, the anterior band of the IGHLC fans out to support the humeral head anteriorly.

Many weight lifting exercises such as the military press, pull-downs, pull-ups, flyes, and pull-overs require the shoulder to assume a position of abduction and external rotation. Also during the squat, the athlete's shoulders are placed into this orientation as he or she grasps the bar that rests across the upper back. This position has been identified as an "at-risk" position for the shoulder, as undo tension may be applied to the IGHLC, resulting in occult or frank injury.[18] Poppen and Walker[44,45] have described the forces occurring across the glenohumeral joint in varying positions of abduction in the scapular plane. With increasing abduction and neutral rotation, the resultant force increases linearly to a maximum of 0.89 times body weight at 90 degrees of abduction and then decreases steadily to 0.4 times body weight at 150 degrees. Interestingly, the shear component of this resultant force peaks at 0.24 times body weight at 60 degrees abduction and is directed cephalad. With increasing abduction, the shear component of the resultant force declines steadily to zero at 150 degrees abduction in neutral rotation. In any given position of abduction, external rotation leads to a redirection of the resultant force toward a more inferior orientation. These data lend support to the concept of abduction/external rotation being an at-risk position for the anteroinferior structures of the glenohumeral joint.

GENERAL CONSIDERATIONS

Most weight lifters experience some degree of pain in their shoulders at some time during their weight lifting activities. This pain is usually mild, the result of postexercise muscle soreness and minor strains, usually resolving with a short period of relative rest, local application of ice, and occasionally over-the-counter anti-inflammatory medications. The athlete most often will treat him- or herself for these mild episodes of shoulder pain and will only seek the assistance of a physician if the pain persists or is of a different character than the usual post-work-out shoulder pain.

It is important to remember when evaluating the weight lifter with shoulder pain that different styles of training may predispose to different types of injuries. Athletes who train or compete with relatively heavy amounts of weight are more subject to significant muscle and tendon strains or rupture, whereas those who use relatively lighter or moderate amounts of weight for more repetitions seem to experience more overuse-type injuries such as tendonitis.

In my experience, exercises that involve the use of a straight bar with the hands held in a fixed position are more strenuous to the shoulder than those that allow the upper extremity more freedom of movement throughout the lift, such as dumbbell exercises. Subtle changes in hand and shoulder position allow the lifter to carry out the movement in the most comfortable and likely safest groove or zone.

SPECIFIC INJURIES

Distal Clavicular Osteolysis

Nontraumatic osteolysis of the distal clavicle is a lesion found almost exclusively in male weight lifters, although other activities that involve repeated minor stress across the acromioclavicular (AC) joint have also been implicated as causative factors.[8,40,52,55] Distal clavicular osteolysis has also been reported after acute trauma to the AC joint.[20,26,33,46,56,57] Although the terms *nontraumatic* and *posttraumatic* are used to describe two different subsets of distal clavicular osteolysis, the distinction is likely only a historical one, as physical, radiographic, and pathologic findings in both conditions are essentially identical. Cahill[8] was the first to describe the association between weight lifting and this condition. Scavenius and Iversen[51] have suggested that the prevalence of distal clavicular osteolysis in weight lifters is approximately 27 percent.

The etiology of this condition is unclear. Madsen[33] postulated a neurologic cause based on his findings of ipsilateral anisocoria in four of seven patients with distal clavicular osteolysis. He thought that a change in the autonomic control of blood vessels on the clavicular side of the joint contributed to the process. Levine et al[26] postulated that the synovium of the joint is primarily involved. In addition to diffuse vascular proliferation, they found villous hyperplasia of the synovium and hypertrophy of fibrocartilage in biopsy specimens of the AC joint in a patient with distal clavicular osteolysis. Scavenius et al[52] thought that destruction of terminal nerve endings and arteries by repeated microtrauma lead to a reduction of the distal clavicles strength, resulting in microfractures. Cahill[8] has suggested that the condition arises as a result of attempts at repair of multiple microfractures of the subchondral plate of the clavicular side of the joint. Aseptic necrosis of the distal clavicle has been found in retrieved surgical specimens.[40] Involvement of the acromial side of the joint has been reported infrequently.[8,26] Distal clavicular osteolysis after acute trauma has been reported in a few female patients.[2,33,40,46] A single case of distal clavicular osteolysis in a female body builder has been reported.[35]

The athlete with distal clavicular osteolysis typically relates a history of the insidious onset of gradually increasing pain fairly well localized to the AC joint, aggravated by heavy pressing-type exercises such as supine straight bar bench press. In my experience, these athletes also experience pain with behind the neck pull-downs and military press, perhaps related to rotation of the clavicle and compression across the AC joint with abduction of the shoulder, resulting from upward scapular rotation. Scavenius et al[52] also noted painful abduction in their series of patients. Also, many patients complain of pain with any throwing motion.

Physical examination demonstrates well-localized tenderness over the AC joint and pain with cross-body abduction. Swelling is usually not present, and most patients have no deformity suggestive of remote AC sprain. The remainder of the shoulder and cervical examination is usually within normal limits.

Radiographic findings progress from early findings of demineralization and subchondral erosion of the distal clavicle to late findings of permanent widening of the AC joint and reconstitution of a smooth distal clavicular cortical surface (Fig. 33-2). Radiographic changes have been reported as early as 2.5 weeks after acute trauma.[26] However, in the weight lifter, several months to years of shoulder pain usually precede any radiographic findings.[8] Technetium-99 bone scan scintigraphy will show increased uptake on the clavicular side of the involved AC joint in all cases and has been suggested by Cahill[8] to be the diagnostic procedure of choice for this condition.

Initial treatment should include relative rest with elimination of aggravating exercises (typically supine bench press, pull-downs, pull-ups, and military press), local ice application, and oral anti-inflammatory medications. Immobilization of the affected extremity has been reported to result in decreased bone loss, cessation of bone resorption, and more rapid reconstitution of the distal clavicle with an associated decrease in clinical symptoms.[26,57] Although this may be helpful in cases of distal clavicular osteolysis after acute trauma if instituted early, I have not found it of benefit in the weight lifting population. Permanent cessation of weight lifting has been shown to result in complete resolution of symptoms after 4 to 6 months, with reconstitution of the distal clavicle and permanent widening of the AC joint resulting.[52]

If symptoms persist after several weeks of the above-mentioned treatment, more structured physical therapy including modalities is instituted. Intra-articular corticosteroid injection is often helpful, with effective symptom relief for up to several months. However, symptoms often return after reinstitution of aggravating exercises.

For those patients who do not respond to a reasonable

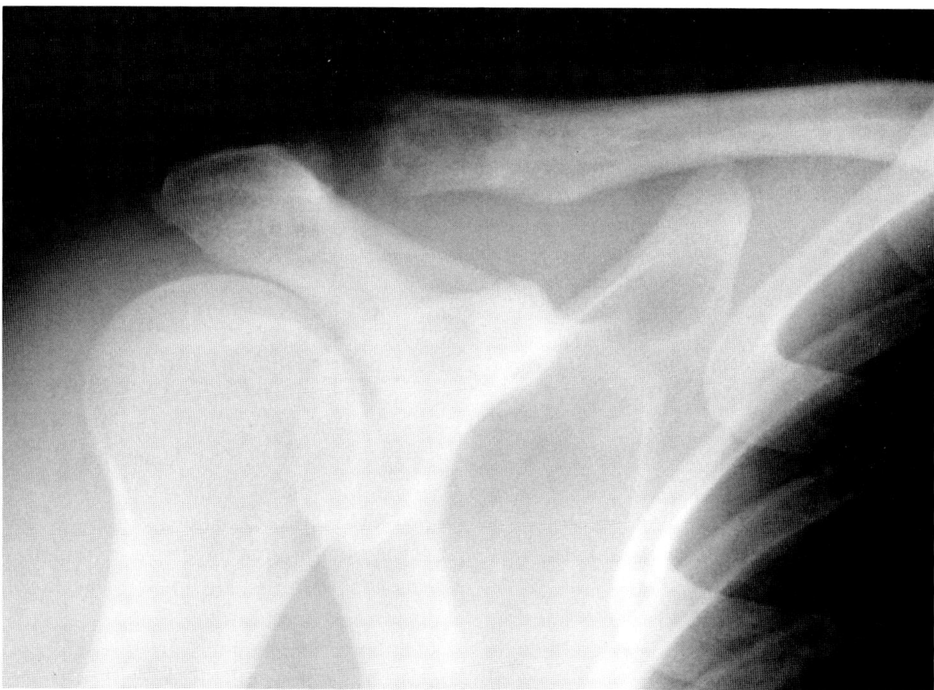

Figure 33-2. Acromioclavicular joint with radiographic evidence of nontraumatic clavicular osteolysis showing two lateral cystic changes at the edge of the clavicle. (Courtesy of Michael Scavenius, M.D.)

trial of nonoperative treatment measures or who cannot modify or curtail their weight lifting activities for various reasons (e.g., professional athlete), open or arthroscopic excision of the distal clavicle is recommended. Distal clavicular excision has been found to be highly effective in relieving symptoms and allowing return to weight lifting.[8,52] Cahill[8] reported that 14 of 19 patients returned to their previous level of sports participation, which included weight lifting as the primary or secondary activity, after open distal clavicular excision. In their original series, Scavenius et al[52] reported four of four competitive weight lifters returned to their preinjury level of activity after open distal clavicular excision. Petersson[43] found no significant difference in results after distal clavicular excision in 50 patients with traumatic and nontraumatic distal clavicular osteolysis. Interestingly, he found no correlation between postoperative radiographic findings of newly formed bone spurs or radiopaque deposits within the AC joint and clinical outcome. Reports of arthroscopic excision of the distal clavicle are limited.[11,16,21] However, early results are favorable in patients with stable AC joints.[11] After open or arthroscopic distal clavicular excision, heavy weight lifting activities should be curtailed for a minimum of 12 weeks. Aggravating exercises such as the supine bench press should be cautiously reinstituted.

Rotator Cuff Injuries

Although not addressed specifically in the peer review literature, impingement-type lesions and full-thickness tears of the rotator cuff do occur in weight lifters at about the same incidence as within the population of heavy laborers involved with repetitive overhead use of the upper extremities. The athlete will typically complain of the gradual onset of increasing anterolateral shoulder pain, aggravated with overhead activities and exercises involving shoulder abduction. Chronic advanced lesions are accompained by rest and night pain. Physical examination demonstrates typical findings characteristic of impingement lesions of the rotator cuff, with greater tuberosity tenderness and impingement signs being present. Crepitance with shoulder rotation is common and may be due to either chronic thickening or dense scarring of the subacromial bursa or a full-thickness tear of the rotator cuff. Weakness with external rotation or abduction is often difficult to demonstrate, even in patients with full-thickness tears due to the strength of the ipsilateral glenohumeral muscles found in these athletes In patients with associated AC disease, selective injections of local anesthetic are often helpful in isolating the primary source of pain, which may be secondary to both processes.

Because of the relatively high tolerance to pain and the difficulty in demonstrating weakness of the rotator cuff, the diagnosis of a full-thickness rotator cuff tear in these patients, based on history and physical examination alone, is often difficult. Imaging studies such as arthrogram, ultrasound, or magnetic resonance imaging (MRI) are very helpful. Due to the invasiveness of the arthrogram and technical limitations of the ultrasound (due to the typical thickness of the deltoid musculature in these individuals), MRI is the imaging procedure of choice in this population. Treatment of impingement tendinitis/tendinosis in these patients consists of relative rest with avoidance of aggravating activities or exercises. I have my patients eliminate all straight bar exercises from their program and substitute with dumbbells, cable exercises, or high-quality machines. As a general rule while performing an exercise, the athlete should always be able to see his or her hands while looking straight ahead. Also, local ice or physical therapy modalities are used. Institution of a rotator cuff and scapular rotator concentric and eccentric progressive exercise program is also recommended. Oral anti-inflammatory agents are generally helpful as well.

If after 6 weeks of this program no progress is noted, consideration is given to subacromial corticosteroid injection. However, because of the difficulty in diagnosing with certainty a full-thickness rotator cuff tear in these patients and my hesitancy to inject a torn rotator cuff, I usually proceed with MRI before corticosteroid injection. If the MRI demonstrates changes consistent with impingement tendinitis or tendinosis, subacromial corticosteroid injection is carried out, followed by 2 weeks of "rest" for the rotator cuff, during which time range of motion and general light strengthening exercises are performed. Further modifications in the weight lifting program are made as needed, and physical therapy is continued. Patients with acute tendinitis of the cuff typically respond better to this course of treatment than do those with chronic tendinosis. Most patients achieve a significant reduction in their pain for a variable period of time with this program, and many, usually those with acute tendinitis, achieve long-lasting results. For those who do not, and wish to continue weight lifting, arthroscopic subacromial decompression is recommended. After surgery, heavy weights are avoided for 12 weeks. Results of arthroscopic decompression in weight lifters have yet to be reported in the peer review literature. In my experience, most athletes return to weight lifting, although their program often is modified, as outlined above.

If the MRI demonstrates a full-thickness rotator cuff tear, I favor open subacromial decompression and repair of the rotator cuff to a trough in bone. An arthroscopic decompression followed by a "mini-open" lateral repair is possible but, in my experience, is extremely technically demanding due to the thickness of the deltoid muscle in these patients and the propensity for these tears to be slightly anterior to the location of the more typical chronic attrition-type tear seen in older patients. After surgery, passive range of motion is initiated immediately, and at 6 weeks, active motion with terminal stretch is begun. Ten weeks after surgery, light strengthening exercises for the rotator cuff and scapular rotators are instituted and continued for another 2 to 3 months. Patiens are allowed to return to a modified weight lifting program 6 months after surgery. Results of repair of full-thickness rotator cuff tears in weight lifters have not been reported in the peer review literature.

An unfused acromial apophysis, or os acromiale, can be responsible for impingement lesions of the rotator cuff in weight lifters. This developmental anomaly has been found in 2.7 percent of the general population and occurs bilaterally 62 percent of the time.[27] Os acromiale has been shown to be associated with tears of the rotator cuff.[39] In the weight lifter, contraction of the deltoid results in depression of the unfused bony fragment, effectively narrowing the subacromial space. An axillary radiograph is essential for accurate diagnosis (Fig. 33-3). Treatment for patients with impingement lesions secondary to os acromiale is essentially the same as to that for patients without the anomaly.

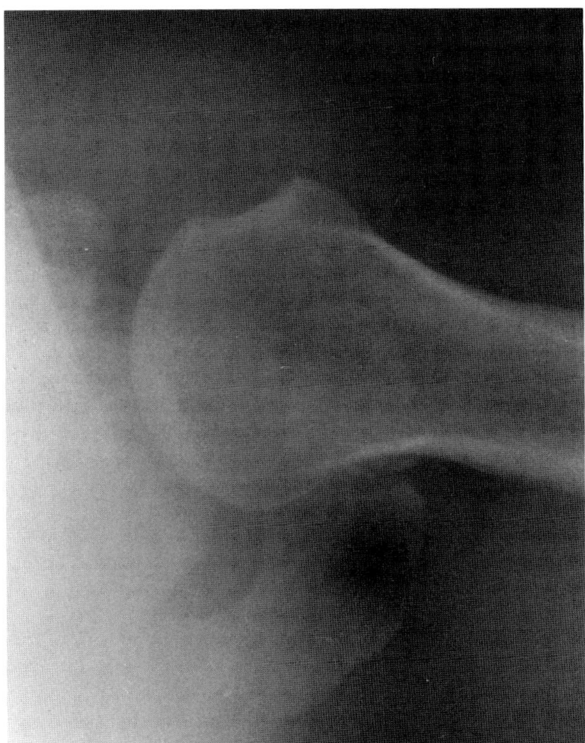

Figure 33-3. Axillary radiograph of a weight lifter's shoulder demonstrating a meso os acromiale.

Although attempts at fusion of the ununited site through various methods may be undertaken at the time of subacromial decompression or rotator cuff repair, recent data suggest that better results can be obtained with a modified subacromial decompression without fusion or excision of the ununited fragment.[4]

Muscle and Tendon Ruptures

Complete ruptures of muscles about the shoulder during weight lifting are relatively uncommon injuries and are the result of tensile failure of either the musculotendinous junction or the tendinous insertion of the muscle secondary to application of excessive force. The muscle most commonly ruptured during weight lifting is the pectoralis major. Marmor et al[34] in 1961 reported the first case of pectoralis major rupture in a weight lifter who was performing a bench press at the time of injury. Since Marmor's report, 27 other cases of pectoralis major rupture in weight lifters have been reported in the English peer review literature.[3,24,29,30,36,61,63] By far, the most common site of rupture is the distal extent of the sternal head of the muscle, either near or at its insertion into the humerus. These injuries occur almost exclusively during the bench press, although the series of Kretzler and Richardson[24] includes two injuries sustained during "flyes" (a dumbbell exercise performed supine on a flat bench involving cross-body adduction) and McEntire et al[36] reported a case occurring during a push press (a straight bar bell exercise involving pressing a weight straight up overhead).

Wolfe et al[61] reported a cadaveric study of a simulated bench press, demonstrating that the short inferior fibers of the pectoralis major lengthened disproportionately during the last 30 degrees of humeral extension during this exercise. These authors proposed that because of the mechanical disadvantage that these fibers incur during the final eccentric phase of this exercise, application of excessive force to these maximally stretched fibers in this position results in rupture.

The weight lifter with pectoralis major rupture presents typically with a history of an acute onset of severe searing anterior axillary pain experienced while bench pressing an excessive amount of weight, usually during a one repetition maximal attempt. A loud snap or tear, similar to the sound made by Velcro, is often heard across the gym. There is usually no history of pre-existing disease such as chronic tendinosis. Physical examination demonstrates local tenderness at the site of rupture; a palpable defect in the tendon in the axilla is usually present and can be accentuated by resisted adduction of the abducted extremity. Lack of a palpable defect, however, is not a reliable sign of an intact pectoralis major tendon.[63] Swelling and ecchymosis are often diffuse and extensive, involving the axilla and anterior chest wall. In the most common distal ruptures, the proximal muscle belly retracts a short distance medially, resulting in a visible and palpable bulge on the anterior chest wall and thinning of the axillary fold. Several authors have pointed out the importance of examining these patients with the arm in an abducted position.[3,36]

Although history and physical examination usually result in accurate diagnosis, MRI has been shown to be helpful in determining the location and extent of the tear and thus may be a useful diagnostic and preoperative planning tool.[38]

Recommended treatment for complete ruptures of the pectoralis major tendon in weight lifters is acute anatomic surgical repair to its humeral attachment. Satisfactory results have been reported using nonabsorbable suture passed through drill holes.[3,24,29,30,34,36,61,63] The use of suture anchors has recently been reported to lead to acceptable results as well.[38] Surgical repair has been shown to restore near-normal strength and cosmesis in most cases, whereas nonoperative treatment always leaves the patient with residual weakness and some deformity.[3,24,29,30,34,36,61,63] In the series of Zeman et al,[63] two of the three weight lifters included elected nonoperative treatment and could not return to their previous level of activity. The one patient who underwent repair noted a full return of strength and function. Wolfe et al[61] used isokinetic testing to demonstrate that shoulder torque and work produced by the affected extremity that has undergone surgical repair of a ruptured pectoralis major tendon is comparable with the unaffected contralateral side. Furthermore, the same testing of shoulders treated nonoperatively demonstrated marked deficits in these same parameters.

Delayed repair of chronic ruptures has also been reported in weight lifters. Strength and function return are comparable with results reported in acute repairs; however, cosmetic results are not as favorable.[24]

After surgical repair, light strengthening can be instituted at 6 to 8 weeks and heavier training commenced at 12 weeks. Patients should be cautioned regarding excessive humeral extension during the bench press or other exercises, at this is the position of risk for the repair.

Although reported infrequently in weight lifters, rupture of the distal insertion of the biceps tendon does occur, usually as a result of excessive force applied to a fully extended elbow, such as occurs during the power lifting dead lift or Olympic lifts (the snatch and the clean-and-jerk).[10] As with pectoralis rupture, the muscle is fully contracted in a lengthened position at the time of rupture, with rupture occurring at or near the insertion. Patients report an acute tearing sensation in the distal upper arm while performing typically a one repetition maximal lift of very heavy weight. Physical examination acutely demonstrates local tenderness, swelling, ecchymosis, and usually a visible deformity and palpable defect in the distal upper arm.

Weakness in flexion in supination is evident. MRI may be a useful study, especially in chronic injuries.

Recommended treatment for acute distal biceps rupture in weight lifters is surgical repair of the tendon to bone, followed by immobilization in flexion for 4 to 6 weeks. Heavy weight lifting is avoided for 3 months.

Ruptures of the proximal long head of the biceps tendon may also occur in weight lifters. This injury is less common than the distal rupture and usually occurs in the middle-aged or older athlete with pre-existing concomitant subacromial disease. The patient's vocation and activity level determine whether surgical repair is indicated. I recommend tenodesis proximally in patients who wish to remain active weight lifters or whose vocation or other activities require strenuous use of the involved extremity.

Traumatic acute rupture of the rotator cuff has not been reported to have occurred during a weight lifting exercise.

Nerve Injuries

Injury to peripheral nerves about the shoulder as a result of weight lifting is an uncommon occurrence. Published reports are limited to isolated cases of suprascapular and long thoracic nerve damage.[1,6,12,14,17,22,31,41,58,62] The anatomy of the suprascapular nerve has been well documented[5,19,37,47,48,60] and has been discussed in detail in another part of this text. The relatively fixed position of the nerve as it passes beneath the transverse scapular ligament and around the scapular spine at the level of the spinoglenoid notch makes it susceptible to injury at these levels as a result of friction, stretching, or kinking that can occur with repetitive scapular movement. Rengachary et al[47] used the term *sling effect* to describe the phenomenon of kinking of the nerve against the transverse ligament with shoulder depression, retraction, and hyperabduction. Most reported cases of suprascapular nerve injury as a result of weight lifting are postulated to have resulted from this type of mechanism.[1,6,13,31] Suprascapular nerve compression by ganglion cysts has also been reported in weight lifters.[14,41,62]

The athlete typically relates a history of the insidious onset of diffuse aching posterior shoulder pain, without any single initiating event, although a recent increase in weight lifting intensity, frequency, or duration is sometimes noted. Weakness is not a universal complaint; however, weakness of external rotation is always noted on physical examination. Other physical findings can include muscular atrophy, especially of the infraspinous fossa. Patients with ganglion cysts usually have palpable tenderness but rarely is the mass palpable. Patients with traction-type injury are less likely to demonstrate local tenderness. Electrodiagnostic studies, including electromyography (EMG) and nerve conduction studies (NCS), are very helpful in determining the site and extent of the lesion. MRI has been shown to be a useful diagnostic tool as well, especially in cases of ganglion cyst compression.[13,53]

Treatment of these injuries is somewhat controversial, and long-term results are variable. Ganzhorn et al[14] were the first to publish a case of isolated injury to the infraspinous branch of the suprascapular nerve. The injury was sustained

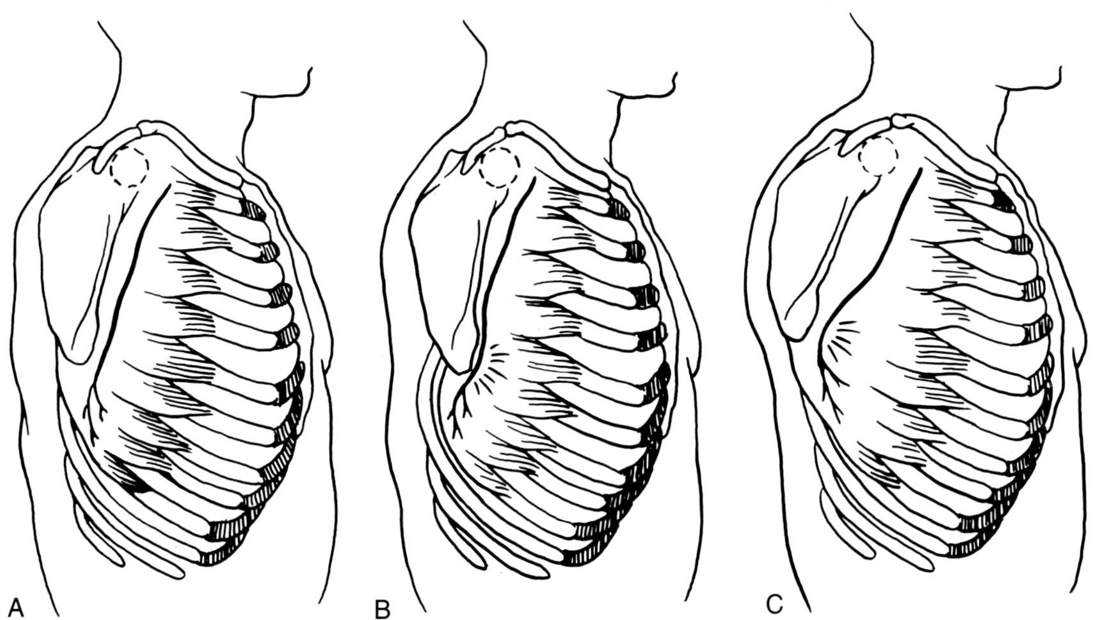

Figure 33-4. Course of the long thoracic nerve. (**A**) In normal circumstances, serratus anterior is inactive. (**B**) Anterior movement in the scapula may result in compression of the nerve. (**C**) Winging of scapula may cause traction on nerve. (From Kauppila,[23] with permission.)

by a weight lifter who noticed painless atrophy of his infraspinous fossa. Surgery was elected, and at the time of the procedure, a ganglion cyst was found to be compressing the nerve of the level of the spinoglenoid notch. No return of musclc bulk or function was noted 18 months after surgery.

Nevaiser et al[41] reported complete clinical and electrical recovery after excision of a ganglion cyst causing suprascapular nerve compression in the supraspinous fossa in a weight lifter The two weight lifters included in Black and Lombardo's series[6] both experienced full recovery from traction-type suprascapular nerve injuries with nonoperative course of treatment. Both patients returned to full weight lifting 6 to 9 months after diagnosis. The series of Liveson et al[31] includes one weight lifter with a traction-type suprascapular nerve injury who gave up weight lifting and experienced "full" recovery within 12 months. Agre et al[1] reported complete clinical and electrical recovery in one weight lifter who underwent decompression of the nerve at the level of the suprascapular notch for a traction-type injury.

In patients with traction-type injuries to the suprascapular nerve, weight lifting activities should be curtailed and a rehabilitation program consisting of physical therapy modalities and exercises initiated. Consideration is given to the use of oral anti-inflammatory agents. Occasionally, oral corticosteroid preparations may be helpful. Baseline EMG and NCS are essential. If no improvement is seen after 3 months of nonoperative therapy, repeat electrodiagnostic studies are performed. If no change or progression of the lesion is noted, surgical decompression at the appropriate level is indicated. Both the suprascapular and the spinoglenoid notch may be accessed from a posterior approach, either through a transverse incision paralleling the lateral extent of the scapular spine or vertical incision just medial to the glenohumeral joint line. In patients with MRI evidence of ganglion cyst compression of the nerve, I recommend early surgical decompression from a posterior approach. After surgery, active range of motion exercises and light use of the extremity are allowed as pain permits. Light rotator cuff, scapular rotator, and glenohumeral muscle strengthening is initiated at 2 weeks and progresses as tolerated. Heavy weight lifting is discouraged for 3 months.

Injury to the long thoracic nerve as a result of weight lifting has been reported and is likely secondary to compression of the nerve by the inferior border of the scapula during forceful contraction of the serratus anterior[23] (Fig. 33-4). Such contraction occurs during supine heavy pressing exercises such as the bench press. Pronounced scapular protraction also occurs during the overhead pressing phase of the clean-and-jerk and the snatch exercises (Fig. 33-5). Injury can occur suddenly or insidiously. Patients present

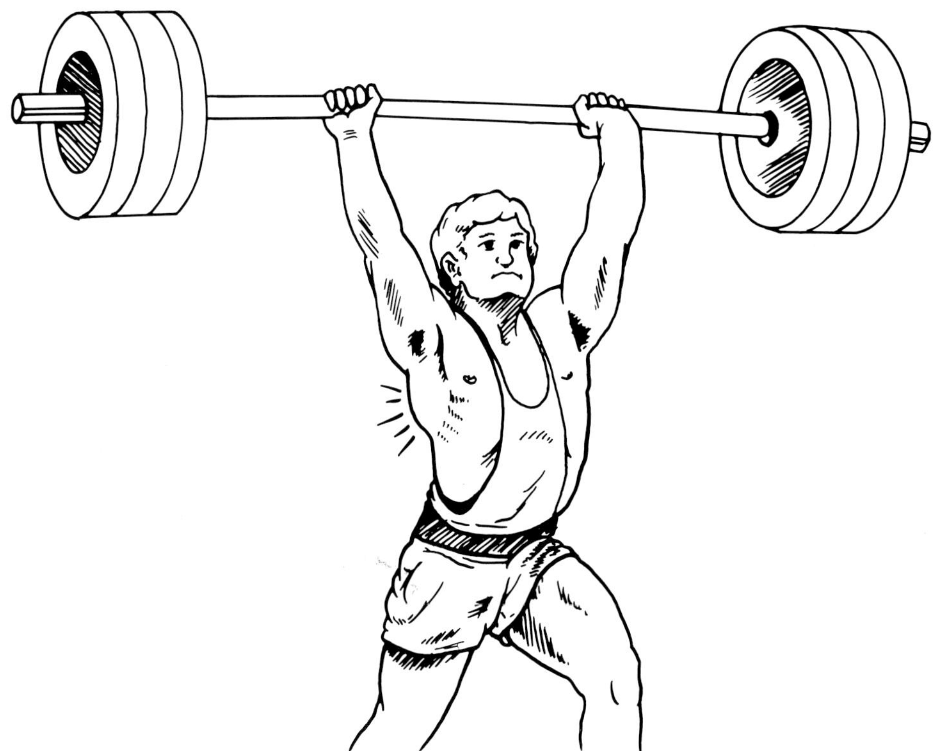

Figure 33-5. The serratus anterior strongly protracts the scapula during the jerk. (Adapted from Kulund et al,[25] with permission.)

with poorly localized shoulder pain and demonstrate significant scapular winging and difficulty in elevating the arm above horizontal. Rotator cuff impingement signs may develop secondarily in long-standing cases.

Treatment for this injury is nonoperative and involves relative rest of the serratus anterior (refraining from weight lifting) and institution of a physical therapy program designed to maintain range of motion and strengthen the other scapular rotators, specifically the rhomboideus and the trapezius. Rotator cuff exercises are also initiated. Recovery is variable, with most patients regaining near full function within 6 to 24 months.[12,17] Residual winging and difficulty with endurance activities may persist, however.[12,17]

Instability

Occult anterior instability of the glenohumeral joint is a recognized cause of shoulder pain in weight lifters.[9,15,18] The diagnosis is a difficult one to make in this group of athletes, as it is in others, and often is one of exclusion. Typically, the athlete relates a history of posterior shoulder

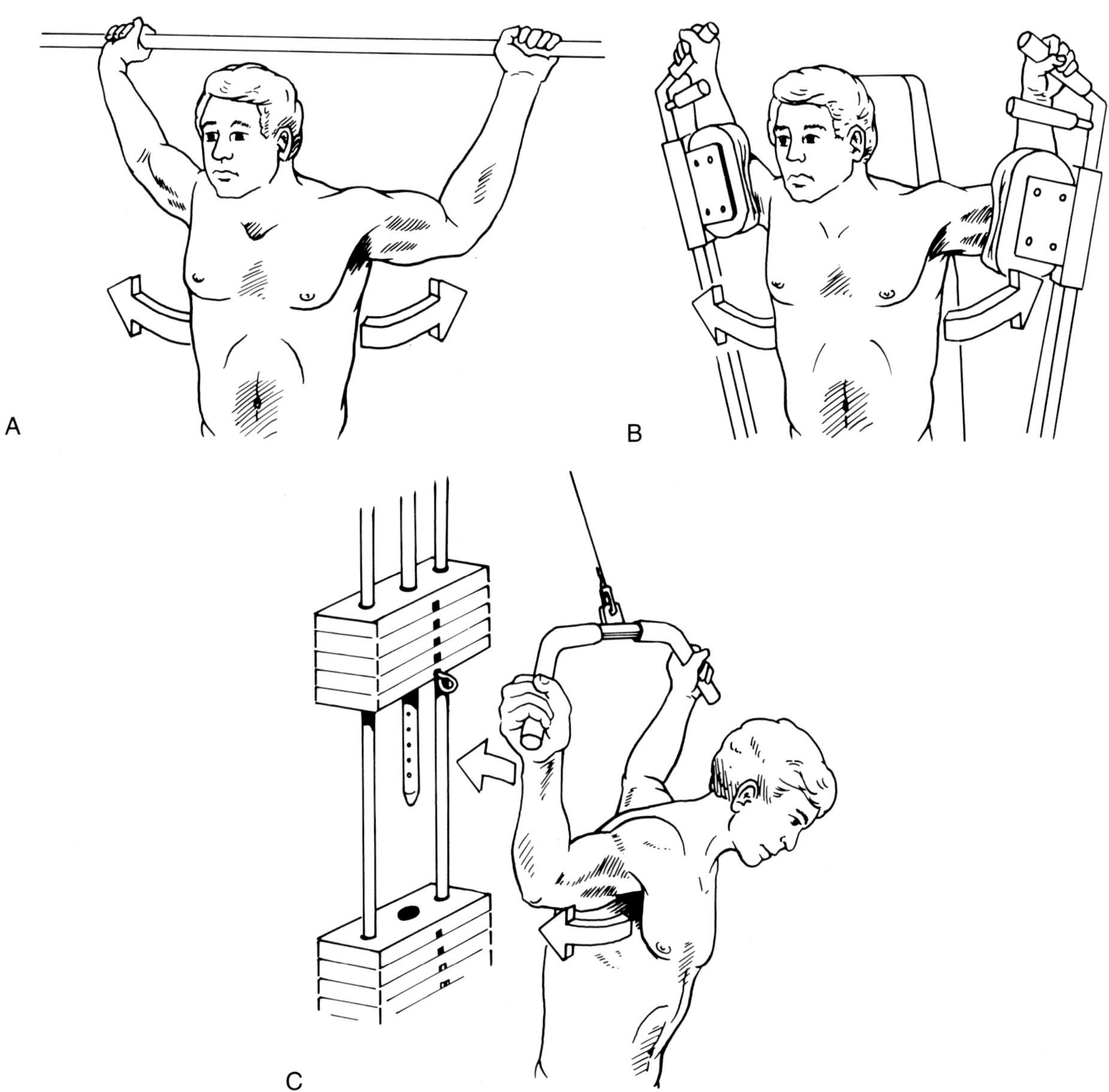

Figure 33-6. (**A–C**) Weight lifting maneuvers producing forced abduction, extension, and external rotation; the at-risk position of the shoulder. (From Gross et al,[18] with permission.)

pain experienced while performing exercises that place the arm in an abducted externally rotated and extended position (Fig. 33-6). A history of frank dislocation is extremely rare, and most patients have no sense of instability of the shoulder. Physical examination is usually unremarkable except for the finding of symptom reproduction with abduction, external rotation, and extension of the affected shoulder. Fully 100 percent of the 20 weight lifters in the series of Gross et al[18] demonstrated this finding. Garth et al[15] have reported a similar experience in a group of "noncontact" athletes that included nine weight lifters. Imaging studies may be helpful in making an accurate diagnosis. Garth et al[15] found that apical oblique projection radiographs demonstrated "small Hill-Sachs lesions" in 23 of their 28 patients, often apparent merely as subtle radiolucency. Also, using this same projection, two shoulders demonstrated bony changes of the anterior glenoid rim consistent with a Bankart-type lesion. Interestingly, neither of these patients had concomitant Hill-Sachs lesions. Gross et al[18] found radiographs to be less useful, with only 4 of 23 shoulders demonstrating "mild Hill-Sachs lesions."

Initial treatment consists of elimination of exercises that place the affected extremity in abduction, external rotation, and extension. Gross et al[18] recommended modifying the three at-risk exercises they identified. I prefer to eliminate those three exercises and substitute dumbbell military press performed anterior to the coronal plane for the straight bar military press; dumbbell flies performed anterior to the coronal plane for flies performed on a fixed arc machine; and lateral pull-downs anterior to the coronal plane for those performed behind the neck. Pull-overs and pull-ups are eliminated completely.

Physical therapy modalities and oral anti-inflammatory agents are used as needed to decrease pain and inflammation. Rehabilitation exercises emphasizing concentric and eccentric strengthening of all the rotator cuff and scapular rotators are instituted. This program is followed for 3 months, with modifications made as needed. Many athletes respond well to this nonoperative program but often are unable to return to performing the at-risk exercises and, in fact, should be counseled against trying to do so. Gross et al[18] found that 13 shoulders in 10 of their 20 patients responded to nonoperative treatment and returned to weight lifting. Ten shoulders in 10 patients in that same series eventually came to surgery, which consisted of an arthroscopic evaluation in all cases. Examination under anesthesia demonstrated anterior instability in 9 of these 10 shoulders; no other instability was noted. Hill-Sachs lesions were visualized in all nine unstable shoulders. Eight of these nine unstable shoulders were found to have anteroinferior capsular/ligamentous separations, and all underwent arthroscopic-assisted modified Bankart repair using a multiple suture technique. After surgery, all 10 patients returned to weight lifting using modified techniques at 4 months postoperatively, and all reported complete resolution of symptoms and satisfaction with their outcome.

REFERENCES

1. Arge JC, Ash N, Cameron MC, House J: Suprascapular neuropathy after intensive progressive resistive exercise: case report. Arch Phys Med Rehabil 68:236, 1987
2. Allen WC: Post-traumatic osteolysis of the distal clavicle. Postgrad Med 41:73, 1967
3. Bakalim G: Rupture of the pectoralis major muscle: a case report. Acta Orthop Scand 36:274, 1965
4. Barallat JA, Brittis DA, Self EB, Flatow EL: The surgical treatment of an unfused acromial epiphysis in association with a tear of the rotator cuff. Paper presented at the 9th Open Meeting of the American Shoulder and Elbow Surgeons, San Francisco, 1993
5. Bigliani LU, Dalsey RM, McCann PD, April EW: An anatomical study of the suprascapular nerve. Arthroscopy 6:301, 1990
6. Black KP, Lombardo JA: Suprascapular nerve injuries with isolated paralysis of the infraspinatus. Am J Sports Med 18:225, 1990
7. Brady TA, Cahill BR, Bodnar LM: Weight training-related injuries in the high school athlete. Am J Sports Med 10:1, 1982
8. Cahill BR: Osteolysis of the distal part of the clavicle in male athletes. J Bone Joint Surg [Am] 64:1053, 1982
9. Cordasco FA, Steinmann S, Flatow EL, Bigliani LU: Arthroscopic treatment of glenoid labral tears. Am J Sports Med 21:425, 1993
10. D'Alessandro DF, Sheilds LL, Tibone JE, Chandler RW: Repair of distal biceps tendon rupture in athletes. Am J Sports Med 21:114, 1993
11. Duralde X, Flatow EL, Pollock RG, Nicholson GP: Arthroscopic resection of the distal clavicle: factors associated with success. Paper presented at the annual meeting of the American Academy of Orthopaedic Surgeons, San Francisco, 1993
12. Foo CL, Swann M: Isolated paralysis of the serratus anterior. J Bone Joint Surg [Br] 65:552, 1993
13. Fritz RC, Helms CA, Steinbach LS, Genant HK: Suprascapular nerve entrapment: evaluation with MR imaging. Radiology 182:437, 1992
14. Ganzhorn RW, Hocker JT, Horowitz M, Switzer HE: Suprascapular-nerve entrapment: a case report. J Bone Joint Surgery [Am] 63:492, 1981
15. Garth WP, Allman FL, Armstrong WS: Occult anterior subluxations of the shoulder in noncontact sports. Am J Sports Med 15:579, 1987
16. Gartsman GM: Arthroscopic resection of the acromioclavicular joint. Am J Sports Med 21:71, 1993
17. Gregg JR, Labosky D, Harty M et al: Serratus anterior paralysis in the young athlete. J Bone Joint Surg [Am] 61:825, 1979
18. Gross ML, Brenner SL, Esformes I, Sonzogni JJ: Anterior shoulder instability in weight lifters. Am J Sports Med 21:599, 1993
19. Horiguchi M: The cutaneous branch of some human suprascapular nerves. J Anat 130:191, 1980

20. Jacobs P: Post-traumatic osteolysis of the outer end of the clavicle. J Bone Joint Surg [Br] 46:705, 1964
21. Jerosch J, Castro WHM, Halm HFH, Rondhuis JJ: Arthroscopic Mumford procedure: surgical technique and short term results. Paper presented at the annual meeting of the American Academy of Orthopaedic Surgeons, San Francisco, 1993
22. Kaspi A, Yanai J, Pick CG, Mann G: Entrapment of the distal suprascapular nerve. Int Orthop 12:273, 1988
23. Kauppila LI: The long thoracic nerve: possible mechanisms of injury based on autopsy study. J Shoulder Elbow Surg 2:244, 1993
24. Kretzler HH, Richardson AB: Rupture of the pectoralis major muscle. Am J Sports Med 17:453, 1989
25. Kulund DN, Dewey JB, Brubaker CE, Roberts JR: Olympic weight-lifting injuries. Phys Sportsmed 6:111, 1978
26. Levine AH, Pais MJ, Schwartz EE: Posttraumatic osteolysis of the distal clavicle with emphasis on early radiologic changes. AJR 127:781, 1976
27. Liberson F: Os acromiale—a contested anomaly. J Bone Joint Surg [Am] 19:683, 1937
28. Lillegard WA: Strength training for the young athlete. J Back Musculoskel Rehabil 1:29, 1991
29. Lindenbaum BL: Delayed repair of a ruptured pectoralis major muscle. Clin Orthop 109:120, 1975
30. Liu J, Wu J-J, Chang C-Y et al: Avulsion of the pectoralis major tendon. Am J Sports Med 20:366, 1992
31. Liveson JA, Bronson MJ, Pollack MA: Suprascapular nerve lesions at the spinoglenoid notch: report of three cases and review of the literature. J Neurol Neurosurg Psychiatry 54:241, 1991
32. Madsen B: Osteolysis of the acromial end of the clavicle following trauma. Br J Radiol 36:822, 1963
33. Madsen N, McLaughlin T: Kinematic factors influencing performance and injury risk in the bench press exercise. Med Sci Sports 16:376, 1984
34. Marmor L, Bechtol CO, Hall CB: Pectoralis major muscle. J Bone Joint Surg [Am] 43:81, 1961
35. Matthews LS, Simonson BG, Wolock BS: Osteolysis of the distal clavicle in a female body builder—a case report. Am J Sports Med 21:150, 1993
36. McEntire JE, Hess WE, Coleman SS: Rupture of the pectoralis major muscle. J Bone Joint Surg [Am] 54:1040, 1972
37. Mestdagh J, Drizenko A, Ghestem P: Anatomical bases of suprascapular nerve syndrome. Anat Clin 3:67, 1981
38. Miller MD, Johnson DL, Fu FH et al: Rupture of the pectoralis major muscle in a collegiate football player: use of magnetic resonance imaging in early diagnosis. Am J Sports Med 21:475, 1993
39. Mudge MK, Wood VE, Frykman GK: Rotator cuff tears associated with os acromiale. J Bone Joint Surg [Am] 66:427, 1984
40. Murphy OB, Bellamy R, Wheeler W, Brower TD: Post-traumatic osteolysis of the distal clavicle. Clin Orthop 109:108, 1975
41. Neviaser TJ, Ain BR, Neviaser RJ: Suprascapular nerve denervation secondary to attenuation by a ganglionic cyst. J Bone Surg [Am] 68:627, 1986
42. O'Brien SJ, Neves MC, Arnoczky SP et al: The anatomy and histology of the inferior glenohumeral ligament complex of the shoulder. Am J Sports Med 18:449, 1990
43 Petersson CJ: Resection of the lateral end of the clavicle. Acta Orthop Scand 54:904, 1983
44. Poppen NK, Walker PS: Normal and abnormal motion of the shoulder. J Bone Joint Surg [Am] 58:195, 1976
45. Poppen NK, Walker PS: Forces at the glenohumeral joint in abduction. Clin Orthop 135:165, 1978
46. Quinn SF, Glass TA: Posttraumatic osteolysis of the clavicle. South Med J 76:307, 1983
47. Rengachary SS, Burr D, Lucas S et al: Suprascapular entrapment neuropath: a clinical, anatomical, and comparative study. Part 2: anatomical study. Neurosurgery 5:447, 1979
48. Rengachary SS, Neff JP, Singer PA Brackett CE: Suprascapular entrapment neuropathy: a clinical, anatomical, and comparative study. Part I: clinical study. Neurosurgery 5:441, 1979
49. Requa RK, DeAvilla LN, Garrick JG: Injuries in adult fitness activities. Am J Sports Med 21:461, 1993
50. Rians CB, Weltman A, Cahill B: Strength training for prepubescent males: is it safe. Am J Sports Med 15:483, 1987
51. Scavenius M, Iversen BF: Nontraumatic clavicular osteolysis in weight lifters. Am J Sports Med 20:463, 1992
52. Scavenius M, Iversen BF, Sturup J: Resection of the lateral end of the clavicle following osteolysis, with emphasis on non-traumatic osteolysis of the acromial end of the clavicle in athletes. Injury 18:261, 1987
53. Schickendantz MS, Ho CP: Suprascapular nerve compression by a ganglion cyst: diagnosis by magnetic resonance imaging. J Shoulder Elbow Surg 2:110, 1993
54. Schwartz RE, O'Brien SJ, Warren RF, Torzilli PA: Capsular restraints to anterior-posterior motion of the shoulder, abstracted. Orthop Trans 12:727, 1988
55. Seymour EQ: Osteolysis of the clavicular tip associated with repeated minor trauma to the shoulder. Radiology 123:56, 1977
56. Smart MJ: Traumatic osteolysis of the distal ends of the clavicles. J Can Assoc Radiol 23:264, 1972
57. Stahl F: Considerations on post-traumatic absorption of the outer end of the clavicle. Acta Orthop Scand 23:9, 1954
58. Vastamaki M, Kauppila LI: Etiologic factors in isolated paralysis of the serratus anterior muscle: a report of 197 cases. J Shoulder Elbow Surg 2:241, 1993
59. Warner JJP, Deng XH, Warren RF, Torzilli PA: Static capsuloligamentous restraints to superior-inferior translation of the glenohumeral joint. Am J Sports Med 20:675, 1992
60. Warner JJP, Krushell RJ, Masquelet A, Gerber C: Anatomy and relationships of the suprascapular nerve: anatomical constraints to mobilization of the supraspinatus and infraspinatus muscles in the management of massive rotator-cuff tears. J Bone Joint Surg [Am] 74:36, 1992
61. Wolfe SW, Wickiewicz TL, Cavanaugh JT: Ruptures of the pectoralis major muscle: an anatomic and clinical analysis. Am J Sports Med 20:587, 1992
62. Zeiss J, Woldenberg LS, Saddemi SR, Ebraheim NA: MRI of suprascapular neuropathy in a weight lifter. J CAT 17:303, 1993
63. Zeman SC, Rosenfeld RT, Lipscomb PR: Tears of the pectoralis major muscle. Am J Sports Med 7:343, 1979

Index

Page numbers followed by f *represent figures; those followed by* t *represent tables.*

B

D

E

F

G

K

L

M

N

O

P

T

U

V

W

Y